Clinical Decisions
in Medical Retinal Disease

Clinical Decisions in Medical Retinal Disease

William S. Tasman, M.D.

Ophthalmologist-in-Chief,
Wills Eye Hospital;
Professor and Chairman,
Department of Ophthalmology,
Jefferson Medical College
of Thomas Jefferson University,
Philadelphia, Pennsylvania

with 313 illustrations and 38 color plates

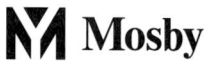 Mosby

St. Louis Baltimore Berlin Boston Carlsbad Chicago London Madrid
Naples New York Philadelphia Sydney Tokyo Toronto

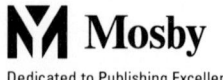
Dedicated to Publishing Excellence

Editor: Laurel Craven
Developmental Editor: Dana Battaglia
Project Manager: John Rogers
Manuscript Editor: George B. Stericker, Jr.
Designer: Renée Duenow
Manufacturing Supervisor: Karen Lewis

Copyright © 1994 by Mosby–Year Book, Inc.

All rights reserved. No part of this publication may be reproduced, stored in a retrieval system, or transmitted, in any form or by any means, electronic, mechanical, photocopying, recording, or otherwise, without prior written permission from the publisher. Printed in the United States of America.

Permission to photocopy or reproduce solely for internal or personal use is permitted for libraries or other users registered with the Copyright Clearance Center, provided that the base fee of $4.00 per chapter plus $.10 per page is paid directly to the Copyright Clearance Center, 21 Congress Street, Salem, MA 01970. This consent does not extend to other kinds of copying, such as copying for general distribution, for advertising or promotional purposes, for creating new collected works, or for resale.

Printed in the United States of America
Composition by the Clarinda Company
Printing/Binding by Maple Vail Book Mfg Group

Mosby–Year Book, Inc.
11830 Westline Industrial Drive
St. Louis, MO 63416

Library of Congress Cataloging-in-Publication Data

Clinical decisions in medical retinal disease / [edited by] William S. Tasman.
   p. cm.
  Includes bibliographical references and index
  1. Retina—Blood vessels—Diseases. 2. Macula lutea—Diseases.
I. Tasman, William, 1929-
  [DNLM: 1. Retinal Diseases—diagnosis. 2. Retinal Diseases—therapy.
  3. Diagnosis, Differential. WW 270 C641 1994]
RE551.C565 1994
617.7′3—dc20
DNLM/DLC
for Library of Congress   94-267
                                                                      CIP

94 95 96 97 98 / 9 8 7 6 5 4 3 2 1

Contributors

Emad B. Abboud, M.D.
Ophthalmologist, Retina-Vitreous Division, King Khaled Eye Specialist Hospital; Clinical Assistant Professor, Ophthalmology, King Saud University, Riyadh, Saudi Arabia

William H. Annesley, Jr., M.D., F.A.C.S.
Member and Past Director, Retina Service, Wills Eye Hospital, Philadelphia; Emeritus Member (Past Chief), Division of Ophthalmology, Department of Surgery, Lankenau Hospital, Wynnewood, Pennsylvania

James J. Augsburger, M.D.
Associate Clinical Professor of Ophthalmology, Oncology Unit, Retina Service, Wills Eye Hospital, Jefferson Medical College of Thomas Jefferson University, Philadelphia, Pennsylvania

William E. Benson, M.D.
Director, Retina Service, Wills Eye Hospital; Professor, Department of Ophthalmology, Thomas Jefferson University Hospital, Philadelphia, Pennsylvania

Alan C. Bird, M.D., F.R.C.S., F.R.C.Ophth
Professor of Ophthalmology, Department of Clinical Science, Institute of Ophthalmology, Moorfields Eye Hospital, London, England

Gary C. Brown, M.D.
Professor of Ophthalmology, Thomas Jefferson University; Director, Retina Vascular Unit, Wills Eye Hospital, Philadelphia, Pennsylvania

Jay S. Duker, M.D.
Director, Vitreoretinal Service, Ophthalmology, New England Medical Center; Associate Professor of Ophthalmology, Tufts University, Boston, Massachusetts

Jay L. Federman, M.D.
Professor of Ophthalmology, Department of Ophthalmology, Jefferson Medical College of Thomas Jefferson University; Co-Director of Retina Service and Research, Wills Eye Hospital, Philadelphia, Pennsylvania

David H. Fischer, M.D.
Associate Surgeon, Director of Uveitis Unit, Retina/Vitreous, Wills Eye Hospital, Philadelphia; Associate Surgeon, Retina/Vitreous, Lankenau Hospital, Wynnewood, Pennsylvania

Richard E. Goldberg, M.D., F.A.C.S.
Attending Surgeon, Retina Service, Wills Eye Hospital; Clinical Professor of Ophthalmology Jefferson Medical College of Thomas Jefferson University, Philadelphia, Pennsylvania

Robert C. Kleiner, M.D.
Assistant Surgeon, Retina Service, Wills Eye Hospital, Philadelphia, Pennsylvania

Alfred C. Lucier, M.D.
Associate Professor, Department of Ophthalmology, Jefferson Medical College of Thomas Jefferson University; Attending Surgeon, Retina Service, Wills Eye Hospital, Philadelphia, Pennsylvania

Joseph I. Maguire, M.D.
Assistant Surgeon, Retina Service, Wills Eye Hospital, Philadelphia, Pennsylvania

J. Arch McNamara, M.D.
Associate Surgeon, Retina Service, Wills Eye Hospital; Assistant Professor of Ophthalmology, Jefferson Medical College of Thomas Jefferson University, Philadelphia, Pennsylvania

Eric P. Shakin, M.D.
Clinical Instructor, Department of Ophthalmology, Jefferson Medical College of Thomas Jefferson University; Assistant Surgeon, Retina Service, Wills Eye Hospital, Philadelphia, Pennsylvania

Carol L. Shields, M.D.
Associate Surgeon, Ocular Oncology Service, Wills Eye Hospital; Associate Professor, Department of Ophthalmology, Jefferson Medical College of Thomas Jefferson University, Philadelphia, Pennsylvania

Jerry A. Shields, M.D.
Oncology Service, Wills Eye Hospital; Professor of Ophthalmology, Jefferson Medical College of Thomas Jefferson University, Philadelphia, Pennsylvania

Arunan Sivalingam, M.D.
Instructor, Ophthalmology Jefferson Medical College of Thomas Jefferson University Hospital; Assistant Surgeon, Wills Eye Hospital, Philadelphia, Pennsylvania

William S. Tasman, M.D.
Ophthalmologist-in-Chief, Wills Eye Hospital; Professor and Chairman, Department of Ophthalmology, Jefferson Medical College of Thomas Jefferson University, Philadelphia, Pennsylvania

James F. Vander, M.D.
Assistant Surgeon, Wills Eye Hospital; Assistant Professor, Department of Ophthalmology, Thomas Jefferson University, Philadelphia, Pennsylvania

Foreword

It is a great honor and pleasure, indeed, for a European coming from the Netherlands, the land where Dr. Tasman's roots are, to write this foreword to *Clinical Decisions in Medical Retinal Disease.*

Dr. William Tasman and his coauthors have succeeded in writing a very timely and concise book on the many interesting entities in the exciting and expanding field of medical retina. Many ophthalmologists throughout the world will be delighted to read the various chapters reflecting the high quality of eye care administered in Philadelphia's Wills Eye Hospital.

Relatively new are the excellent chapters on viral retinopathies, which, unfortunately, have become a serious concern in current ophthalmic practice. The management of retinopathy of prematurity, among others, has also considerably improved during the last years, and this is reflected in this book. Hopefully, more and even better therapeutic approaches will soon find their way into preserving the function and structure of one of our most sensitive and precious structures, the retina. Undoubtedly the subspecialty "medical retina" remains, from an intellectual point of view, one of the most challenging fields in ophthalmology.

I congratulate the authors on this successful and stimulating undertaking.

Professor August F. Deutman
Institute of Ophthalmology,
Nijmegan, Netherlands

Preface

The purpose of this book is to present a practical and useful volume that will help all ophthalmologists, whether in training or in practice, to manage patients with macular and retinovascular diseases. Originally it was planned to have each of the chapters formatted in a clinical-decision manner, but it became apparent that this subject in many cases did not lend itself to that type of presentation. Thus, the chapters are generally arranged in traditional fashion, with presentations of current findings and discussions of differential diagnosis and treatment.

The project is the result of a conjoint effort by members of the Retina Service of the Wills Eye Hospital. Currently all but three of the authors are active members of the Wills Retina Service. The three exceptions are Doctors Emad Abboud and Jay Duker and Professor Alan Bird of the Moorfields Eye Hospital London, England. However, all three of these gentlemen are extensions of the Wills family. Doctors Abboud and Duker had their vitreoretinal training at Wills, and Dr. Duker was a Wills resident and co–chief resident as well. Dr. Abboud is currently a vitreoretinal surgeon at the King Khaled Eye Hospital in Riyadh, Saudi Arabia, and Dr. Duker heads the Vitreoretinal Service at Tufts New England Medical Center.

Professor Bird is world renowned, and Wills is fortunate indeed to count this outstanding clinician and research scientist among its very best friends. He has visited us innumerable times, and many of our residents and fellows have had their lives enriched by his tutelage during electives or fellowship training. His generosity and willingness to prepare a chapter on Inherited Outer Retinal Dystrophies, a subject in which he has been a pioneer investigator, we believe has provided us with the crown jewel of the book.

Finally, we are indebted as well to another close friend of the Wills, Professor August Deutman, who, like Professor Bird, has visited with us on many occasions. Professor Deutman was kind enough to review our manuscript and to write the Foreword.

William S. Tasman, M.D.

Contents

PART I
Normal Retinal Anatomy and Function

1 Fluorescein Angiography: Principles and Interpretation, 3
Jay L. Federman

PART II
Macular Disease

2 Inherited Outer Retinal Dystrophies, 29
Alan C. Bird

3 Age-Related Macular Degeneration, 78
Joseph I. Maguire, William H. Annesley, Jr.

4 Choroidal Neovascularization Associated with Myopic Macular Degeneration, 95
James F. Vander

5 Central Serous Retinopathy, 103
Joesph I. Maguire

6 Idiopathic Macular Holes, 117
James F. Vander

7 Macular Dystrophies, 125
Eric P. Shakin

PART III
Retinal Vascular Disease

8 Treatment of Nonproliferative Diabetic Retinopathy, 141
William E. Benson

9 Treatment of Proliferative Diabetic Retinopathy, 152
William E. Benson

10 Retinal Arterial Obstructive Disease, 163
Gary C. Brown

11 Central Retinal Vein Obstruction, 175
Arunan Sivalingam

12 Branch Retinal Vein Occlusion, 182
J. Arch McNamara

13 Hypertension, 190
Eric P. Shakin, Alfred C. Lucier

14 Idiopathic Parafoveal Telangiectasis, 198
Robert C. Kleiner

15 Coats' Disease, 204
WIlliam S. Tasman

16 Hemoglobinopathies, 211
Richard E. Goldberg

17 Retinopathy of Prematurity, 224
J. Arch McNamara

18 Acquired Retinal Macroaneurysms, 253
James F. Vander

19 Radiation Retinopathy, 261
James J. Augsburger

20 Ocular Ischemic Syndrome, 276
Gary C. Brown

PART IV
Inflammatory Disease

21 Ocular Toxoplasmosis, 289
David H. Fischer

22 Ocular Toxocariasis, 304
Carol L. Shields, Jerry A. Shields

23 Cytomegalovirus Infections of the Retina: Retinal and Ophthalmologic Manifestations of AIDS, 320
Emad B. Abboud

24 Acute Retinal Necrosis (ARN) Syndrome, 332
Jay S. Duker

25 Pars Planitis, 339
James F. Vander

26 Diffuse Unilateral Subacute Neuroretinitis, 345
Arunan Sivalingam

27 Sarcoidosis of the Posterior Segment, 348
Jay S. Duker

COLOR PLATES

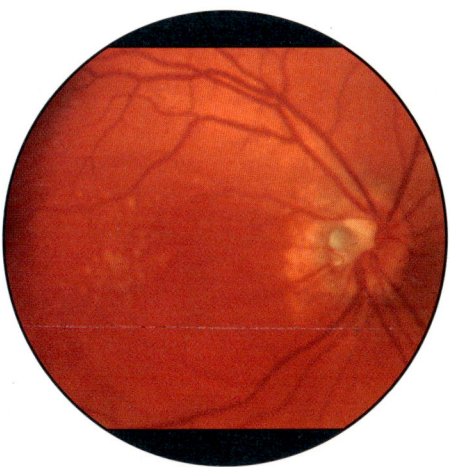

Plate 1 Congenital pit of the optic nerve. A serous macular elevation of the sensory retina frequently accompanies temporal optic nerve pits. The presence of retinic precipitates is sometimes noted.

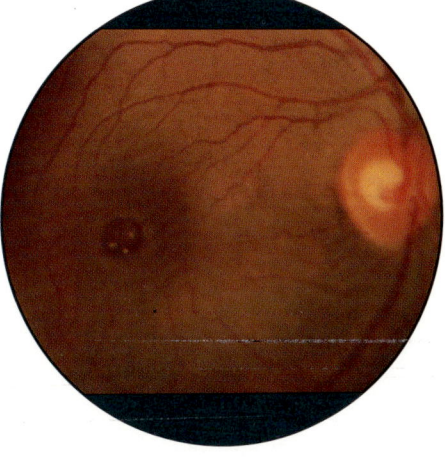

Plate 2 Yellow flecks within the base of a macular hole at the level of the RPE.

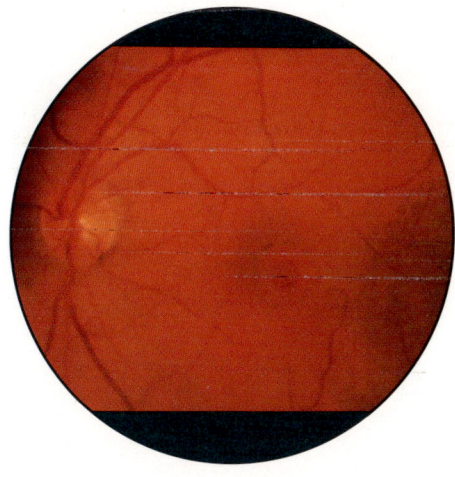

Plate 3 Cuff of subretinal fluid surrounding a macular hole.

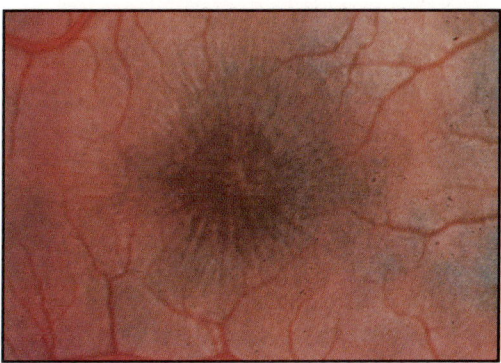

Plate 4 X-linked retinoschisis.

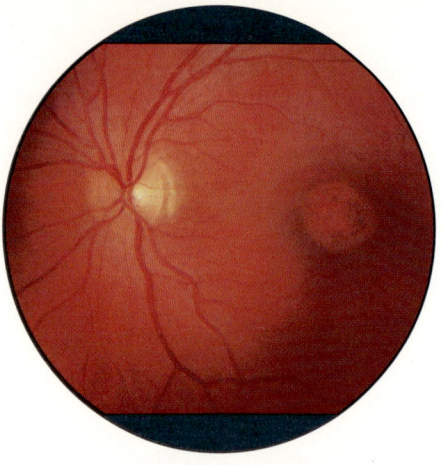

Plate 5 Cone dystrophy demonstrating a bull's-eye effect.

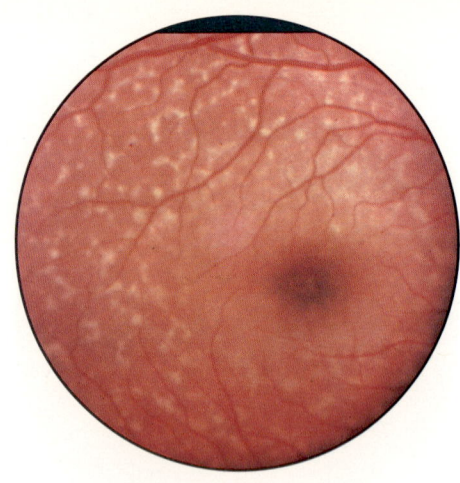

Plate 6 Fundus flavimaculatus demonstrating parafoveal flecks.

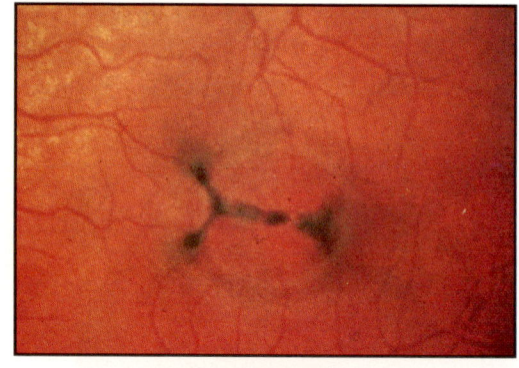

Plate 7 Butterfly pattern dystrophy.

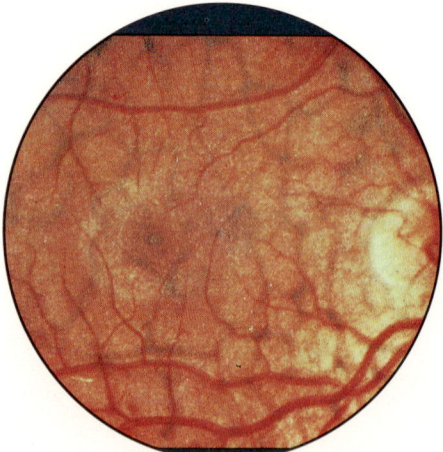

Plate 8 Reticular pattern dystrophy.

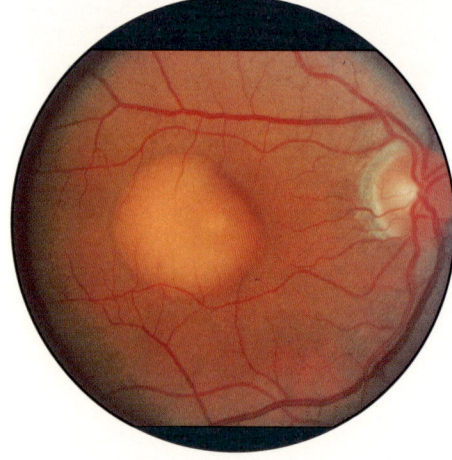

Plate 9 Right eye with vitelliform dystrophy in the vitelliform stage.

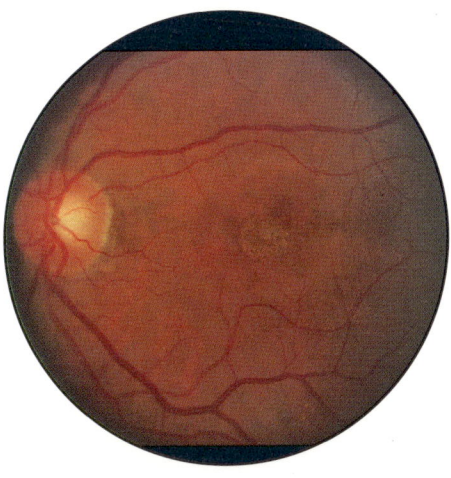

Plate 10 Left eye with vitelliform dystrophy in the vitelleruptive/atrophic maculopathy stage.

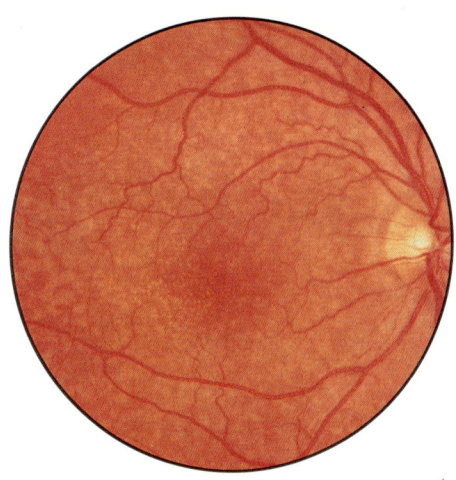

Plate 11 Dominant drusen.

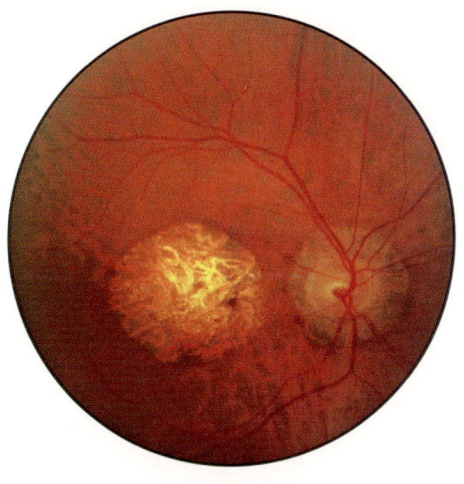

Plate 12 Central areolar choroidal dystrophy.

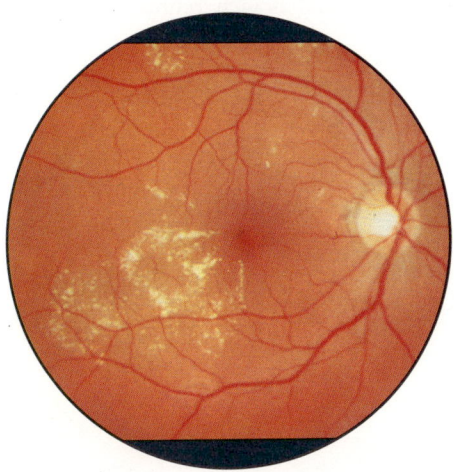

Plate 13 Right eye of a 42-year-old man with diabetes. There is nonproliferative diabetic retinopathy with a circinate ring of hard exudates invading the center of the foveal avascular zone.

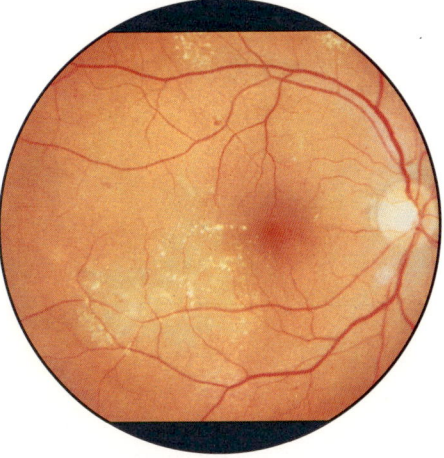

Plate 14 Eight months later there is less macular edema. The hard exudates have resolved. Visual acuity improved to 20/30.

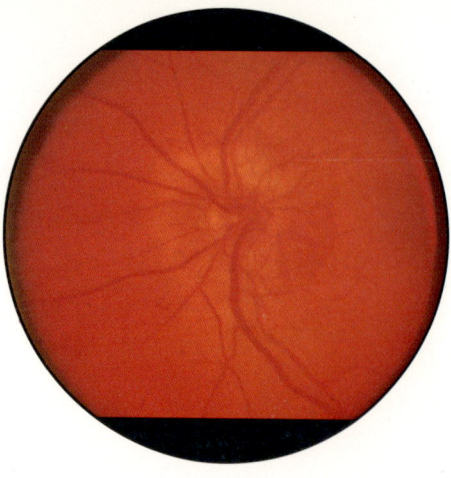

Plate 15 Neovascularization of the optic disc.

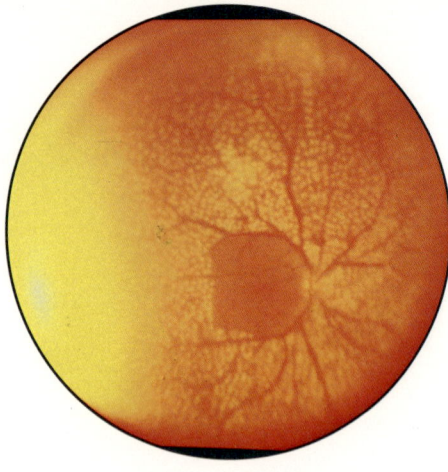

Plate 16 Complete panretinal photocoagulation. The treatment extends two disc diameters from the center of the macula to the periphery.

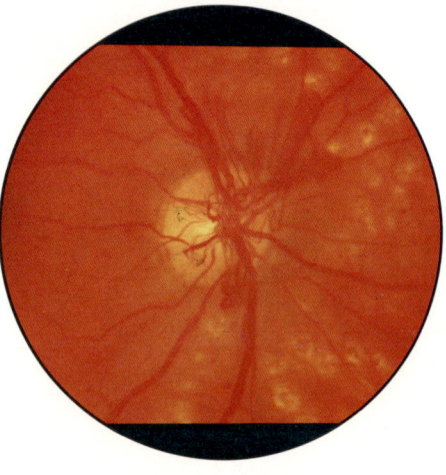

Plate 17 Persistent neovascularization of the disk despite complete panretinal photocoagulation.

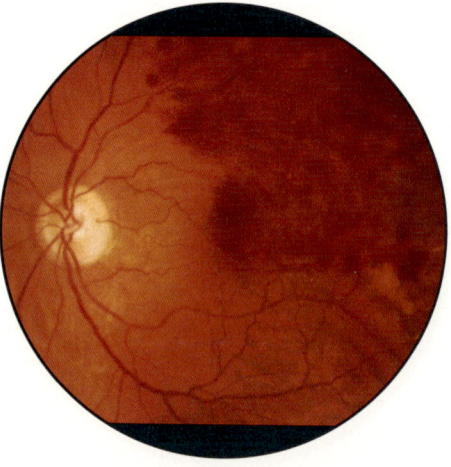

Plate 18 Typical appearance of nonischemic superotemporal branch retinal vein occlusion.

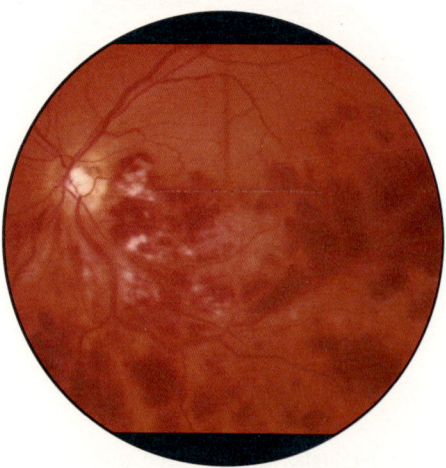

Plate 19 Ischemic superotemporal branch retinal vein occlusion. Note the multiple nerve fiber layer infarcts.

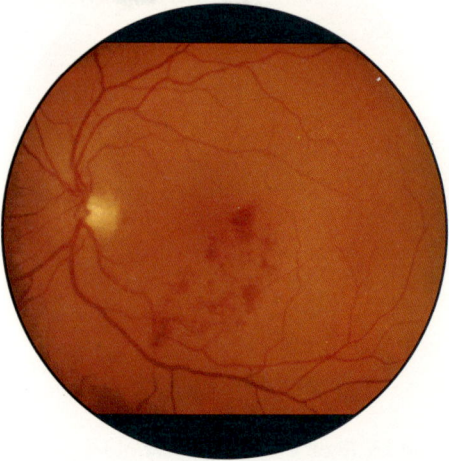

Plate 20 Small macular branch retinal vein occlusion.

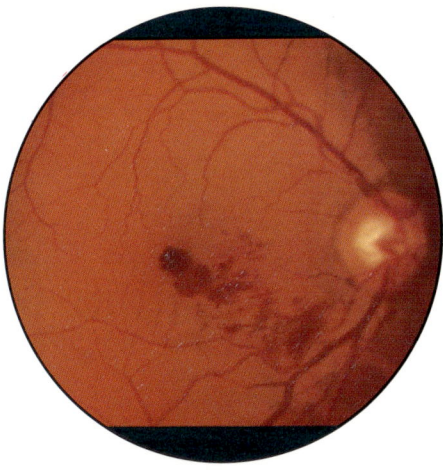 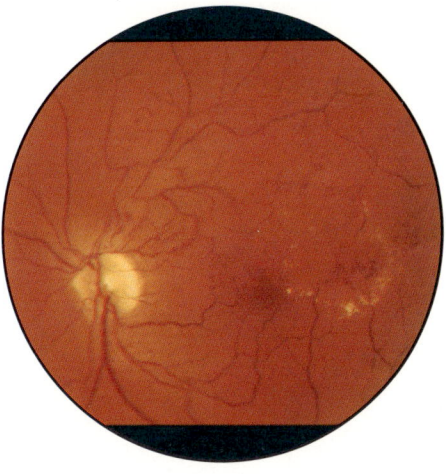

Plate 21 Branch retinal vein occlusion with macular hemorrhage.

Plate 22 Chronic branch retinal vein occlusion with collateral vessel formation across the horizontal raphe both temporal and nasal to the fovea.

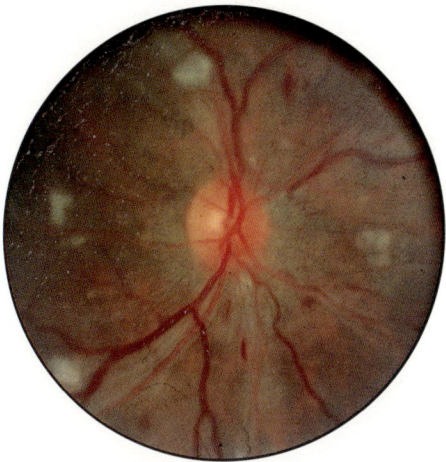 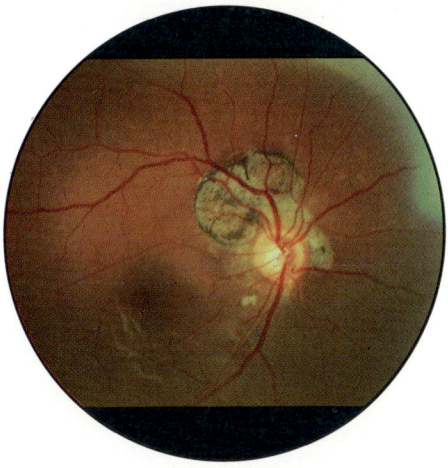

Plate 23 Hypertensive retinopathy demonstrating hemorrhages and nerve fiber layer infarcts.

Plate 24 Healed Elschnig spots in a patient who has recovered from an episode of malignant hypertension.

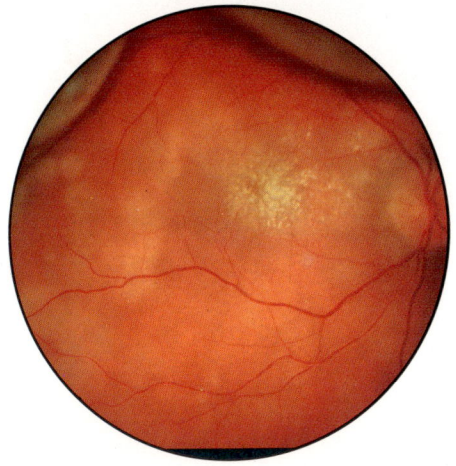

Plate 25 Serous retinal detachment in pregnancy-induced hypertension.

Courtesy James Augsburger, M.D.

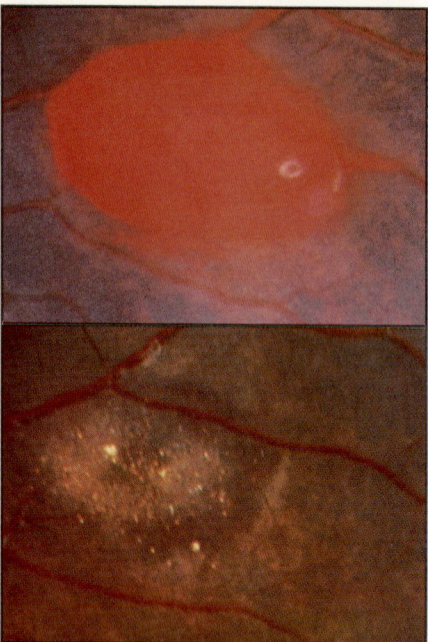

Plate 26 Evolution of salmon patch hemorrhage *(top),* evolving over time to iridescent deposits *(bottom).*

From Gagliano DA, Goldberg MF: *Arch Ophthalmol* 107:1814-1815, 1989.

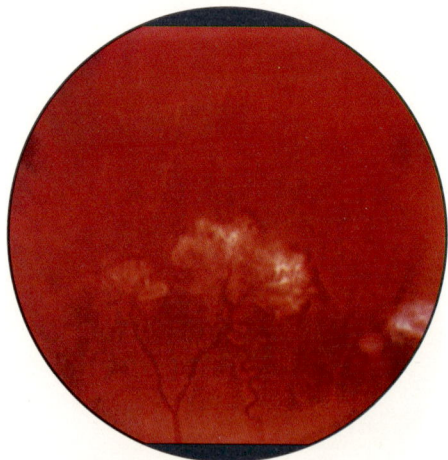

Plate 27 Peripheral neovascular proliferation ("sea fan") in a patient with proliferative sickle cell retinopathy (PSR).

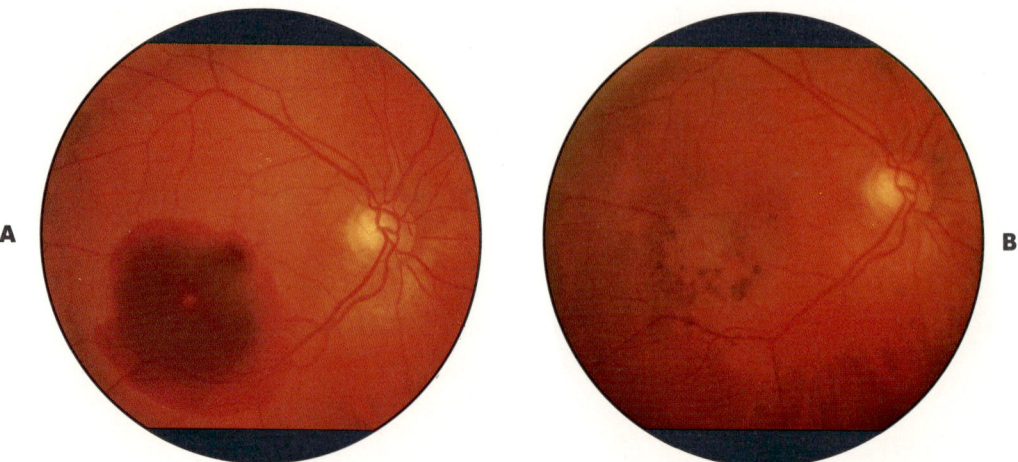

Plate 28 A, Large subretinal hemorrhage from a retinal arterial macroaneurysm that has reduced vision to counting fingers. **B,** Six months later the blood has resorbed but extensive RPE alteration can be seen clinically.

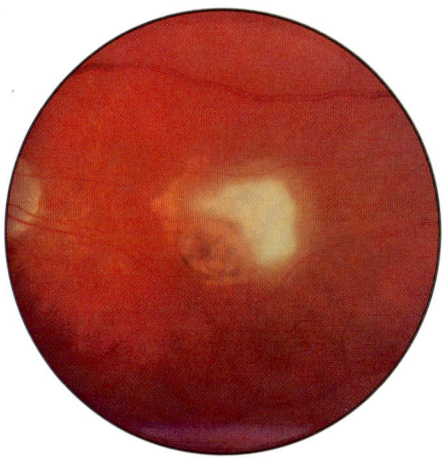
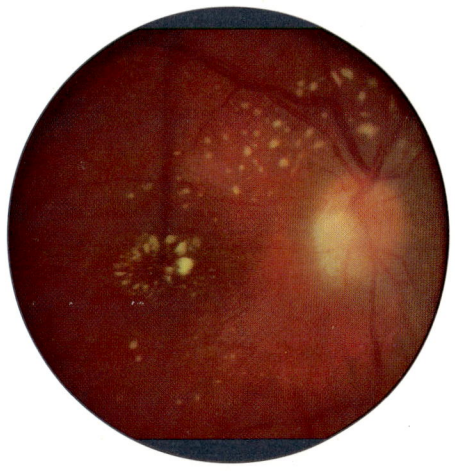

Plate 29 This central macular scar, just inferior to a superotemporal fluffy retinal exudate, is the characteristic macular lesion of recurrent ocular toxoplasmosis. Associated with central photopsia, worsening of central vision, and spots and floaters, it is almost pathognomonic of a recurrent ocular toxoplasmic infection.

Plate 30 This optic nerve has a fluffy lesion of juxtapapillary retinitis with secondary serous fluid leakage. Note the punctate exudates involving the superior portion of the macula and a central macular scar.

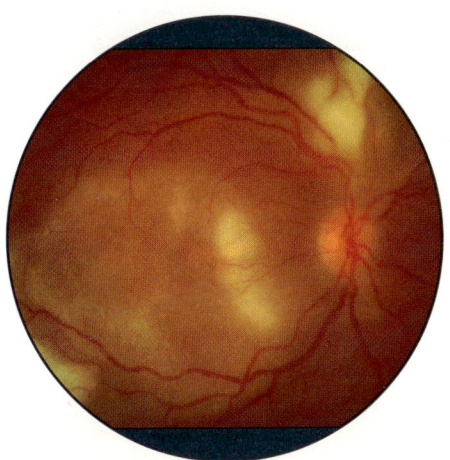
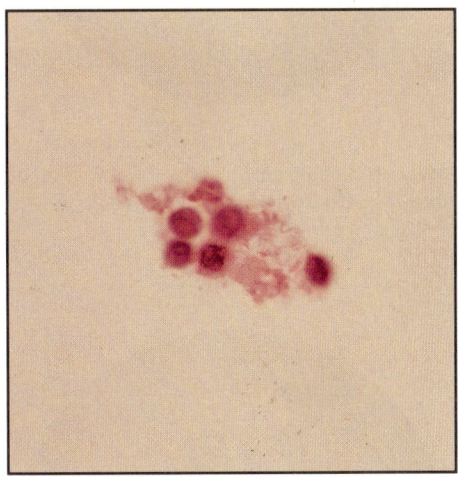

Plate 31 Retinal and subretinal infiltrates involving the macular region in a post–bone marrow transplant patient treated for leukemia with immunosuppressive drugs. Visual function in the macular region had been diminished for 2 to 3 months.

Plate 32 Fine needle aspiration biopsy of the yellowish exudate in Plate 31. Note the toxoplasmic cysts. Treatment with specific antitoxoplasmic agents brought about prompt resolution.

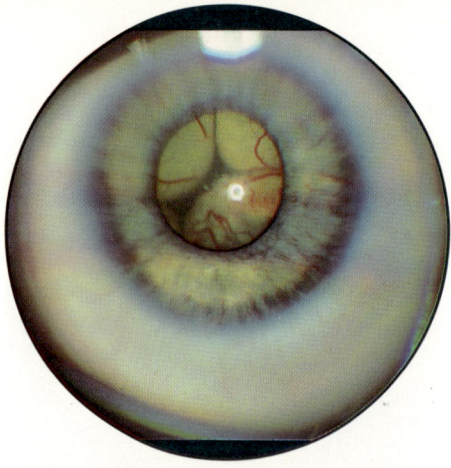

Plate 33 Total bullous retinal detachment in advanced Coats' disease.

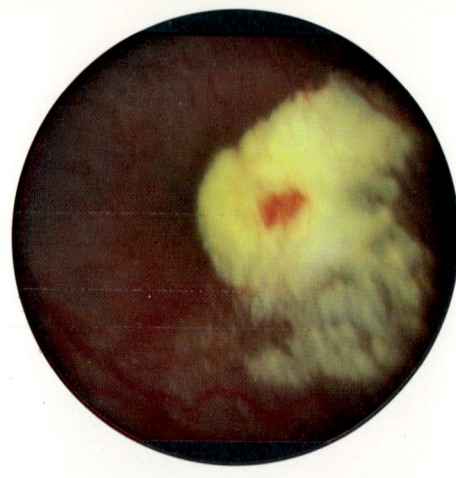

Plate 34 Exudation in the macular area before cryotherapy.

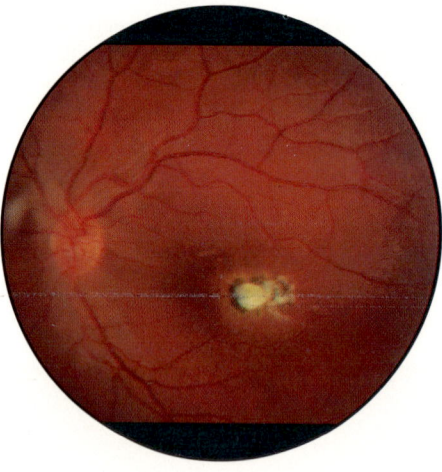

Plate 35 Twelve years after cryotherapy, exudate in the posterior pole of the patient shown in Plate 34 has not recurred.

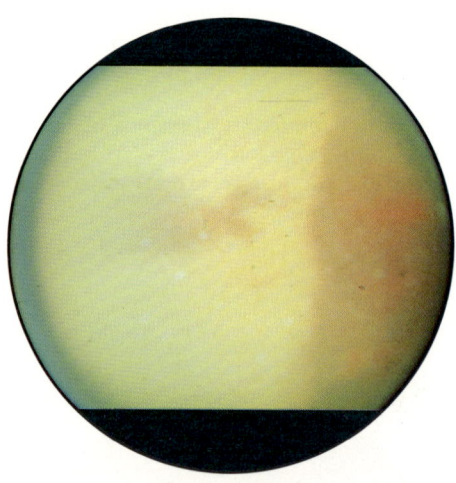

Plate 36 Typical peripheral retinitis in a patient with acute retinal necrosis. Note the dense whitening with a well-defined border between active and uninvolved retina.

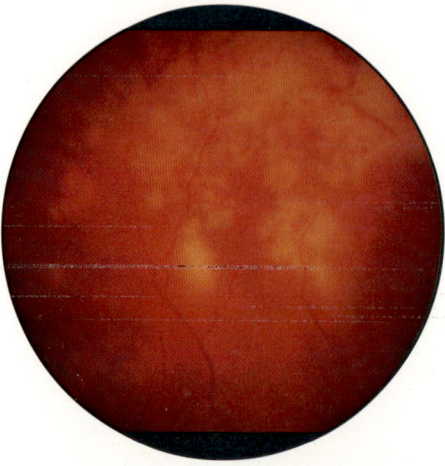

Plate 37 New satellite lesions of acute retinal necrosis approaching the posterior pole. Superiorly the necrosis was confluent.

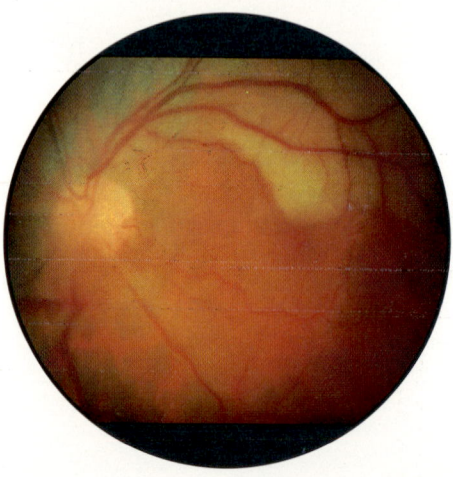

Plate 38 Branch retinal arterial obstruction associated with acute retinal necrosis.

Courtesy Robert Sergott, M.D.

PART I

Normal Retinal Anatomy and Function

1

Fluorescein Angiography: Principles and Interpretation

Jay L. Federman

The structural and functional integrity of the ocular tissue and vasculature is among the most important indicators of many ophthalmic disease processes. Direct visualization provides a great deal of valuable information; however, fluorescein angiography enables the clinician to supplement anatomic impressions with evidence of altered fluid dynamics in the iris, retina, and choroid and to discern structural changes in the retinal pigment epithelium.

Fluorescein angiography has been in clinical use for more than 30 years.[1,2] With each passing year it has become an increasingly refined, accurate, and invaluable tool, not only in the diagnosis and treatment of ocular disease but also for studying the basic functional anatomy of the eye.[3,4]

The results obtained from fluorescein angiography are the function of five basic factors: the physical and chemical properties of fluorescein dye, the anatomy of the human eye, the proficiency of the photographers, the sophistication of the recording equipment, and (most critically) the skill of the professional at correctly interpreting the information and relating it to other clinical findings.

FLUORESCEIN DYE

Historical Perspective

The phenomenon of fluorescence in excited crystalline substances was extensively studied during the midnineteenth century. In 1871 the German chemist Adolf von Baeyer[5] first synthesized fluorescein, a xanthene dye that eventually proved useful in the diagnosis of corneal abrasions, ulcers, and other disorders.[6,7] In 1882 Paul Ehrlich[8] noted that fluorescein parenterally administered to rabbits was detectable in the anterior chamber of the eye as a vertical yellow-green line. Many subsequent angioscopic studies of the animal fundus following intravenous injection of fluorescein or other dyes were carried out by various investigators until 1955, when MacClean and Maumenee[9] employed fluorescein dye in living human subjects. In January 1960 Novotny and Alvis[10,11] took the first human fluorescein angiogram, and they were the ones who developed the basic photographic system required for sequential documentation of flow through the fundus.[12] Publication of these reports launched a revolution in the approach to understanding and treating posterior segment disease.

Chemical and Physical Properties

Sodium fluorescein ($C_{20}H_{10}Na_2$) is a stable, highly water-soluble, pharmacologically inert, and complex organic molecule with a molecular weight of 376.27.[6,13,14]

Luminescence is the emission of light through means other than incandescence. Certain materials, when stimulated by light, subsequently reemit light of a longer wavelength and lower energy level, either slowly (as in phosphorescence) or almost instantaneously (as in fluorescence, in which decay occurs on time scales in the range of 10^{-8} second).[6,13]

Sodium fluorescein molecules preferentially absorb light at wavelengths from 465 to 490 nm, in the blue region of the visible spectrum, and emit light in the yellow-green range at 520 to 530 nm.[13-17] In the bloodstream, binding of sodium fluorescein to red blood cells and serum protein greatly reduces the amount of free fluorescein available for excitation,[14] but it also more narrowly limits the absorption and emission wavelengths to 465 nm and 525 nm respectively.[17,18] This wider and cleaner distinction between excitation and emission frequencies facilitates their separation by filters during the photographic process.[17,18]

Sodium fluorescein is a practical and convenient diagnostic tool. It is inexpensive, water soluble, pharmacologically inert, and relatively safe. It fluoresces at normal blood pH, and absorbs and emits light within the visible range of the spectrum, permitting the use of standard photographic equipment and supplies.[6,13,14,16] Physiologically the sodium fluorescein molecule is small enough to diffuse rapidly within fluid compartments yet sufficiently large not to pass through the tight endothelial junctions of intact retinal blood vessels and the zonula occludens of the retinal pigment epithelium.[13,14,16] The visible distribution of fluorescein in the posterior segment thus becomes a valuable indicator of the functional integrity of the blood retinal barrier.

Administration

A solution of 10% sodium fluorescein (5 ml) is injected intravenously. Some investigators have obtained equally satisfactory results, with fewer adverse effects, using smaller quantities of a 25% solution[16] or even smaller injections (2 ml) of the standard 10% solution.[19]

The patient is seated comfortably at the fundus camera, and fluorescein is rapidly injected via an antecubital vein. One must check proper placement and avoid extravasation, since the alkaline fluorescein solution is irritating and may cause severe local pain or even necrosis of overlying skin.[20,21]

Fluorescein first appears in the eye as faint patchy regions of fluorescence in the choroid approximately 12 to 15 seconds following intravenous administration (Figs. 1-1 to 1-3), and the dye is evenly distributed throughout the blood after 3 to 5 minutes. It is then rapidly cleared from the system, primarily through the kidneys,[14,16,22] and elimination is mostly complete by the end of 1 hour.

When intravenous administration is not feasible, fluorescein can be given

Fluorescein angiography: principles and interpretation

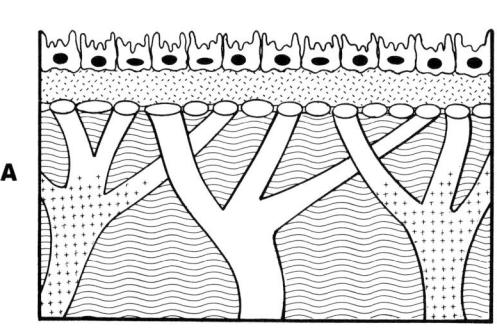
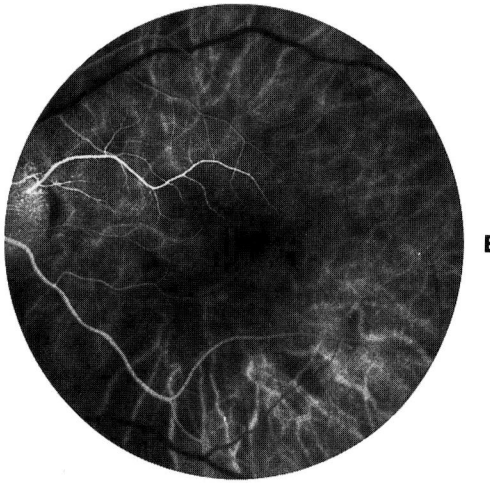

Figure 1-1 Early filling of large and medium-sized choroidal arterioles with fluorescein. **A,** The fluorescein *(black crosses)* has not reached the level of the choriocapillaris at this stage. **B,** Earliest phase of the fluorescein study.

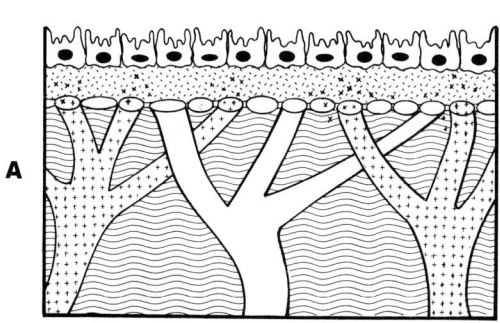
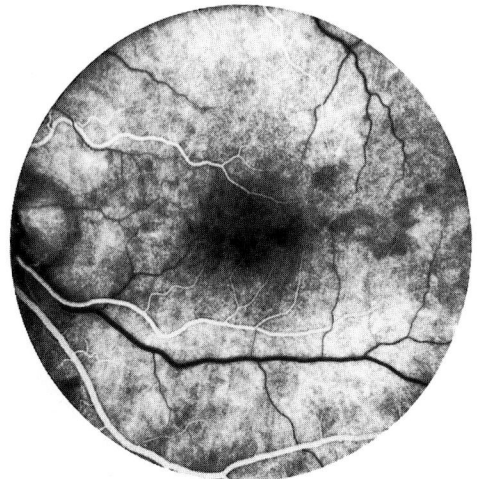
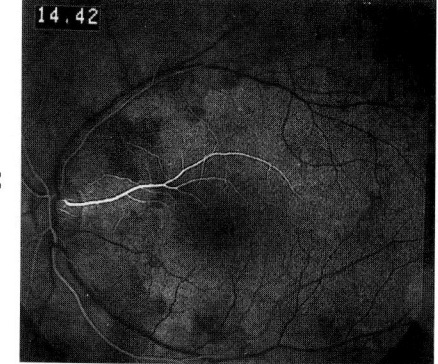

Figure 1-2 Early filling of the choriocapillaris with fluorescein. **A,** The fluorescein *(black crosses)* flows in a patchy manner from the efferent side of the circulation. Some is beginning to leak into the extravascular space near Bruch's membrane. **B,** Medium-sized and smaller arterioles are seen leading to patches of fluorescein-filled choriocapillaris. **C,** A cilioretinal artery usually fills at the same time that an early choroidal flush is seen.

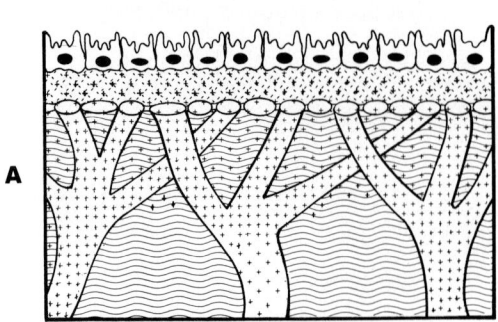 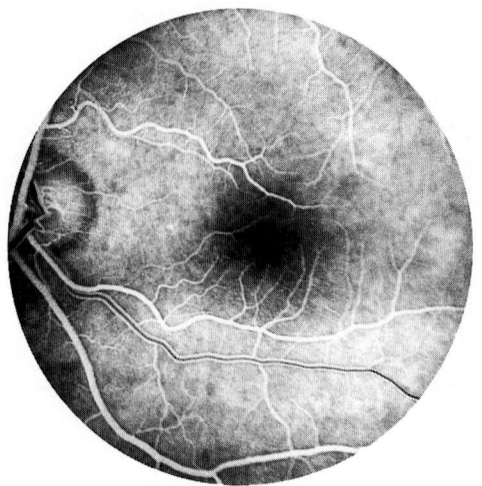

Figure 1-3 Complete filling of the choriocapillaris with fluorescein. **A,** The fluorescein *(black crosses)* has now begun to leak into the extravascular choroidal stroma. An extravascular flush appears in Bruch's membrane and the inner choroidal layers. **B,** Same eye as in Figure 1-12, *B,* a few seconds later in the study. More diffuse filling of the choriocapillaris now largely obscures the earlier patchy distribution. Leakage from the capillaries into the extravascular component of the inner choroid and Bruch's membrane contributes to the diffuse and more uniform fluorescence.

orally. It is relatively poorly absorbed through the gastrointestinal tract, however, and provides a low early serum concentration that is adequate for demonstrating cystoid maculopathy and other blood–retinal barrier disorders but not for detailed anatomic studies or evaluation of blood flow velocities.[23,24,25]

Toxicity

Fluorescein is a remarkably safe diagnostic compound, though as with any internally administered substance there is some risk of side effects. Transient nausea and occasional vomiting 30 to 60 seconds after administration are the most common reactions, experienced in fewer than 5% of patients.[26] Moderate adverse reactions, occurring in fewer than 1% of patients, include thrombophlebitis, nerve palsy, syncope, temperature elevation, and localized tissue necrosis.[20,26] There is a very low incidence of severe potentially life-threatening reactions such as laryngeal edema, bronchospasm, anaphylaxis, circulatory shock, and myocardial infarction. Yannuzzi et al.[26] have reported a single death among 220,000 fluorescein angiography studies surveyed. The incidence of reported adverse reactions appears to be lower when fluorescein is administered by the oral route, although severe allergic reactions may still occur.[27] There are no reports of fetal complications resulting from fluorescein angiography; however, many physicians try to avoid the use of this, as of any other drug substance, during pregnancy.

Prophylaxis for possible adverse reactions is controversial. An intradermal skin test has been recommended[28] when toxicity is suspected. Despite the rarity of severe adverse reactions, oxygen and an emergency tray should always be readily available during fluorescein administration.

Patients should be cautioned before the procedure of minor inevitable side effects such as red afterimages from the camera flash and discoloration of skin and urine from fluorescein for up to several days after the procedure. Physicians should be aware that the presence of residual fluorescein may cause short-term alterations in the results of clinical serum laboratory tests.[29]

ANATOMIC CONSIDERATIONS

The actual distribution, and thus visibility, of fluorescein in the eye during angiography is determined by the functional anatomy of the normal and pathologic ocular vasculature. There are two distinct vascular systems in the ocular fundus: retinal and choroidal. Between them lies the retinal pigment epithelium (RPE), an opaque cell monolayer anterior to the choroid that normally largely obscures its vasculature. Pathologic alteration of the structure and pigmentation of the RPE affects the pattern of choroidal fluorescence perceptible during angiographic studies. Familiarity with the anatomy and interaction of these anatomic layers is the key to accurate interpretation of fluorescein angiograms.

Choroid

The choroid is a layer composed of vasculature and connective tissue, about 0.25 mm thick on average, that nourishes the RPE and outer retina. The choroidal circulation is completely independent of the retinal circulation. It is supplied by the long and short posterior and recurrent anterior ciliary arteries and is drained by the four midperipheral vortex veins. The choroidal capillary system, the choriocapillaris, is located innermost, its basement membrane forming the outer layer of Bruch's membrane, and has a lobular pattern, with central arterioles feeding capillary beds drained by peripheral venules.

The walls of the choroidal capillaries are extremely thin, with multiple fenestrations permitting passive fluid transport from the capillary lumen to the surrounding extravascular space. The fluorescein molecule is sufficiently small to pass readily and rapidly out of the choriocapillaris, but it does not pass through the zonula occludens of the overlying retinal pigment epithelium.

Fluorescein dye appears as a patchy choroidal filling across the posterior fundus within a few seconds, often before it reaches the retinal circulation (Fig. 1-1). The presence of fluorescein in the choroidal vasculature is difficult to study because of extravascular leakage and rapid retinal filling and because, in all but patients with albinism or an exceedingly pale RPE, the features are partially obscured by the overlying pigmented tissues.[6]

Retinal Pigment Epithelium

The retinal pigment epithelium (RPE) is a single layer of pigmented cuboidal cells whose apical portions are intermingled with the photoreceptors and whose basal portions are attached to Bruch's membrane. It serves important metabolic functions for the overlying photoreceptors and forms a structural barrier between the sensory retina and choroid that, under normal circumstances, fluorescein dye will not cross.[30,31]

Because of the presence of pigmented melanosomes, the RPE serves as an optical barrier. Pigment density is not uniform across the whole retina but is distributed in a characteristic gradient across the fundus of any normal eye. Pigmentation is greatest in the foveomacular region, where pigment epithelial cells are tall, columnar, and densely packed, and least in regions anterior to the equator, where these cells are flatter and more cuboidal, with a resulting sparsity of pigment granules.

Retina

For purposes of the present discussion, the important characteristics of the retina are its functional architecture and its light absorption and transmission properties. The retina is a thin transparent tissue perfused by the central retinal artery and, in about 32% of eyes, by an additional cilioretinal artery. The cilioretinal artery, when present, fills at the same time as the choroid.[32] Unlike the choroid, the retinal capillary bed is nonfenestrated and there is virtually no extracellular space between the densely packed retinal cells. As a result, the retinal vasculature constitutes a "closed system" that stands out in stark optical contrast to the surrounding tissue.

When interpreting fluorescein angiograms, it is important to remember that the outer nuclear and plexiform retinal layers have a high concentration of yellow xanthophyll pigment, particularly in the macula, a region about two disc diameters in size surrounding (but not including) the fovea. Selective absorption of light at the blue excitation frequency by this pigment produces a relatively darker macular background in fluorescein angiography.[16]

PHOTOGRAPHIC EQUIPMENT

The progression of fluorescein dye through the eye is recorded using special motorized fundus cameras and video equipment designed to take rapid sequential photographs at intervals of less than 1 second.

Light is passed through an appropriate filter to produce a narrow band of blue excitatory light corresponding to the absorption peak of sodium fluorescein. The dye distributed throughout the ocular vasculature and extracellular space then emits light of a longer (yellow-green) wavelength, which can be photographed through a second filter that selectively blocks reflected blue light. The sodium fluorescein excitation and emission curves are in close juxtaposition and may even overlap, which can lead to a phenomenon called pseudofluorescence if the filters employed are not carefully selected. Most modern angiography filters are well matched to minimize transmission curve overlaps, although one should be aware of this potential source of error.

Another possible cause of confusion is "autofluorescence" by certain ocular structures following illumination with blue light.[14,16,33] Best's vitelliform lesions, lipofuscin over choroidal melanomas, flecks associated with fundus flavimaculatus, and optic nerve head drusen are all pathologic conditions that may autofluoresce even in the absence of fluorescein dye in the eye.[34] There is also a degree of autofluorescence in normal ocular structures, including the sclera, retina, lens, and Descemet's membrane.[14] Recent work[35] indicates that the autofluorescence of the lens may serve as a reliable indicator of metabolic control in diabetics.

INTERPRETATION

Fluorescein angiography is a valuable adjunct to diagnosis that supports and enhances, but does not replace, standard clinical examination. One exception to this rule is found in patients with dense asteroid hyalosis obscuring the posterior pole. Because only the yellow-green fluorescent light emitted from the dye is detected, and not reflected incident light, the angiographic detail may be vastly superior to the results of white light ophthalmoscopy, wherein reflection from asteroid bodies hampers visualization.[36]

One of the great advantages of fluorescein angiography is that it documents both the static functional anatomy and the fluid dynamics of the eye. It is important to review negatives or contact sheets in appropriate sequential order.

Fluorescein studies are typically divided into four phases: prefilling, transit, recirculation, and late.

The *prefilling* phase occurs after administration but before fluorescein dye enters the circulation of the eye. Angiograms taken during the prefilling phase are useful controls to establish background levels of pseudofluorescence or autofluorescence that might otherwise lead to interpretation errors.

The *transit* phase corresponds to the first complete passage of fluorescein-bearing blood through the choroidal and retinal vasculature, and occurs within about 30 seconds of dye injection. Following perfusion of the choroid and choriocapillaris, there are three functional subdivisions of the transit phase: the arterial phase, which corresponds to complete arterial filling, the capillary (or arteriovenous) phase, which culminates in the first evidence of laminar venous flow, and the venous filling (or laminar) phase, which occurs as the veins completely fill and the arteries begin to empty of dye.

The *recirculation* phase corresponds to the first return of fluorescein-bearing blood to the eye after its passage through the general circulation, and is complete about 3 minutes into the study. Most fluorescein is removed from the blood in a single passage through the kidneys; thus recirculation fluorescence is considerably dimmer than transit fluorescence. Early staining or leakage is generally noted during this stage of the study.

The *late* (or elimination) phase represents the complete removal of fluorescein dye from the circulation, leaving only spots of residual leakage and late staining. For all practical purposes, elimination is virtually complete 30 minutes after administration.

In any isolated portion of the ocular vasculature one can observe this sequence of distinct phases, although because circulation time varies in different regions of the retina, there is considerable overlap of phases. Interpretation of the overall fundus fluorescein pattern involves both the additive features of the three superimposed tissue layers—choroid, retinal pigment epithelium, and retina—and the spatial distribution of these features across the fundus.

NORMAL ANGIOGRAPHIC PATTERN

Fluorescein enters the choroidal vasculature through the posterior ciliary arteries. In a very lightly pigmented fundus, filling of large choroidal arterioles may be faintly perceived (Fig. 1-1), although in general the first discernible presence of fluorescein is the patchy background "choroidal flush" corresponding

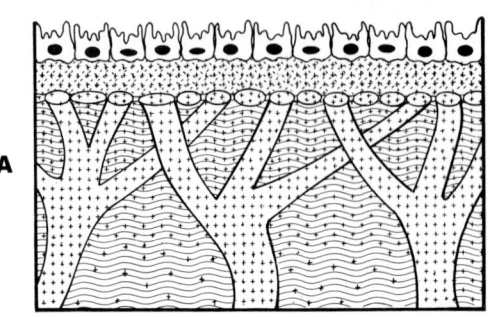 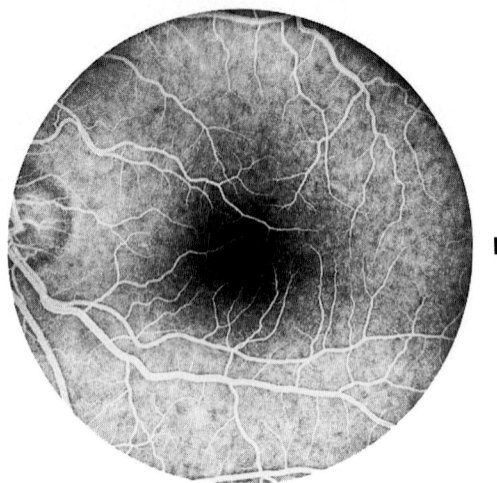

Figure 1-4 Complete filling of intravascular and extravascular components of the inner choroid. **A,** Dense equilibrated concentrations of fluorescein *(black crosses)* fill the choroidal vessels and inner choroidal extravascular space. The extravascular concentration in the outer choroid is lower. All choroidal detail is now completely obscured by the dense evenly distributed dye. **B,** Same eye as in Figure 1-13, *B,* a few seconds later in the study. The intravascular and extravascular components of the inner choroid are now evenly filled with dye, completely obscuring all choroidal detail.

to perfusion of the choriocapillaris[37,38] (Fig. 1-2, *A* and *B*). The cilioretinal artery, when present, fills at the same time (Fig. 1-2, *C*).

The choroidal sequence cannot be followed in the foveomacular region, where it is masked by the densely pigmented overlying RPE and by the highly localized macular concentration of xanthophyll pigment in the sensory retina.[16] Choriocapillaris perfusion is first and most clearly observed at the posterior pole, where the larger choroidal vessels progressively deliver fluorescein to separate and irregular choroidal regions. By focusing attention deep to the RPE early in the study, one may briefly discern these feeding vessels before their outlines are obscured by the choroidal flush, which rapidly intensifies and spreads anteriorly toward the ora serrata. (See Figures 1-1 to 1-4.)

Because of the capillary fenestrations in the choriocapillaris, intravascular choroidal fluorescein rapidly leaks into the extravascular space (Fig. 1-2, *A*), beginning at the inner choroidal layers directly below Bruch's membrane (Fig. 1-3, *A*). Fluorescein diffuses throughout the inner choroidal layers, rapidly reaching equilibrium between the intravascular and extravascular compartments and including the inner scleral fibers (Fig. 1-4, *A*). During the somewhat later venous filling phase of the study extravascular fluorescein begins to appear, to a lesser extent, in the stroma of the outer choroid (Fig. 1-4).

As the study progresses, the process of choroidal perfusion is reversed. The combined result of dye leakage, elimination, and distribution through the entire blood volume is that the intravascular fluorescein concentration quickly drops below the extravascular concentration. Beginning in the inner choroidal layers, the medium-sized choroidal vessels are darkly silhouetted against the still fluorescent extravascular background (Fig. 1-5).

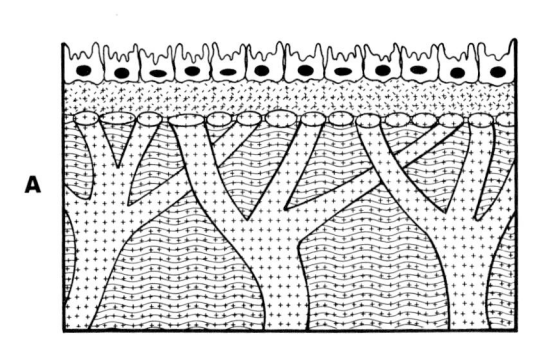

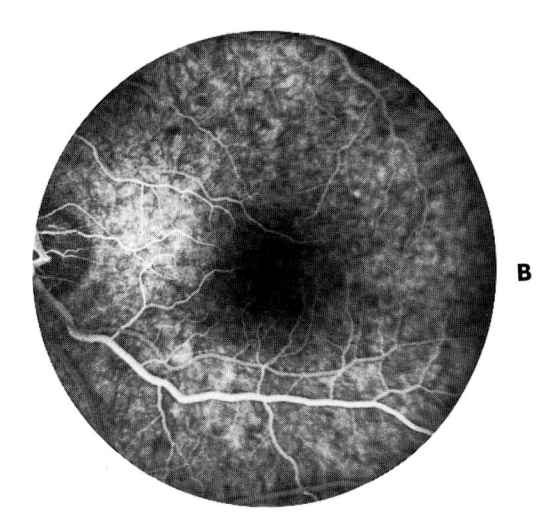

Fluorescein angiography: principles and interpretation 11

Figure 1-5 Visualization of medium-sized choroidal vessels. **A,** As fluorescein recirculates and is diluted through the entire blood volume, the intravascular choroidal concentration *(black crosses)* drops below the extravascular concentration. The concentration in the outer choroidal extravascular space is the same as within the entire choroidal intravascular space. Since the concentration is greater in the inner choroidal layers, medium-sized vessels within the inner and middle choroid can be visualized during the early phases of the study. **B,** Medium-sized choroidal vessels stand out in dark relief against the more concentrated dye in the extravascular inner choroidal space.

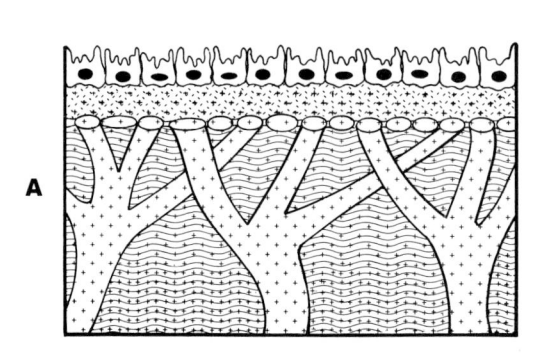

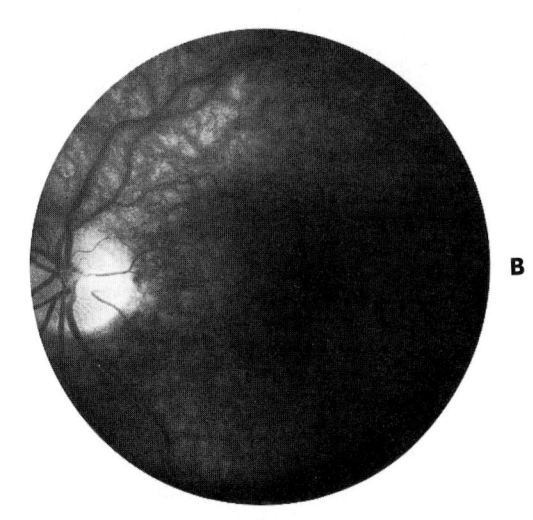

Figure 1-6 Visualization of large choroidal vessels. **A,** As the recirculation phase progresses, fluorescein concentrations *(black crosses)* in the inner and outer choroid are equal. In the later and elimination phases the extravascular concentration in the inner choroid continues to drop below that in the more slowly purged outer choroid layers. Large vessels in the outer choroid layers are surrounded by extravascular regions with much higher fluorescein concentrations. **B,** Large vessels in the outer choroid layers stand out in dark relief against the more concentrated extravascular fluorescein.

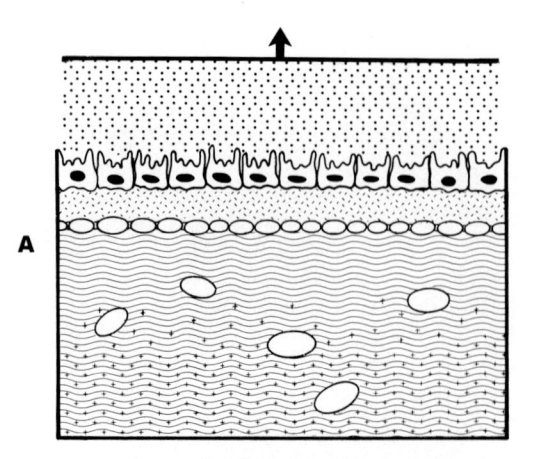

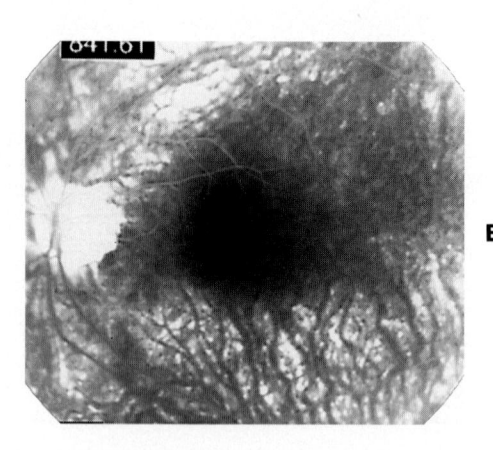

Figure 1-7 Hyperfluorescence in a patient with a lightly pigmented fundus. **A,** Dye in the outer choroidal extravascular space during the late elimination phase. Fluorescein *(black crosses)* from the outer choroidal layers readily passes through the depigmented retinal pigment epithelium. **B,** Late elimination phase in the lightly pigmented fundus, showing the choroidal vasculature, now emptied of fluorescein, standing out in dark relief against the extravascular fluorescence of the outer choroid layers.

Over time, fluorescein leaks back into the choroidal vessels from, successively, the choriocapillaris, outer choroid, and inner scleral layers. During the later stages of this process the extravascular fluorescein concentration is greater in the outer choroid than in the inner choroid, and large vessels stand out in dark relief (Fig. 1-6). Even in the late phase, when fluorescein has been effectively purged from the vasculature, residual extravascular dye in the outer choroidal and inner scleral layers leaves patterns of choroidal fluorescence (Fig. 1-7).

The zonula occludens of the retinal pigment epithelium prevents diffusion or transport of fluorescein directly from the choroid to the outer retinal layers. Approximately 1 second after the choroidal flush, fluorescence is perceived in the central column of large arterioles, and rapidly increases in intensity, filling the arterioles completely. Vessels have a larger apparent diameter than with ophthalmoscopy or standard photography, since the entire vascular lumen is revealed rather than the dense central column alone.

Fluorescein next crosses the capillary network, revealing fine details of its structure in the perifoveal region where background choroidal fluorescence is masked by the densely pigmented RPE. As dye then enters the venous system, the veins take on a columnar appearance caused by early laminar flow, which gives way to a more confluent appearance as the concentration and uniformity of dye distribution increase.[16] Because the time required for arteriovenous transit is determined by the distance the dye must flow, the process is significantly faster in the macula than at the fundus periphery.

ABNORMAL ANGIOGRAPHIC PATTERNS

Abnormal fluorescein angiographic patterns result from disruption of the normal functional relationships between the various structures in the eye. The terms "hyperfluorescence" and "hypofluorescence" refer to departures from the normal pattern of fluorescence in the eye, and can be related to various ocular pathologies.

Hyperfluorescence may correspond to (1) the presence of fluorescein in a location where it is not normally found, (2) an abnormally high concentration of fluorescein in an appropriate location, and/or (3) abnormal visibility of a normal dye distribution and concentration because of defects in overlying structures that would ordinarily obscure it.

Keeping in mind the optical and functional anatomy of the various tissue layers helps determine the probable cause of hyperfluorescence. For example, the presence of dye in abnormal locations is not usually implicated in choroidal hyperfluorescence. Since, as was discussed above, fluorescein rapidly diffuses throughout the intravascular and extravascular choroidal compartments, fluorescence is normally expected everywhere in the choroid, although its transmission depends on the integrity of other structures. Consequently, choroidal hyperfluorescence most often corresponds to high relative concentrations of dye or to pathologic defects in overlying tissue layers.

Hypofluorescence may be caused by (1) the complete absence of fluorescein in a location where it is normally found, (2) an abnormally low concentration of fluorescein in some region, and/or (3) the abnormally obstructed visibility of light from normal dye distribution and concentration because of overlying pathology.

Hyperfluorescence

An excellent example of hyperfluorescence caused by the accumulation of dye in an abnormal location is found in focal detachment of the retinal pigment epithelium (Fig. 1-8). Dye-containing fluid that accumulates between the RPE and Bruch's membrane in the region of the serous detachment produces a hyperfluorescent patch with sharp and abrupt borders.

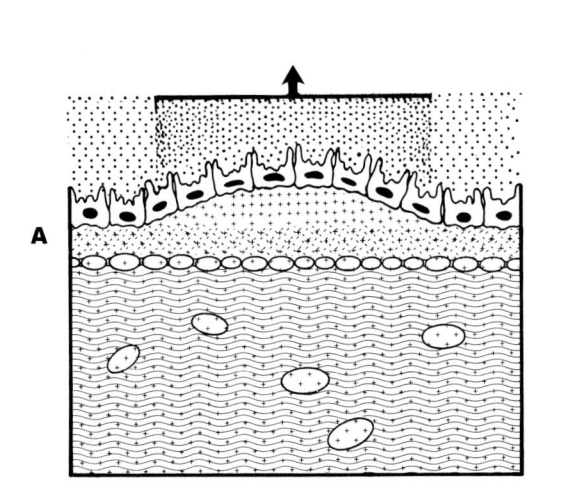

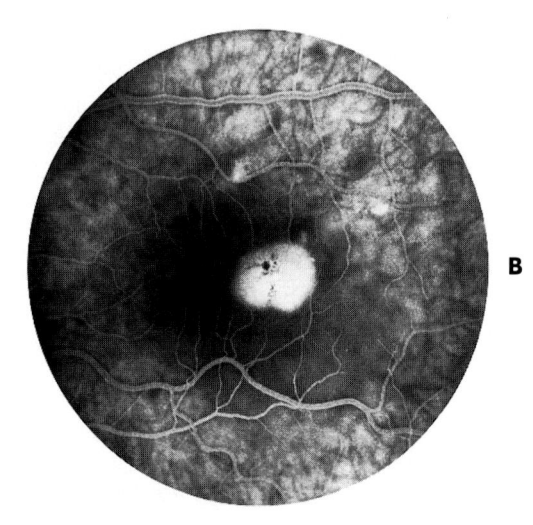

Figure 1-8 Hyperfluorescence in a patient with retinal pigment epithelium detachment. **A,** Accumulation of fluorescein *(black crosses)* in a localized serous detachment of the RPE. **B,** This localized area of hyperfluorescence has resulted from an accumulation of dye under the RPE.

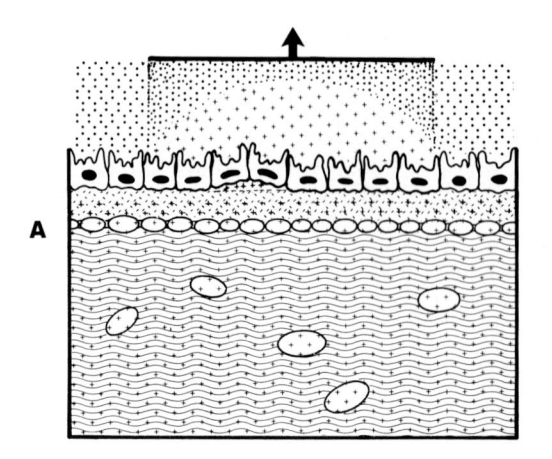

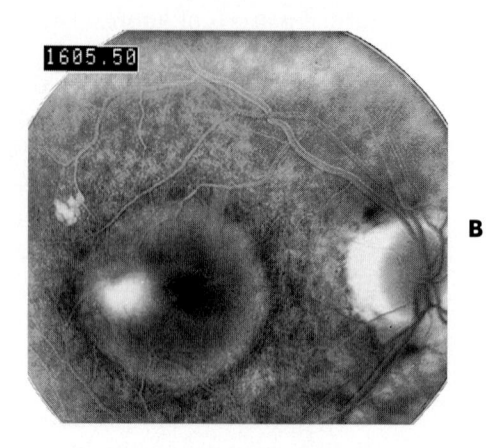

Figure 1-9 Hyperfluorescence in a patient with central serous chorioretinopathy. **A**, Accumulation of fluorescein *(black crosses)* between the neurosensory retina and the retinal pigment epithelium. A small focal detachment of the RPE has also filled with fluorescein. **B**, Area of hyperfluorescence corresponding to serous detachment of neurosensory retina that has filled with fluorescein. Within this region lies a smaller, more hyperfluorescent site corresponding to a small focal detachment of the RPE.

In central serous chorioretinopathy, dye accumulates between the neurosensory retina and the RPE to produce a diffuse region of hyperfluorescence. The diffuse borders of the hyperfluorescent region (Fig. 1-9, *B*), as contrasted with those in simple RPE detachment (Fig. 1-8, *B*), may reflect differences in the strength of attachment of photoreceptors to the RPE and of the RPE to Bruch's membrane, leading to different overlapping regions of dye accumulation.

In ocular histoplasmosis, nodular elevation of the RPE by choroidal neovascular membranes may cause choroidal hyperfluorescence (Fig. 1-10, *A* and *B*). In early stages of this disease very early phase angiograms reveal neovascular tufts filled with fluorescein. During later phases of the study dye leaks from the vascular loops to the surrounding tissue and may cause staining of the RPE (Fig. 1-10, *C* and *D*).

Another example of hyperfluorescence that can be seen in the choroid is caused by a localized increase in the concentration of dye. Choroidal hemangiomas demonstrate hyperfluorescence at very early phases of angiographic studies (Fig. 1-11, *A* and *B*). These highly vascular tumors fill with fluorescein dye at the same time as the choroidal vessels, and then the intensity drops off by the later phases of the study, leaving a fainter residual extravascular fluorescence (Fig. 1-11, *C* and *D*).

Solid tumors such as choroidal melanomas or metastatic lesions show hyperfluorescence caused by elevated fluorescein dye concentrations in the uveal stroma near the tumor site (Figs. 1-12 and 1-13). The increased vascularity of these tumors results in early-phase hyperfluorescence of vessels. Fluorescein then leaks into the extravascular space (Figs. 1-12, *A,* and 1-13, *A*), possibly penetrating slowly between the densely packed solid tumor cells. Fluorescein must also leak through defects in the overlying RPE to stain the subretinal space and retinal tissue, creating late hyperfluorescence. The peak of hyperfluores-

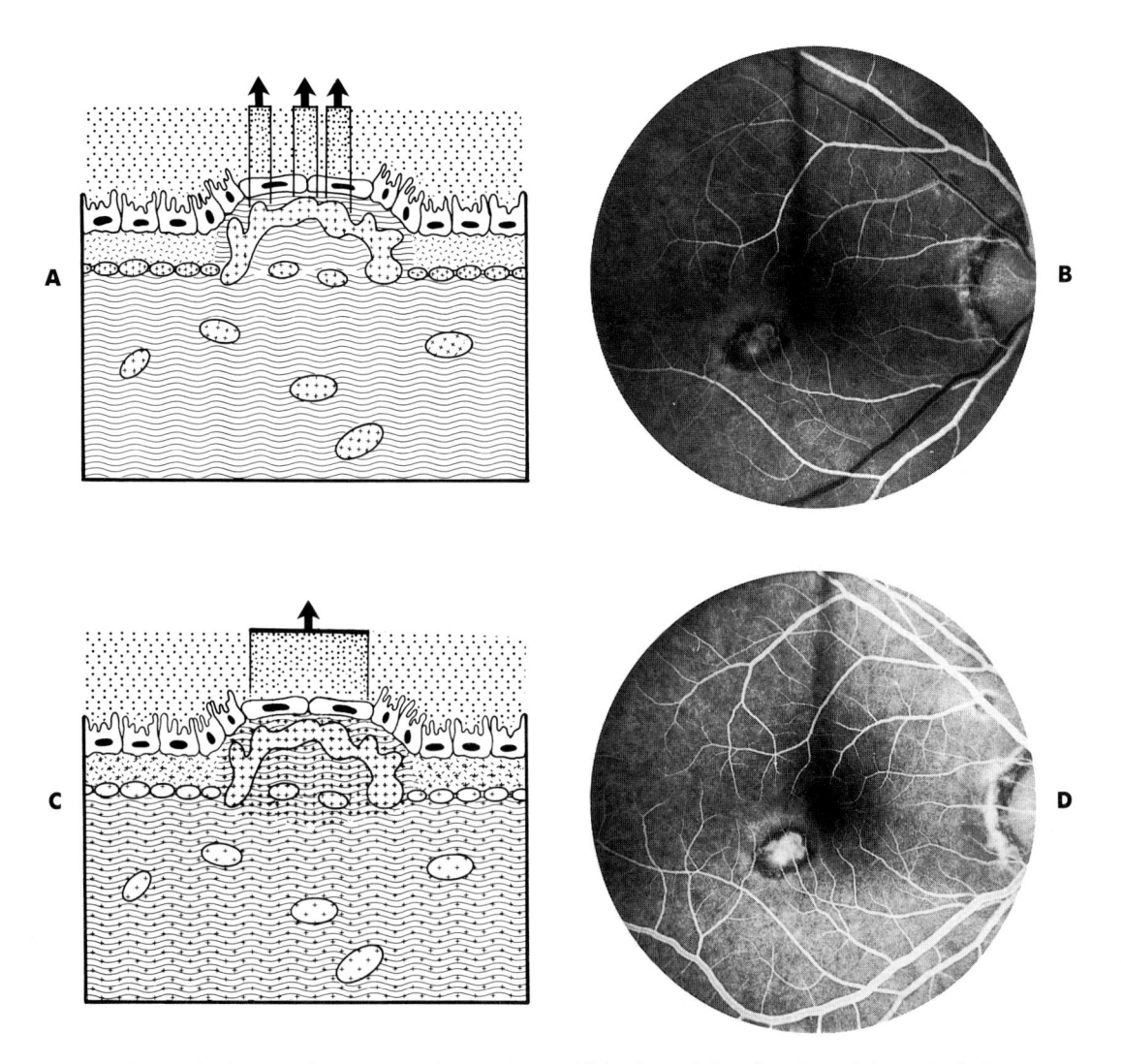

Figure 1-10 Hyperfluorescence in a patient with early nodular elevation of the retinal pigment epithelium secondary to presumed ocular histoplasmosis. **A**, Early filling of neovascular tuft with fluorescein *(black crosses)* within nodular elevation of the RPE. **B**, Early filling of a neovascular tuft with fluorescein within a nodular elevation of the RPE. **C**, Later phase of the study with leakage of fluorescein *(black crosses)* from the intravascular component of the nodular elevation of the retinal pigment epithelium into the extravascular space. Heavily concentrated fluorescein now fills the nodule uniformly. **D**, Nodular elevation of the RPE completely filled with fluorescein.

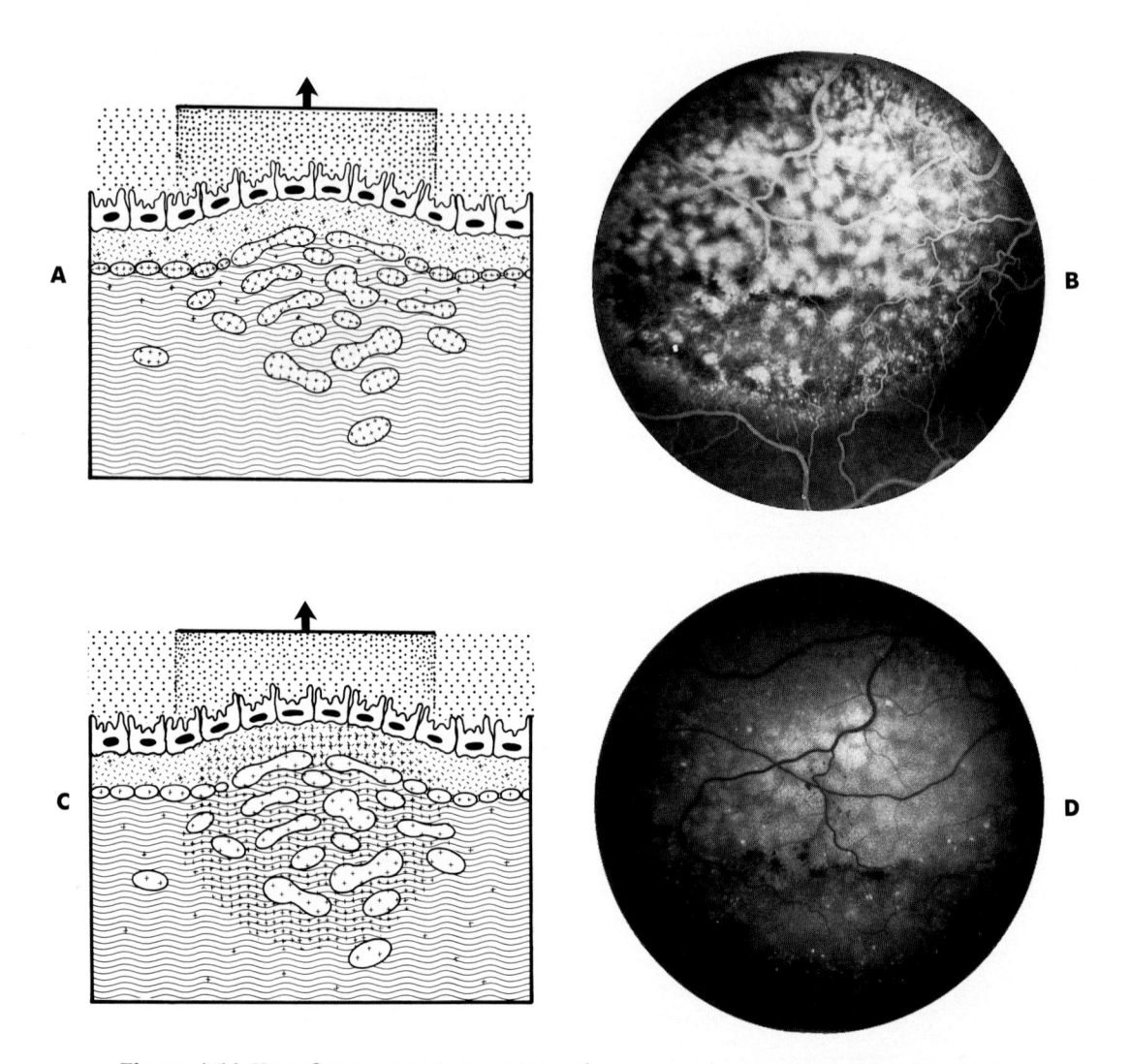

Figure 1-11 Hyperfluorescence in a patient with cavernous hemangioma of the choroid. **A**, Fluorescein *(black crosses)* fills the intravascular component of the tumor during the very early phases of the study. Note its greater concentration within the area of the lesion. **B**, Very early hyperfluorescence of the tumor. At this phase the hyperfluorescence is principally from intravascular tumor components as the dye leaks into walls of the abnormal vessels and surrounding tissue. **C**, Later phase of the study showing a greater concentration of fluorescein *(black crosses)* in the extravascular components of the lesion than in the vessels themselves. Note the microcystic spaces in the RPE and the RPE breakdown. **D**, Very late phase of the study showing hyperfluorescence caused by fluorescein accumulating in the extravascular tumor components. Note the cystic areas of degeneration of the overlying retina and the pinpoint areas of hyperfluorescence (probably related to microcystic changes in the overlying RPE).

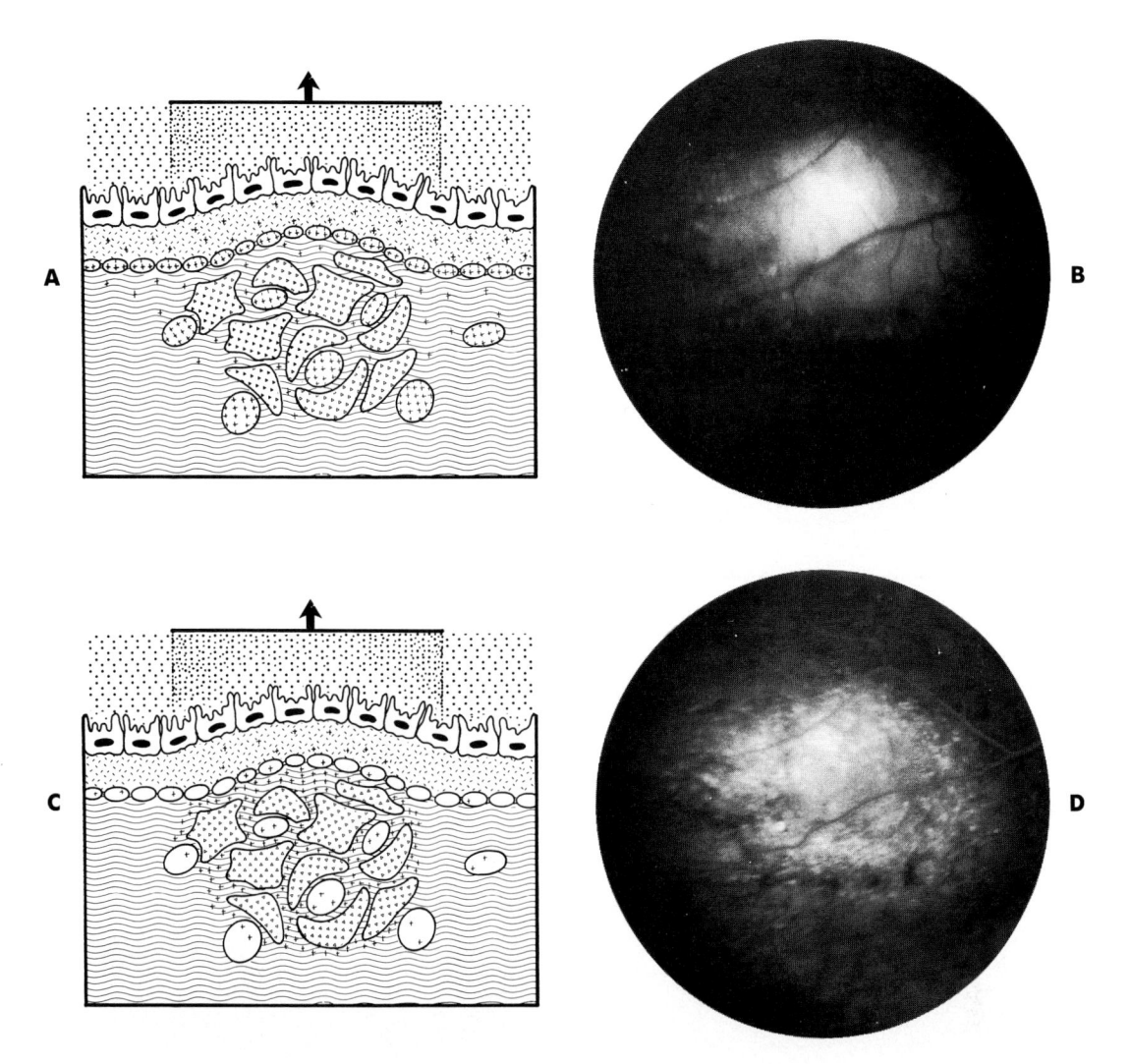

Figure 1-12 Hyperfluorescence in a patient with choroidal melanoma. **A,** The mass of tumor cells is more highly vascularized than the surrounding choroidal tissue. In this midphase of the study fluorescein *(black crosses)* accumulates in the tumor vessels, with some leakage into the extravascular space. Except for the intravascular tumor component, there is greater concentration of dye within the lesion than within the surrounding choroid. Hyperfluorescence of the tumor is also attributable possibly to increased transmission through the abnormal melanosomes (*clear circles* within the tumor cells) and probably to secondary degenerative RPE changes (not shown). **B,** Midfilling of the melanoma. In the early study phases fluorescence from the melanoma stems from filling of the tumor intravascular space. As the study progresses, tumor hyperfluorescence increases because of continuing fluorescein accumulation in the extravascular space (seen here). Increased transmission also has resulted from possibly abnormal pigment granules and RPE defects. **C,** Greater extravascular stroma fluorescein concentration *(black crosses)* in the tumor than in choroidal tissue. It is not known whether fluorescein is actually taken up by the melanoma cells or simply surrounds them. This is very late in the elimination phase, when most fluorescein has been removed from the intravascular and extravascular spaces. **D,** Late phases of the fluorescein study, showing hyperfluorescence of the melanoma from dye remaining in the extravascular stroma of the tumor. Hyperfluorescence is probably caused by a combination of the relatively high concentration of fluorescein and its increased transmission through abnormal pigment granules and RPE defects into the overlying cystically degenerated RPE and retina.

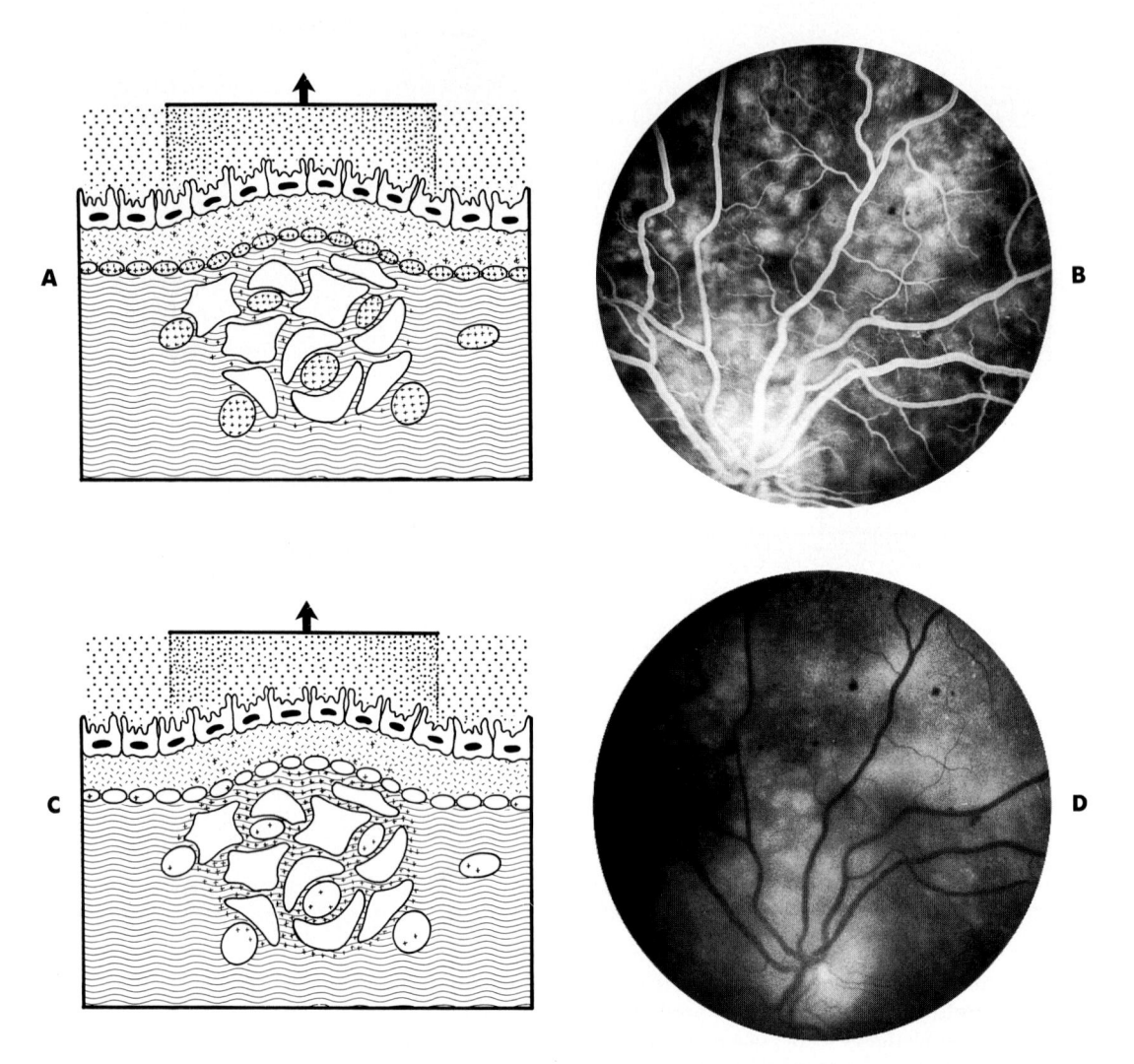

Figure 1-13 Hyperfluorescence in a patient with metastatic choroidal tumor. **A,** Neoplastic cells in a localized area within the choroid. In early phases of the study, when fluorescein *(black crosses)* is found predominantly in the intravascular spaces, the tumor (which is more vascular than the surrounding choroid) shows hyperfluorescence. This effect may be enhanced by secondary retinal pigment epithelium defects (not shown). **B,** Early fluorescence arising mostly from the intravascular component of the tumor. **C,** Metastatic choroidal tumor cells with increased vascular supply. The concentration of fluorescein *(black crosses)* in the extravascular stroma of the tumor is greater than within the intravascular space. Hyperfluorescence may be enhanced by the absence of pigment granules within the lesion and by secondary RPE degenerative changes (not shown). **D,** Hyperfluorescence is due to fluorescein remaining in the extravascular component of the tumor after dye has been eliminated from the surrounding choroid and possibly leaked into and beyond the degenerating RPE into overlying tissues.

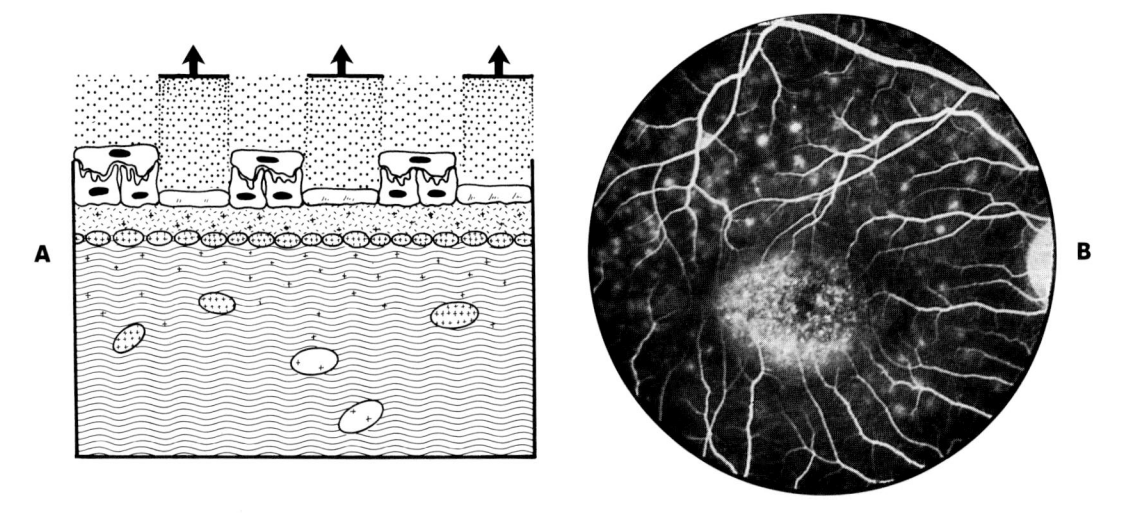

Figure 1-14 Hyperfluorescence in heredodegeneration of the retinal pigment epithelium. **A,** Areas where the RPE is attenuated with adjacent hyperpigmentation from the uptake of pigment granules by macrophages or hyperplastic pigmented epithelial cells. Early phases of the study show fluorescein *(black crosses)* within the choroidal vasculature and beginning to leak into the inner choroidal extravascular space. Hyperfluorescence results from this increased transmission through areas of the defective RPE. **B,** Transmission in the early phases of choroidal fluorescence through RPE defects. Blockage of the underlying background choroidal fluorescence by adjacent focal areas of hyperpigmentation can also be seen. This patient has both macular and diffuse changes throughout the midperiphery.

cence generally appears and passes later with these tumors than with choroidal hemangiomas, in which extravascular diffusion is more rapid.

Hyperfluorescence caused by normal choroidal fluorescence transmitted with abnormal intensity through RPE defects may be a contributing factor to the angiographic image of tumors and is also found in various other pathologic conditions. The decreased melanosome population associated with albinism leads to generalized fundus hyperfluorescence (see Fig. 1-7). In degenerative diseases that affect the RPE there may be focal nonpigmented regions intermingled with hyperpigmented areas. During the early phases of angiographic studies the choroidal fluorescence is transmitted through the RPE defects[39] (Fig. 1-14). Adjacent hyperpigmented regions block the background choroidal fluorescence. A similar picture is seen with drusen, where thinning of the RPE may occur, resulting in early-phase transmission followed by later-phase staining[40] (Fig. 1-15).

Hypofluorescence

The absence of fluorescein in a location where it is normally found may be attributable to either a lack of perfusion or the absence of tissue itself. In patients with a coloboma there is early-phase hypofluorescence because the choriocapillaris is missing. Only the large vessels of the choroidal vasculature fluoresce and are clearly visible without the obstruction of an overlying RPE (Fig. 1-16, *A* and *B*). In very late stages of the study secondary hyperfluorescence of the

Text continued on p. 24.

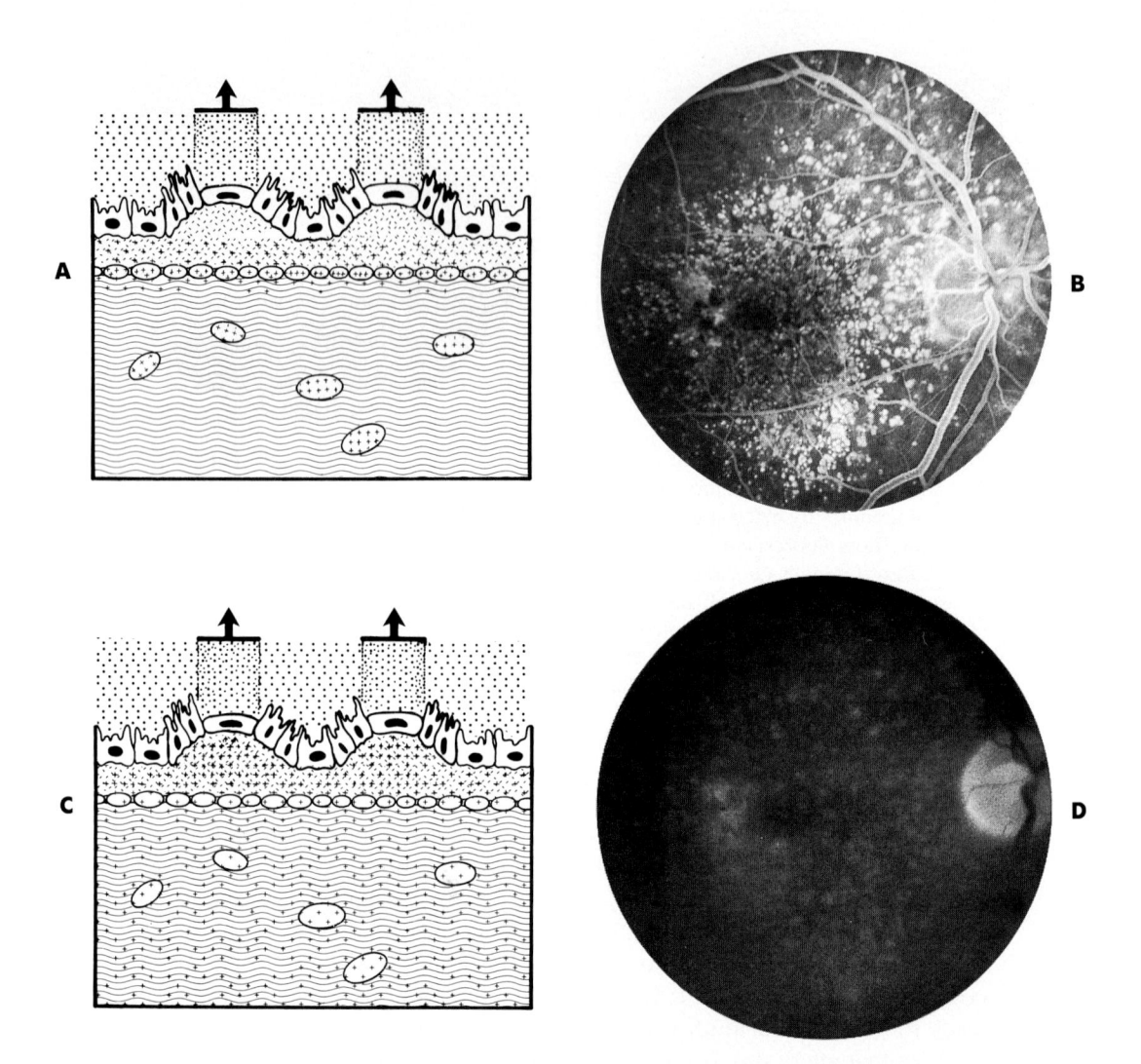

Figure 1-15 Hyperfluorescence in a patient with multiple drusen. **A,** The accumulation of material forming the drusen in the inner layers of Bruch's membrane elevates the RPE, causing thinning of the overlying pigment epithelium, with a concentration of pigment at the edges of the drusen. During early phases, when the inner choroid fluorescein concentration *(black crosses)* is high, there is increased transmission of choroidal fluorescence through the thinned RPE at the peaks of the drusen. The hyperfluorescent plateau is ringed by a relatively hypofluorescent border corresponding to the more pigmented edges of the drusen. **B,** Transmission of normal background choroidal fluorescence through a thinned RPE overlying the drusen in the posterior pole. **C,** In later phases the fluorescein *(black dots)* accumulates within the drusen. Hyperfluorescence is secondary to transmission through the thinned RPE and greater dye concentration within the drusen. **D,** Hyperfluorescence of drusen in the late phases is due to transmission of background choroidal fluorescence and the increased concentration of fluorescein within drusen.

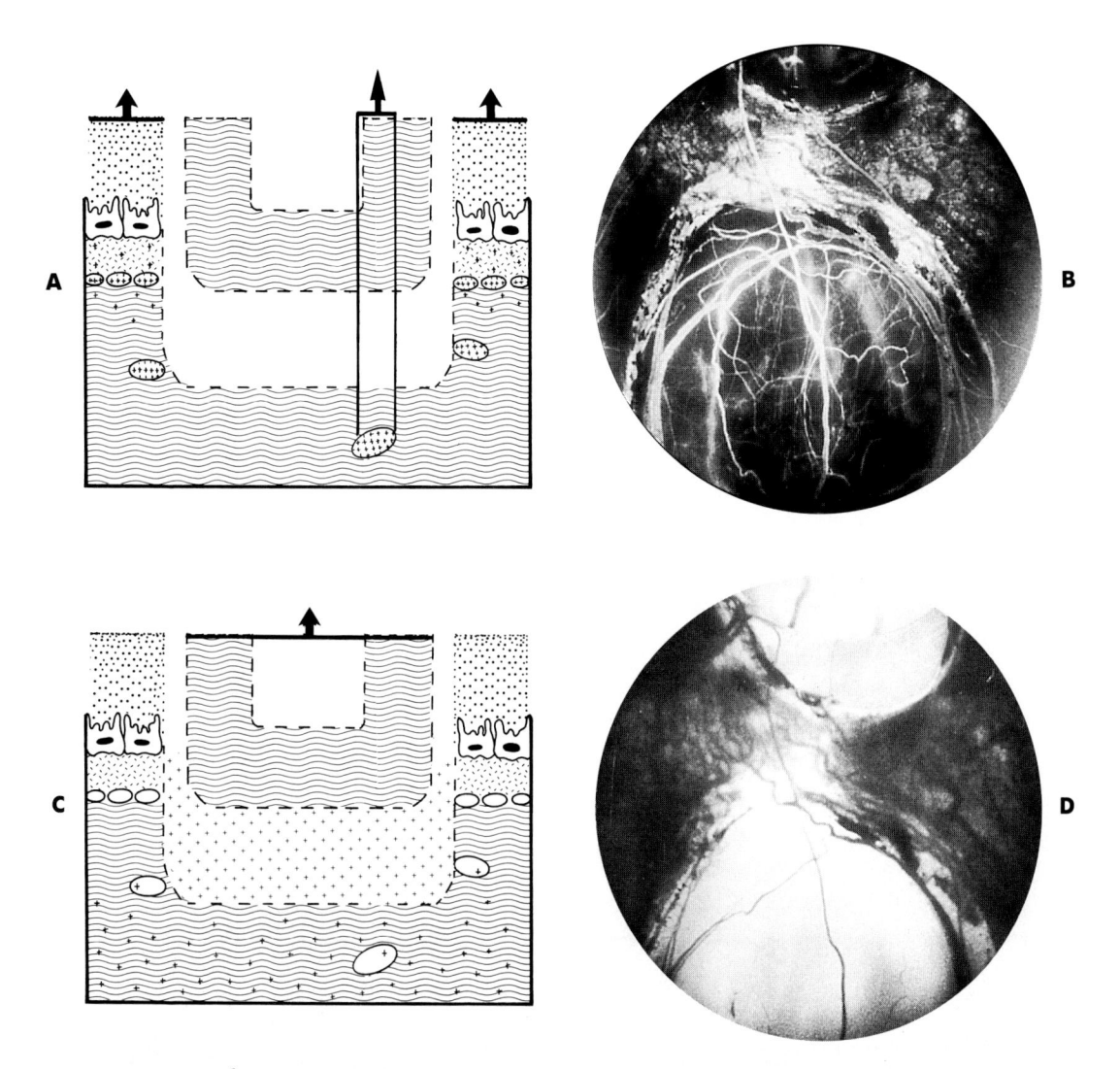

Fluorescein angiography: principles and interpretation

Figure 1-16 Hypofluorescence in a patient with coloboma involving the retinal pigment epithelium and inner choroidal layers. **A,** The tumor infiltrates the RPE, Bruch's membrane, choriocapillaris, and inner choroidal layers (which are absent in this diagram). In the early filling phase, fluorescein *(black crosses)* accumulates in the choriocapillaris on each side of this region but little is detected within the area of the coloboma except in the large outer choroidal vessels. **B,** During early phases the coloboma is hypofluorescent because fluorescein is absent in this area. Deep choroidal vessels filled with dye transmit fluorescence. The surrounding region of relative hyperfluorescence is due to the accumulation of fluorescein within adjacent normal inner choroid layers. **C,** In late phases, fluorescein *(black crosses)* remains in the outer choroidal extravascular space. In contrast to the early phases, the area of the coloboma shows relative hyperfluorescence because transmission is unobstructed by the RPE and inner choroid layers. **D,** In late phases the coloboma shows a relative hyperfluorescence because dye is transmitted from the outer choroid layers through the absent RPE and inner choroid layers.

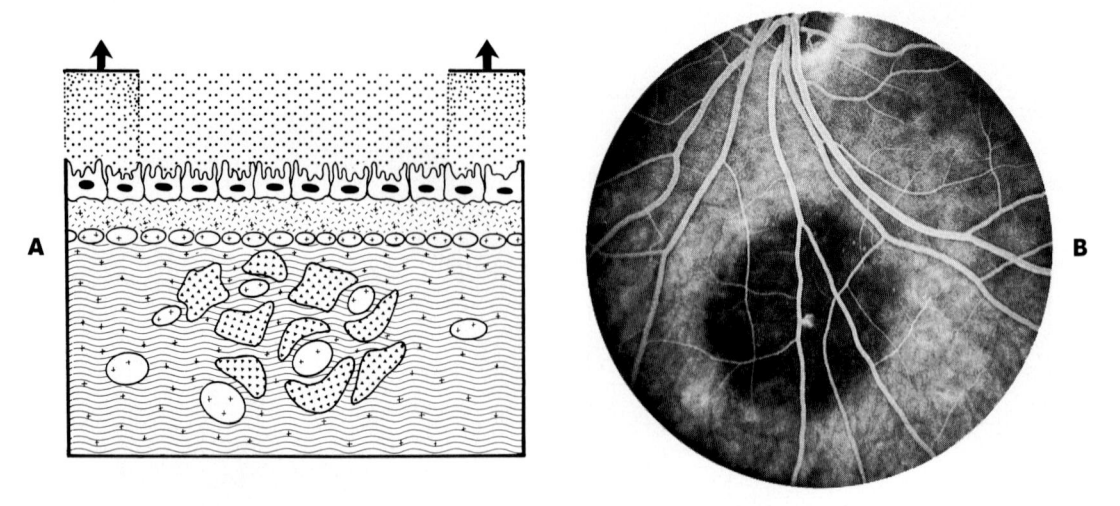

Figure 1-17 Hypofluorescence in a patient with choroidal nevus. **A,** The fluorescein concentration *(black crosses)* may be lower between comparatively densely packed nevus cells than in the surrounding choroidal intravascular and extravascular spaces. Some combination of the lower relative nevus dye concentration and obstruction or absorption of fluorescence by nevus pigment granules leads to the hypofluorescence. **B,** In the early phases hypofluorescence is exaggerated by surrounding normal background choroidal fluorescence.

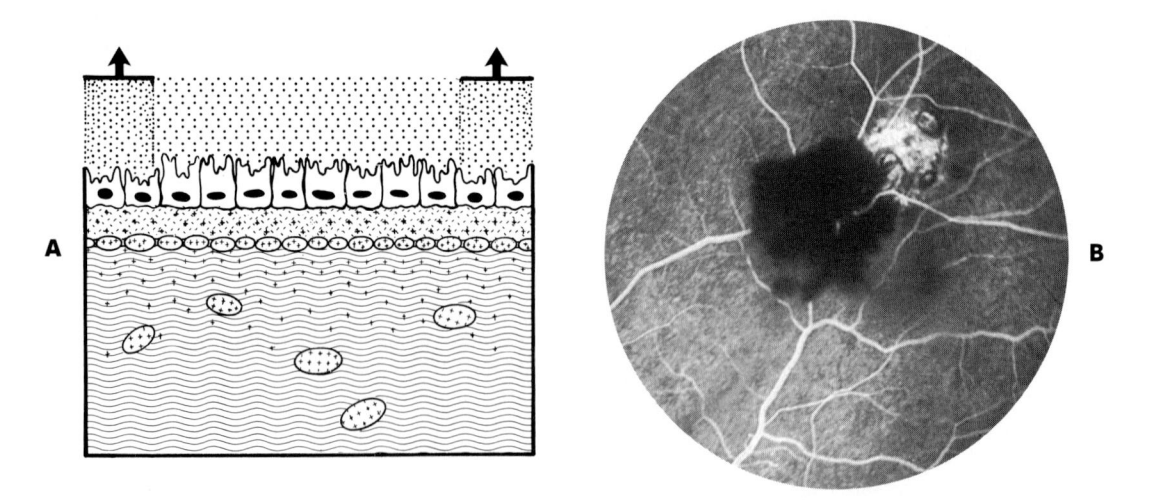

Figure 1-18 Hypofluorescence in a patient with focal hypertrophy of the retinal pigment epithelium. **A,** Increased pigment concentration within the region of RPE hypertrophy. Fluorescein transmission *(black crosses)* from the inner choroidal layers is obscured by the densely pigmented hypertrophied RPE. **B,** Hypofluorescent area corresponding to hypertrophy of the RPE. The greater pigment density in the hypertrophied RPE blocks transmission of the normal choroidal fluorescence.

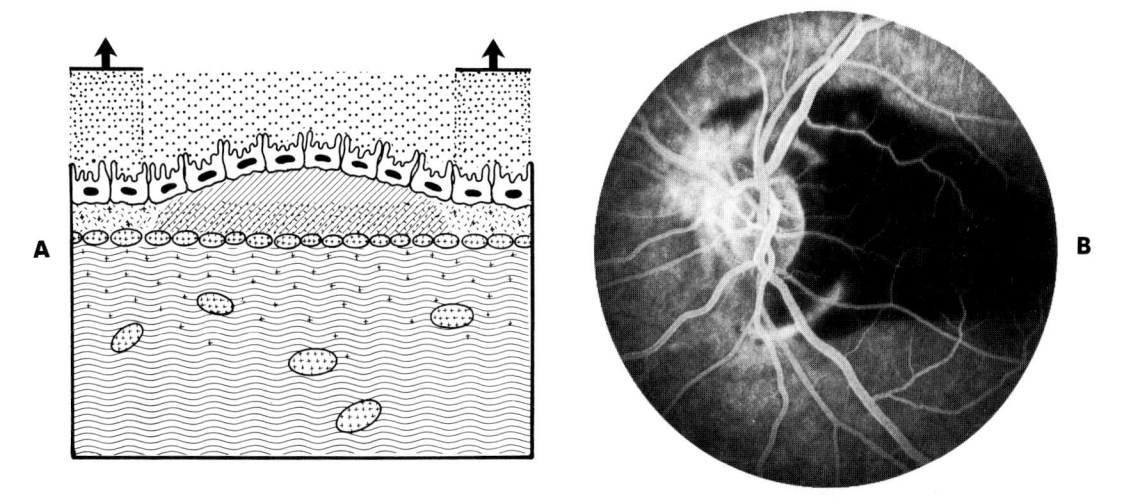

Fluorescein angiography: principles and interpretation

Figure 1-19 Hypofluorescence in a patient with hemorrhage under the retinal pigment epithelium. **A,** Hemorrhagic detachment of the RPE. There is normal fluorescein perfusion *(black crosses)* of the intravascular and extravascular choroidal spaces, but transmission is blocked by an overlying hemorrhagic RPE detachment. **B,** The corresponding hypofluorescent area is due to blockage or obscuration of the normal choroidal fluorescence by hemorrhagic detachment of the RPE.

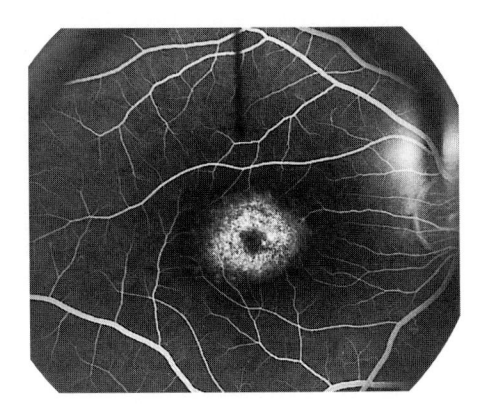

Figure 1-20 Absence of the normal background choroidal fluorescence in a patient with Stargardt's disease (so called "silent choroid").

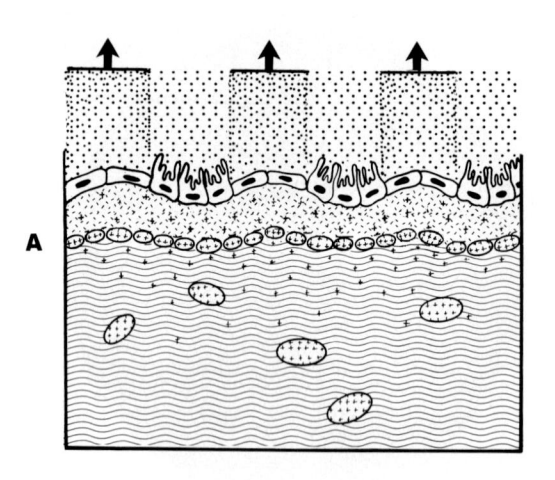

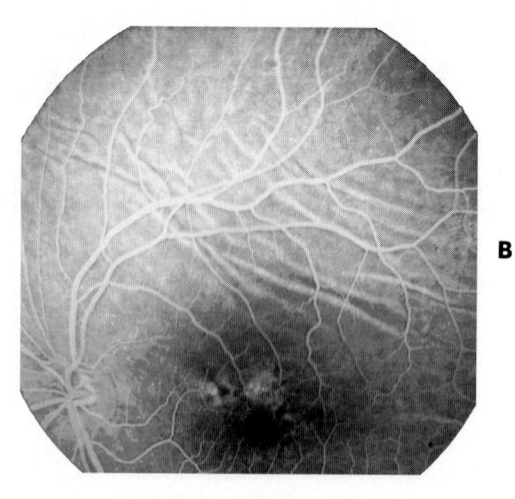

Figure 1-21 Hypofluorescence in a patient with choroidal folds. **A,** Folding of the inner choroid layers involving the retinal pigment epithelium. The pigment cells overlying the peaks of the folds are thinner than those along the edges, which are crowded together at the base of the folds. This results in alternating regions of higher and lower transmission of choroidal fluorescence. The fluorescein *(black crosses)* perfusion of the intravascular and extravascular choroidal spaces is normal. **B,** Linear areas of hyperfluorescence alternating with areas of hypofluorescence.

coloboma results from scleral staining and transmission from the outer choroidal layers through the region devoid of RPE (Fig. 1-16, *C* and *D*).

Hypofluorescence can also be secondary to a relative decrease in dye concentration. A choroidal nevus is hypofluorescent, presumably because the crowded cells of the nevus displace fluorescein dye (Fig. 1-17). Transmission may be further reduced by pigment granules within the nevus cells, a phenomenon that also accounts for hypofluorescence in patients with focal hypertrophy of the RPE (Fig. 1-18).

In several other pathologic conditions hypofluorescence is caused by blocked transmission of choroidal fluorescence. Hemorrhagic detachment of the RPE produces a corresponding region of hypofluorescence (Fig. 1-19). In Stargardt's disease lipofuscin accumulation in the RPE may completely obscure normal background fluorescence (Fig. 1-20).

At angiography patients with choroidal folds exhibit distinctive alternating light and dark areas[41] (Fig. 1-21). These hyperfluorescent and hypofluorescent regions correspond, respectively, to the peaks of the choroidal folds, where the RPE pigment concentration is least and transmission is greatest, and to the troughs, where pigment concentration is greatest and transmission is correspondingly poor.

References

1. Blacharski PA: Twenty-five years of fluorescein angiography, *Arch Ophthalmol* 103:1301-1302, 1985.
2. Alvis DL: Twenty-fifth anniversary of fluorescein angiography, *Arch Ophthalmol* 103:1269, 1985.

3. Patz A, Finkelstein D, Fine SL, et al: The role of fluorescein angiography in national collaborative studies, *Ophthalmology* 93:1466-1470, 1986.
4. Singerman LJ: Fluorescein angiography: practical role in the office management of macular diseases, *Ophthalmology* 93:1209-1215, 1986.
5. Von Baeyer A: Über ein neue Klasse von Farbstoffen, *Ber Dtsch Chem Ges* 4:555, 1871.
6. Nielson NV: The normal fundus fluorescein angiogram and the normal fundus photograph, *Acta Ophthalmol [Suppl]* 180:1-30, 1986.
7. Passmore JW, King JH: Vital staining of conjunctiva and cornea, *Arch Ophthalmol* 53:568-574, 1955.
8. Ehrlich P: Über provisirte Fluorescenzerscheinungen am Auge, *Dtsch Med Wochenschr* 8:21, 1882.
9. MacClean AL, Maumenee AE: Hemangioma of the choroid, *Trans Am Ophthalmol Soc* 47:171-194, 1959.
10. Novotny HR, Alvis DL: A method of photographing fluorescence in circulating blood of the human eye, U.S. Air Force School of Aviation Medicine, Aerospace Medical Center, Brooks Air Force Base, *Technical report* 60-82, 1960.
11. Novotny HR, Alvis DL: A method of photographing fluorescence in circulating blood in the human retina, *Circulation* 24:82-86, 1961.
12. Tredici TJ: History of fluorescein angiography corrected, *Arch Ophthalmol* 104:21-22, 1986.
13. Wolfe DR: Fluorescein angiography: basic science and engineering, *Ophthalmology* 93:1617-1620, 1986.
14. Romanchuk KG: Fluorescein: physiochemical factors affecting its fluorescence, *Surv Ophthalmol* 26:269-283, 1982.
15. Christy RW, Pytte A: *The structure of matter: an introduction to modern physics,* New York, 1965, WA Benjamin, pp 291-306.
16. Berkow JW, Kelly JS, Orth DH: *Fluorescein angiography: a guide to the interpretation of fluorescein angiograms,* Chicago, 1984, American Academy of Ophthalmology.
17. Delori FC, Ben-Sira I: Excitation and emission spectra of fluorescein dye in the human ocular fundus, *Invest Ophthalmol* 14:487-492, 1975.
18. Wessing A: Fluorescein angiography of the retina: textbook and atlas (translated by von Noorden GK), St Louis, 1969, Mosby, p 14.
19. Nasrallah FP, Jalkh AE, Trempe CL, et al: Low-dose fluorescein angiography, *Am J Ophthalmol* 105:690, 1988.
20. Kratz RP, Mazzocco TR, Davidson B: A case report of skin necrosis following infiltration with I.V. fluorescein, *Ann Ophthalmol* 12:654-656, 1980.
21. Schatz H: Sloughing of skin following fluorescein extravasation, *Ann Ophthalmol* 10:625, 1978.
22. Webb JM, Fonda M, Brower EA: Metabolism and excretion patterns of fluorescein and certain halogenated fluorescein dyes in rats, *J Pharmacol Exp Ther* 137:141-147, 1962.
23. Kelley JS, Kincaid M, Hoover RE, et al: Retinal fluorograms using oral fluorescein, *Ophthalmology* 87:805-811, 1980.
24. Ghose S, Nayak BK: Role of oral fluorescein in the diagnosis of early papilloedema in children, *Br J Ophthalmol* 71:910-915, 1987.
25. Nayak BK, Ghose S: A method for fundus evaluation in children with oral fluorescein, *Br J Ophthalmol* 71:907-909, 1987.
26. Yannuzzi LA, Rohrer KT, Tindel LJ, et al: Fluorescein angiography complication survey, *Ophthalmology* 93:611-619, 1986.
27. Kinsella FP, Mooney DJ: Anaphylaxis following oral fluorescein angiography, *Am J Ophthalmol* 106:745-746, 1988.
28. Stein MR, Parker CW: Reactions following intravenous fluorescein, *Am J Ophthalmol* 72:861-868, 1971.
29. Bloom JN, Herman DC, Elin RJ, et al: Intravenous fluorescein interference with clinical laboratory tests, *Am J Ophthalmol* 108:375-379, 1989.
30. Grayson MC, Laties AM: Ocular localization of sodium fluorescein: effects of administration in rabbit and monkey, *Arch Ophthalmol* 85:600-603, 1971.

31. Ota M, Tsukahara I: Fluorescein microscopic studies on fundus fluorescein angiograph, *Acta Soc Ophthalmol Jpn* 75:1856-1862, 1971.
32. Justice J, Lehmann RP: Cilioretinal arteries, *Arch Ophthalmol* 94:1355-1358, 1976.
33. Schatz H, Burton TC, Yannuzzi LA, Rabb MF: *Interpretation of fundus fluorescein angiography,* St Louis, 1978, Mosby, p 8.
34. Miller SA: Fluorescence in Best's vitelliform dystrophy, lipofuscin, and fundus flavimaculatus, *Br J Ophthalmol* 62:256-260, 1978.
35. Larsen M, Kjer B, Bendtson I, et al: Lens fluorescence in relation to metabolic control of insulin-dependent diabetes mellitus, *Arch Ophthalmol* 107:59-62, 1989.
36. Schatz H, Burton TC, Yannuzzi LA, Rabb MF: *Op. cit.* ref 33, p 84.
37. Archer D, Krill AE, Newell FW: Fluorescein studies of normal choroidal circulation, *Am J Ophthalmol* 69:543-554, 1970.
38. Hyvarinen L, Maumenee AE: Interpretation of choroidal fluorescence, In Proceedings of the International Symposium on Fluorescein Angiography, Albi France, 1969, pp 183-188.
39. Krill AE, Newell FW, Chishti MI: Fluorescein studies in diseases affecting the pigment epithelium, *Trans Am Ophthalmol Soc* 66:269-317, 1968.
40. Gass JD: Drusen and disciform macular detachment and degeneration, *Arch Ophthalmol* 90:206-217, 1973.
41. Newell FW: Choroidal folds: the seventh Harry Searls Gradle memorial lecture, *Am J Ophthalmol* 90:206-217, 1973.

PART II

Macular Disease

2

Inherited Outer Retinal Dystrophies

Alan C. Bird

RETINAL PHOTORECEPTOR DYSTROPHIES

Retinal receptor dystrophies comprise a variety of disparate genetically determined conditions that differ from one to another in their mode of inheritance, their pattern of visual loss, and their ophthalmoscopic appearances. Over the past few years, as a result of research by clinicians, biochemists, cell biologists, and molecular biologists, an increasing number of distinct disorders have been recognized within this heterogeneous group and some clues as to their pathogeneses have emerged. Recently a number of nosologic entities have been identified by detection of point mutations causing outer retinal dystrophies both autosomal dominant and autosomal recessive. In addition, in other conditions the locus of the abnormal gene has been defined. These discoveries are already having a profound impact on clinical management and the effect is likely to increase greatly in the near future.

It is possible to subdivide photoreceptor dystrophies into groups depending on their clinical features. Some cause symptoms early in disease, indicating a primary loss of rod function, and examination reveals defective vision in the midzone of the visual field with morphologic changes in the postequatorial fundus (Fig. 2-1); most of the diseases in this category are known collectively as retinitis pigmentosa (RP). Other disorders, with loss of cone function and morphologic changes in the central fundus, are known as macular degenerations or cone dystrophies. This subdivision into "peripheral degenerations" (in which the rods may be the primary target of disease) and "central degenerations" (in which the cones may be the cells initially affected) is superficially attractive. However, the function of both rod and cone systems is compromised in most if not all progressive disorders, even in the early stages of the disease. The photoreceptor dystrophies, therefore, comprise a spectrum of diseases ranging from predominant rod dystrophies to predominant cone dystrophies with disorders intermediate between the two in which there is varying involvement of the rod and cone systems. Despite these reservations, photoreceptor dystrophies will be considered in two broad categories: peripheral (typified by RP) and central.

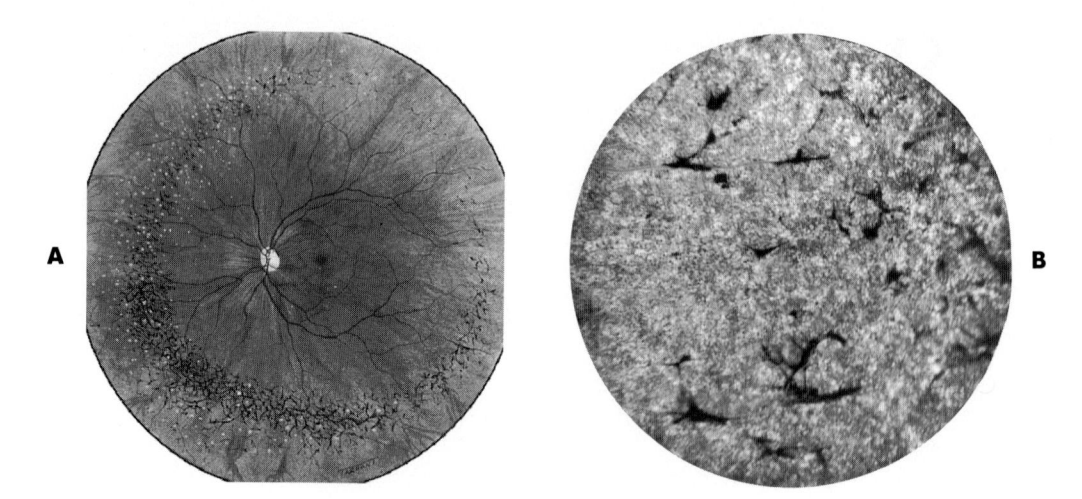

Figure 2-1 A, Fundus painting showing typical bone spicule pigmentation of the midperipheral retina in a patient with autosomal dominant retinitis pigmentosa. **B,** Fluorescein angiogram demonstrating irregular pigmentation at the level of the pigment epithelium with intraretinal pigment highlighted against the choroidal fluorescence.

Peripheral Receptor Dystrophies

To gain a better understanding of these diseases, attempts have been made to subdivide the retinal dystrophies into purer samples of disease on the basis of inheritance, fundus appearance, and functional loss. It is tempting to assume that differences in the phenotype of any inherited condition reflect the influence of different genes or different mutations on the same gene. However, in some instances the differences may be due to observation of the same disorder at different stages of evolution, or of different phenotypic expression of the same genetic disorder. Identification of genetic heterogeneity depends on studies in which comparison is made of inter- and intrafamilial variation of disease. If a characteristic is identified consistently in one family but is absent in another, it is reasonable to assume genetic heterogeneity. This has largely limited clinical studies to extensive families with autosomal dominant and X-linked disease.

Retinitis Pigmentosa. RP is a solitary manifestation of several genetically determined disorders characterized by loss of dark adaptation and progressive reduction of peripheral visual fields early in the disease, leading eventually to impairment of central vision.

Clinical genetic studies. RP may be inherited as an autosomal dominant, autosomal recessive, or X-linked trait. In a large series of cases[1] the frequency of simplex (sporadic) disease in families with RP is at present 52% (Jay M, personal communication), a figure slightly larger than that published 10 years previously (42%). Other authors[2-6] have found a similar high frequency of simplex cases. Autosomal dominant disease causes between 10% and 25% of cases, and X-linked 5% to 18% in different series.[1-6]

Functional studies. By careful studies of visual function some success has been achieved in establishing a subdivision of RP. In some disorders the target cells have been identified, and the characteristics of functional loss indicate the nature of the disease mechanism.

Two broad categories of autosomal dominant RP have been identified[7-9] that are designated as type I or "diffuse" and type II or "regional" forms. The functional characteristics are consistent within families, indicating genetic heterogeneity. In families with diffuse RP, affected members show widespread loss of rod function with relatively well-preserved cone function at some stage in the evolution of their disease. Those with regional RP show variations in the state of rod and cone function, with severe losses of both systems in some regions and near normal function in others. In regional RP, loss of rhodopsin accounts for the reduction of sensitivity, but in diffuse RP there is more rhodopsin than would be predicted if reduced light absorption by visual pigment were responsible for the sensitivity loss.[10] These findings suggest that in regional RP the loss of rod function is due to photoreceptor cell death, short outer segments, or a combination of the two, whereas in diffuse RP this cannot be the case. The two subtypes can usually be distinguished clinically by history alone.[9] In the diffuse form, night blindness is consistently reported within the first decade of life and symptoms of visual field loss by day follow some 20 years later. Pigmentation is often sparse until late in the disease, which may reflect the lack of cell death at least in the first few years of disease. By contrast, in the regional form night blindness and trouble by day occur simultaneously and the age of onset is variable even within the same family. Pigmentation is seen much earlier in regional RP than in the diffuse form.

Additional variants have been identified in autosomal dominant disease in which the distribution is different from the usual pattern of preferential involvement in the midperiphery throughout 360 degrees of the fundus. Sector RP[11,12] is characterized by retinal atrophy restricted to part of the fundus, and gross field loss is confined to the area of visual field corresponding to the involved retina. The lower half of the fundus is usually affected, with loss of visual function in the upper field,[13] but rarely does the disease affect only the superior,[14] nasal,[15] or temporal[16] fundus. In most reported cases[11,12,17-19] with limited sector involvement, inheritance has been autosomal dominant and the distribution of disease was common to affected members of the family. A similar pattern of disease also appears, however, in patients with relatives who have involvement of the whole fundus,[20] and some are heterozygous for X-linked RP[20,21] (Fig. 2-2). By fluorescein angiography minor changes are often found to be more widespread than might be appreciated by ophthalmoscopy with white light, and the sector of RP may be an area of maximum disease rather than of exclusive involvement.[20,21] In typical sector RP, rod and cone ERGs show mild reduction in amplitude with normal cone implicit times.[7,22,23] This pattern of disease is common to all affected members within a family, irrespective of age, suggesting that the disease, in contrast to other forms of autosomal dominant RP, is nonprogressive or progresses very slowly.

Paravenous pigmented chorioretinal atrophy has been described in several reports. There is atrophy of the retinal pigment epithelium underlying the retinal veins that usually extends from the optic disc with pigment around the retinal veins. In most cases the disorder is described[24-26] as an isolated phenomenon that may be of inflammatory origin. However, reports exist with familial involvement—a mother and son,[27] a father and son,[28] and three brothers.[26] It has been shown to be so variable in its severity within a family that the presence of affected relatives cannot be excluded without undertaking a family

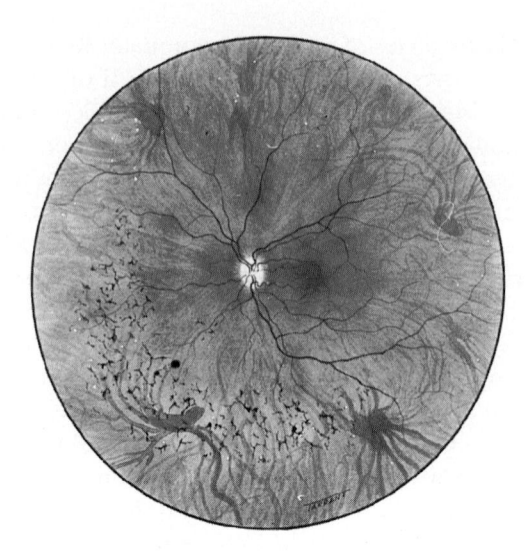

Figure 2-2 Fundus painting of the sectoral distribution of retinitis pigmentosa. This patient is heterozygous for X-linked retinitis pigmentosa.

survey. Most authors take the view that this condition may be genetically determined but that phenocopies exist. Rapid progression, slow progression, and stable visual function have been described,[26,28,29] and the disorder may also be asymmetric.[27,30]

Well-defined atrophy radiating from the optic disc but not following the blood vessels has also been described, as an autosomal dominant disorder. This was first observed in an Icelandic family[31] and was called choroiditis striata. In a further report on the same family[32] the term "helicoid peripapillary chorioretinal degeneration" was used. Several reports[31-36] have followed that appear to concern families exclusively from Iceland and Switzerland, implying the possibility that only two families exist. The disorder is believed to be slowly progressive, and the visual loss is quite variable and associated with refractive error (which is often the reason for ascertainment).[32,33]

No good explanation exists for the regional predilection of disease in any of these conditions. It is tempting to ascribe the inferior involvement to higher lighting levels of the inferior than of the superior retina,[37] but this is unproven and it would not account for the different distributions of disease between families.

In some families there is slow recovery from bleach.[38,39] Cone adaptation and the early part of the recovery of rod sensitivity follow the normal time course, but the later phase of rod adaptation is markedly prolonged.

The expressivity in some families is highly variable such that about 70% of members with the abnormal gene have moderate to severe disease whereas the remainder are asymptomatic but with mild fundus abnormalities and electrophysiologic changes indicating the presence of the abnormal gene.[40] In these families there appears to be bimodal expression of disease, although the factors that modulate gene expression are unknown.

Specific clinical subtypes have also been recognized with autosomal recessive RP. Since its original description,[41] Leber's amaurosis has been considered a distinct disease. In one study[42] it appears to be a monofactorial autosomal recessive affection, but in another[43] several forms of the disease appeared to exist some of which were indistinguishable from autosomal recessive retinitis pigmentosa of early onset. These disorders associated with the name of Leber present a unique problem clinically in which visual loss identified in infancy is due to retinal degeneration with a normal fundus. The diagnosis is usually dependent on identification of a severely reduced ERG. In terms of pathogenesis some may be considered to represent severe forms of autosomal recessive disease. It is possible that individuals with poor vision from birth may have a maturation failure of the retina rather than degeneration of fully developed photoreceptor cells.

RP has been described with preservation of the retinal pigment epithelium adjacent to the retinal arterioles,[44,45] and unlike many patients with RP these persons are consistently hypermetropic.

A further variant comprises night blindness and variably reduced visual acuity associated with restricted pigmentation in the ocular fundus, cystoid macular changes resembling macular schisis, and distinctive electroretinographic abnormalities.[46] The rod ERG is unrecordable, maximal stimulus evokes a large response with prolonged implicit time of the b-wave, photopic and scotopic reactions are of similar magnitude, and the response is much larger when produced by short- than by long-wavelength light. The last attribute is known as the enhanced S cone response. At least in some respects this disorder resembles the Goldmann-Favre syndrome,[47] and it is not yet clear whether this represents a single disorder with variable expressivity.

As early as 1914, Diem[48] reported abnormal fundus reflexes in females heterozygous for X-linked RP, but during subsequent years similar phenomena were reported in other genetic forms of RP[49] and were referred to as "tapetal reflexes." An abnormal tapetal reflex has been reported to be the most common expression of the heterozygous state in X-linked disease.[50-56] However, Schappert-Kimmijser[57] could identify this abnormal reflex in females of only one family out of eight and concluded that, although it is a useful sign when present, its absence does not indicate a normal genotype. The presence of a tapetal reflex in women heterozygous for the abnormal gene in some families but not others[57] may serve to differentiate X-linked RP into two categories on clinical grounds, an observation in keeping with recent genomic studies that indicate the existence of at least two loci for X-linked RP.

Attempts have been made to subdivide X-linked RP on the basis of differential affliction of heterozygotes. Only a few of the early reports of families with X-linked disease described retinal degeneration in females,[58,59] but profound visual loss in heterozygotes was reported by McKenzie[60] in New Zealand. In 1960 Kobayashi[61] described a family with even more severe involvement of the female members, five heterozygous females having RP, 11 having some stigmas of the disease, and at least four being normal. No accurate comparative analysis was made of the severity of disease between affected men and affected women, although it was stated that the females were more mildly affected than the males. From this information, he concluded that there were three separate X-linked conditions: X-linked recessive, X-linked intermediate, and X-linked dominant RP. Subsequent experience, however,[21,62] has indicated that there is considerable intrafamilial variation in the severity of the disease among heterozygotes and that no justification exists for separating X-linked RP into different categories on the basis of severity of the disease in women.

Unilateral RP was reported as early as 1865 by Pedralgia,[63] and the ophthalmoscopic observations were corroborated by histologic examination 25 years later by Deutschman.[64] In 1952 François and Verriest[65] reviewed the 56 unilateral cases reported up to that time and concluded that only 10 had the typical ophthalmoscopic appearance of RP and were strictly unilateral. Subsequent reports[66,67] have shown that, in some cases, minor changes can be demonstrated in the unaffected fellow eye by sophisticated examination. Furthermore, Carr and Siegel[67] thought that the lesions in cases described by them and by some previous authors were due to vascular disease and were not heritable. In no case of unilateral RP has a family history of eye disease been identified, although in one patient[68] the parents were consanguineous. Most workers take the view that there is no good evidence that unilateral RP represents a heritable condition.

Electrophysiologic studies. Soon after the introduction of the electroretinogram (ERG) into clinical practice, its amplitude was found to be reduced in RP[69-71] and it was shown[71-73] that some patients with relatively good visual function had unrecordable ERGs. Riggs[73] stated that receptor cell death alone was insufficient to account for the absence of an ERG and suggested that peripheral receptor degeneration caused short-circuiting between the retina and the choroid so potentials generated in the retina could not be recorded by a distant corneal electrode. He quoted observations by Bush[74] in support of this hypothesis—that multiple perforations of the retina caused extinction of the ERG by electrical short-circuiting without causing massive retinal destruction. It became evident, however, that with better recording systems and averaging techniques, ERG potentials can be recorded in many cases.[75,76] These observations suggest that the reduction of the ERG in RP is due to retinal dysfunction alone.

Using a homogeneous light stimulus and an adapting background illumination, workers have undertaken qualitative analysis of the ERG in different forms of RP. It has been postulated[77] that diminution of the ERG potential in the presence of normal latency implies a reduced population of normal receptors whereas a prolonged implicit time implies widespread receptor dysfunction. The ERG varies in different forms of RP. For example, in patients of a single pedigree with dominantly inherited disease the rod ERG component was of reduced amplitude and latency whereas the cone component was normal. In another family with dominantly inherited RP with reduced penetrance, the cone responses were also abnormal.[78] This finding supports the concept that the difference in penetrance signifies distinct forms of autosomal dominant RP and the differences in influence of the diseases on retinal function imply the presence of different pathogenic mechanisms within this genetic group of RP. In X-linked disease both cone and rod responses are delayed and reduced.[79]

The early receptor potential, which has a short latent period,[80-82] results from the photochemical reaction induced by light falling on the outer segments[83,84] and depends on the concentration of visual pigment,[81] the orientation of the outer segments,[83,84] and their morphology.[81] The early receptor potential is reduced early in X-linked disease and in dominant RP[85,86] and is considered to be caused by a reduction in visual pigment content of the outer segments in the early stages of these conditions.

The light-induced rise in ocular potential as recorded by electrooculography (EOG) has also been shown[87,88] to be reduced or abolished early in RP, when the clinical diagnosis may be in doubt. The response is believed to be due to ion movement by the retinal pigment epithelium in response to changes in the ionic content of the extracellular space of the outer retina that occur with changes in the state of the photoreceptor cation channels. No variation has been recorded between one form of RP and another, and the changes in the EOG merely reflect the severity of the receptor defect.

Genomic studies. The first RP gene to be localized was one for X-linked disease; a probe, L1.28,[89] was used that mapped to the short arm near the centromere at Xp11. Subsequent studies [90,91] have supported the original observation. The first indication of a second locus resulted from the identification of a deletion at Xp21 in a child with RP, Duchenne's muscular dystrophy, and X-linked chronic granulomatous disease[93]; this locus is telomeric to that of L1.28. Localization of a gene linked with RP to this distal site was confirmed by other studies.[94,95] There is no wide agreement on the clinical differences between diseases transmitted at the two loci, although, with one exception,[96] heterozygotes in whom a tapetal reflex is seen seem to belong to families in which the gene is at the more telomeric locus. The possibility of more than one abnormal allele at each locus has not been excluded; and the fact that not all families with disease transmitted at the telomeric site have a tapetal reflex would support this view.

In 1989 a locus for autosomal dominant RP was identified on the long arm of chromosome 3.[97] Three candidate genes exist close to the proposed site, and within a short time a proline-histidine mutation was detected at codon 23 of the rhodopsin gene.[98] Since then many genomic defects have been detected in the rhodopsin gene, and it appears[37,39,40,99-112] that this gene accounts for about 30% of autosomal dominant RP. Most of the substitutions seem to be peculiar to a single family, although some, notably a mutation at codon 347, have been found in many parts of the world. The proline-histidine mutation at codon 23 was identified in a proportion of apparently unrelated subjects in the United States but not in other countries. There is now evidence that the RP patients with this mutation may form part of one large pedigree.

In several families with autosomal dominant RP there is no linkage with markers in the long arm of chromosome 3,[113,114] confirming the heterogeneity of dominant disease, and it has now been shown[115-119] that genes other than that for rhodopsin may be responsible for the autosomal dominant disease. One of these is the gene for the glycoprotein peripherin-rds, which is of particular interest since it is a mutation in this gene that is responsible for the retinal degeneration occurring in *rds**-mice.[120,121] Peripherin is localized to the outer segment disc membranes of both rods and cones and is thought[122-124] to be essential for the assembly, orientation, and physical stability of the outer segment discs of retinal photoreceptors.

Recently mutations have been identified as responsible for recessive disease. A stop sequence at codon 249 in exon 4 of the rhodopsin gene caused no symptoms or fundus changes in the heterozygous state although the ERG potentials

---

*Abnormal genes are designated by *italicized* letters. Human genes are shown by capital letters; animal genes by lower case letters.

were reduced to 50% of normal. Patients homozygous for the mutation had retinitis pigmentosa.[125] Mutations in the gene coding for the beta subunit of phosphodiesterase (β-PDE) have also been recorded as causing autosomal recessive RP.[126] Five different mutations were found in the first 5 of the 22 exons. One case appeared to be heterozygous for two different mutations. These findings are of particular interest in that a mutation in the β-*PDE* gene is responsible for retinal degeneration in the *rd*-mouse.

Choroideremia. Choroideremia was recorded as a distinct condition by Mauthner,[127] and its inheritance was recognized as X-linked in 1942.[128-130] Apart from its inheritance the distinctive feature of this disorder is diffuse progressive atrophy of the retinal pigment epithelium and choriocapillaris.

The symptoms in affected men are identical to those of RP, with loss of dark adaptation and peripheral fields early progressing to leave a small central field. Visual acuity is maintained at a good level until late in disease, often well into the sixth decade of life. Electrophysiologic responses are severely depressed in early disease, as they are in RP.

In males the fundus shows loss of the retinal pigment epithelium, resulting in a blond fundus as early as 2 years of age, followed by the appearance of fine granular subretinal pigment deposits in the midequatorial region. By the third decade there are multifocal areas of loss of the retinal pigment epithelium with concurrent underlying choriocapillaris atrophy in a typically scalloped pattern, becoming more widespread and slowly progressing to a generalized confluent loss of retinal pigment epithelium and choriocapillaris (Fig. 2-3). The disease progresses until a small area of choriocapillaris and pigment epithelium survives at the fovea,[129] and eventually even this is lost. Fluorescein angiographic studies demonstrate well the loss of pigment in the pigment epithelium and the associated loss of choriocapillaris. Histopathologic examination has confirmed the extensive chorioretinal atrophy[131,132] as well as the epiretinal membrane formation and vascular endothelial cell abnormalities.[133]

The heterozygous females almost always have abnormal fundi with changes in the pigment epithelium (Fig. 2-3), but functional loss is unusual in the young and mild later in life. The most common appearance is of midperipheral pigmentation localized deep in the retina and associated with spotty areas of pigment epithelial atrophy. There may be pigment clumping that is linear in distribution. Occasionally, focal areas of choroidal atrophy are seen around the optic disc or in the midperiphery. These fundus changes are usually stationary, although progression has been noted.[130] Microscopic examination demonstrates abnormalities of the pigment epithelium only,[134] widespread malformation of the outer receptor segments and patches of retinal atrophy,[135] and short or absent photoreceptor outer segments in much of the equatorial region, with irregular thickness and pigmentation of the retinal pigment epithelium and areas of profound atrophy in the equatorial region.[136]

Choroideremia is a distinct entity within the group of outer retinal dystrophies, in which it appears that the retinal pigment epithelium is primarily affected rather than the choroid as the name implies. The choroideremia locus was been mapped to band q21 on the X chromosome,[137] and DNA clones that span Xq21 deletions in patients with the disease have been isolated.[138] In some of the patients with microdeletions, mental retardation and deafness have been reported,[139-142] but despite the size of the deletion, the choroideremia remains

Figure 2-3 A, Fundus in advanced choroideremia showing almost total loss of pigment within the choroid and retinal pigment epithelium. **B,** Fluorescein angiogram showing widespread loss of the choriocapillaris. **C,** Posterior pole in a patient heterozygous for choroideremia. Note the irregularity of the retinal pigment epithelium.

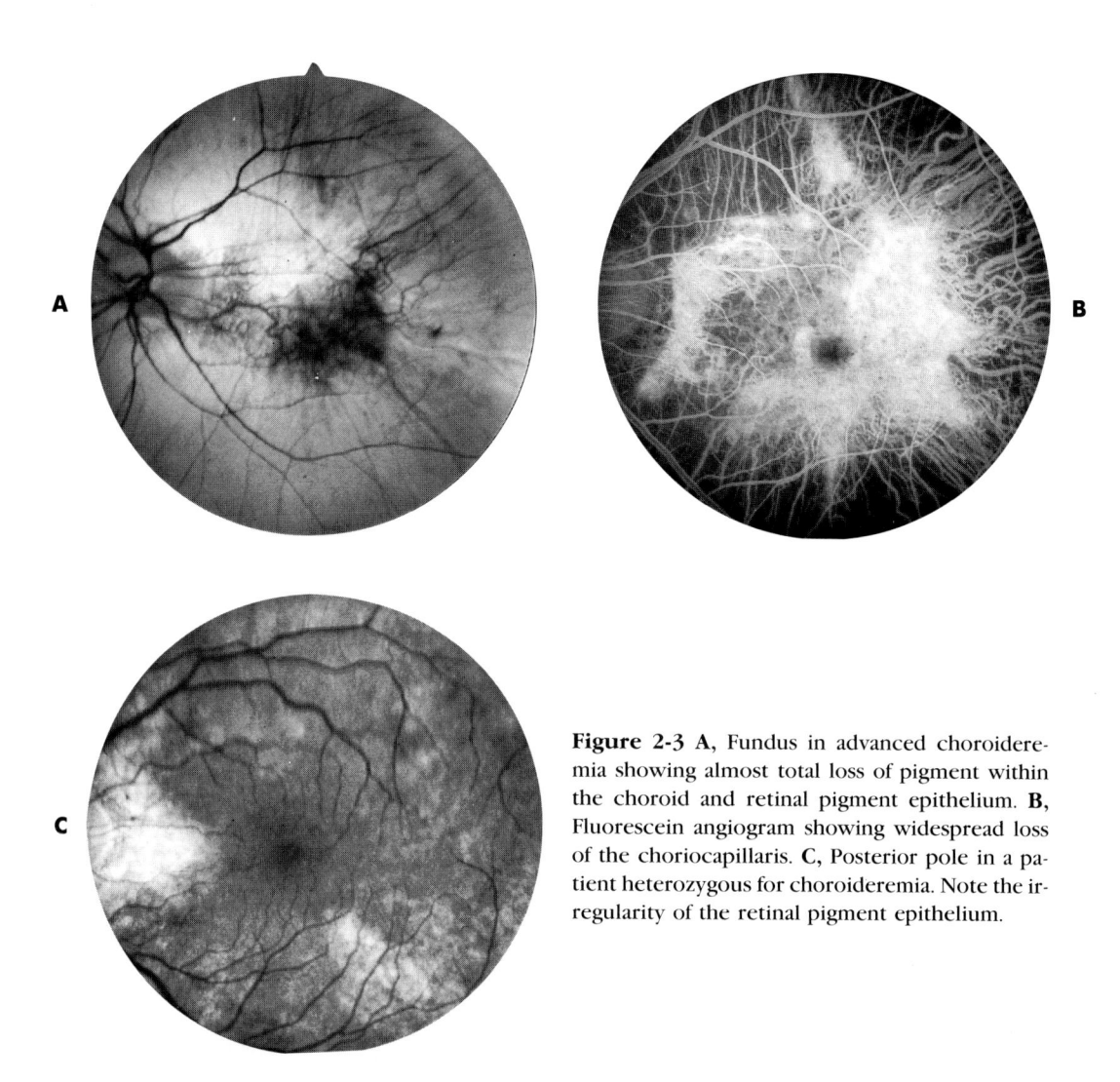

remarkably constant in clinical expression. Subsequently the gene has been sequenced and identified, encoding one component of rab garonylgaronyl transferase,[143,144] and the activity of garonylgaronyl transferase has been demonstrated to be low in cells derived from patients with choroideremia.[145] This complex enzyme activates rab proteins, which themselves are believed to be important in causing fusion of vesicles in the cellular cytoplasm.[146]

How the enzyme deficiency causes choroideremia, and in particular induces defective function only in the retina, is not clear but several possible mechanisms have been postulated.[145] It is likely that the prominent choroidal atrophy is a secondary response to pigment epithelial cell loss. It cannot even be assumed that the primary metabolic abnormality resides within the retinal pigment epithelial cell. Choroidal atrophy is not unique to choroideremia, since it has been identified in about half the eyes with RP subject to histopathologic study, but profound atrophy early is unlike RP and signifies a pathogenic process different from those in other outer retinal diseases.

Bietti's Crystalline Dystrophy. A unique fundus appearance was reported by Bietti[147] in three patients, two of whom were brothers, who had crystals in the retina and in the peripheral cornea. There was progressive atrophy of the retina with prominent atrophy of the pigment epithelium and choroid. As the atrophy supervened, the intraretinal crystals disappeared. The pattern of retinal functional loss was similar to that of RP, with the initial symptoms usually appearing in the third or fourth decade of life. Autosomal recessive inheritance was established by Hu,[148] and crystals were described in patients heterozygous for the abnormal gene by Richards et al.[149] Patients with a similar fundus appearance but without corneal changes have been described and are considered to represent the same disorder.[150-152] No systemic biochemical disorder has been identified, although the corneal crystals resemble cholesterol or cholesterol ester, suggesting that Bietti's crystalline dystrophy may be due to a systemic abnormality of lipid metabolism.[153] This conclusion is supported by the finding of crystals in lymphocytes.

Central Retinal Dystrophies

A number of genetically determined disorders can cause progressive loss of visual function associated with cones—loss of visual acuity, color vision, and central visual field as well as diffuse poor vision in bright light.

Specific disorders (e.g., Best's disease and Sorsby's fundus dystrophy) can be identified as single nosologic entities, but the remainder include groups of disorders that cannot be clearly distinguished one from another. Although they have been subdivided with respect to inheritance and the appearance of the fundus, no satisfactory categorization has been devised and it is likely that each subdivision contains more than one condition. Most disorders fall into two broad subdivisions, fundus flavimaculatus and bull's-eye maculopathy or cone dystrophy, that can be identified on the basis of fundus appearance; however, the distinction may not be absolute. In some disorders both clinical and histopathologic observations imply that the major changes may occur at the level of the retinal pigment epithelium, with good visual function at least for a period, whereas in others the photoreceptor cells appear to be affected initially. These are described in detail in Chapter 20, and only the aspects relevant to counseling and the pathogenic concepts of disease will be addressed.

Best's Disease. The autosomal dominant mode of inheritance of this disorder was first suggested by Best[154] and was substantiated later by further observations on the same family.[155-157]

The typical lesion of Best's disease is a round yellow deposit at the macula[154] (Fig. 2-4) that may be identified within a short time of birth[158] or may develop later in a previously normal fundus.[159,160] On rare occasions the macular disease is not seen until later life[161]; the lesion may be extramacular, the disease asymmetric, or the fundus entirely normal.[134,159-162] Godel et al.[162] state that about half those with the abnormal gene have a normal or near-normal fundus appearance and normal vision. The rise in ocular potential induced by light is always reduced in subjects with the abnormal gene for Best's disease, whatever their clinical status.[159,163] The universal reduction of the light-induced rise in ocular potential, even in patients with normal fundi, indicates a widespread dysfunction of the photoreceptor/pigment epithelial complex that has possibly been present from birth. Thus the distribution of the abnormal gene

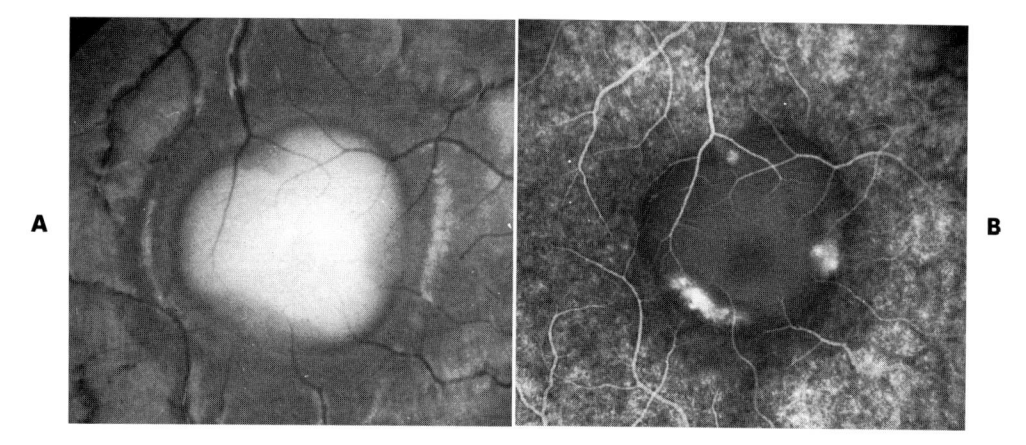

Figure 2-4 A, Posterior pole of a patient with Best's disease. Note the typical pale lesion at the fovea. **B,** fluorescein angiogram showing focal hyperfluorescence at the perimeter of the lesion. This implies the possibility of choroidal new vessels.

in a family cannot be identified by clinical examination but can be achieved only by electrooculography.

Histopathologic studies[164] imply that the abnormal material accumulates initially at the level of the pigment epithelium and that the deposits seen clinically are probably between Bruch's membrane and the pigment epithelium. In patients with advanced disease, histopathology has shown extensive atrophy of the receptors in the macular area.[165,166] There was also, in slightly less advanced cases, widespread abnormality of the retinal pigment epithelial cells in which an excessive amount of lipofuscin had accumulated.[164,167,168] In one case an accumulation of heterogeneous material between Bruch's membrane and the pigment epithelium at the fovea was believed to represent the location of a previtelliform lesion. This material appeared to be derived from degenerating pigment epithelial cells. Despite the fact that the abnormalities of structure and electrical response to light were documented many years ago, the pathogenic relationship between the two is unknown.

The locus of the abnormal gene has been identified on chromosome 11, but the gene is as yet unknown.[169]

Adult Vitelliform Macular Dystrophy. Adult vitelliform macular dystrophy was first described by Gass[170] as a peculiar foveomacular disease. Although series have been reported in which there was no evidence of familial involvement, this condition is now generally regarded as being transmitted as an autosomal dominant trait.[170-173]

The disorder is characterized by focal, round or oval, subretinal yellowish foveal lesions, often with one or more pigment spots on the anterior surface at the level of the pigment epithelium. The lesions may vary in size but are typically one third to one half a disc diameter, bilateral, and symmetric. Patients usually present in the fourth or fifth decade of life and tend to have minimal visual symptoms.[174] The disease differs from vitelliform macular dystrophy (Best's disease) in that its foveal lesions are smaller, it presents at a later age, it does not demonstrate evolutionary changes of the foveal lesion, and the light-

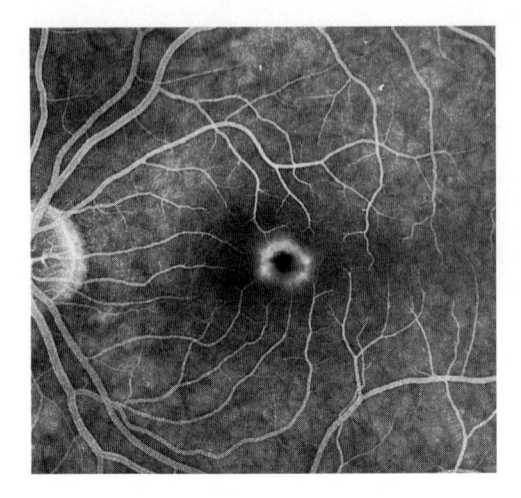

Figure 2-5 Fluorescein angiogram of a patient with adult vitelliform macular dystrophy showing a small foveal lesion with central hypofluorescence and surrounding hyperfluorescence.

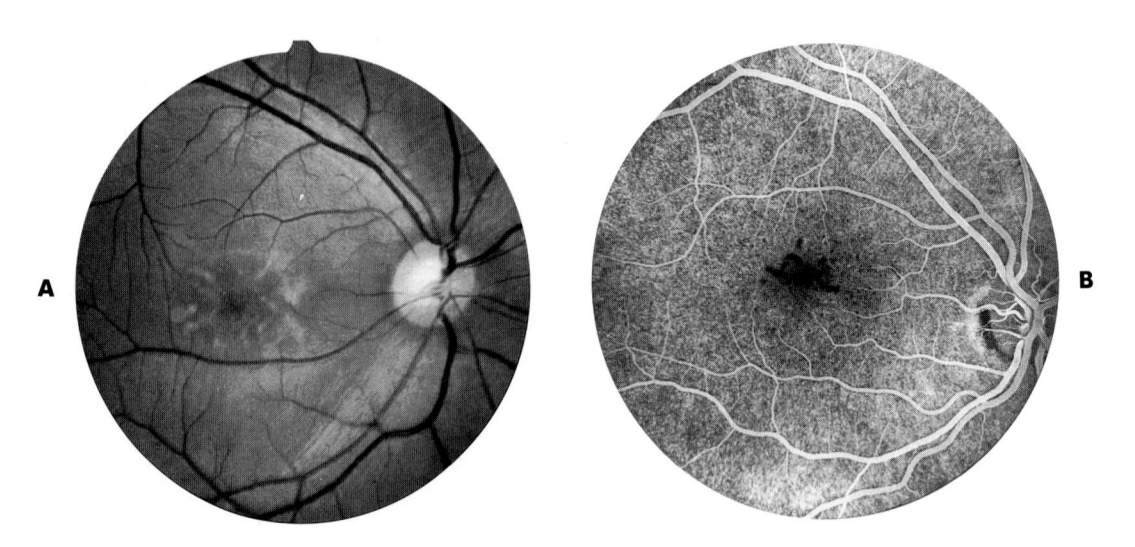

Figure 2-6 A, Posterior pole of a patient with dominantly inherited pattern dystrophy. Note the linear deposition of material at the level of the pigment epithelium/Bruch's membrane. **B,** Fluorescein angiogram of another patient with autosomal dominant disease demonstrating fundus pulverilentus with central linear hypofluorescence.

induced rise in ocular potential is rarely absent. Because of the variation in age of onset and severity, the distribution of the abnormal gene within a family cannot be established with certainty by clinical survey of the family.

The histopathologic reports of this condition[170,174] show loss of the retinal pigment epithelium and disruption of photoreceptors at the fovea. Perhaps of greater significance is the intense autofluorescence seen in the intact retinal pigment epithelium outside the fovea, implying that accumulation of lipofuscin at this site is central to the pathogenesis of the disorder.

A mutation in the *peripherin/RDS* gene, a stop sequence at codon 258, has been found in one patient with a retinal degeneration similar in appearance to adult vitelliform macular dystrophy,[175] but there is no evidence that all families have such a mutation (Fig. 2-5).

Pattern Dystrophies. In 1970 five members of a family from Holland were described[176] with a unique fundus appearance consisting of a linear pattern of hyperpigmentation at the macula. The pigment appeared to be in the pigment epithelium, and fluorescein angiography showed granular hyperpigmentation of the remaining pigment epithelium at the posterior pole. The disorder caused few symptoms since the worst visual acuity was 0.8. The most striking feature was a universal reduction of the light-induced rise in ocular potential to 130% or lower in the presence of good visual function. It was concluded that there was diffuse dysfunction of the retinal pigment epithelium with little associated visual deficit since no indication of rod dysfunction as gauged by the electroretinogram was found and no abnormality of color vision. In this respect butterfly-shaped dystrophy is similar to Best's disease. The original pedigree is suggestive of autosomal dominant inheritance; in the original communication the disease was identified in only two generations, but large pedigrees have subsequently been published.[177]

A number of families are described in the literature[178,179] with autosomal dominant disease characterized by linear or irregular changes of pigment at the level of the retinal pigment (Fig. 2-6) epithelium with considerable variability within each family. Some members have had macroreticular change, and others fundus pulverilentus with an appearance of butterfly dystrophy as described by Deutmann or macular lesions.[180-183] The deposits at the level of the pigment epithelium may be pale or dark and may or may not be linear.[184] In all families the light-induced rise in ocular potential may be depressed, and the condition is compatible with retention of good acuity throughout life. It is now believed that pattern dystrophy represents one or more than one nosologic entity with variable expressivity. The problem may be resolved by comparison between families or by genomic analysis.

In one family with a pattern dystrophy a mutation has been detected in the *peripherin/RDS* gene.[185]

Sorsby's Fundus Dystrophy (Pseudoinflammatory Macular Dystrophy). Sorsby et al.[186] first reported an autosomal dominant disorder in which there was bilateral central visual loss in the fifth decade of life from subretinal neovascularization (Fig. 2-7) with progressive atrophy of the peripheral retina and choroid leading to loss of ambulatory vision by the seventh decade in most cases. Subsequent reports[187-192] have shown that the disease is fully penetrant and the abnormal phenotype becomes evident in the third decade of life. Patients have difficulty passing from light to dark and have slow recovery of sen-

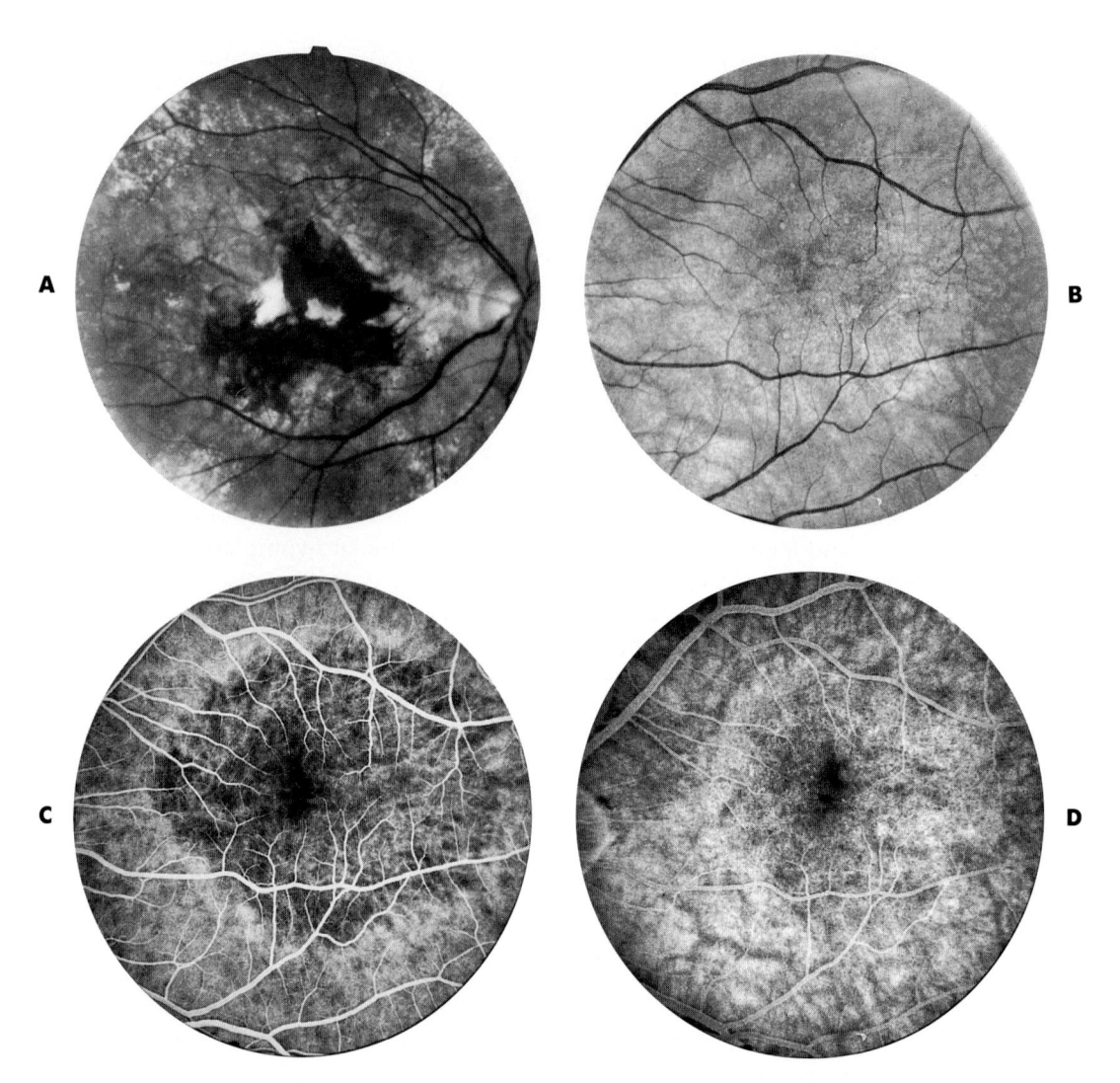

Figure 2-7 A, Hypertrophic pigmented lesion in the retina of a patient from a family with Sorby's fundus dystrophy. Note the drusen at the perimeter of the posterior pole. **B,** Pale discoloration of the posterior pole in a 40-year-old man. Fluorescein angiograms demonstrate slow filling of the central choriocapillaris, **C,** and late subtle hypofluorescence corresponding to the area of slow perfusion, **D.**

sitivity and rhodopsin following bleach. The fundi show drusen, yellow deposits, and slow filling of the choroid at fluorescein angiography (Fig. 2-7).

A light and electron microscopic study of the eyes of one patient[193] showed a 30 μm thick deposit within Bruch's membrane that stained positive for lipids. In addition, the patient had gross loss of the outer retina, a discontinuous retinal pigment epithelium, and atrophy of the choriocapillaris.

Autosomal Dominant Drusen. Drusen of Bruch's membrane were first demonstrated microscopically by Wedl[194] in 1854 and clinically by Donders[195] in 1855. Historically the diagnosis of dominantly inherited drusen has often been

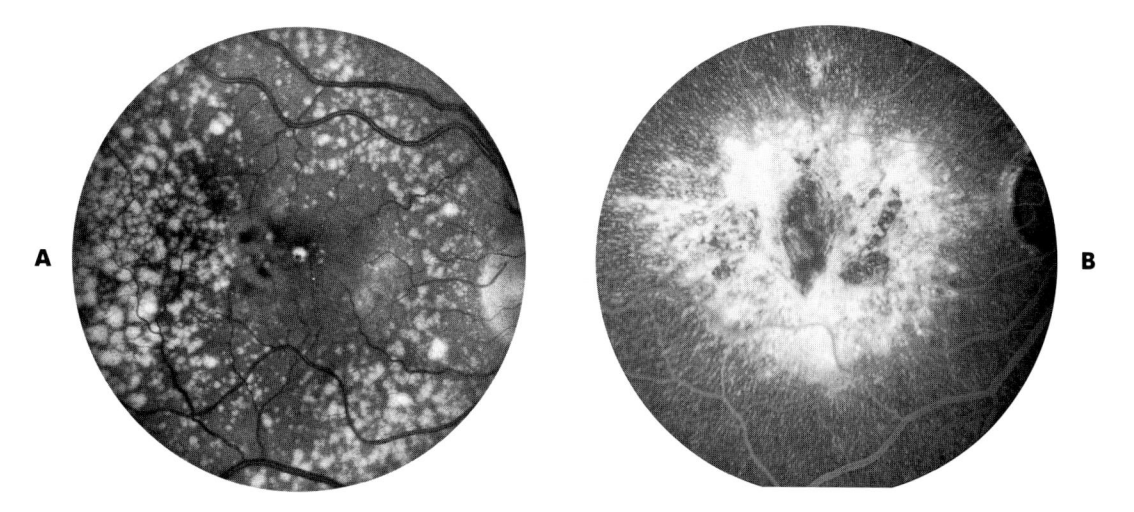

Figure 2-8 A, Doyne's honeycomb dystrophy. Note the predominantly large drusen in the posterior pole. **B,** Fluorescein angiogram of *malattia levantinese* showing a central density of material with small radially oriented drusen.

made in patients in whom the drusen appeared at a relatively early age. These have included Hutchinson-Tay choroiditis,[196] guttata choroiditis,[197,198] Holthouse-Batten superficial chorioretinitis,[199] Doyne's honeycomb retinal degeneration,[200-202] familial choroiditis,[203] *malattia levantinese,*[204] and crystalline retinal degeneration.[205] However, neither Hutchinson and Tay[196] nor Holthouse and Batten[199] reported sufficient evidence to indicate that they were describing a genetically determined disorder. By contrast, in Doyne's honeycomb dystrophy and *malattia levantinese* there is good evidence of dominant inheritance.

The view that the various manifestations of drusen in the posterior pole represent the same disorder has been a popular one in recent decades.[206-209] However, the patterns of drusen in Doyne's honeycomb dystrophy and *malattia levantinese* (Fig. 2-8) are constant with families and differ from each other. In the latter there are small drusen in the peripheral macula distributed in a typical radial pattern with larger confluent drusen centrally. The small drusen have the clinical and angiographic appearance[204,210] of "basal laminar drusen" as described by Gass.[211] None of Doyne's original families or their descendants were noted to have radially oriented basal laminar drusen.[200-202] Based on the presence of radial basal laminar drusen, several families reported in the literature to have a Doyne-type "colloid degeneration" might be more properly described as having *mallatia levantinese.*[212-213]

In both disorders visual acuity remains good until middle life. In Doyne's honeycomb dystrophy geographic atrophy may supervene at any time thereafter. In *mallatia levantinese* either geographic atrophy or occult choroidal neovascularization may supervene.

Central Areolar Choroidal Sclerosis. A dominantly inherited dystrophy with well-defined atrophy of the outer retina, retinal pigment epithelium, and inner choroid has been described by Sorsby[214] (Fig. 2-9). Initially the choriocapillaris was thought to be affected primarily in central areolar choroidal

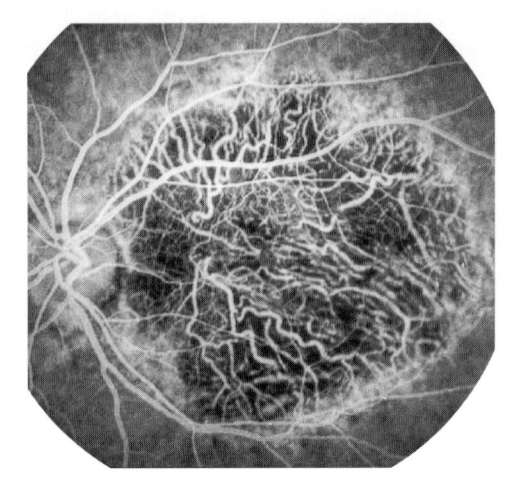

Figure 2-9 Fluorescein angiogram of a case of dominantly inherited macular dystrophy (Sorsby), which is well defined. There is, within the affected area, a loss of both the pigment epithelium and the inner choroid. This patient was found to have a mutation at codon 172 of peripherin.

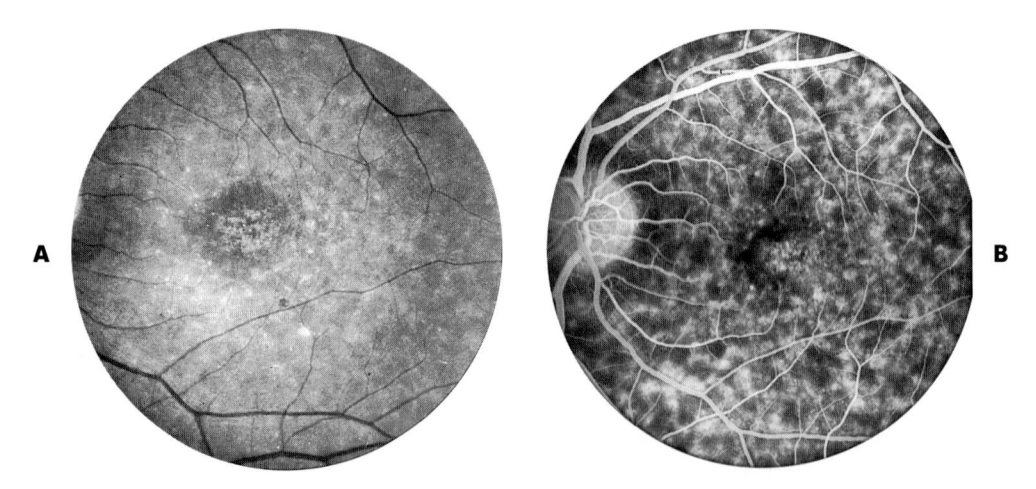

Fig. 2-10 A, Deposition of white material at the level of the retinal pigment epithelium/Bruch's membrane in a patient with fundus flavimaculatus. **B,** The angiogram shows hypofluorescence around the nerve head with irregular hypofluorescence throughout the posterior pole.

atrophy[214-216] because atrophy of the choroid at the macula was apparently the initial or at least the most prominent ophthalmoscopic change when the patient was first seen. However, Ashton[217] demonstrated that the major choroidal blood vessels were normal in a case of central areolar choroidal sclerosis by histopathologic examination and thus the target cell of disease was uncertain.

Two mutations in the *RDS* gene have recently been reported[175] to cause a macular dystrophy closely resembling this condition. The mutations are in codon 172. In two families arginine was substituted by tryptophan, and in one other by glutamine. In each there were symptoms of difficulty in passing from light to dark in the third decade of life and retinal pigment epithelial changes centered at the fovea and extending outside the posterior pole were identifiable by this time. Profound atrophy of the outer retinal and inner choroid occurred during the next three decades at a variable rate. Peripheral rod function was normal. The diseases were qualitatively similar with the mutations but were more severe with the Arg-172-Trp substitution.

Fundus Flavimaculatus. This broad category comprises diseases in which there is deposition of white material at the level of the pigment epithelium (Fig. 2-10). The terms "Stargardt's disease"[218,219] and "fundus flavimaculatus"[220,221] have been used to denote these disorders, but there is no evidence that they describe separate conditions. Most cases show autosomal recessive inheritance as first described by Stargardt, although autosomal dominant forms are occasionally seen.[222,223] The conditions usually cause rapid loss of central vision during a 6-month period in the first 15 years of life; however, in some cases good visual acuity is maintained until the age of 50 years.

With visual loss, confluent atrophy of the outer retina pigment epithelium and choriocapillaris occurs at the fovea, and this area grows slowly during the rest of the patient's life. The white "fishtail" flecks occupy the remaining part of the posterior pole, with characteristic sparing of the peripapillary region. These lesions can be identified at the time of initial visual loss and resolve as additional ones appear elsewhere.[224]

At fluorescein angiography the choroid appears normal in some patients but it is not seen in the majority.[223,225-227] It seems likely that the lack of choroidal fluorescence signifies an even deposition of abnormal material at the level of the pigment epithelium that absorbs blue-green light.[228] This conclusion has been supported by histopathologic studies[228-230] in which it has been demonstrated that the retinal pigment epithelial cells were packed with lipofuscin and melanolipofuscin. These changes start to develop in childhood.[231] At the site of previous white lesions, atrophy of the pigment epithelium occurs and fluorescein angiography shows multifocal hyperfluorescence corresponding to the areas of pigment epithelial atrophy.[224]

Bull's-Eye Dystrophies (including cone and cone-rod dystrophies). The typical fundus changes in this group of cone and cone-rod dystrophies consist of one or more concentric rings of pigment epithelial change around the fovea that give rise to a characteristic appearance at fluorescein angiography. Visual loss may occur any time during the second to fifth decades of life and, once started, progresses slowly.[232] There may or may not be white deposits at the level of the pigment epithelium. The phenomenon of dark choroid is also seen in some families with bull's-eye dystrophy[223,225,226] (Fig. 2-11).

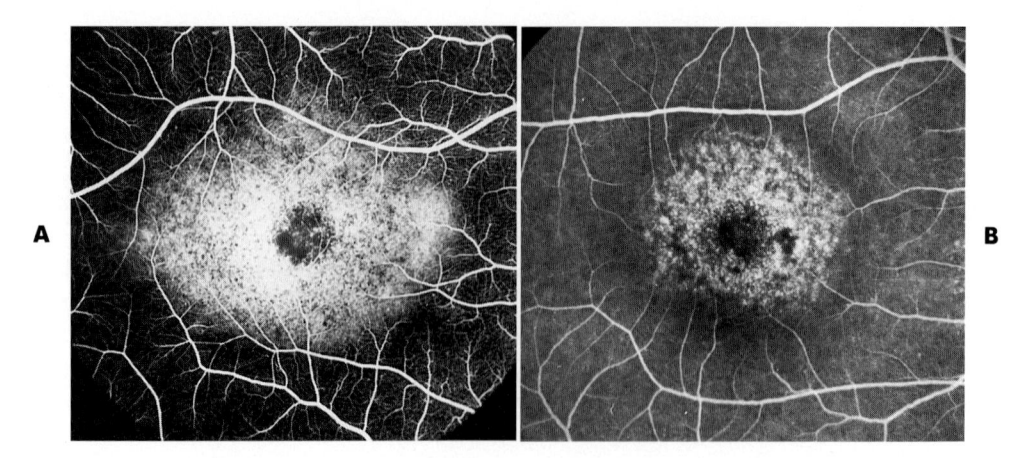

Figure 2-11 Fluorescein angiogram of two patients with bull's-eye dystrophy. Note the light, **A**, and dark, **B**, choroids.

These disorders can be transmitted as autosomal dominant,[233-240] autosomal recessive,[240,241] or X-linked.[242-245] Even within the different genetic forms of cone dystrophy there is heterogeneity. Such lesions may occur with disease restricted to the central region, or generalized cone loss, in which case reduced visual acuity is associated with photophobia and defective of color vision. In dominant cone dystrophies there is one recently described form with early and nearly complete absence of blue cone function but with a blue-sensitive visual pigment locus indistinguishable from normal.[237-239] In a family with X-linked cone dystrophy accompanied by loss of red cone function, a 6.5 kilobase deletion within the red cone pigment gene was found.[244] Heterogeneity is further indicated by the presence of peripheral retinal degeneration in some conditions, for which the term "cone-rod dystrophy" is used, and there is evidence[246,247] that this group also includes several disease entities. The different categories can be distinguished one from another on the basis of ERG testing. Drug-induced phenocopies occur[248,249]; and comparable dystrophies have also been described in the Pierre-Marie type of hereditary ataxia,[250] in fucosidosis,[251] and in amelogenesis imperfecta.[252]

There is considerable doubt as to whether the fundus changes of fundus flavimaculatus and bull's-eye dystrophy indicate that the disorders are clearly separated into two broad groups. Studies of fundus appearance show that in some families the changes are constant but in others the bull's-eye dystrophy may be seen in early disease and flavimaculatus lesions seen later.

North Carolina Dystrophy. This condition was well characterized in a large family from North Carolina,[253] and several reports have followed.[254-256] It is likely that previous reports from Europe[257,258] described the same condition. It is dominantly inherited and appears to be fully penetrant although variable in its expressivity. It may cause profound atrophy of the outer retina and choroid at the macula in early life (Fig. 2-12) despite the fact that visual acuity can be remarkably good. There may be drusen-like deposits, however, only in the posterior pole. The disorder is widely believed not to be progressive.[256] In some families there is the consistent presence of skeletal abnormalities of the extrem-

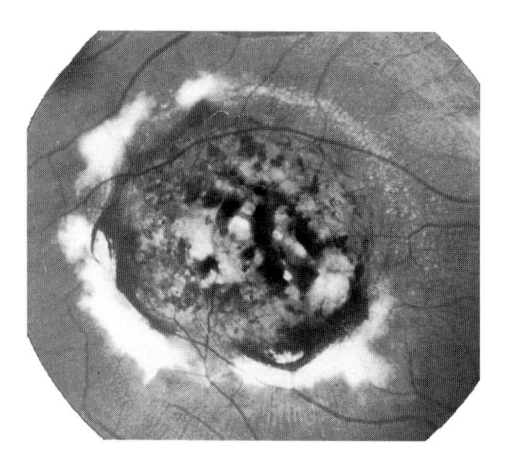

Figure 2-12 North Carolina macular dystrophy showing profound and well-defined atrophy in the posterior pole with some hypopigmentation in the affected area and hypertrophic fibrous tissue around the perimeter of the lesion.

ities,[259,260] implying that more than one disorder may cause the fundus lesion. The abnormal gene has been localized to the short arm of chromosome 6 in at least one family (6p),[261] but the gene has yet to be identified.

CONGENITAL RECEPTOR DEFECTS

Several conditions have been recognized in which there is a genetically determined nonprogressive visual defect that may be related to either the cone or the rod systems.

Cone Defects

Defective Color Vision. Defects in color vision have been classified on the basis of the concept that color vision is determined by three classes of cones: red-sensitive, green-sensitive, and blue-sensitive. The basis for this classification has been confirmed by the sequencing of the three cone pigment genes.[262] If color-matching tests demonstrate that one of the three systems is defective but present (trichromats), the terms "protanomaly" (red), "deuteranomaly" (green), and "tritanomaly" (blue) are used; and if one is functionally absent (dichromats), the suffix *-anopia* replaces *-anomaly*.

Deuteranomaly, deuteranopia, protanopia, and protanomaly are X-linked conditions[263]: deuteranomaly is found in about 5% of the population of Western Europe and North America; and deuteranopia, protanomaly, and protanopia in each about 1%. Tritanomaly and tritanopia, which are inherited as autosomal dominant disorders, are much less common, affecting between 0.002% and 0.007% of the population.[264]

Individuals with these abnormalities of color vision have normal visual acuity, and anomalous trichromats are often unaware of their condition. Apart from the color defect, the eye is normal.

The molecular genetic basis of the red and green color defects has now been demonstrated.[265,266] Abnormalities of the red and green pigment genes to differing degrees occur in deuteranopia, deuteranomaly, protanopia, and protanomaly. People with deuteranopia have been found to possess a normal red pigment gene but no green pigment gene(s). Those with protanopia lack a normal red pigment gene, which is replaced by a hybrid red-green pigment gene. Deuteranomalous and protanomalous trichromats have hybrid red-green genes.

Monochromatism. Patients suffering from monochromatism have absent or markedly impaired color vision. In complete rod monochromatism there is little evidence of cone function; thus visual acuity is poor, the patient has nystagmus, and extreme photophobia is characteristic. The fundi show no gross abnormality, although the foveolas may appear abnormal and changes in the central pigment epithelium are sometimes identified.[263] The dark adaptation curve is typically monophasic, fusion frequency is very low, and the photopic (cone) ERG is absent but the scotopic (rod) ERG is normal. Rod monochromatism is an autosomal recessive trait.

Blue cone monochromatism presents in a similar fashion to complete rod monochromatism, except that there appears to be an intact blue cone system and the inheritance is X linked.[267] The gene for this form of monochromatism maps to Xq28, and it is possible that this rare disorder results from alterations of the red and green pigment genes, or from their deletion.[268]

An incomplete form of rod monochromatism has been described[269-271] in which the symptoms are less severe, visual acuity is better, and photophobia and nystagmus may be absent. In another form of monochromatism there is absence of central cones.[260]

Four eyes from individuals with monochromatism have been examined histopathologically.[272-275] They showed a change at the fovea with a reduced number of cones and an abnormality of those that remained.

Rod Defects

Congenital Stationary Night Blindness. Congenital stationary night blindness (CSNB) is characterized by a normal fundus appearance, the absence of rod dark adaptation (monophasic dark adaptation curve), and a lack of progression. It may be inherited as an autosomal dominant, autosomal recessive, or X-linked trait.

The most widely reported form of CSNB is an autosomal dominant disorder.[276] Patients appear to have normal cone function but little rod function. Visual acuity, color vision, and photopic visual fields are normal or at most mildly abnormal, and dark adaptation shows only a cone segment that may be abnormally prolonged[277]; there is no shift from cone to rod characteristics in the dark adaptation curve, and the ERG shows no prolongation of the b-wave implicit time between the photopic and scotopic records. Fundus reflectometry, however, indicates a normal concentration of bleachable rhodopsin in one case,[278] and histologic studies[279] have shown no structural abnormalities either in the retina as a whole or in the rods in particular.

The majority of patients with autosomal recessive and X-linked CSNB, and occasional patients with autosomal dominant CSNB, have an ERG with a near normal a-wave and a substantially reduced b-wave on testing under scotopic conditions (negative ERG).[280,281] With increasing intensity of the test stimulus the amplitude of the a-wave increases but that of the b-wave is unchanged.[282] These patients could be further divided into two groups: one lacking rod function (complete type) and the other with some rod function (incomplete type). Patients with the complete type are myopic; those with the incomplete type may be hyperopic or myopic. Although complete and incomplete CSNB did not coexist in any of the families reported by Miyake et al.,[283] others [284,285] have found patients with both complete and incomplete CSNB within the same X-linked pedigrees. This led Pearce et al.[285] to propose that X-linked CSNB is a single clinical entity manifesting a wide variation in clinical expression. It has also been suggested[286,287] that incomplete CSNB and Åland Island eye disease may be the same condition.

Myopia is almost always associated with the X-linked form of CSNB, when visual acuity is reduced and nystagmus may be present. Carriers of X-linked CSNB are not night blind but may show abnormal oscillatory potentials on ERG.[288,289] Myopia also occurs in cases of autosomal recessive CSNB that have abnormal vision and, again, the patients may have nystagmus.[134] These forms of CSNB may present in infancy with blindness.[290]

The complete form of X-linked CSNB has been assigned to Xp11.3[291,292] or Xp11.22.[293] A mutation in the rhodopsin gene has now been identified in autosomal recessive CSNB.[294] It is believed that the mutant rhodopsin may create noise by activating transducin in the absence of light, causing profound reduction in sensitivity of the scotopic system.

Light and electron microscopic studies of one eye with CSNB and a negative ERG showed a normal arrangement of discs of rod outer segments and normal synaptic ends of the photoreceptors. It was suggested that the cause in this case of CSNB might be related to mechanisms inhibitory to cells of the bipolar layer.[295] The absence of rod-cone interaction, together with an absent scotopic b-wave, also implies that the defect is in the midretinal layers.[296]

Prolonged Dark Adaptation. Three distinct conditions have been described in which the final threshold of dark adaptation is normal but the rod phase is abnormally prolonged; the defect in each appears to be static.

Oguchi's disease. This autosomal recessively inherited disorder with prolonged dark adaptation was first reported in Japan in 1907,[297] and most subsequent reported cases have come from the same country, although non-Japanese patients have also been described.[298,299] In most patients defective night vision is the only complaint, visual acuity being normal. The characteristic feature of this condition is the abnormal coloration of the light-adapted fundus, the abnormal white or cream-colored appearance being derived from the inner limiting membrane and presumably from the footplates of Mueller cells. The abnormal color resolves over a period of 8½ hours in darkness and has been termed the "Mizuo-Nakamura phenomenon" after the authors who provided the first description.[300,301] Dark adaptation is characteristically slow, and a final rod threshold may be attained only after several hours, and even then may be slightly elevated.[302]

Histopathologic examination has been undertaken on three eyes. An excess of cones compared to rods, together with an abnormal layer of material between the receptors and pigment epithelium, was reported by Oguchi.[303] Parallel histologic studies on the other half of the same eye by another investigator[304] failed to confirm this additional layer. It was then considered that an abundance of round lipofuscin granules confined to the apical portion of the pigment cells was the characteristic feature. Histopathologic and electron

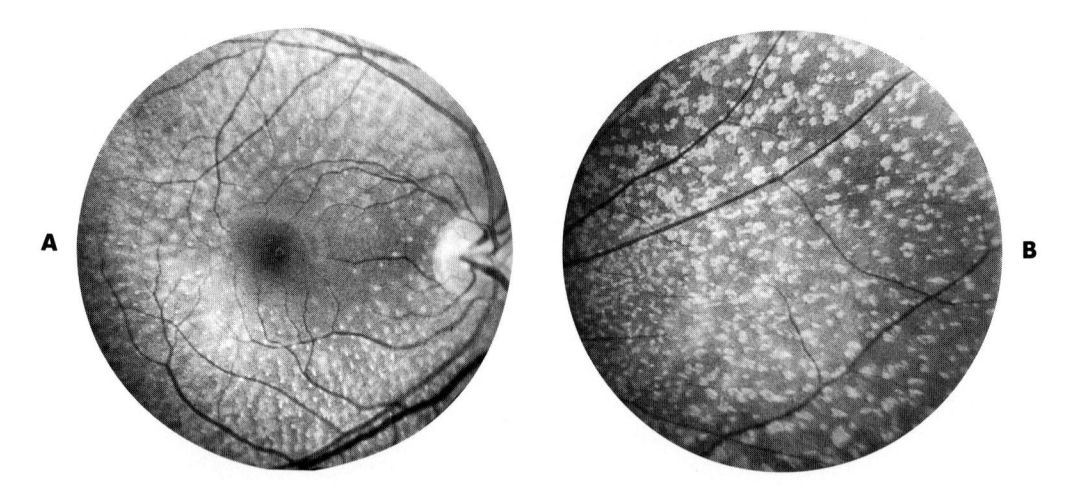

Figure 2-13 A, Posterior pole and **B,** peripheral retina in fundus albipunctatus showing white lesions at the level of the retinal pigment epithelium/Bruch's membrane. They are small and round in the posterior pole but become larger and more irregular in the peripheral fundus.

microscopic study of another eye more recently[305] supported the view that there was an abnormal layer between the outer segments of the photoreceptors and the pigment epithelial cells. However, the constituents were normal components of the retina, consisting of lipofuscin granules and protrusions of the pigment epithelium with complex interdigitations of the outer segments. There was no abnormal cone distribution. A third histologic study[306] is open to question since the patient had reduced vision with retinal pigmentary changes and both parents had RP. On electrophysiologic testing, both the a-wave of the ERG and the light rise in the standing potential of the eye were normal but the scotopic b-wave of the ERG was severely depressed even in the fully dark-adapted eye.[281,307]

The pathogenesis of Oguchi's disease is not understood. Rhodopsin regeneration is normal.[307] These observations imply that the primary abnormality is unrelated to light catch and rhodopsin bleaching but is related to other systems of transduction. From electrophysiologic results the region of bipolar cells appears to be the earliest stage in the visual pathway exhibiting signs of defective function. Because the abnormal reflex arises from the inner limiting membrane (at which site the major cellular component is the footplate of Mueller cells) and the Mueller cells are the source of the b-wave, it is likely that these cells are primarily at fault as suggested by de Jong et al.[178] Unfortunately, these histopathologic studies did not report on the state of the Mueller cells.

Fundus albipunctatus. Fundus albipunctatus is a static autosomal recessive condition in which the only symptoms are related to defective dark adaptation.[308] It should not be confused with albipunctate dystrophy (retinitis punctata albescens), which is progressive and represents a variant of RP. The fundus shows widespread distribution of uniform-sized almost white dots at the level of the pigment epithelium, most dense in the post-equatorial fundus (Fig. 2-13); the macula may or may not be involved. Changes in the distribution of the white dots have been described,[309] as has their changing from flecks in childhood to relatively permanent punctate dots that increase in number over the years.[310] Diffuse changes in the pigment epithelium are unusual. Fluorescein angiography shows punctate hyperfluorescence that does not, however, correspond to the punctate white dots.[310] Although fundus albipunctatus usually involves both eyes, unilateral disease has been reported.[311]

Typically, visual acuity and the visual fields are normal, but minor loss of field has been described.[309] In a majority of cases, the dark adaptation of both cones and rods is markedly prolonged[281,309-312] and there is delay in the acquisition of scotopic ERG thresholds.[281,312-314] Variation from this pattern has been described in which the dark adaptation and ERG are normal[314,315] or dark adaptation shows a cone segment only.[316] It is not clear whether this variation implies various degrees of severity of a single disease or several disorders that share the fundus abnormality.

Studies of rhodopsin kinetics[317] have shown slow rhodopsin regeneration that parallels dark adaptation. This implies that, in contrast to Oguchi's disease, the sensory defect is due to abnormal photopigment kinetics in fundus albipunctatus.

Fleck retina of Kandori. This rare condition, in which there is prolonged dark adaptation giving rise to difficulty with night vision but no other symptoms, has been described only in Japan.[318] Dark adaptation shows a prolonged rod phase reaching normal thresholds within 40 minutes. The fundus presents large irregular white lesions at the level of the pigment epithelium that are most concentrated in the equatorial region. The photopic ERG is normal, and a prolonged interval of dark adaptation is needed to reach scotopic potentials.

PATHOGENESIS OF PHOTORECEPTOR DYSTROPHIES
General Considerations

Many questions are amenable to investigation concerning the site of expression of disease and the factors that determine its form and the severity of dysfunction. Hereditary disorders are caused by defects in the genetic code, which, in turn, result in an abnormal amino acid composition of specific proteins. If a defective protein is coded by a gene whose activity is confined to a single cell type, the primary effect will be localized in that cell, even though secondary effects may occur in other cells. For example, the mutation may either reside in the photoreceptor cell, giving rise to the observed degeneration, or be expressed in a support tissue, leading to the same consequences. Alternatively, a systemic metabolic abnormality may result in the degeneration of a specific cell type, such as visual cells, by depriving them of vital metabolites.

In autosomal dominant disease the abnormality is produced in the heterozygous state. It is not known whether the disease is due to the product of the abnormal gene or a shortage of product from the normal gene. That there is great variation of disease in humans because of different mutations on the same gene implies that both mechanisms are important. The first is shown by the observation[319] that mice transfected with a mutant rhodopsin gene develop retinal degeneration. The second possibility[320] is illustrated in the rds-mouse, in which transgenic rescue is achieved by insertion of a normal peripherin/rds gene on a rhodopsin promoter. Retinal changes in the heterozygous *rds*-mouse are compatible with this concept.[321] The relevance of this model to human disease is illustrated by the finding of mutations in the peripherin gene in autosomal dominant retinal dystrophies.[116-119,175,185]

The identification of mutations on the rhodopsin and peripherin genes allows investigation of pathogenic mechanisms involved. It is fortunate that much was known concerning the structure and function of both proteins before the discovery of these mutations.

Rhodopsin. Rhodopsin is an intrinsic protein of rod disk membranes, and its activation by light to the photoexcited form (R*) is the first step in the enzyme amplification cascade of vertebrate phototransduction. Thus, specific functional and structural domains are inherent in the three-dimensional topography of the molecule to enable (1) effective quantum capture and (2) appropriate energy transfer kinetics and pathways for conformational alterations, thereby leading to (3) the unmasking of receptor sites for information transfer to cytoplasmic proteins. More generalized considerations will include appropriate folding and incorporation into membranes during its synthesis and stabilization on transfer to the disk membrane.

The basic membrane topography of the rhodopsin molecule is known, but details of structural reorganization during photostimulation and consequent alterations in receptor unmasking are rudimentary. Therefore it is not possible to predict at present the subtle alterations in function that should be induced by a mutational change in amino acid residues. Generalizations can be made, however. The rhodopsin molecule consists of 348 amino acid residues with two asparagine-linked oligosacchride side chains. Peptide folding results in the embedding of seven predominantly α-helices in the disc bilayer with interconnecting hydrophilic segments protruding from the membranous surface.[322-328] A lysine residue (no. 296) situated at the midpoint of the seventh helix is the attachment site for the 11-*cis* retinal chromophore. 11-*cis* Retinal also interacts with the other helices, and since all seven are aligned in a plane perpendicular to the disc surface, they effectively form a cage around the chromophore.[327,329,330] Photon absorption by 11-*cis* retinal causes isomerization of the chromophore to the all-trans form with simultaneous rearrangement of the helices. This conformation change in rhodopsin exposes a binding site (residues 231 to 252) for the G-protein, transduction, on the cytoplasmic surface,[331] the first step in signal amplification and activation of the enzymic cascade leading to visual transduciton.[332] On the cytoplasmic surface the carboxy terminal contains many serines and threonines, which on formation of R* are phosphorylated by a rhodopsin kinase. The ensuing binding of arrestin to phosphorylated rhodopsin blocks the further activation of transduction; this is therefore one of the termination steps in visual transduction. Also important for structural stability of rhodopsin are the two highly conserved cysteines on the intradistal surface.[333]

How a specific mutation would alter the dynamic stability of the resting molecule or influence cytoplasmic interactions of R* are as yet unclear. Nevertheless, certain generalizations can be made. Mutations in the hydrophobic regions or near the oligosaccharide attachment sites may interfere with initial folding and glycosylation, which would disturb membrane incorporation of the newly synthesized protein. Thus it would be expected that newly formed rhodopsin would accumulate in the inner segment.

In the families with autosomal dominant RP showing mutations of the rhodopsin gene on chromosome 3, different patterns of retinal dysfunction have been demonstrated with different mutations.* In three mutations, proline to leucine at codon 347, lysine to glutamic acid at codon 296 (i.e., the binding site for retinal), and an isoleucine deletion at codon 255 or 256, functional loss compatible with diffuse (type I) autosomal dominant RP was identified. With all three mutations poor night vision was consistently noted in early life and rod ERGs were severely reduced or unmeasurable. In those with measurable visual function, psychophysical testing showed rod function to be severely affected throughout the retina (with threshold elevations of more than 3 log units), even in younger individuals, whereas loss of cone function varied widely between families and was less widespread and less severe than loss of rod function. In one of the most severely affected families (Lys-296-Glu) there was little visual function after the age of 30 years in most members. With the isoleucine deletion at codon 256, cone function was limited to the central 10 degrees by the age of 25 years but little further loss occurred thereafter. Cone function was retained over most of the visual field until middle life in the 347 mutations despite widespread and severe early loss of rod function.

The functional abnormalities in families with mutations Thr-17-Arg, Pro-23-His, Thr-58-Arg, Gly-106-Arg, and Gua-182-Ade are qualitatively similar with altitudinal distribution of the disease and appear to be constant within the families.[37,39,105-110] This characteristic of the disease is in marked contrast with that seen in patients with other rhodopsin mutations examined to date. Rod sensitivity is severely depressed in the superior field but is nearly normal in the inferior field. Loss of cone sensitivity closely follows that of the rods. In this respect the pattern of disease resembles regional (type II) RP.

An additional striking finding in these families with sectorial-type RP is a characteristic abnormality in one component of the kinetics of dark adaptation following exposure to a bright light. Before bleaching, measurements made in the relatively intact portion of the visual field show mild threshold elevations of approximately 1 log unit. Following light adaptation there is a marked delay in the recovery of sensitivity. The initial portion of recovery mediated by cones and rods is normal. However by 1 hour, when in normal subjects the recovery of sensitivity is complete, these patients show residual threshold elevations of 1 to 2 log units from the prebleach values. Even after nearly 2 hours thresholds are still elevated by more than 1 log unit. In two subjects it was found[39] that the time course of this slow recovery of sensitivity was on the order of at least 80 to 120 hours. When a model based on primate data of rod outer segment length and turnover was used, it was calculated that the delayed phase of the recovery of rod sensitivity following strong light adaptation could be due in part to the formation of new disc membranes with a normal concentration of rhodopsin rather than in situ regeneration of photopigment.[39] The model requires that the outer segments be short as a result of RP and that a major portion of the outer segment be shed following strong light adaptation.

These observations show that there are both quantitative and qualitative dif-

---

*References 37, 39, 40, 105-112.

ferences in RP consequent upon mutations in the rhodopsin gene. Also important is the fact that some forms of RP have been shown for the first time to be due to defects of metabolic systems that are limited to rod photoreceptors, and yet it is evident that a loss of photopic function is consistently found in these disorders. No explanation exists to account for cone cell death. It possibly occurs as a result of either the release of endotoxins by dying rods or the cones, being metabolically dependent on the presence of rods. Thus the loss of cone function, although important to the patient, is but a secondary effect.

The mechanism by which alteration of the amino acid sequence in the rhodopsin molecule may influence rod photoreceptor function is unclear. Some observations on the behavior of the abnormal protein in the laboratory allow predictions to be made concerning possible effects of the mutation on metabolic systems. More general concepts can be formulated on the basis of recently identified mechanisms of protein formation and the cellular handling of abnormal proteins produced by mutant genes. It is known, for example, that abnormal proteins may or may not pass from the rough endoplasmic reticulum to the Golgi apparatus and that this depends on the influence of the mutation on molecular folding.[334] Proteins that do not pass on may be destroyed or may accumulate in the rough endoplasmic reticulum and, in turn, interfere with cell function.[335-338] From these considerations it is predictable that the nature of cell dysfunction would depend on the site of expression of the abnormal protein. If the protein is incorporated into the outer segment, it may generate physical instability of the membrane if glycosylation on the N-terminal or the disulfide bond between the cysteine residues 110 and 187 is abnormal.[331,339] Transduction efficiency may be reduced by mutations near the C-terminal, causing a reduction in sensitivity because of the reduced signal. It has been shown[340] that rhodopsin with a mutation at amino acid 296, which is the binding site for retinal, fails to form a complex with 11-*cis* retinal and reacts constantly with transducin. It might be predicted from this observation that the retina would act as if it were in constant lighting and would not dark adapt. These possibilities can be distinguished one from another by clinical testing. The interaction of the abnormal with the normal protein may also influence function.

The fate of protein produced by rhodopsin genes with mutations found in human RP has been investigated.[341,342] COS and 293S cells were transfected with various mutant rhodopsin genes. The abnormal proteins were then divided into distinct classes according to their behavior compared to normal.[342] In class I mutations rhodopsin was expressed normally on the plasma membrane and bound 11-*cis* retinal, creating a chromophore with an absorbance spectrum similar to that of rhodopsin. Class II showed little if any ability to form a pigment when exposed to 11-*cis* retinal, inefficient transport to the plasma membrane, and low levels of cell surface localization. However, in no instance was expression on the plasma membrane absent. In a similar experiment[343] mutant rhodopsin was prepared by site-directed mutagenesis and COS cells were transfected and incubated in the presence of 11-*cis* retinal. There was no binding of 11-*cis* retinal with the 68-72 deletion. Binding did occur with Thr-58-Arg, Arg-137-Leu, and Arg-135-Trp mutations, however, giving rise to a pigment with a λ max of 500 nm. Although light caused conversion to meta-rhodopsin II, when incubated with GDP and transducin there was defective activation.

Several of the mutations were identical to those found in forms of RP in which the functional deficit has been characterized. Pro-347-Leu was designated as biochemical class I, and the same mutation in humans causes diffuse RP. The mutations Pro-23-His, Thr-358-Arg, and Gly-106-Trp were designated as biochemical class II and in humans have been associated with regional RP, characterized by altitudinal distribution of disease and slow recovery from strong light adaptation. The information to date shows striking confirmation of the fundamental difference in mechanism for the RP types, which may be confirmed by functional studies in the other mutations.

Peripherin. Even more striking is the realization that RP and macular dystrophy may be due to mutations in the *RDS* gene.* The RP is of early onset and not obviously different from that seen with rhodopsin mutations, with one exception: it simulates retinitis punctata albescens.[119] Two families with a form of macular dystrophy were shown[175] to have a tryptophan substitution for arginine at codon 172 and another family with almost identical disease to have a glutamine substitution at the same codon. A mutation resulting in a stop codon at position 258 has been identified in a family with a retinal degeneration similar in appearance to adult vitelliform macular dystrophy,[175] and a mutation at codon 168 has caused a pattern dystrophy.[185] These findings demonstrate that some forms of autosomal dominant RP and dominantly inherited macular dystrophies are caused by mutations in the same *(RDS)* gene. The variability of phenotype caused by mutations at different codons suggests that the functional significance of certain amino acids to cones and rods may be different.

The current knowledge of the putative function of peripherin-rds provides a potential explanation for diseases being different from different mutations of the *RDS* gene. Peripherin has an amino acid sequence of 346 amino acids with four transmembrane hydrophobic domains and two putative N-linked glycosylation sites.[122] One of these is conserved across four species and is thought to be important to the protein's function in stabilizing photoreceptor outer segment membranes.[123,124,344] Immunohistochemical studies have shown that the protein is limited to the membranes of outer segments in both rods and cones although there is disagreement over its precise location. One study using a polyvalent antibody to a short peptide sequence near the carboxyl terminus[123] implied that the protein was distributed over the entire length of the outer segment disc membrane. It was suggested that covalent bonding between peripherin molecules was responsible for the maintenance of the parallel arrangement of outer segment membranes. By contrast, a separate study using a monoclonal antibody to purified photoreceptor discs[124] showed that labeling was confined to the rims of the outer segment, implying that the primary function of the protein was to stabilize the unfavorable thermodynamic bend at the disc rim. To explain these different findings, it was hypothesized[123] that the epitopes available for antibody binding may differ at the disc rim when compared to other parts of the disc membrane. Regardless of the precise mechanism, the general belief is that peripherin is important to the structural stability of the outer segment disc membrane.

Recently it has been shown[345] that peripherin may bind noncovalently to

---
*References 117-119, 175, 185.

ROM1, a protein structurally related to peripherin. ROM1 has been located on the disc rims of rod outer segments but has not been identified in cones. It has been proposed that the formation and stability of the bend in the disc membrane in rods are dependent on the association between peripherin and ROM1. However, the absence of ROM1 in cones implies that differences exist between the precise mechanisms by which peripherin stabilizes outer segment membranes in the two classes of photoreceptor. In rods the association between peripherin and ROM1 may be important whereas in cones peripherin may bind to a different membrane protein or may act alone. If the binding sites were different in rods and cones, constancy of one amino acid in the peripherin molecule might be important to rods only, and a mutation causing an abnormality at this site would cause a dystrophy falling within the category of RP (in which rods were the target cell of disease with relative preservation of cones). Conversely, a different mutation on the *RDS* gene might disrupt the metabolism or structure either of cones alone (causing macular dystrophy) or of both rods and cones. It appears that the presence of arginine at 172 is important to the structure and function of cones but not of rods.[175] No data exist at present to explain the apparent preferential loss of central cones as opposed to peripheral cones, or peripheral rods as opposed to paracentral rods.[175]

The disorders associated with a stop sequence at codon 258 and the mutation at codon 167 are different from the others with mutations in the *RDS* gene in that there is little evidence of functional loss and the changes in the ocular fundus are apparently at the level of the retinal pigment epithelium. It is possible that these mutations produce metabolic changes similar to those seen in the mouse heterozygous for the abnormal *rds* gene, in which there is a 10 kB insert in the gene at codon 238.[123] In the homozygous rds-mouse *(rds/rds)* a relatively high–molecular weight mRNA is produced, demonstrating that the whole insert is transcribed.[123] It is unlikely, however, that the mutant protein is expressed, since the mRNA does not appear to leave the nucleus. As a consequence outer segment discs are not formed, the disc membrane being discharged as small vesicles into the subretinal space.[346-349] Predictably, only half the normal amount of protein would be available in the heterozygous state *(rds/+)* as a result of expression of the normal gene. The photoreceptor outer segment would develop but contain long lengths of disc membrane[321] compatible with having less than the normal quantity of peripherin/rds. However, the ERG is well preserved and 50% of the photoreceptors survive after 18 months of life,[321,350] which is close to the life expectancy of the mouse. The outer segments appear to be unstable, and the retinal pigment epithelium contains large and abnormal phagosomes.[350] Such a situation may exist in some patients with adult vitelliform macular degeneration, since the mutations are close. As in the heterozygous *rds*-mouse it is likely that the photoreceptors receive only half the normal quantity of peripherin-rds and that the abnormal protein does not pass into the outer segment. If the homology is close, it would be understandable that excessive shedding of the photoreceptor outer segments over many years would cause change in the retinal pigment epithelium but little photoreceptor dysfunction. A similar situation may pertain in pattern dystrophies. Assuming this reasoning is correct, a primary photoreceptor disease causes changes that are recognizable clinically only at the level of the retinal pigment epithelium.

MANAGEMENT

Patients can expect an account of the implications concerning the visual prognosis and genetic implications of their retinal dystrophy. This demands that a precise diagnosis be made with respect to the classification of disease and its inheritance.

Identification of disease. The type of retinal dystrophy is frequently identifiable on the basis of history and physical signs. The distinction between a stationary condition such as stationary night blindness or rod monochromatism and progressive disease such as retinitis pigmentosa or macular dystrophy is usually evident if a reliable history is available. The fundus changes are rarely difficult to define in well-established disease.

Additional testing may be necessary to identify the presence or absence of disease. In recent-onset RP and Leber's amaurosis, confirmation of the functional loss may be dependent on demonstrating profound loss of amplitudes of the ERG. The nature of the ERG abnormalities may also indicate the nature of the condition. Loss of b-wave with a relatively well preserved a-wave is characteristic of X-linked retinoschisis, autosomal recessive and X-linked CSNB, and Oguchi's disease. The ability to give an accurate prognosis may be helped by recording amplitude of loss. A bull's eye lesion at the macula may indicate loss of central cones, loss of cones throughout the fundus or the initial indication of a cone/rod dystrophy—each having different implications for vision from the others. The distinction can be made easily with ERGs.

Documentation of visual field loss may be important in assessing the degree of disability and the suitability and safety of a subject for certain activities such as driving, but it is relatively unhelpful in establishing the diagnosis.

Fluorescein angiography has been advocated for defining the extent of retinal pigment epithelial abnormality in RP although it is unusual for it to provide new information. It may be useful for the detection of macular edema if visual acuity is reduced and there is no obvious atrophy of the outer retina at the fovea. Although cystoid edema may be easy to recognize, diffuse edema is hard to confirm by ophthalmoscopy alone. The distinction between macular retinoschisis and cystoid edema may not be evident without angiography.

There are few forms of retinal dystrophy for which treatment will modify the course of the primary disorder,[351-358] and it clearly is important to identify these disorders. Abetalipoproteinemia can be diagnosed on the basis of the clinical presentation of malabsorption in infancy and low levels of cholesterol and β-lipoproteins in blood. The diagnosis of gyrate atrophy of the retina and choroid can be established by recognition of the typical fundus appearance as well as the demonstration of raised blood ornithine and low or absent cellular orthinine aminotransferase activity. Refsum's syndrome usually presents with visual loss alone, other deficits appearing some years later. This accounts for the long delays in making the diagnosis after presentation to ophthalmologists.[356] The vast majority of patients have symptoms by the age of 30 years and present to the ophthalmologist by the age of 40. The only other physical deficits likely to be present in early disease are anosmia, hearing loss, and short terminal phalanges (affecting mainly the thumbs) but many will have visual loss alone. It is justified to exclude the condition by measuring plasma levels of phytanic acid in patients having symptoms in the first 30 years of life and without evidence of dominant or X-linked inheritance.

Identification of inheritance. When transmission can be identified through several generations, the recognition of X-linked or autosomal dominant inheritance is usually simple. As with other disorders, parental consanguinity may indicate the possibility of autosomal recessive inheritance. The inheritance may be evident if the pattern of disease is distinctive and indicative of a single nosologic entity with known inheritance. Such a situation is illustrated by choroideremia and gyrate atrophy, which are X-linked and autosomal recessive respectively.

When faced with a sporadic case without distinctive changes, one may find the problem of identifying the genetic form of the disease more difficult. Until fairly recently it was commonly assumed that patients with simplex RP had autosomal recessive disease. However, the excess of males over females in this group implies that a number have X-linked disease.[1,360] Failure to recognize X-linked disease can occur if heterozygous females are asymptomatic and affected male relatives are not known to the proband. Alternatively, the disease may be autosomal dominant as a result of a new mutation although this is probably uncommon.[1] Finally, the possibility of a phenocopy cannot be ignored despite there being good evidence that such cases are rarely diagnosed as RP.[1]

The genetic status may be established by detailed inquiry of the family regarding the means by which affected relatives previously unknown to the patient are identified. This is particularly the case in X-linked disease. Further genetic information may be obtained by examining asymptomatic relatives, which may reveal females heterozygous for X-linked disease or evidence of dominant disease if the disorder is mild or has variable expressivity. Certain diagnoses (e.g., as adult vitelliform degeneration and pattern dystrophies) are rarely proven without a family survey. If there is reasonable suspicion of Best's disease, EOG testing may be necessary to confirm the diagnosis and document the distribution of the gene within the family.

It has been suggested[360] that the severity of the disease may be used as a guide to the likely inheritance of RP. In general, X-linked RP and autosomal recessive RP are severe and of early onset whereas dominant disease is milder. Thus severe disease in a female may indicate autosomal recessive, and mild disease in a male autosomal dominant, disease. Mild disease in a female is compatible with either the heterozygous state of X-linked disease or the autosomal dominant disease, but severe disease in a male suggests X-linked or autosomal recessive disease. However, there are many simplex cases with mild disease, implying that recessive disease may not be severe.

Treatment. In only three conditions has treatment been shown to reduce the speed of visual loss by modifying the primary disorder. The treatment of *abetalipoproteinemia* by restricting lipid intake and giving vitamin A and E supplementation is effective in preventing the occurrence of retinal degeneration if initiated early in life.[351] Treatment is monitored by the regular measurement of retinal function and of serum vitamin A levels. In patients with *gyrate atrophy* dietary restriction of arginine intake reduces plasma ornithine levels to normal or near-normal.[352-354] There is evidence[352,353] that this treatment influences the progress of the disease, although this is not universal experience.[354] In addition, it is difficult to persuade patents to maintain their diet over long periods. In a very small proportion of subjects vitamin B_6 supplementation modifies the levels of serum ornithine by enhancing ornithine aminotransferase activity, although the influence of this treatment on functional loss is not recorded.[355] In *Refsum's syndrome* the mainstay of treatment is dietary, restricting the intake of phytanic acid and unbound phytol but maintaining sufficient caloric intake to prevent release of endogenous phytanic acid from the fat stores.[356-358] At the time of diagnosis or during severe exacerbations, plasmapheresis may be used to lower the levels of phytanic acid rapidly, which may prevent fatal sequelae. It is implied that the visual prognosis may be improved by treatment, but this has yet to be proven.

Recently a controlled trial of treatment of RP[361] has shown that the rate of reduction of the cone ERG may be slowed by supplementing vitamin A intake with 15,000 units of vitamin A palmitate per day. Surprisingly, adding vitamin E appeared to be positively harmful on the basis of cone ERG. As a consequence the authors recommended that patients with RP take vitamin A supplements regularly. Excluded from the trial were patients under the age of 18 years and those with Usher's type I syndrome, thus no statement could be made with respect to these patients, and treatment was not recommended for pregnant women. On theoretic grounds there is no reason why other forms of vitamin A (e.g., the vitamin A acetate) should not be as effective. Some doubt has been expressed as to the relevance of these findings to the potential for treatment to modify vision, and some[362] have taken the view that firm recommendations should await additional data concerning visual function.

Although modification of the primary disorder is not feasible in the majority of conditions, help may be achieved by treating the secondary consequences of general dystrophies. Macular edema is a frequent association of RP and may cause significant additional loss of visual function. It has been shown[363-365] to respond to carbonic anhydrase inhibitors, with reduction of the edema and improvement of visual acuity and visual fields. For any patient with loss of central vision but no atrophy of the central retina, treatment is worth considering. Whether it is necessary to undertake fluorescein angiography before treatment is uncertain, since the edema is often hard to prove at angiography and it often takes several days to recover vision after angiography. Over half those with proven edema respond to treatment, although no guidelines have been identified to indicate who will respond. It is reasonable to give a 4-week trial of treatment before deciding whether a response has occurred. If there is no response, treatment should be be withdrawn. If vision improves, the patient should be asked to titrate the level of treatment against the therapeutic effect.

Cataract is also common in RP, and posterior subcapsular opacities are particularly disturbing since they are near the nodal point of the eye; surgery may lead to major improvement in visual function.[366] Some idea of the potential vision following surgery can be acquired by excluding changes at the fovea through clinical examination: potential acuity meter measurement of visual acuity may be helpful. It is wise to avoid excessive exposure of the fundus to light during surgery.

Optical devices are helpful and vary from simple to complex (e.g., lens to closed circuit television).[367,368] Poor vision in bright light is a common problem and tinted glasses may be helpful. Apart from blue cone monochromatism, red or red/brown glasses are the most effective and should be dark enough to relieve photphobia; in rod monochromatism a density giving rise to less than 10% transmission may be necessary. Apart from improving immediate function, it is possible that avoiding prolonged exposure to bright light alters the course of the disorder (especially if light toxicity hastens visual loss in retinal dystrophies), but this is unproven. Image intensifiers have been assessed[369,370] in the management of subjects with poor night vision. Although function was improved, they have not become widely used.

Counseling. Counseling is important in the management of patients with retinal dystrophies since, with rare exception, there is no effective treatment by which the primary disorder can be modified. Both the prospect of visual loss and the genetic implications of the diagnosis may generate major psychologic problems for the patient and the family.[371] Many of the problems can be overcome, however, by giving adequate support, which may continue over a prolonged period before total rehabilitation is achieved.[372] There are particular difficulties in the blind child, in whom learning deficits are superimposed on the sensory handicap and can be overcome only with considerable education support.[373,374] Although provision of additional help may not be the primary responsibility of the ophthalmologist, the clinician who first recognizes the problem is responsible for apprising the patient of the diagnosis and may be crucial to initiating additional support. The ophthalmologist may also be in a good position to assess whether the help given is adequate and to ensure that support is rendered for a long as necessary.

IMPLICATIONS OF ADVANCES IN MOLECULAR BIOLOGY

The recent advances in molecular biology whereby specific genomic defects have been identified in retinal dystrophies have already had an impact on clinical management and are advancing our understanding of the pathogenesis of the disease. It is to be hoped that this work will eventually lead to therapy for patients with retinal dystrophies.

Disease Mechanisms

Identification of the genomic defect and demonstration of the influence of abnormal proteins on cell function render the findings of clinical investigation much more significant. In the past the functional deficits of retinal dystrophies were valuable in distinguishing one disorder from another or at least in identifying categories of disease. It is now possible to relate these characteristics to putative disease mechanisms and to generate hypotheses that are amenable to testing in the laboratory. It is also the case that observations are possible in humans, particularly with respect to detailed recording of functional loss in patients with retinal dystrophies, that cannot be made in animals. Thus the results of clinical and laboratory studies are relevant one to the other.

Although there are both quantitative and qualitative differences in functional loss between families, the severity of disease varies considerably within families. Analysis of the variation within families should allow assessment of the potential effect of mechanisms influencing phenotypic expression of abnormal genes by genomic imprinting and allelic competition.[375,376]

The initial subdivision of retinal dystrophies was achieved on the basis of their patterns of inheritance; morphologic and functional studies have added to our understanding of this complex group of disorders. The recent identification of a number of mutations in the rhodopsin and peripherin genes is at present being correlated with clinical and functional abnormalities, and we can expect, in the near future, to find other genes responsible for further members of this group of disorders. The mechanism by which alteration of the amino acid sequence in rhodopsin or peripherin molecules may influence photoreceptor function is unclear, but much may depend on the site of expression of the abnormal protein. The recognition that a disease affecting the retinal pigment epithelium is due to a gene expressed in photoreceptor cells has already led to a change in our appreciation of potential disease processes. More sophisticated visual testing is required to correlate the genotype with the phenotypic expression of the disease. The generation of transgenic mice carrying a specific human mutation should accelerate our understanding of functional aberrations and, more important, the mechanisms that lead to eventual death of the photoreceptor. Although there has been a rapid advance in our understanding of the disease mechanisms in RP, there is every prospect that the expansion of knowledge will accelerate in the next few years, particularly with continued and increasing collaboration between clinicians and basic scientists.

Impact on Clinical Management

The considerable advances so far achieved have not yet brought any great advance in therapy, although some effects on clinical management have become evident. Genetic counseling in a family is undoubtedly simplified if the genomic abnormality is known. The distribution of an abnormal gene in a family can be documented with almost 100% certainty, and the genetic status of a subject can be established at any age and any stage of the disease. Furthermore, advice on visual prognosis can be made on a firmer basis if single nosologic entities are identified by genomic studies.

Eugenic management is also possible as a consequence of these discoveries. Selective termination of pregnancy may be requested by patients in a small number of conditions in which the disease is severe. Selective implantation of normal embryos following in vitro fertilization is also now feasible. These management techniques have been initiated in severe diseases like cystic fibrosis. Population screening has also been initiated for cystic fibrosis, by which it is proposed to identify the distribution of the mutant genes within the population.[376-379] Whether this would ever be feasible or desirable for retinal dystrophies is not clear; to some extent this would depend on the number of genes involved.

In addition, it is to be hoped that with the knowledge that will accrue from extension of current studies, it may eventually be possible to offer effective treatment to the patient with retinitis pigmentosa. The rescue of the retina in *rd*- and *rds*-mouse by insertion of normal genes[320,380] is impressive, although there are major differences between insertion of genes into the ovum on the one hand and into a nondividing photoreceptor cell on the other. The techniques of grafting retinal pigment epithelium (RPE) and photoreceptor cells, and whole retina, are still in their infancy[381-384]; but these forms of management may one day be feasible. The preservation of retinal function in the Royal College of Surgeons rat by intravitreal injection of growth factors is impressive, although there is no evidence to date that a homologous situation exists in humans.[387]

CONCLUSIONS

The management of retinal dystrophies now requires a team of workers with a variety of disciplines. Advice is dependent on establishing the ophthalmic diagnosis in the first instance, which may involve clinical, psychophysical, and electrophysiologic evaluation. The inheritance can be established only if the family is well known to the patient; the pedigree may be constructed by the patient on the basis of memory or inquiries within the family. Failing this, the help of genetic services may be needed to search other sources of information (e.g., registrations of births, marriages, and deaths as well as censuses and parish records). Examination of relatives at risk of having the abnormal gene but who are asymptomatic is often helpful. In addition, the mutation may be sought by molecular biologists.

It is essential that the patient understand the advice given, which may require an experience in counseling. The patient has the problem of coping with the deficit, and this may be hampered initially by depression and potential guilt feelings, which frequently accompany the presence of inherited disease within a family. To overcome these problems, prolonged counseling may be needed. Finally, optical and social help may be provided, which calls for further expertise.

Although a cure is not available for inherited retinal dystrophies, management of patients is extremely complex; and considerable help can be given that will in the majority of cases be initiated by the ophthalmologist.

References

1. Jay M: On the heredity of retinitis pigmentosa, *Br J Ophthalmol* 7:405-416, 1982.
2. Fishman GA: Retinitis pigmentosa: genetic percentages, *Arch Ophthalmol* 96:822-826, 1978.
3. Pearlman JT: Mathematical models of retinitis pigmentosa: a study of the rate of progress in the different genetic forms, *Trans Am Ophthalmol Soc* 77:643-656, 1979.
4. Hu D: Genetic aspects of retinitis pigmentosa in China, *Am J Med Genet* 12:51-56, 1982.
5. Boughman JA, Fishman GA: A genetic analysis of retinitis pigmentosa, *Br J Ophthalmol* 66:405-416, 1983.
6. Heckenlively JR: 1987. Quoted in Heckenlively JR: *Retinitis pigmentosa,* Philadelphia, 1988, JB Lippincott, p 21.
7. Massof RW, Finkelstein D: Two forms of autosomal dominant primary retinitis pigmentosa, *Doc Ophthalmol* 51:289-346, 1981.
8. Arden GB, Carter RM, Hogg CR, et al: Rod and cone activity in patients with dominantly inherited retinitis pigmentosa: comparison between psychophysical and electroretinographic measurements, *Br J Ophthalmol* 67:405-418, 1983.
9. Lyness AL, Ernst W, Quinlan MP, et al: A clinical, psychophysical, and electroretinographic survey of patients with autosomal dominant retinitis pigmentosa, *Br J Ophthalmol* 69:326-339, 1985.
10. Kemp CM, Jacobson SG, Faulkner DJ: Two types of visual dysfunction in autosomal dominant retinitis pigmentosa, *Invest Ophthalmol Vis Sci* 29:1235-1241, 1988.
11. Bietti GB: Su alcune forme atipiche o rare di degenerazione retinica (degenerazioni tappeto-retiniche e quadri morbosi similari), *Boll Oculist* 16:1159-1241, 1937.
12. Haase W, Hellner KA: Über familiäre bilaterale sektorenförmige Retinopathia pigmentosa, *Klin Monatsbl Augenheilkd* 147:365-375, 1965.
13. Fledelius H, Simonsen SE: A family with bilateral symmetrical sectorial pigmentary retinal lesion, *Acta Ophthalmol* 48:14-22, 1970.
14. Ragnetti E: An atypical form of retinitis pigmentosa, *Boll Oculist* 41:617-625, 1962.
15. Vukovich V: Das ERG bei Retinitis pigmentosa (Retinopathia pigmentosa) mit bitemporalen Gesichtsfeldausfall, *Albrecht von Graefes Arch Klin Exp Ophthalmol* 161:27-32, 1959.
16. Alezzandrini A: Retinitis pigmentosa in symmetric quadrants, *Am J Ophthalmol* 60:1160, 1965.

17. Hommer K: Das Elektroretinogramm bei sektorenförmiger Retinitis pigmentosa (Retinopathia pigmentosa), *Albrecht von Graefes Arch Klin Exp Ophthalmol* 161:16-26, 1959.
18. Kuper J: Familiäre sektorenförmige Retinitis pigmentosa, *Klin Monatsbl Augenheilk* 136:97-102, 1960.
19. Lisch K: Isolierte Entwicklungsstörungen, *Med Monatsschr* 14:720-725, 1960.
20. Krill AE, Archer DB, Martin D: Sector retinitis pigmentosa, *Am J Ophthalmol* 69:977-987, 1970.
21. Bird AC: X-linked retinitis pigmentosa, *Br J Ophthalmol* 59:177-199, 1975.
22. Berson EL, Howard J: Temporal aspects of the electroretinogram in sector retinitis pigmentosa, *Arch Ophthalmol* 48:653-665, 1971.
23. Fulton AB, Hansen RM: The relationship of rhodopsin and scotopic retinal sensitivity in sector retinitis pigmentosa, *Am J Ophthalmol* 105:132-140, 1988.
24. Haustrate FM, Oosterhuis JA: Pigmented paravenous retinochoroidal atrophy (PPRA), *Doc Ophthalmol* 63:209-237, 1986.
25. Foxman SG, Heckenlively JR, Sinclair SH: Rubeola retinopathy and pigmented paravenous retinochoroidal atrophy, *Am J Ophthalmol* 99:605-606, 1985.
26. Noble KG, Carr RE: Pigmented paravenous chorioretinal atrophy, *Am J Ophthalmol* 90:338-344, 1983.
27. Traboulsi EI, Maumenee IH: Hereditary pigmented paravenous chorioretinal atrophy, *Arch Ophthalmol* 104:1636-1640, 1986.
28. Skalka HW: Hereditary pigmented paravenous retinochoroidal atrophy, *Am J Ophthalmol* 87:286-291, 1979.
29. Lessel MR, Thaler A, Heilig P: ERG and EOG in progressive paravenous retinochoroidal atrophy, *Doc Ophthalmol* 62:25-30, 1986.
30. Cheung DS: Pigmented paravenous chorioretinal atrophy, *Am J Ophthalmol* 97:113, 1984.
31. Sveinsson K: Choroiditis areata, *Acta Ophthalmol* 17:73-79, 1939.
32. Sveinsson K: Helicoid peripapillary chorio-retinal degeneration, *Acta Ophthalmol* 57:69-75, 1979.
33. Magnusson L: Atrophia areata, a variant of peripapillary chorioretinal degeneration, *Acta Ophthalmol* 59:659-664, 1981.
34. Rubino A: Su una paralitica anomalia bilaterale alle e simmetrica dello strato pigmento retinico, *Boll Ocul* 19:318, 1940.
35. Franceschetti A: A curious affection of the ocular fundus: helicoid peripapillary chorioretinal degeneration, its relation to pigmented paravenous chorioretinal degeneration, *Doc Ophthalmol* 16:81-110, 1962.
36. Brazitikos PD, Safran AB: Helicoid peripapillary chorioretinal degeneration, *Am J Ophthalmol* 109:290-294, 1990.
37. Heckenlively, JR, Rodriguez JA, Daiger SP: Autosomal dominant sectoral retinitis pigmentosa: two families with transversion mutation in codon 23 of rhodopsin, *Arch Ophthalmol* 109:84-91, 1991.
38. Alexander KR, Fishman GA: Prolonged rod adaptation in retinitis pigmentosa, *Br J Ophthalmol* 68:561-569, 1984.
39. Moore AT, Fitzke FW, Kemp CM, et al: Abnormal dark adaptation kinetics in autosomal dominant sector retinitis pigmentosa due to rod opsin mutation, *Br J Ophthalmol* 76:465-469, 1992.
40. Moore AT, Fitzke F, Jay M, et al: Autosomal dominant retinitis pigmentosa with apparent incomplete penetrance: a clinical, electrophysiological, psychophysical and molecular biological study, *Br J Ophthalmol* 77:473-479, 1993.
41. Leber T: Über anomale Formen der retinitis pigmentosa, *Arch Ophthalmol* 17(1):314-341, 1971.
42. Alstrom CH, Olson O: Heredo-retinopathia congenitalis monohybrida recessive autosomalis, *Hereditas* 43:1-178, 1957.
43. Henkes HE, Verduin PC: Dysgenesis or abiotrophy? A differentiation with the help of the electroretinogram (ERG) and electroculogram (EOG) in Leber's congenital amaurosis, *Ophthalmologica* 145:144-160, 1963.

44. Heckenlively JR: Preserved para-arteriole retinal pigment epithelium (PPRPE) in retinitis pigmentosa, *Br J Ophthalmol* 66:26-31, 1982.
45. Porta A, Pierrottet C, Aschero M, Orzalesi N: Preserved para-arteriole retinal pigment epithelium retinitis pigmentosa, *Am J Ophthalmol* 113:161-164, 1992.
46. Marmor MF, Jacobson SG, Foerster MH, et al: Diagnostic findings of a new syndrome with night blindness, maculopathy, and enhanced S-cone sensitivity, *Am J Ophthalmol* 110:124-134, 1990.
47. Favre M: A propos de deux cas de dégénérescence hyaloïdéo-rétinienne, *Ophthalmologica* 135:337-361, 1958.
48. Diem M: Retinitis punctata albescens et pigmentosa, *Klin Monatsbl Augenheilkd* 53:371-379, 1914.
49. Mann I: *Developmental abnormalities of the eye,* Cambridge, 1937, Cambridge University Press, Figure 105.
50. Falls HF, Cotterman CW: Choroido-retinal degeneration: a sex-linked form in which heterozygous women exhibit a tapetal-like reflex, *Arch Ophthalmol* 40:685-703, 1948.
51. Weiner RL, Falls HF: Intermediate sex-linked retinitis pigmentosa, *Arch Ophthalmol* 53:539-553, 1955.
52. François J: Chorioretinal degeneration of retinitis pigmentosa of intermediate sex-linked heredity, *Doc Ophthalmol* 16:111-127, 1962.
53. Ricci A, Ammann F, Franceschetti A: Reflet tapéto-réversible (phénomène de Mizuo inverse) chez des conductrices de rétinopathie pigmentaire récessive liée au sexe, *Bull Mem Soc Fr Ophtalmol* 76:31-35, 1963.
54. Hussels I: Une famille atteinte de rétinopathie pigmentaire lié au sexe, de maladie de Parkinson et d'autres troubles neuro-psychiatriques, *J Gon Hum* 16:106-155, 1967.
55. Warburg M, Simonsen SE: Sex-linked recessive retinitis pigmentosa, *Acta Ophthalmol (Copenh)* 46:494-499, 1968.
56. Krill AE: X-chromosomal linked diseases affecting the eye: status of the heterozygote female, *Trans Am Ophthalmol Soc* 67:535-608, 1969.
57. Schappert-Kimmijser J: Les dégénérescences tapéto-rétiniennes du type X chromosomal aux Pays-Bas, *Bull Mem Soc Fr Ophtalmol* 76:122-129, 1963.
58. McQuarrie MD: Two pedigrees of hereditary blindness in man, *J Genet* 30:147-153, 1935.
59. Janssen O: Zur Erbbiologie der Retinitis pigmentosa (inaugural dissertation), Münster in Westfalen, 1938.
60. McKenzie DS: The inheritance of retinitis pigmentosa in one family, *Trans Ophthalmol Soc NZ* 5:79-82, 1951.
61. Kobayashi VA: Genetic study on retinitis pigmentosa, *Jpn J Ophthalmol* 7:82-88, 1960.
62. Berson EL, Gouras PL, Bunkel RD, Myrianthopoulos NC: Rod and cone responses in sex-linked retinitis pigmentosa, *Arch Ophthalmol* 81:215-225, 1969.
63. Pedralgia C: Klinische Beobachtungen: Retinitis pigmentosa, *Klin Monatsbl Augenheilkd* 3:114-117, 1865.
64. Deutschman R: Einseitige typische Retinitis pigmentosa mit pathologisch anatomischem Befund, *Beitr Augenheilkd* 1:69-80, 1891.
65. François J, Verriest G: Rétinopathie pigmentaire unilatérale, *Ophthalmologica* 124:65-88, 1952.
66. Kolb H, Galloway NR: Three cases of unilateral pigmentary degeneration, *Br J Ophthalmol* 48:471-479, 1964.
67. Carr RE, Siegel IM: Unilateral retinitis pigmentosa, *Arch Ophthalmol* 90:21-26, 1973.
68. Cordier J, Reny A, Seigneur JB: Rétinite pigmentaire unilatérale, *Bull Soc Ophtalmol Fr* 66:224-227, 1966.
69. Armington JC: Electrical responses of the light adapted eye, *J Opt Soc Am* 43:450-456, 1953.
70. Bjork A, Karp G: The electroretinogram in retinitis pigmentosa, *Acta Ophthalmol* 29:361-371, 1951.
71. Dodt F, Wadenstein L: The use of flicker electroretinography in the human eye, *Acta Ophthalmol* 32:165-180, 1954.

72. François J: L'Electrorétinographie dans les dégénérescences tapéto-rétiniennes périphériques et centrales, *Ann Ocul* 185:842-856, 1952.
73. Riggs LA: Electroretinography in cases of night blindness, *Am J Ophthalmol* 38:70-78, 1954.
74. Bush NR: The electrical responses of the eye before and after perforation of the retina. (MD thesis), Brown University, 1951.
75. Armington JC, Gouras P, Tepas DL, Gunkel R: Detection of the electroretinogram in retinitis pigmentosa, *Exp Eye Res* 1:74-80, 1961.
76. Henkes HE, van der Tweel L, van der Gon JJ: Selective amplication of the electroretinogram, *Ophthalmologica* 132:140-150, 1956.
77. Berson EL, Gouras P, Hoff M: Temporal aspects of the electroretinogram, *Arch Ophthalmol* 81:207-214, 1969.
78. Berson EL, Gouras P, Gunkel RD, Myrianthopoulos NC: Dominant retinitis pigmentosa with reduce penetrance, *Arch Ophthalmol* 81:226-235, 1969.
79. Berson EL, Gouras P, Gunkel RD, Myrianthopoulos NC: Rod and cone responses in sex-linked retinitis pigmentosa, *Arch Ophthalmol* 81:215-225, 1969.
80. Brown KT, Murakami MA: A new receptor potential of the monkey retina with no detectable latency, *Nature* 201:626-628, 1964.
81. Arden BB, Ikeda H: Effects of hereditary degeneration of the retina on the early receptor potential and the corneo-fundal potential of the rat eye, *Vis Res* 6:121-184, 1966.
82. Cone RA: Early receptor potentials of the vertebrate retina, *Nature* 204:736-739, 1964.
83. Brindley GA, Gardner-Medwin AR: The origin of the early receptor potential of the retina, *J Physiol* 182:105-191, 1966.
84. Cone RA, Brown PK: Dependence of the early receptor potential on the orientation of rhodopsin, *Science* 156:536, 1967.
85. Berson EL, Goldstein EB: The early receptor potential in sex-linked retinitis pigmentosa, *Invest Ophthalmol* 9:58-63, 1970.
86. Berson, EL, Goldstein EB: Recovery of the human early receptor potential during dark adapation in hereditary retinal disease, *Vis Res* 10:219-226, 1970.
87. Arden GB, Barrada A: Analysis of the electro-oculograms of a series of normal subjects, *Br J Ophthalmol* 46:468-482, 1962.
88. Arden GB, Kolb H: Electrophysiological investigations in retinal metabolic disease: their range and application, *Exp Eye Res* 3:334-347, 1964.
89. Bhattacharya SS, Wright AF, Clayton JF, et al: Close genetic linkage between X-linked retinitis pigmentosa and a restriction fragments length polymorphism identifed by recombinant DNA probe L1.28, *Nature* 309:253-255, 1984.
90. Friedrich U, Warburg M, Wieacker P, et al: X-linked retinitis pigmentosa: linkage with the centromere and a cloned DNA sequence from the proximal short arm of the X chromosome, *Hum Genet* 71:93-99, 1985.
91. Mukai S, Dryja TP, Bruns GAP, et al: Linkage between the X-linked retinitis pigmentosa locus and the L1.28 locus, *Am J Ophthalmol* 100:225-229, 1985.
92. Wright AF, Bhattacharya SS, Clayton JF, et al: Linkage relationships between X-linked retinitis pigmentosa and six short arm markers: exclusion of the disease locus from Xp21, *Am J Hum Gen* 41:635-644, 1987.
93. Francke U, Ochs HD, De Martinville B, et al: Minor Xp21 chromosome deletion in a male associated with expression of Duchenne muscular dystrophy and McLeod syndrome, *Am J Hum Genet* 37:250-267, 1985.
94. Nussbaum RL, Lewis RA, Lesko JG, Ferrell R: Mapping ophthalmological disease. II. Linkage of relationship of X-linked retinitis pigmentosa to X chromosome short arm markers, *Hum Genet* 70:45-50, 1985.
95. Denton MJ, Chen J-D, Serravalle S, et al: Analysis of linkage relationships of X-linked retinitis pigmentosa with the following Xp loci: L1.28, OTC, 754, XJ1.1, pERT 87, and C7, *Hum Genet* 78:60-64, 1988.
96. Jacobson SG, Roman AJ, Cideciyan AV, et al: X-linked retinitis pigmentosa: functional phenotype of an RP2 genotype, *Invest Ophthalmol Vis Sci* 33:3481-3492, 1992.

97. McWilliams P, Farrar GJ, Kenna P, et al: Autosomal dominant retinitis pigmentosa (ADRP): localization of an ADRP gene to the long arm of chromosome 3, *Genomics* 5:619-622, 1989.
98. Dryja TP, McGee T, Reichel E, et al: A point mutation of the rhodopsin gene in one form of retinitis pigmentosa, *Nature* 343:364-366, 1990.
99. Dryja TP, McGee T, Hahn LB, et al: Mutations within the rhodopsin gene in patients with autosomal dominant retinitis pigmentosa, *N Engl J Med* 323:1302-1307, 1990.
100. Dryja TP, Hahn LB, Cowley GS, et al: Mutation spectrum of the rhodopsin gene among patients with autosomal dominant retinitis pigmentosa, *Proc Natl Acad Sci USA* 88:9370-9374, 1991.
101. Sung CH, Davenport CM, Hennessey JC, et al: Rhodopsin mutations in autosomal dominant retinitis pigmentosa, *Proc Natl Acad Sci USA* 88:6481-6485, 1991.
102. Keen TJ, Inglehearn CF, Lester DH, et al: Autosomal dominant retinitis pigmentosa: four new mutations in rhodopsin, one of them in the retinal attachment site, *Genomics* 11:199-205, 1991.
103. Inglehearn CF, Bashir R, Lester DH, et al: A 3-bp deletion in the rhodopsin gene in a family with autosomal dominant retinitis pigmentosa, *Am J Hum Genet* 48:26-30, 1991.
104. Sheffield VC, Fishman GA, Kimura A: Identification of novel rhodopsin mutations associated with retinitis pigmentosa using GC-clamped denaturing gradient gel electrophoresis, *Am J Hum Genet* 49:699-706, 1991.
105. Fishman GA, Stone EM, Gilbert LD, et al: Ocular findings associated with a rhodopsin gene codon 58 transversion mutation in autosomal dominant retinitis pigmentosa, *Arch Ophthalmol* 109:1387-1393, 1991.
106. Fishman GA, Stone EM, Sheffield VC, et al: Ocular findings associated with rhodopsin gene codon 17 and codon 182 transition mutations in dominant retinitis pigmentosa, *Arch Ophthalmol* 110:54-62, 1992.
107. Jacobson SG, Kemp CM, Sung CH, Nathans J: Retinal function and rhodopsin levels in autosomal dominant retinitis pigmentosa with rhodopsin mutations, *Am J Ophthalmol* 112:256-271, 1991.
108. Kemp CM, Jacobson SG, Roman AJ, et al: Abnormal rod adaptation in autosomal dominant retinitis pigmentosa with Pro-23-His rhodopsin mutation, *Am J Ophthalmol* 113:165-174, 1992.
109. Richards JE, Kuo CY, Boehnke M, Sieving PA: Rhodopsin Thr58Arg mutation in a family with autosomal dominant retinitis pigmentosa, *Ophthalmology* 98:1797-1805, 1991.
110. Stone EM, Kimura Ae, Nichols BE, et al: Regional distribution of retinal degeneration in patients with the proline to histidine mutation in codon 23 of the rhodopsin gene, *Ophthalmology* 98:1806-1813, 1991.
111. Fishman GA, Vandenberg K, Stone EM, et al: Ocular findings associated with rhodopsin gene codon 267 and codon 190 mutations in dominant retinitis pigmentosa, *Arch Ophthalmol* 108:152-158, 1992.
112. Kim RY, Al-Maghtheh M, Fitzke FW, et al: Dominant retinitis pigmentosa associated with two rhodopsin mutations. *Arch Ophthalmol.* 111:1518-1525, 1993.
113. Lester DH, Inglehearn CF, Bashir R, et al: Linkage to D3S47 (C17) in one large dominant retinitis family and exclusion in another: confirmation of genetic heterogeneity, *Am J Hum Genet* 47:536-541, 1990.
114. Blanton SH, Cottingham AW, Giesenschlag N, et al: Further evidence of exclusion of linkage between type II autosomal dominant retinitis pigmentosa (ADRP) and D3S47 on 3g, *Genomics* 8:179-181, 1990.
115. Blanton SH, Heckenlively JR, Cottingham AW, et al: Linkage mapping of autosomal dominant retinitis pigmentosa (RP1) to the pericentric region of human chromosome 8, *Genomics* 11:857-869, 1991.
116. Farrar GJ, Jordan SA, Kenna P: Autosomal dominant retinitis pigmentosa: localization of a disease gene (RP6) to the short arm of chromosome 6, *Genomics* 11:870-874, 1991.
117. Farrar GJ, Kenna P, Jordan SA, et al: A three-base-pair deletion in the peripherin-RDS gene in one form of retinitis pigmentosa, *Nature* 354:478-480, 1991.

118. Kajiwara K, Hahn LB, Mukai S, et al: Mutations in the human retinal degeneration slow gene in autosomal dominant retinitis pigmentosa, *Nature* 354:480-483, 1991.
119. Kajiwara K, Sandberg MA, Berson EL, Dryja TP: A null mutation in the human peripherin/RDS gene in a family with autosomal dominant retinitis punctata albescens, *Nat Genet* 3:208-12, 1993.
120. Travis GH, Brennan MB, Danielson PE, et al: Identification of a photoreceptor-specific mRNA encoded by the gene responsible for retinal degeneration slow (rds), *Nature* 338:70-73, 1989.
121. Connell G, Bascom R, Molday L, et al: Photoreceptor peripherin is the normal product of the gene responsible for retinal degeneration in the rods mouse, *Proc Nat Acad Sci USA.* 88:723-726, 1991.
122. Connell G, Molday RS: Molecular cloning, primary structure and orientation of the vertebrate photoreceptor cell protein peripherin in the rod disc membrane, *Biochemistry* 29:4691-4698, 1990.
123. Travis G, Sutcliffe JG, Bok D: The retinal degeneration slow (rds) gene product is a photoreceptor disc membrane associated glycoprotein, *Neuron* 6:61-70, 1991.
124. Arokawa K, Molday MM, Molday RS, Williams DS: Localization of peripherin/rds in the disk membranes of cone and rod photoreceptors; relationship to disk membrane morphogenesis and retinal degeneration, *J Cell Biol* 116:659-667, 1992.
125. Rosenfeld P, Cowley GS, McGee TL, et al: A null mutation in the rhodopsin gene causes rod photoreceptor dysfunction and autosomal recessive retinitis pigmentosa, *Nat Genet* 1:209-213, 1992.
126. McLaughlin ME, Sandberg MA, Berson EL, Dryja TP: Recessive mutations in the gene encoding the beta subunit of phosphodiesterase in patients with retinitis pigmentosa, *Nat Genet* 4:130-134, 1993.
127. Mauthner L: 1971. Quoted in Duke-Elder S: *System of ophthalmology,* St Louis, 1964, Mosby, vol III, part 2, p 619.
128. Goedbloed J: Mode of inheritance in choroideraemia, *Ophthalmologica* 104:308-315, 1942.
129. Waardenburg PJ: Choroideremia als Erbmerkmal, *Acta Ophthalmol* 20:235-274, 1942.
130. McCulloch C, McCulloch RJP: A hereditary and clinical study of choroideremia, *Trans Am Acad Ophthalmol Otolaryngol* 52:160-190, 1948.
131. Rafuse EV, McCulloch C: Choroideraemia, a pathological report, *Can J Ophthalmol* 3:347-352, 1968.
132. McCulloch C: Choroideraemia: a clinical and pathological review, *Trans Am Ophthalmol Soc* 67:142-195, 1969.
133. Cameron JD, Fine BS, Shapiro I: Histopathological observations in choroideremia with emphasis on vascular changes of the uveal tract, *Ophthalmology* 94:187-196, 1987.
134. Krill AE: *Hereditary retinal and choroidal diseases,* Hagerstown Md, 1977, Harper & Row.
135. Ghosh M, McCulloch C, Parker JA: Pathological study in a female carrier of choroideremia, *Can J Ophthalmol* 23:181-186, 1988.
136. Flannery JG, Bird AC, Farber DB, et al: A histopathologic study of a choroideremia carrier, *Invest Ophthalmol Vis Sci* 31:229-236, 1990.
137. Nussbaum RL, Lewis RA, Lesko JG, Ferrell R: Choroideremia is linked to the restriction fragment length polymorphism DXYS1 at Xq13-21, *Am J Hum Genet* 37:473-481, 1985.
138. Cremers FP, van de Pol DJ, Diergaarde PJ, et al: Physical fine mapping of the choroideremia locus using Xq21 deletions associated with complex syndromes, *Genomics* 4:41-46, 1989.
139. Hodgson SV, Robertson ME, Fear CN, et al: Prenatal diagnosis of X-linked choroideremia with mental retardation, associated with a cytologically detectable chromosome deletion, *Hum Genet* 75:286-290, 1987.
140. Rosenberg T, Niebuhr E, Yang HM, et al: Choroideremia, congenital deafness, and mental retardation in a family with an X chromosomal deletion, *Ophthal Paed Genet* 8:139-143, 1987.

141. Cremers FPM, van de Pol DJR, van Kerkhoff LPM, et al: Cloning of a gene that is rearranged in patients with choroideraemia, *Nature* 347:674-677, 1990.
142. Merry DE, Lesko JG, Sosnoski DM, et al: Choroideremia and deafness with stapes fixation: a contiguous gene deletion syndrome in Xq21, *Am J Hum Genet* 45:530-540, 1989.
143. Merry DE, Jänne PA, Landers JE, et al: Isolation of a candidate gene for choroideremia, *Proc Natl Acad Sci USA* 89:2135-2181, 1992.
144. Seabra MC, Brown MS, Slaughter CA, et al: Purification of component A of Rab geranylgeranyl transferase: possible identity with the choroideremia gene product, *Cell* 70:1049-1057, 1992.
145. Seabra MC, Brown MS, Goldstein JL: Retinal degeneration in choroideremia: deficiency of RAb geranylgeranyl transferase, *Science* 259:337-381, 1993.
146. Seabra MC, Goldstein JL, Südhof TC, Brown MS: Rab geranylgeranyl transferase: a multisubunit enzyme that prenylates GTP-binding proteins terminating in Cys-X-Cys or Cys-Cys, *J Biol Chem* 267:14497-14503, 1992.
147. Bietti G: Über familiäres Vorkommen von "retinitis punctata albescens" (verbunden mit "dystrophia marginalis cristallinea cornea"), Glitzern des Glascörpers und anderen degenerativen Augenveränderungen, *Klin Monatsbl Augenheilkd* 99:737-756, 1937.
148. Hu D-N: Ophthalmic genetics in China, *Ophthal Paediatr Genet* 2:39-45, 1983.
149. Richards BW, Brodstein DE, Nussbaum JJ, et al: Autosomal dominant crystalline dystrophy, *Ophthalmology* 98:568-665, 1991.
150. François J, De Laey JJ: Bietti's crystalline fundus dystrophy, *Klin Monatsbl Augenheilkd* 170:353-362, 1970.
151. Welch RB: Bietti's tapetoretinal degeneration with marginal corneal dystrophy: crystalline retinopathy, *Trans Am Ophthalmol Soc* 75:164-179, 1977.
152. Hayasaka S, Okuyama S: Crystalline retinopathy, *Retina* 4:177-181, 1984.
153. Wilson DJ, Weleber RG, Klein ML, et al: Bietti's crystalline dystrophy: a clinicopathologic correlative study, *Arch Ophthalmol* 107:213-221, 1989.
154. Best F: Über eine hereditäre Maculaaffektion: Beitrag zur Vererbungslehre, *Z Augenheilkd* 13:199-212, 1905.
155. Vossius A: *Graefes Arch Ophthalmol* 105:1050, 1921. Quoted in Duke-Elder S: *System of ophthalmology,* Vol X, *Diseases of the retina,* St Louis, 1967, Mosby, p 632.
156. Weisel G: Beitrag Zur Bestschen hereditären Maculaerkrankung (dissertation), Geissen (1922). Quoted in Duke-Elder S: *System of ophthalmology,* Vol X, *Diseases of the retina,* St Louis, 1967, Mosby, p 632.
157. Jung EE: Über eine Sippe mit angeborener Maculadegeneration, *Ber Dtsch Ophthalmol Ges* 51:81, 1936. Quoted in Duke-Elder S: *System of ophthalmology,* Vol X, *Diseases of the retina,* St Louis, 1967, Mosby, p 632.
158. Barkman Y: A clinical study of a central tapetoretinal degeneration, *Acta Ophthalmol* 39:663-671, 1961.
159. Deutman AF: *The hereditary dystrophies of the posterior pole of the eye,* Assen Netherlands, 1971, Van Gorcum.
160. Barricks ME: Vitelliform lesions developing in normal fundi, *Am J Ophthalmol* 83:324-327, 1977.
161. Mohler CW, Fine SL: Long-term evaluation of patients with Best's vitelliform dystrophy, *Ophthalmology* 88:688-692, 1981.
162. Godel V, Chaine G, Regenbogen L, Coscas G: Best's vitelliform macular dystrophy, *Acta Ophthalmol Suppl (Copenh),* 175:1-31, 1986.
163. Deutman AF: Electro-oculography in families with vitelliform dystrophy of the fovea, *Arch Ophthalmol* 81:305-316, 1969.
164. O'Gorman S, Flaherty WA, Fishman GA, Berson EL: Histopathologic findings in Best's vitelliform macular dystrophy, *Arch Ophthalmol* 106:1261-1268, 1988.
165. McFarland CB: Heredodegeneration of macular lutea: study of clinical and pathological aspects, *Arch Ophthalmol* 53:224-228, 1955.
166. Anderson S: Quoted in Krill AE: *Hereditary and choroidal diseases,* New York, 1977, Harper & Row, p 697.

167. Frangieh GT, Green R, Fine SL: A histopathological study of Best's macular dystrophy, *Arch Ophthalmol* 100:1115-1121, 1982.
168. Weingeist TA, Kobrin JL, Watzke RC: Histopathology of Best's macular dystrophy, *Arch Ophthalmol* 100:1108-1114, 1982.
169. Stone EM, Nichols BE, Streb LM, et al: Genetic linkage of vitelliform macular degeneration (Best's disease) to chromosome 11q13, *Nat Genet* 1:246-250, 1992.
170. Gass JDM: A clinicopathologic study of a peculiar foveomacular dystrophy, *Trans Am Ophthalmol Soc* 72:139-156, 1974.
171. Vine AK, Schatz H: Adult-onset foveomacular pigment epithelial dystrophy, *Am J Ophthalmol* 89:680-691, 1980.
172. Kingham JD, Lochen GP: Vitelliform macular degeneration, *Am J Ophthalmol* 84:526-531, 1977.
173. Brecher R, Bird AC: Adult vitelliform macular dystrophy, *Eye* 4:210-215, 1990.
174. Patrinely JR, Lewis RA, Font RL: Foveomacular vitelliform macular dystrophy, adult type: a clinicopathological study including electron microscopic observations, *Ophthalmology* 92:1712-1718, 1985.
175. Wells J, Wroblewski J, Keen J, et al: Mutations in the human retinal degeneration slow (rds) gene can cause either retinitis pigmentosa or macular dystrophy, *Nat Genet* 3:213-217, 1992.
176. Deutman AF, van Bloomestein JDA, Henkes HE, et al: Butterfly shaped pigment dystrophy of the fovea, *Arch Ophthalmol* 83:558-569, 1970.
177. Prensky JG, Bresnic GH: Butterfly-shaped macular dystrophy in four generations, *Arch Ophthalmol* 101:1198-1203, 1983.
178. de Jong PT, Zrenner E, van Meel GJ, et al: Mizuo phemomenon in X-linked retinoschisis: pathogenesis of the Mizuo phenomenon, *Arch Ophthalmol* 109:1104-1108, 1991.
179. Watzke RC, Folk JC, Lang RM: Pattern dystrophy of the retinal pigment epithelium, *Ophthalmology* 66:1400-1406, 1981.
180. Guiffre G, Lodata G: Vitelliform dystrophy and pattern dystrophy of the retinal pigment epithelium: concomitant presence in a family, *Br J Ophthalmol* 70:526-532, 1988.
181. Guiffre G: Autosomal dominant pattern dystrophy of the retinal pigment epithelium, *Retina* 8:169-173, 1988.
182. Gutman I, Walsh JB, Henkind P: Vitelliform macular dystrophy and butterfly-shaped epithelial dystrophy, *Br J Ophthalmol* 66:170-173, 1982.
183. De Jong PTVM, Delleman JW: Pigment epithelial pattern dystrophy, *Arch Ophthalmol* 3:1416-1421, 1982.
184. Cortin P, Archer D, Maumenee IH: A patterned macular dystrophy with yellow plaques and atrophic changes, *Br J Ophthalmol* 64:127-134, 1980.
185. Nichols BE, Sheffield VC, Vandenburgh K, et al: Butterfly-shaped pigment dystrophy of the fovea caused by a point mutation in codon 167 of the RDS gene, *Nat Genet* 3:202-207, 1993.
186. Sorsby A, Mason MEJ, Gardener N: A fundus dystrophy with unusual features, *Br J Ophthalmol* 33:67-97, 1949.
187. Hoskin A, Bird AC, Schmi K: Sorsby's pseudoinflammatory macular dystrophy, *Br J Ophthalmol* 65:859-865, 1981.
188. Capon MRC, Polkinghorne PJ, Fitzke FW, Bird AC: Sorsby's pseudoinflammatory macula dystrophy: Sorsby's fundus dystrophies, *Eye* 2:114-122, 1988.
189. Polkinghorne PJ, Capon MRC, Berninger T, et al: Sorsby's fundus dystrophy: a clinical study, *Ophthalmology* 96:1763-1768, 1989.
190. Hamilton WK, Ewing CC, Ives EJ, Carruthers JD: Sorsby's fundus dystrophy, *Ophthalmology* 96:1755-1762, 1989.
191. Carr RE, Mittl RN, Noble KG: Choroidal abiotrophies, *Trans Am Acad Ophthalmol Otolaryngol* 79:796-816, 1975.
192. Steinmetz RL, Polkinghorne PC, Fitzke FW, et al: Abnormal dark adaptation and rhodopsin kinetics in Sorsby's fundus dystrophy, *Invest Ophthalmol Vis Sci* 33:1633-1636, 1992.

193. Capon MRC, Marshall J, Krafft JI, et al: Sorsby's fundus dystrophy: a light and electron microscopic study, *Ophthalmology* 96:1769-1777, 1989.
194. Wedl C: *Rudiments of pathological history,* London, 1854, George Busk, p 282.
195. Donders FC: Beiträge zür pathologischen Anatomie des Auges, *Graefes Arch Ophthalmol* 1:106-118, 1855.
196. Hutchinson J, Tay W: Symmetrical central chorioretinal disease occuring in senile persons, *R Lond Ophthalmol Hosp Rep* 8:231-244, 1875.
197. Clarke E: Tay's "gutta choroiditis," *Proc R Soc Med* 25(12):59-60, 1932.
198. Juler H: Guttata choroiditis, *Trans Ophthalmol Soc UK* 13:143, 1893.
199. Holthouse EH, Batten RD: A case of superficial chorioretinitis of peculiar form and doubtful causation, *Trans Ophthalmol Soc UK* 17:62-63, 1897.
200. Doyne RW: Peculiar condition of choroiditis occurring in several members of the same family, *Trans Ophthalmol Soc UK* 19:71, 1899.
201. Tree M: Familial hyaline dystrophy in the fundus oculi or Doyne's family honeycomb choroiditis, *Br J Ophthalmol* 21:65-91, 1937.
202. Pearce WG: Doyne's honeycomb retinal degeneration: clinical and genetic features, *Br J Ophthalmol* 52:73-78, 1968.
203. Doyne RW: A note on family choroiditis, *Trans Ophthalmol Soc UK* 30:93-95, 1910.
204. Klainguti R: Die tapeto-retinal Degeneration im Kanton Tessin, *Klin Monatsbl Augenheilkd* 89:253-254, 1932.
205. Evans PJ: Five cases of familial retinal abiotrophy, *Trans Ophthalmol Soc UK* 70:96, 1950.
206. Forni S, Babel J: Étude clinique et histologique de la malattia levantinese. Affection appartenant au groupe des dégénérescences hyalines du pole posterieur, *Ophthalmologica* 143:313-322, 1962.
207. François J, Deweer JP: Dégénérescence maculaire sénile et hérédité, *Ann Ocul* 185:136-154, 1952.
208. Deutman AF, Jansen LM: Dominantly inherited drusen of Bruch's membrane, *Br J Ophthalmol* 54:373-382, 1970.
209. Gass JDM: Drusen and disciform macular detachment and degeneration, *Arch Ophthalmol* 90:206-217, 1973.
210. Scarpatetti A, Forni S, Niemeyer G: Die Netzhautfunktion bei Malattia levantinese (dominant Drusen), *Klin Monatsbl Augenheilkd* 172:590-597, 1978.
211. Gass JDM: Adult vitelliform macular detachment occurring in patients with basal laminar drusen, *Am J Ophthalmol* 99:445-459, 1985.
212. Alper MG, Alfano JA: Honeycomb colloid degeneration of the retina, *Arch Ophthalmol* 49:392-399, 1953.
213. Pajtas J: A case of Doyne's honeycomb choroidits, *Cesk Oftamol* 6:282-286, 1950.
214. Sorsby A: Choroidal angiosclerosis with special reference to its hereditary character, *Br J Ophthalmol* 23:433-444, 1939.
215. Sorsby A, Crick RP: Central areolar choroidal sclerosis, *Br J Ophthalmol* 37:129-139, 1953.
216. Noble KG: Central areolar choroidal dystrophy, *Am J Ophthalmol* 84:310-318, 1977.
217. Ashton N: Central areolar choroidal sclerosis: a histopathological study, *Br J Ophthalmol* 37:140-147, 1953.
218. Stargardt K: Über familiäre, progressive Degeneration in der Makulagegend des Auges, *Graefes Arch Klin Exp Ophthalmol* 71:534-550, 1909.
219. Stargardt K: Über familiäre, progressive Degeneration in der Makulagegend des Auges, *Z Augenheilkd* 30:95-116, 1913.
220. Franceschetti A: Über tapeto-retinale Degeneration in Kindesalter. In *Entwicklung und Fortschritte in der Augenheilkunde,* Stuttgart, 1963, Enke, p 107.
221. Franceschetti A, François J: Fundus flavimaculatus, *Arch Ophthalmol* 25:505-530, 1965.
222. Cibis GN, Morey M, Harris DJ: Dominantly inherited macular dystrophy with flecks (Stargardt), *Arch Ophthalmol* 98:1785-1789, 1980.

223. Uliss AE, Moore AT, Bird AC: The dark choroid in posterior retinal dystrophies, *Ophthalmology* 95:1423-1427, 1987.
224. Hadden OB, Gass JDM: Fundus flavimaculatus and Stargardt's disease, *Am J Ophthalmol* 82:527-539, 1976.
225. Bonin P: Le signe du silence choroïdien dans les dégénérescences tapéto-rétiniennes centrales examinées sous fluorescence, *Bull Soc Ophtalmol Fr* 71:348-351, 1971.
226. Fish G, Grey RHB, Sehmi KS, Bird AC: The dark choroid in posterior retinal dystrophies, *Br J Ophthalmol* 65:359-363, 1981.
227. Fishman GA, Farber M, Patel BS, Derlacki DJ: Visual acuity loss in patients with Stargardt's macular dystrophy, *Ophthalmology* 94:809-814, 1987.
228. Eagle RC, Lucier AC, Bernardino JR, Yanof M: Retinal pigment epithelial abnormalities in fundus flavimaculatus; a light and electron microscopic study, *Ophthalmology* 87:1189-1200, 1980.
229. Klien BA, Krill AE: Fundus flavimaculatus: Clinical, functional, and histologic observations, *Am J Ophthalmol* 64:2-23, 1967.
230. Lopez PF, Maumenee IH, de la Cruz Z, Green WR: Autosomal-dominant fundus flavimaculatus. Clinicopathologic correlation, *Ophthalmology* 97:798-809, 1990.
231. Steinmetz RL, Garner A, Maguire JI, Bird AC: Histopathology of incipient fundus flavimaculatus, *Ophthalmology* 98:953-956, 1991.
232. Grey RHB, Blach RK, Barnard WM: Bull's eye maculopathy with early cone degeneration, *Br J Ophthalmol* 61:702-718, 1977.
233. Goodman G, Ripps H, Siegel IM: Cone dysfunction syndromes, *Arch Ophthalmol* 70:214-231, 1963.
234. Berson EL, Gouras PG, Gunkel RD: Progressive cone degeneration, dominantly inherited, *Arch Ophthalmol* 80:77-83, 1968.
235. Krill AE, Deutman AF: Dominant macular degenerations: the cone dystrophies, *Am J Ophthalmol* 73:352-369, 1972.
236. Pearlman JT, Owen GW, Brounley DW, Sheppard JJ: Cone dystrophy with dominant inheritance, *Am J Ophthalmol* 77:293-303, 1974.
237. van Schooneveld MJ, Went LN, Oosterhuis JA: Dominant cone dystrophy starting with blue cone involvement, *Br J Ophthalmol* 75:332-336, 1991.
238. Went LN, van Schooneveld MJ, Oosterhuis JA: Late onset dominant cone dystrophy with early blue cone involvement, *J Med Genet* 29:295-298, 1992.
239. Bresnick GH, Smith VC, Pokorny J: Autosomal dominantly inherited macular dystrophy with preferential short wavelength sensitive cone involvement, *Am J Ophthalmol* 108:265-276, 1989.
240. Gouras P, Eggars HM, MacKay CJ: Cone dystrophy, nyctalopia, and supernormal rod responses: a new retinal degeneration, *Arch Ophthalmol* 101:718-724, 1983.
241. Yagasaki Y, Jacobson SG: Cone-rod dystrophy: phenotypic diversity by retinal function testing, *Arch Ophthalmol* 107:701-708, 1989.
242. Heckenlively JR, Weleber RG: X-linked recessive cone dystrophy with tapetal like sheen: a newly recognized entity with Mizuo-Nakamura phenomenon, *Arch Ophthalmol* 104:1322-1328, 1986.
243. Jacobson DM, Thompson HS, Bartley JA: X-linked progressive cone dystrophy: clinical characteristics of affected males and female carriers, *Ophthalmology* 96:885-895, 1989.
244. Reichel E, Bruce AM, Sandberg MA, Berson EL: An electroretinographic and molecular genetic study of X-linked cone degeneration, *Am J Ophthalmol* 108:540-547, 1989.
245. van Everdingen JAM, Went LN, Keunen JEE, Oosterhuis JA: X-linked progressive cone dystrophy with specific attention to carrier detection, *J Med Genet* 29:291-294, 1992.
246. Pruett RC: Retinitis pigmentosa: clinical observations and correlations, *Trans Am Ophthalmol Soc* 81:693-735, 1983.
247. Szlyk JP, Fishman GA, Alexander KR, et al: Clincial subtypes of cone-rod dystrophies, *Arch Ophthalmol* 111:781-788, 1993.
248. Kearns TP, Hollenhorst RW: Chloroquine retinopathy: evaluation by fluorescein angiography, *Arch Ophthalmol* 76:378-384, 1966.

249. Krill AE, Potts AM, Johanson CE: Chloroquine retinopathy: investigation of discrepancy between dark adaptation and electroretinographic findings in advanced stages, *Am J Ophthalmol* 71:530-543, 1971.
250. Bjork A, Lindbalm V, Wadanstein L; Retinal degeneration in hereditary ataxia, *J Neurol Neurosurg Psychiatry* 19:186-193, 1956.
251. Snodgrass NB: Ocular findings in fucosidosis, *Br J Ophthalmol* 60:508-511, 1976.
252. Jalili IK, Smith NJD: A progressive cone rod dystrophy and amelanogenesis imperfecta: a new syndrome, *J Med Genet* 25:738-740, 1988.
253. Lefler WH, Wadsworth JAC, Sidbury JB: Hereditary macular degeneration and amino-acid uria, *Am J Ophthalmol (Suppl)* 71:224-230, 1971.
254. Frank HR, Landers MB, Williams RJ, Sidbury JB: A new dominant progressive foveal dystrophy, *Am J Ophthalmol* 78:903-916, 1974.
255. Small KW: North Carolina macula dystrophy revisited, *Ophthalmology* 96:1747-1754, 1989.
256. Small KW, Killian J, McLean WC: North Carolina's dominant progressive foveal dystrophy: how progressive is it? *Br J Ophthalmol* 75:401-406, 1991.
257. Clausen W: Zur Frage der Vererbung der Makula-Kolobome, *Klin Monatsbl Augenheilkd* 81:385, 1928.
258. Davenport RC: Bilateral macular coloboma in mother and son, *Proc R Soc Med* 21:109-110, 1927.
259. Sorsby A: Congenital coloboma of the macula, together with an account of the familial occurrence of bilateral coloboma in association with apical dystrophy of the hands and feet, *Br J Ophthalmol* 19:65-90, 1935.
260. Turut P, Chaine G, Puech B, et al: Les dystrophies héréditaires de la macule, *Bull Soc Ophtalmol Fr* (numéro spécial), pp 237-244, 1991.
261. Small KW, Weber JL, Roses A, et al: North Carolina macular dystrophy is assigned to chromosome 6, *Genomics* 13:681-685, 1992.
262. Nathans J, Thomas D, Hogness DS: Molecular genetics of human color vision: the genes encoding blue, green, and red pigments, *Science* 232:193-202, 1986.
263. Waardenburg PJ, Franceschetti A, Klein D: *Genetics and ophthalmology,* Springfield Ill, 1963, Charles C Thomas, vol 2, p 1736.
264. Verriest MG: Recent progress in the study of acquired deficiencies of colour vision, *Bull Soc Ophtalmol Fr* 74:595-620, 1974.
265. Nathans J, Piantandida TP, Eddy RL, et al: Molecular genetics of inherited variation in human color vision, *Science* 232:203-210, 1986.
266. Vollrath D, Nathans J, Davis RW: Tandem array of human visual pigment genes at Xq28, *Science* 240:1669-1672, 1988.
267. Alpern M, Lee GB, Spivey BE: Pi cone monochromatism, *Arch Ophthalmol* 74:334-337, 1965.
268. Lewis RA, Holcomb JD, Bromley WC, et al: Mapping X-linked ophthalmic diseases. III. Provisional assignment of the locus for blue cone monochromacy to Xq28. *Arch Ophthalmol* 105:1055-1059, 1987.
269. Sloan LL, Newhall SM: Comparison of cases of atypical and typical achromatopsia, *Am J Ophthalmol* 25:945, 1942.
270. Siegel IM, Graham CH, Ripps H, Hsia Y: Analysis of photopic and scotopic function in an incomplete achromat, *J Opt Soc Am* 56:699-704, 1966.
271. Krill AE: Incomplete rod-cone degenerations. In Krill AE, Archer D (eds): *Hereditary retinal and choroidal diseases,* Hagerstown Md, 1977, Harper & Row, pp 625-636.
272. Larsen H: Demonstration mikroskopischer Präparate von einem monochromatischen Auge, *Klin Monatsbl Augenheilkd* 67:301-302, 1921.
273. Harrison R, Hoeffnagel D, Hayward JN: Congenital total color blindness: a clinicopathological report, *Arch Ophthalmol* 64:685-692, 1960.
274. Falls HF, Wolter JR, Alpern M: Typical total monochromacy, *Arch Ophthalmol* 74:610-616, 1965.
275. Glickstein M, Heath GG: Receptors in the monochromat eye, *Vis Res* 15:633-636, 1975.

276. Dejean C, Gassenc R: Note sur la généalogie de la famille Nougaret, Vendémian, *Bull Soc Ophtalmol Fr* 1:96-99, 1949.
277. Krill AE, Martin D: Photopic abnormalities in congenital stationary night blindness, *Invest Ophthalmol* 10:625-636, 1971.
278. Carr RE, Ripps H, Siegel IM, Weale RA: Rhodopsin and the electical activity of the retina in congenital night blindness, *Invest Ophthalmol* 5:497-507, 1966.
279. Vaghefi HA, Green R, Kelly JS, et al: Correlation of clinicopathological findings in a patient: congenital night blindness, branch retinal vein occlusion, cilioretinal artery, drusen of the nerve head, and intraretinal pigmented lesion, *Arch Ophthalmol* 96:2079-2104, 1978.
280. Noble KG, Carr RE, Siegel IM: Autosomal dominant congenital stationary night blindness and normal fundus with an electronegative electroretinogram, *Am J Ophthalmol* 109:44-48, 1990.
281. Sharp DM, Arden GB, Kemp CR, et al: Mechanisms and sites of loss of scotopic sensitivity: a clinical analysis of congenital night blindness, *Clin Vis Sci* 5:217-230, 1990.
282. Schubert G, Bornschein H: Beitrag zur Analyse des menschlichen Elektroretinogramms, *Ophthalmologica* 123:396-412, 1952.
283. Miyake Y, Yagasaki K, Horiguchi M, et al: Congenital stationary night blindness with negative electroretinogram: a new classification, *Arch Ophthalmol* 104:1013-1020, 1986.
284. Khouri G, Mets MB, Smith VC, et al: X-linked congenital stationary night blindness: review and report of a family with hyperopia, *Arch Ophthalmol* 106:1417-1422, 1988.
285. Pearce WG, Reedyk M, Coupland SG: Variable expressivity in X-linked congenital stationary night blindness, *Can J Ophthalmol* 25:3-10, 1990.
286. Weleber Rg, Pillers Da, Powell BR, et al: Åland Island eye disease (Forsius-Eriksson syndrome) associated with contiguous deletion syndrome at Xp21: similarity to incomplete congenital stationary night blindness, *Arch Ophthalmol* 107:1170-1179, 1989.
287. Alitalo T, Kruse TA, Forsius H, et al: Localization of the Åland Island eye disease locus to the pericentromeric region of the X chromosome by linkage analysis, *Am J Hum Genet* 48:31-38, 1991.
288. Miyake Y, Kawase Y: Reduced amplitude of oscillatory potentials in female carriers of X-linked recessive congenital stationary night blindness, *Am J Ophthalmol* 98:208-215, 1984.
289. Young RS, Chaparro A, Price J, Walters J: Oscillatory potentials of X-linked carriers of congenital stationary night blindness, *Invest Ophthalmol Vis Sci* 30:806-812, 1989.
290. Weleber RG, Tongue AC: Congenital stationary night blindness presenting as Leber's congenital amaurosis, *Arch Ophthalmol* 105:360-365, 1987.
291. Musarella MA, Weleber RG, Murphey WH, et al: Assignment of the gene for complete X-linked congenital stationary night blindness (CSNB1) to Xp11.3, *Genomics* 5:727-737, 1989.
292. Gal A, Schinzel A, Orth U, et al: Gene of X-chromosomal congenital stationary night blindness is closely linked to DXS7 on Xp, *Hum Genet* 81:315-318, 1989.
293. Bech-Hansen NT, Field LL, Schramm AM, et al: A locus for X-linked congenital stationary night blindness is located on the proximal proton of the short arm of the X chromosome, *Hum Genet* 84:406-408, 1990.
294. Dryja TP, Berson EL, Rao V, Oprian DD: Heterozygous missence mutation in the rhodopsin gene as a cause of stationary night blindness, *Invest Ophthalmol Vis Sci* 34(suppl):1150, 1993.
295. Watanabe I, Taniguchi Y, Morioka K, Kato M: Congenital stationary night blindness with myopia: a clinicopathologic study, *Doc Ophthalmol* 63:55-62, 1986.
296. Siegel IM, Greenstein VC, Seiple WH, Carr RE: Cone function in congenital nyctalopia, *Doc Ophthalmol* 65:307-318, 1987.
297. Oguchi C: Über einen Fall von eigenartiger Hemeralopie, *Nippon Ganka Gakkai Zasshi* 11:123, 1907.
298. Klein BA: A case of so-called Oguchi's disease in the USA, *Am J Ophthalmol* 22:953-955, 1939.

299. Winn S, Tasman W, Spaeth G, et al: Oguchi's disease in Negroes, *Arch Ophthalmol* 81:501-507, 1969.
300. Mizuo A: On new discovery in dark adaptation in Oguchi's disease, *Acta Soc Ophthalmol Jpn* 17:1148-1150, 1913.
301. Nakamura B: Über ein neues Phänomen der Farberveränderung des menschlichen Augenhintergrundes im Zusammenhang mit der fortschreitenden Dunkeladaptation, *Klin Monatsbl Augenheilkd* 65:83-85, 1920.
302. François J, Verriest G: La maladie d'Oguchi, *Bull Soc Belge Ophtalmol* 108:465-506, 1954.
303. Oguchi C: Zur Anatomie der sogenannten Oguchi'schen Krankheit, *Graefes Arch Klin Exp Ophthalmol* 115:234-244, 1925.
304. Yamanaka J: Existiert die Pigmentverschiebung im Retinalepithel im menschlichen Auge? Der erste Sektionsfall von sogenannter Oguchischer Krankheit, *Klin Monatsbl Augenheilkd* 73:742-752, 1924.
305. Kuwabara Y, Ishikara K, Akiya S: Histologic and electron microscopic studies of the retina in Oguchi's disease, *Acta Soc Ophthalmol Jpn* 67:1323-1351, 1963.
306. Yamanaka M: Histologic study of Oguchi's disease: its relationship to pigmentary degeneration of the retina, *Am J Ophthalmol* 68:19-26, 1969.
307. Carr RE, Ripps H: Rhodopsin kinetics and rod adaptation in Oguchi's disease, *Invest Ophthalmol Vis Sci* 6:426-436, 1967.
308. Lauber H: The origin of hyalin formations within the eye, *Ber Dtsch Ophthalmol Gesundht* 44:216-220, 1924.
309. Marmor MF: Defining fundus albipunctatus, *Doc Ophthalmol* 13:227-234, 1977.
310. Marmor MF: Long-term follow-up of the physiologic abnormalities and fundus changes in fundus albipunctatus, *Ophthalmology* 97:380-384, 1990.
311. Henkes HE: Unilateral fundus albipunctatus, *Ophthalmologica* 145:470-480, 1963.
312. Margolis S, Siegel IM, Ripps H: Variable expressivity in fundus albipunctatus, *Ophthalmology* 94:1416-1422, 1987.
313. Smith BF, Ripps HA, Goodman G: Retinitis punctata albescens: a functional and diagnostic evaluation, *Arch Ophthalmol* 61:93-101, 1959.
314. François J, Verriest G, De Rouck A: Les fonctions visuelles dans les dégénérescences tapéto-rétiniennes, *Ophthalmologica* 131(Suppl 43):1-40, 1956.
315. Franceschetti A, Dieterle P, Amman P, Marty F: Une nouvelle forme de fundus albipunctatus cum hemeralopia, *Ophthalmologica* 145:403-410, 1963.
316. Mandelbaum J: Dark adaptation: some physiologic and clinical observations, *Arch Ophthalmol* 26:203-239, 1941.
317. Carr RE, Ripps H, Siegel IM: Visual pigment kinetics and adaptation in fundus albipunctatus, *Doc Ophthalmol Proc Ser* 4:193-204, 1974.
318. Kandori F, Tamai A, Kurimoto S, Fukunaga K: Fleck retina, *Am J Ophthalmol* 73:673-685, 1972.
319. Olsson JE, Gordon JW, Pawlyk BS, et al: Transgenic mice with a rhodopsin mutation (Pro23His): a mouse model of autosomal dominant retinitis pigmentosa, *Neuron* 9:815-830, 1992.
320. Travis G, Lloyd M, Bok D: Complete reveresal of photoreceptor dysplasia in transgenic retinal degeneration slow (rds) mice, *Neuron* 9:113-120, 1992.
321. Hawkins RK, Jansen HG, Sanyal S: Development and degeneration of retina in rds mutant mice: photoreceptor abnormalities in the heterozygotes, *Exp Eye Res* 41:701-720, 1985.
322. Albert AD, Litman BJ: Independent structural domains in the membrane protein bovine rhodopsin, *Biochemistry* 17:3893-3900, 1978.
323. Davison MD, Findlay JBC: Modification of ovine opsin with the photosensitive hydrophobic probe 1-azido-4-[^{125}I]iodobenzene, *Biochem J* 234:413-420, 1986.
324. Hargrave PA: Rhodopsin chemistry, structure, and topography, *Prog Retin Res* 1:1-51, 1982.
325. Applebury ML, Hargrave PA: Molecular biology of the visual pigments, *Vis Res* 26:1881-1895, 1982.

326. Michel-Villaz M, Saibil HR, Chabré M: Orientation of rhodopsin α-helices in retinal rod outer segment membranes studied by infrared linear dichroism, *Proc Natl Acad Sci USA* 76:4405-4408, 1979.

327. Rothschild KJ, Sanches R, Hsiao TL, Clark NA: A spectroscopic study of rhodopsin alpha-helix orientation, *Biophys J* 31:53-64, 1980.

328. Hargrave PA, Fong SL, McDowell JH, et al: The partial primary structure of bovine rhodopsin and its topography in the retinal rod cell disc membrane, *Neurochem Int* 1:231-244, 1980.

329. Honig B, Dinur U, Nakanishi K, et al: An external point-charge model for wavelength regulation in visual pigments, *J Am Chem Soc* 101:7084-7086, 1979.

330. Kakitani H, Kakitani T, Rodman H, Honig B: On the mechanism of wavelength regulation in visual pigments, *Photochem Photobiol* 41:471-479, 1985.

331. Kühn H, Hargrave PA: Light-induced binding of guanosinetriphosphate to bovine photoreceptor membranes: effect of limited proteolysis of the membranes, *Biochemistry* 20:2410-2417, 1981.

332. McNaughton PA: Light response of vertebrate photoreceptors, *Physiol Rev* 70:847-883, 1990.

333. Karnik SS, Sakmar TP, Chen HB, Khorana HG: Cysteine residues 110 and 187 are essential for the formation of correct structure in bovine rhodopsin, *Proc Natl Acad Sci USA* 85:8459-8463, 1988.

334. Lodish HF: Transport of secretory and membrane glycoproteins form the rough endoplasmic reticulum to the Golgi, *J Biol Chem* 263:2107-2110, 1988.

335. Carlson JA, Rogers BB, Sifers RN, et al: Multiple tissues express alpha 1-antitrypsin in transgenic mice and man, *J Clin Invest* 82:26-36, 1988.

336. Klausner RD, Sitia R: Protein degradation in the endoplasmic reticulum, *Cell* 62:611-614, 1990.

337. Lippincott-Shwartz JL, Bonifacio JS, Yuan LC, Klausner RD: Degradation from the endoplasmic reticulum: disposing of newly synthesised protein, *Cell* 54:209-220, 1988.

338. Cheng SH, Gregory RJ, Marshall J, et al: Defective intracellular transport and processing of CFT is the molecular basis of most cystic fibrosis, *Cell* 63:827-834, 1990.

339. Karnik SS, Khorana HG: Assembly and functional rhodopsin requires a disulphide bond between cysteine residues 110 and 187, *J Biol Chem* 265:17520-17524, 1990.

340. Robinson PR, Cohen GB, Zhukovsky EA, Oprian DD: Constitutively active mutants of rhodopsin, *Neuron* 9:719-725, 1992.

341. Doi T, Molday RS, Khorana HG: Role of the intradiscal domain in rhodopsin assembly and function, *Proc Natl Acad Sci USA* 87:4991-4995, 1990.

342. Sung CH, Schneider BG, Agerwal N, et al: Functional heterogeniety on mutant rhodopsin responsible for autosomal retinitis pigmentosa, *Proc Natl Acad Sci USA* 88:8840-8844, 1991.

343. Min KC, Zvyzga TA, Cypess AM, Sakmar TP: Characterization of mutant rhodopsin responsible for autosomal dominant retinitis pigmentosa, *J Biol Chem* 268:9400-9404, 1993.

344. Travis GH, Christerson L, Danielson PE, et al: The human retinal degeneration slow (RDS) gene: chromosome assignment and structure of the mRNA, *Genomics* 10:733-739, 1991.

345. Bascom RA, Manara S, Collins L, et al: Cloning of the cDNA for a novel photoreceptor membrane (rom-1) identifies a disk rim protein family implicated in human retinopathies, *Neuron* 8:1171-1184, 1992.

346. Sanyal S, Jansen H: Absence of receptor outer segments in the retina of rds mutant mice (letter), *Neurosciences* 21:23-26, 1992.

347. Cohen AI: Some cytological and initial biochemical observations of photoreceptors in retinas of rds mice, *Invest Ophthalmol Vis Sci* 24:832-843, 1983.

348. Jansen HG, Sanyal S: Development and degeneration of retina in rds mutant mice: electron microscopy, *J Comp Neurol* 224:71-84, 1984.

349. Usukura J, Bok D: Changes in the localization and content of opsin during retinal development in the rds mutant mouse: immunocytochemistry and immunoassay, *Exp Eye Res* 45:501-515, 1987.

350. Sanyal S, Hawkins RK: Development and degeneration of retina in rds mutant mice. Altered disc shedding pattern in the albino heterozygotes and its relation to light exposure, *Vis Res* 28:1171-1178, 1987.
351. Muller DPR, Lloyd JK, Bird AC: Long-term management of abetalipoproteinaemia: possible role for vitamin E, *Arch Dis Child* 52:209-214, 1977.
352. Kaiser-Kupfer MI, de Monasterio FM, Valle D: Gyrate atrophy of the choroid and retina: improved of visual function by reduction of plasma ornithine by diet, *Science* 210:1128-1131, 1980.
353. Kaiser-Kupfer MI, Caruso RC, Valle D: Gyrate atrophy of the choroid and retina: long-term reduction of ornithine slows retinal degeneration, *Arch Ophthalmol* 109:1539-1548, 1991.
354. Vannas-Sulonen K, Simell O, Sipila I: Gyrate atrophy of the choroid and retina: the ocular disease progresses in juvenile patients despite normal or near normal plasma ornithine concentration, *Ophthalmology* 94:1428-1433, 1991.
355. Weleber RG, Kennaway NG, Buist NRM: Clinical trial of vitamin B6 for gyrate atrophy of the choroid and retina, *Ophthalmology* 88:316-324, 1981.
356. Claridge KG, Gibberd FB, Sidey MC: Refsum disease: the presentation and ophthalmic aspects of Refsum disease in a series of 23 patients, *Eye* 6:371-375, 1992.
357. Gibberd FB, Bilimoria, JD, Page NG, Retsas S: Heredopathia atactica polyneuritiformis (Refsum's disease) treated by diet and plasma-exchange, *Lancet* 1:575-578, 1979.
358. Hansen E, Bachen NI, Flage T: Refsum's disease, eye manifestations in a patient treated with low phytol low phytanic acid diet, *Acta Ophthalmol (Copenh)* 57:899-913, 1979.
359. Nettleship E: On retinitis pigmentosa and allied diseases, *R Lond Ophthalmol Hosp Rep* 17:1-56, 151-166, 333-426, 1907-1908.
360. Jay B, Bird AC: X-linked retinitis pigmentosa, *Tr Am Acad Ophthalmol Otolaryngol* 77:641-651, 1973.
361. Berson EL, Rosner B, Sandberg MA, et al: A randomized trial of vitamin A and vitamin E supplementation for retinitis pigmentosa, *Arch Ophthalmol* 111:761-772, 1993.
362. Massof RW, Finkelstein D: Supplemental vitamin retards loss of ERG in amplitude in retinitis pigmentosa, *Arch Ophthalmol* 111:751-754, 1993.
363. Cox N, Hay E, Bird AC: Treatment of macular edema with acetazolamide, *Arch Ophthalmol* 106:1190-1195, 1988.
364. Fishman GA, Gilbert LD, Fiscella Kimura AE, Jampol LM: Acetazolamide for the treatment of chronic macular edema in retinitis pigmentosa, *Arch Ophthalmol* 107:1445-1452, 1989.
365. Chen J, Fitzke F, Bird AC: Long term effect of acetazolamide in a patient with retinitis pigmentosa, *Invest Ophthalmol Vis Sci* 31:1914-1918, 1990.
366. Heckenlively JR: The frequency of posterior subcapsular cataract in the hereditary retinal degenerations, *Am J Ophthalmol* 93:733-738, 1982.
367. Faye E: *Clinical low vision,* Boston, 1984, Little Brown.
368. Silver J, Gould E, Thomsitt J: The provision of low vision aids to the visually handicapped. *Trans Ophthalmol Soc UK* 94:310-318, 1974.
369. Berson EL, Mehaffy L, Rabin AR: A night vision device as an aid for patients with retinitis pigmenosa, *Trans Ophthalmol Soc UK* 90:112-116, 1973.
370. Morrisette DL, Marmor MF, Goodrich GL: An evaluation of night vision mobility aids, *Ophthalmology* 90:1226-1230, 1983.
371. Pearlman JT, Adams GL, Sloan SH: *Psychiatric problems in ophthalmology,* Springfield Ill, 1977, Charles C Thomas.
372. Conyers M: *Vision for the future: meeting the challenge of sight loss,* London, 1992, Jessica Kingsley.
373. Freeman RD, Goetz E, Richards P, et al: Blind children's early emotional development: do we know enough to help? *Child Care Health Dev* 15:3-28, 1989.
374. Fraiberg S: *Insights from the blind: comparative studies in blind and sighted infants,* New York, 1977, Basic Books, Souvenir Press.
375. Moore T, Haig D: Genomic imprinting in mammalian development: a parental tug of war, *Trend Genet* 7:45-49, 1991.

376. Willison K: Opposite imprinting of the mouse Igf2 and Igf2r genes, *Trends Genet* 7:107-109, 1991.
377. Williamson R: Cystic fibrosis: a strategy for the future, *Adv Exp Med Biol* 290:1-7, 1991.
378. Watson EK, Williamson R, Chapple J: Attitudes to carrier screening for cystic fibrosis: a survey of health care professionals, relatives of sufferers and other members of the public, *Br J Gen Pract* 41:237-240, 1991.
379. Williamson R: Universal community carrier screening for cystic fibrosis? *Nat Genet* 3:195-201, 1993.
380. Flannery J, Lem J, Simon M, et al: Transgenic rescue of the rd/rd mouse, *Invest Ophthalmol Vis Sci* 33(suppl):945, 1992.
381. Lazar E, del Cerro M: A new procedure for multiple intraretinal transplantation into mammalian eyes, *J Neurosci Methods* 43:157-169, 1992.
382. Schuschereba ST, Silverman MS: Retinal cell and photoreceptor transplantation between adult New Zealand red rabbit retinas, *Exp Neurol* 115:95-99, 1992.
383. Yamaguchi K, Yamaguchi K, Young RW, et al: Vitreoretinal surgical technique for transplanting retinal pigment epithelium in rabbit retina, *Jpn J Ophthalmol* 36:142-150, 1992.
384. Banerjee R, Lund RD: A role for microglia in the maintenance of photoreceptors in retinal transplants lacking pigment epithelium, *J Neurocytol* 21:235-243, 1992.
385. Faktorovich EG, Steinberg RH, Yasumura D, et al: Photoreceptor degeneration in inherited retinal dystrophy delayed by basic fibroblast growth factor, *Nature* 347:83-86, 1990.

3

Age-Related Macular Degeneration

Joseph I. Maguire
William H. Annesley, Jr.

Age-related macular degeneration (ARMD) is the leading cause of permanent central visual loss in men and women over the age of 55 years in the United States and Great Britain.[23,41] Although typical cases are easily recognized by the presence of classic clinical findings in elderly patients, an exact definition of this condition is still difficult to articulate. ARMD is characterized by an alteration of the sensory retina, retinal pigment epithelium (RPE), and choroid in the macular region as the eye matures. The Framingham Eye Study[23] defined ARMD as that condition existing when an eye evidenced one of the following with an associated visual loss to 20/30 or less: (1) drusen, (2) macular RPE disturbances, (3) serous or hemorrhage elevation of the neurosensory retina, or (4) perimacular circinate exudates. ARMD, however, has yet defied exact definition since it follows a slow temporal progression during which both clinical and subclinical changes occur within the macular region. At which point these alterations constitute a diagnosis of ARMD is unclear.

Although ARMD has a multitude of clinical presentations, it is frequently divided into two broad categories: nonexudative (or "dry") and exudative (or "wet"). In this chapter we review the pathogenesis, etiology, presenting symptoms, clinical and fluorescein angiographic appearances, and treatment options as well as the long-term prognosis of ARMD.

PATHOGENESIS

The macula is a unique area of metabolic activity and physiologic stress. The photoreceptors and RPE are essentially amitotic structures with close anatomic and metabolic interdependence. As the photoreceptor outer segments (POSs) are exposed to light energy, they are phagocytosed by the pigment epithelium, which then assumes responsibility for the elimination of visual by-products and the renewal of retinal for later return to the photoreceptors as rhodopsin.[16,35,56,71,72] The POSs have a high concentration of long-chain polyunsaturated fatty acids, which imparts great fluidity to rhodopsin molecules in the outer segment cell membranes.[49] In addition, the extremely high blood flow in the choroid contributes a high oxygen tension in the area of the outer retina. This combination of chronic photic exposure, high concentrations of long-chain polyunsaturated fatty acids, and high oxygen tension creates an environment ripe for lipid peroxidation and free radical formation. Such developments can (1) retard the lysosomal degradation, by the RPE, of metabolic by-products created in visual transduction and (2) cause local tissue damage. These long-term metabolic pressures lead to secondary changes in the microarchitecture of the retina, RPE, and choroid, resulting in the ophthalmoscopic and angiographic features found in this disease.

The retinal pigment epithelium's central position between the POSs and the choroid necessitates its ability to assume several physical, biochemical, and metabolic functions.[72] These include maintenance of the blood-retina barrier, transport of metabolites and other factors from the choroid to the retina (and vice-versa), maintenance of retinal adhesion, ionic transport through membrane-specific pumps, and the processing of retinal for use in the molecule rhodopsin. Since in its normal state the RPE is an amitotic cellular monolayer, it depends on self-renewal and not regeneration as found in many epithelial cell layers. Failure in any of its many responsibilities leads to significant changes in the surrounding macular tissues, ultimately causing retinal degeneration.[34,42,71,72]

Over time the RPE does undergo change, and this reduces its effectiveness. The reasons revolve around the increasing difficulty in processing cellular waste. The POS discs are being constantly shed and phagocytosed by the RPE.[72] The phagosomes are then fused with intracellular lysosomes, which process, degrade, and finally eliminate this cellular waste in the direction of Bruch's membrane. The accumulation of nondegradable lipofucsin within the individual RPE cells, however, slowly increases with age.[4,16,18,35] This is especially so in the macular region.[16] The increasing volume of cellular waste within the RPE cytoplasm eventually leads to decreased metabolic efficiency and progressive cell failure.

Increases of lipofucsin within the RPE are temporally associated with the accumulation of various materials at the level of the RPE basal lamina and Bruch's membrane. The changes in Bruch's membrane (BM) begin in the macula as early as the second decade of life.* Feeney-Burns and Ellersieck,[17] Hogan,[35] Killingsworth,[39] and others have reported on the accumulation and secondary thickening of BM by a wide range of substance—including various forms of collagen, granular and vesicular debris, and mineralized deposits. These deposits have been noted in all layers of BM. Pauleikhoff, Sheraidah, Bird, and Marshall have likewise shown[30,49,53,54,63] the progressive accumulation of neutral and polar lipids as a function of age and that the severity of these changes increases dramatically beyond the sixth decade of life. They postulate that the accumulation of both polar and nonpolar lipids could be responsible for interrupting the normal transport of water, essential metabolites, and various modifiers of cellular activity within the macula. The relative concentrations of these lipids might partially explain the protean clinical manifestations of ARMD.

---

*References 11, 17, 32, 43, 54, 57, 63.

ETIOLOGY

Although advancing age is a leading associated factor in the development of ARMD, the exact etiology of the condition is still unknown despite the consensus that it is certainly multifactorial.[15,19,66,67] Contributing factors such as ethnic background, heredity, photic exposure, diet, and vitamin and rare element deficiencies as well as hypertension and smoking have all been implicated.* Prospective evaluation of vitamins, antioxidants, and rare elements is ongoing to determine their long-term value in the prevention or delay of senescent retinal alterations.[15]

SYMPTOMS

The symptoms of ARMD range from profound loss of visual acuity to no visual complaints whatsoever. Changes in visual symptoms are dependent on the variety and severity of an individual eye's involvement. Nonexudative forms of ARMD such as drusen and RPE alterations are frequently asymptomatic. Larger drusen may lead to mild focal distortion or atrophy, producing central and paracentral scotomas.

Exudative forms of ARMD frequently cause the acute or subacute onset of visual blurring, central scotomas, and metamorphopsia. Metamorphopsia may give the perception that images are smaller (i.e., micropsia) or larger (macropsia) than they really are. The changes often appear as alterations in straight lines or surfaces, which now seem curved to the involved eye. Amsler grids are effective in testing the central 20 degrees of visual field and often reveal early changes possibly overlooked by the individual with good bilateral vision.

Nonexudative Degeneration

The ophthamoscopic features of nonexudative ARMD classically include (1) drusen and (2) atrophy with pigmentary alterations. Exudative changes—including hemorrhage, hard exudate formation, and serous fluid in the subretinal or sub-RPE space—are absent. Although these findings can be present in alternate macular conditions as well as in younger individuals, their presence with advancing age usually indicates ARMD.

Drusen. Drusen are typically focal, round, white to yellow deposits found at clinical examination in or deep to the RPE. Early drusen may be very subtle and require indirect illumination at biomicroscopic examination. They have a predisposition for the macular area, particularly the parafoveal location, but may frequently be seen in the periphery as well.[1,25,52,57-59] At histologic examination they appear as eosinophilic accumulations between the inner collagenous zone of Bruch's membrane and the basal lamina of the RPE, and this position can interfere with normal cellular interactions, sometimes leading to the presence of pigmentary changes on their surfaces [6,28,29] (Fig. 3-1). Alternatively, the clinical appearance of drusen has also been associated with lipoidal degeneration of, or apoptosis in, individual RPE cells. Although their exact origin is unproven, it is thought[14,22,36,37] that they represent the end stage metabolic by-products of visual transduction that have been processed and then eliminated by the RPE.

---

*References 15, 19, 31, 51, 66, 67.

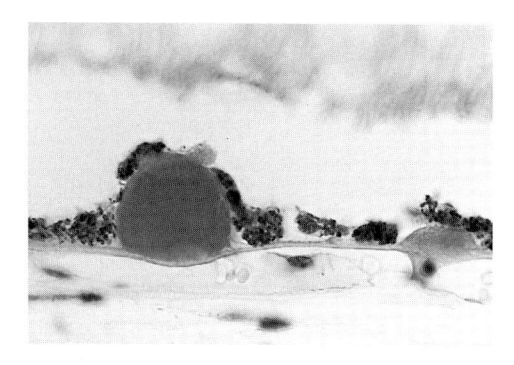

Figure 3-1 Light microscopy of drusen. Note the eosinophilic dome-shaped elevations between Bruch's membrane and the pigment epithelial basal lamina. The RPE is also attenuated on the surfaces of the larger drusen.

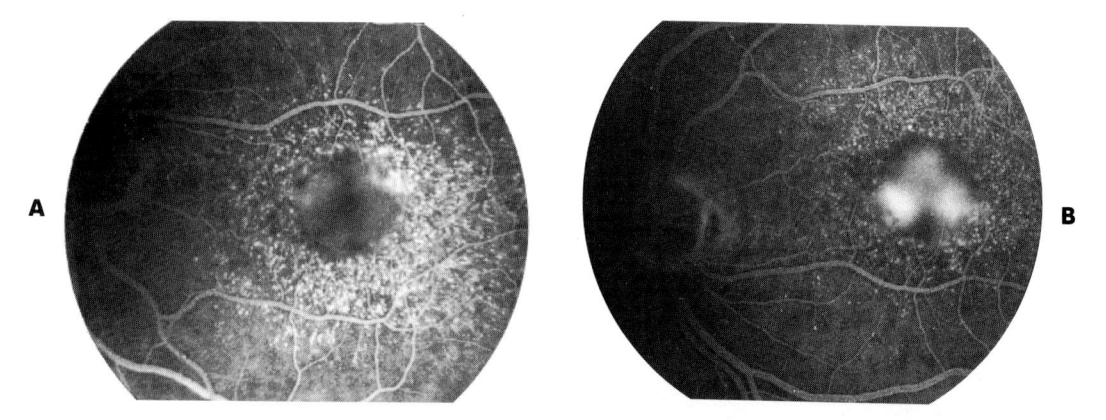

Figure 3-2 Fluorescein angiogram of basal laminar drusen. **A,** The punctate excrescences show early fluorescence, giving a "stars-in the-sky" appearance. **B,** Some eyes will develop accumulations of sub–sensory retinal fluid, giving a vitelliform appearance.

Descriptive terminology regarding drusen can be misleading and confusing. For example, drusen present in individuals with ARMD, including nonexudative ARMD, are known as exudative or typical drusen. In addition, the term "drusen" is used in other conditions not necessarily associated with senescence (i.e., cuticular or basal laminar drusen). Gass et al.[26] have described basal laminar drusen as multiple, small, focal yellow deposits deep to the retina that transmit fluorescein in the early angiographic stages giving a "stars-in-the-sky" appearance. They are often found in early and midlife, predisposing those affected to a yellow exudative detachment of the macula unassociated with choroidal neovascularization and the development of typical drusen in later years (Fig. 3-2). These changes, unlike the typical drusen, have been found histologically[57] to represent nodular excrescences of the RPE basal lamina. Similar-sounding terms such as "basal laminar deposits" and "basal linear deposits" refer, respectively, to histologically noted accumulations of widely spaced collagen between

Figure 3-3 Hard drusen. These small discrete lesions at the level of the RPE have sharp borders with little elevation.

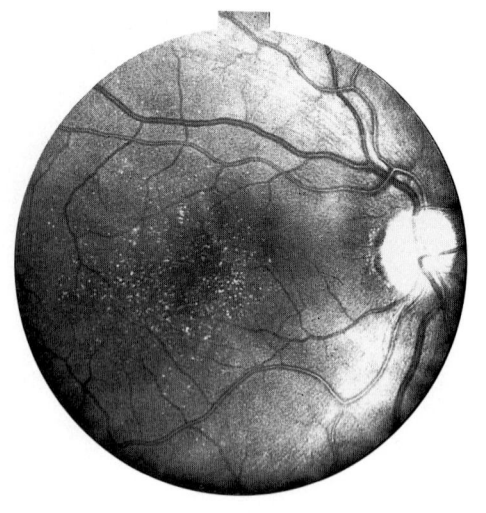

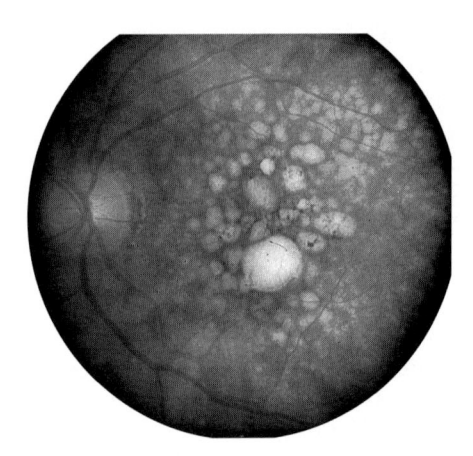

Figure 3-4 Soft drusen. These large, amorphous, yellow to white accumulations at the level of the RPE tend to coalesce and enlarge, sometimes appearing as solid pigment epithelial detachments.

Figure 3-5 Regressed drusen with associated calcification and atrophy.

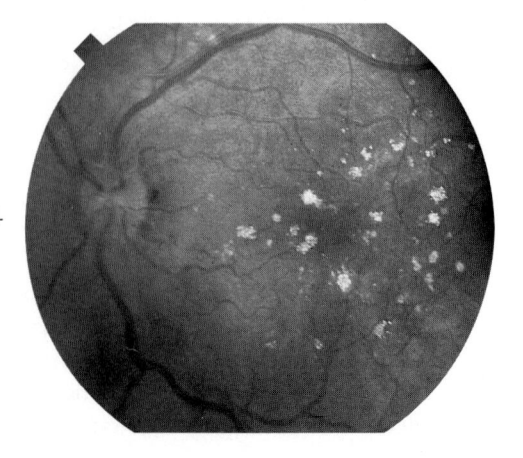

the RPE and its basement membrane and to lipid-laden material external to the RPE basement membrane.[21,29,38,43] They are not forms of drusen.

Exudative drusen include hard and soft varieties. Differentiation between them is made purely on clinical grounds. Hard drusen are small discrete nodules that appear flat and have sharp borders (Fig. 3-3). Soft drusen tend to be larger and more amorphous and to have borders that are less well defined. They frequently exhibit confluence with surrounding drusen and have a more notable elevation at biomicroscopic evaluation (Fig. 3-4). Not only are exudative drusen important as clinical markers for dry forms of the disease, their characteristics serve as predictors of future risk in the development of exudative forms of the disease. Greater confluence of drusen in individuals less than 75 years of age, more pronounced pigmentary changes, and a relatively increased hyperfluorescence have all been associated with the heightened risk of choroidal neovascular membrane (CNVM) formation.[1,6,7,25,61,64]

The natural course of drusen is variable. Progressive enlargement, calcification, spontaneous resolution, resolution with secondary atrophy, pigment epithelial detachment, and secondary neovascularization have all been reported[25,61,64] (Fig. 3-5). Laser treatment with secondary resolution of drusen has also been noted by several authors[13,70]; but since drusen represent a ubiquitous finding in the aging population, their therapeutic advantage and impact on long-term visual function are unclear.

Atrophy. Although most significant visual loss secondary to ARMD is from complications related to choroidal neovascularization, 10% to 20% of visual morbidity is related to nonexudative changes that result in retinal atrophy.[23]

Geographic atrophy typically evolves over a several-year period with a subtle and gradual loss of visual function. Initially, fine granular pigmentary changes appear in the parafoveal region.[2] These then progress to focal well-demarcated areas of atrophy involving the retina, RPE, and choriocapillaris (Fig. 3-6, *A*). As time passes, discrete parafoveal atrophic foci coalesce to form a petalloid ap-

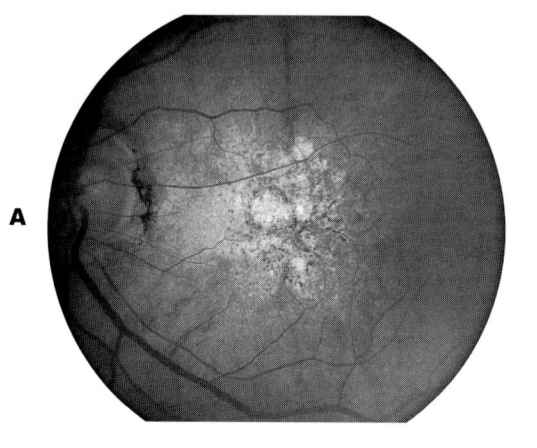

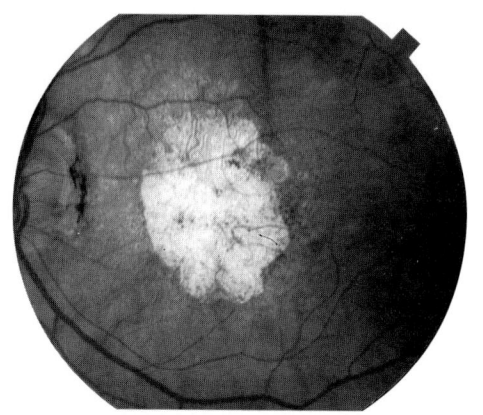

Figure 3-6 Geographic atrophy. Initial pigmentation implies photoreceptor and pigment epithelial dysfunction near the fovea. **A,** Progression results in the development of well-demarcated areas of parafoveal atrophy involving the retina, RPE, and choriocapillaris. **B,** The fovea is initially spared. As time progresses, parafoveal areas of atrophy will coalesce into a large area of central atrophy involving the fovea itself.

pearance that initially spares the fovea itself.[48,59,60] End stage changes, however, eventually involve fixation and are indistinguishable from the central areolar sclerosis seen in several other entities (including Best's and Stargardt's disease, chloroquine toxicity, and cone dystrophy) (Fig. 3-6, *B*). The pathogenesis of such changes is unclear. Some authors[34,42] believe that the segmental appearance of geographic atrophy indicates closure of the choriocapillaris lobules with secondary retinal effects. The documented survival of RPE and photoreceptors above areas of absent choriocapillaris, however, indicates a probable primary dysfunction of the RPE with secondary loss of photoreceptors and choroid.

Exudative Degeneration

"Exudative macular degeneration" is a term that encompasses several clinical presentations involving the presence of fluid and/or hemorrhage in the macular region. It implies the presence of choroidal neovascularization, but this is not invariably so as evidenced by serous detachment of the RPE.

Pigment Epithelial Detachments. A pigment epithelial detachment (PED) represents a discrete separation of the RPE and its basal lamina from the underlying Bruch's membrane. It is typically a smooth dome-shaped orange to yellow elevation that displaces the RPE and sensory retina (Fig. 3-7, *A*). Angiographically it fills early and evenly with fluorescein and its fluorescence persists beyond the recirculation phase (Fig. 3-7, *B* and *C*). Its pathogenesis and natural course are dependent on its variable clinical and fluorescein angiographic appearances, which have allowed PEDs to be placed in several categories for better prediction of their long-term visual prognoses.

Casswell et al.[11a] divided them into five categories depending on their fluorescein angiographic appearance: early hyperfluorescent, late fluorescent, drusenlike, irregular fluorescent, and mixed. Similarly Poliner et al.[54a] distinguished between PEDs based on the clinical presence or absence of serous fluid, hemorrhage, exudate, or proven choroidal neovascularization at fluorescein angiography. Essentially, they divided PEDs into drusen-type, a serous variety (i.e., without angiographic or clinical evidence of neovascularization), and a type with clinical and/or fluorescein evidence of neovascularization. Solid PEDs from large drusen had the best long-term visual prognosis; those with evidence of exudative changes did poorly.

Natural Course. More than 50% of eyes with pigment epithelial detachments caused by age-related disease develop visual acuity of 20/200 or less within 36 to 50 months.[11a,54a] This is independent of initial clinical findings or subsequent complicating factors like choroidal neovascularization or pigment epithelial tear formation.

Pigment epithelial detachments follow one of four outcomes;
1. Spontaneous resolution

    This occurs most commonly in the drusen-type and serous variety of PEDs. It frequently has pigmentary alterations and/or atrophy with poor vision.[11a] Flattening may be secondary to RPE cell death, with resultant failure of the pigment epithelium's pump function.

2. Choroidal neovascular membrane formation

    Serous PEDs whose diagnosis is supported by fluorescein angiography develop secondary neovascularization in nearly 25% of eyes within 1 year and in almost 50% within 3 years. The presence of subretinal fluid at ini-

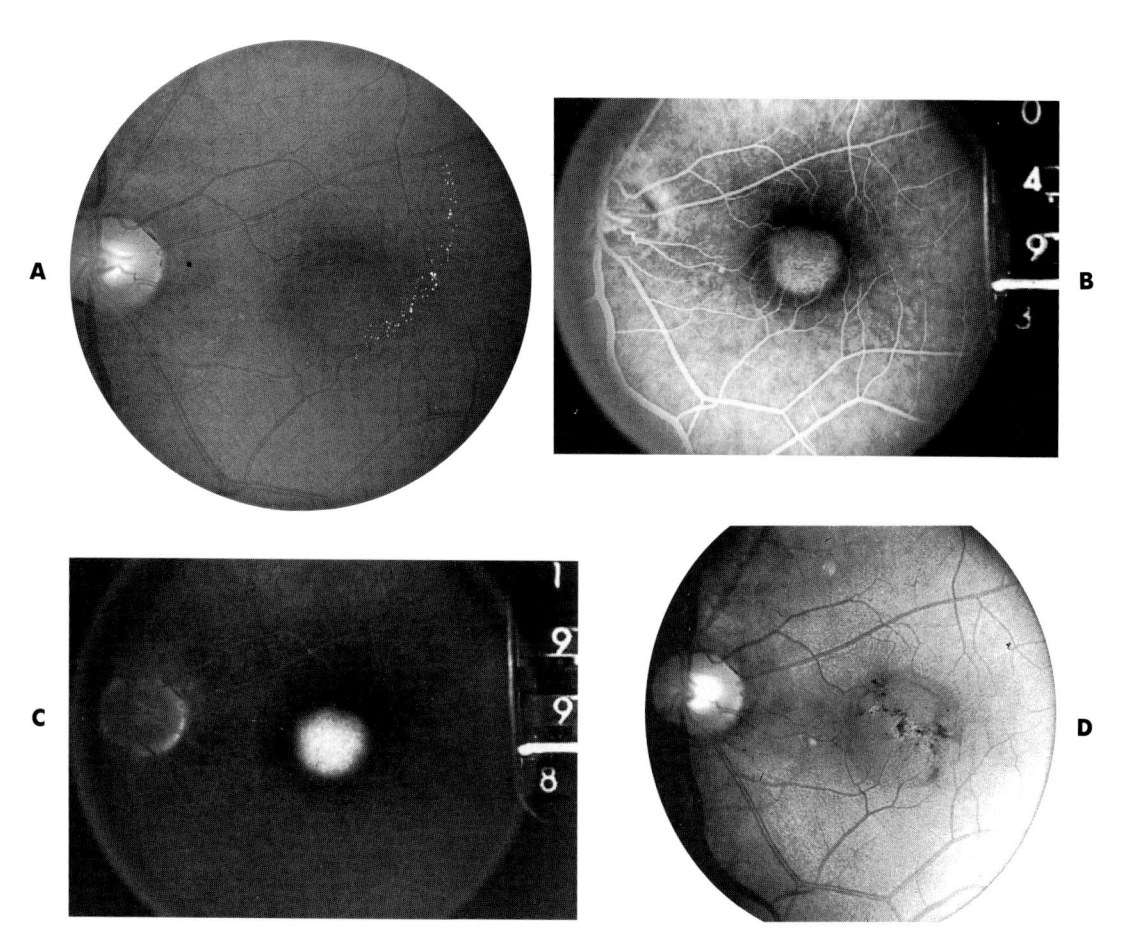

Figure 3-7 Serous pigment epithelial detachment. **A,** Discrete dome-shaped macular lesion without associated hemorrhage or exudate. **B,** Fluorescein angiogram showing early diffuse filling of the PED. **C,** Dye uniformly diffuses and maintains fluorescence after resolution of the background fluorescence. **D,** Two years later the PED is essentially unchanged with the exception of overlying pigmentary changes.

tial examination, a larger PED size, an older mean patient age, and late or irregular fluorescence of the PED are all associated with the increased risk of neovascularization.[14a,54a] PEDs with neovascularization eventually proceed to disciform scars, with nearly 90% of patients developing a final visual acuity of 20/200 or less.[11a,54a]

3. Pigment epithelial tears

Tears or rips of the pigment epithelium, first described by Hoskin et al.[35a] in 1981, represent a cleavage of the pigment epithelial monolayer at the edge of a PED with resultant retraction toward its center. They occur in at least 10% of eyes, with resultant poor vision in most cases if the fovea is involved.[11a] They frequently occur spontaneously, within a few months before being diagnosed, but have also been observed[11a,62] during the application of laser photocoagulation. Clinically they often lead to significant flattening of a PED, with a sharp demarcation existing be-

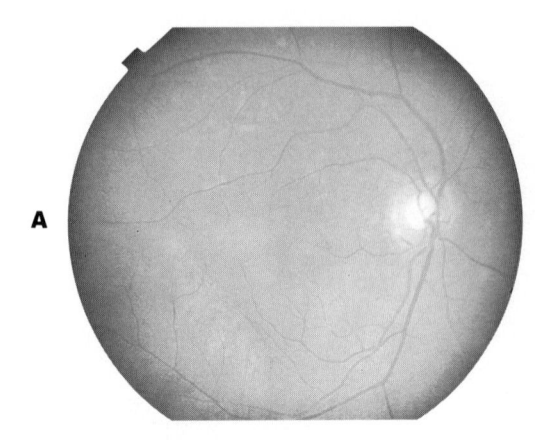

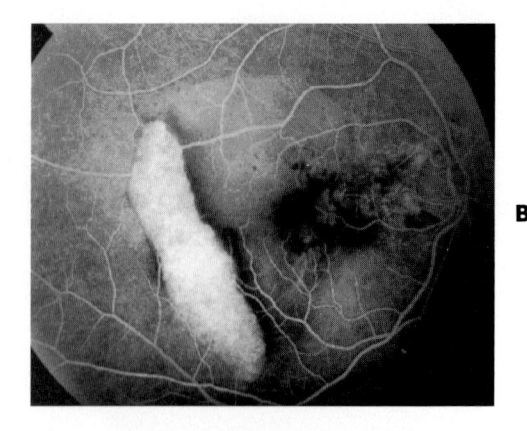

Figure 3-8 Pigment epithelial tear. **A,** Temporal to the fovea, which forms a vertical demarcation made up of retracted pigment epithelium sharply contrasted by the exposed choroid. **B,** Fluorescein angiogram showing the area of absent pigment epithelium. Note the detachment nasal to the tear.

tween the edge of the retracted epithelium and the exposed adjacent choroid (Fig. 3-8). Schoeppner et al.[62] have reported a risk of PED and tear formation in over 80% of contralateral eyes within 3 years of initial eye involvement.

4. No change

The Moorfields Macular Study Group[50a] reported that nearly half of all eyes with PEDs remain unchanged for a follow-up period of 18 months, maintaining their initially documented visual acuities during this period. This group included drusen-type and early fluorescent or serous PEDs[11a] (Fig. 3-7, *D*).

Treatment. Several authors reporting their experiences with laser photocoagulation of PEDs have had only limited success. The Moorfields Macular Study Group[50] conducted a randomized prospective study of laser photocoagulation in eyes with PEDs and no angiographic evidence of neovascularization. Their treatment technique included the application of laser in a grid pattern over the surface of the involved pigment epithelium with avoidance of the fovea itself. Despite successful flattening of the PED in many cases, visual function did not improve and frequently worsened.[50]

Successful laser photocoagulation of PEDs associated with contiguous choroidal neovascularization has been reported to be successful in the improvement or stabilization of vision in several retrospective studies.[47] These PEDs frequently have a notched or kidney bean appearance, with the CNVM residing in this notch. Treatment theoretically eliminates at least one source of the elevation without diffusely injuring the pigment epithelium itself (Fig. 3-9). The advent of digitalized photographic techniques and indocyanine green angiography has added to the number of PEDs treated with photocoagulation because of the increased resolution of CNVMs in patients who were previously thought to have serous PED or occult neovascularization with fluorescein angiography alone.[55,73]

Age-related macular degeneration 87

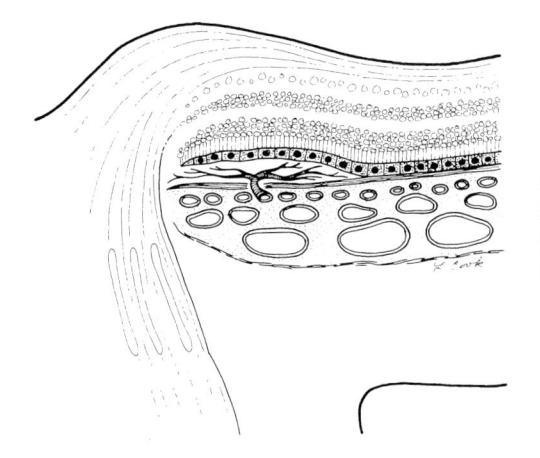

Figure 3-9 Choroidal neovascular membrane formation. Choroidal vessels gain entrance to the subretinal or subretinal pigment epithelial space via defects in Bruch's membrane.

Figure 3-10 Disciform scar. End stage development of a fibrotic subretinal scar results in permanent alteration of the macular anatomy, with a loss of central acuity.

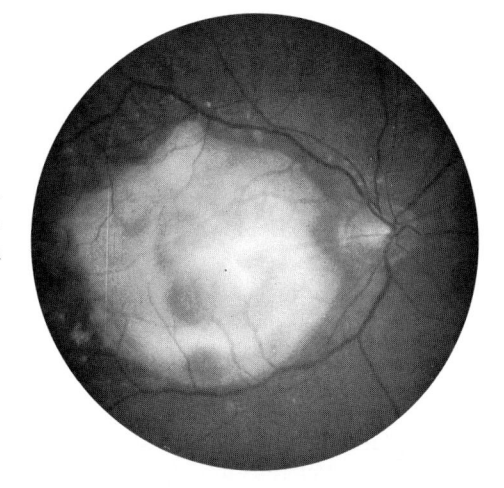

Choroidal Neovascularization

Choroidal neovascular membrane (CNVM) formation is the classic presentation of exudative ARMD. It represents the abnormal growth of new vessels that originate in the choroid, penetrate Bruch's membrane and spread beneath the RPE and/or sensory retina. Although age-related fractures within Bruch's membrane allow vessel spread, the impetus for this growth is unclear and may depend on the relative balance of various growth and inflammatory factors in the macular region, which act as stimuli and antagonists to vascular growth.[55,73]

Teeters and Bird[64a] first documented the association between fluorescein angiographic findings and the clinical appearance of the macula in ARMD. Choroidal neovascular membrane formation has two basic angiographic patterns: well-defined and occult. Both can lead to one of several clinical appearances—including disciform scar, PED, massive subretinal or choroidal hemorrhage, and vitreous hemorrhage (Fig. 3-10). Although neovascularization itself may not be responsible for visual loss, the secondary decompensation of these vessels with exudation and frank hemorrhage eventually disrupts the normal extracellular milieu leading to retinal cell death and consequent visual loss.

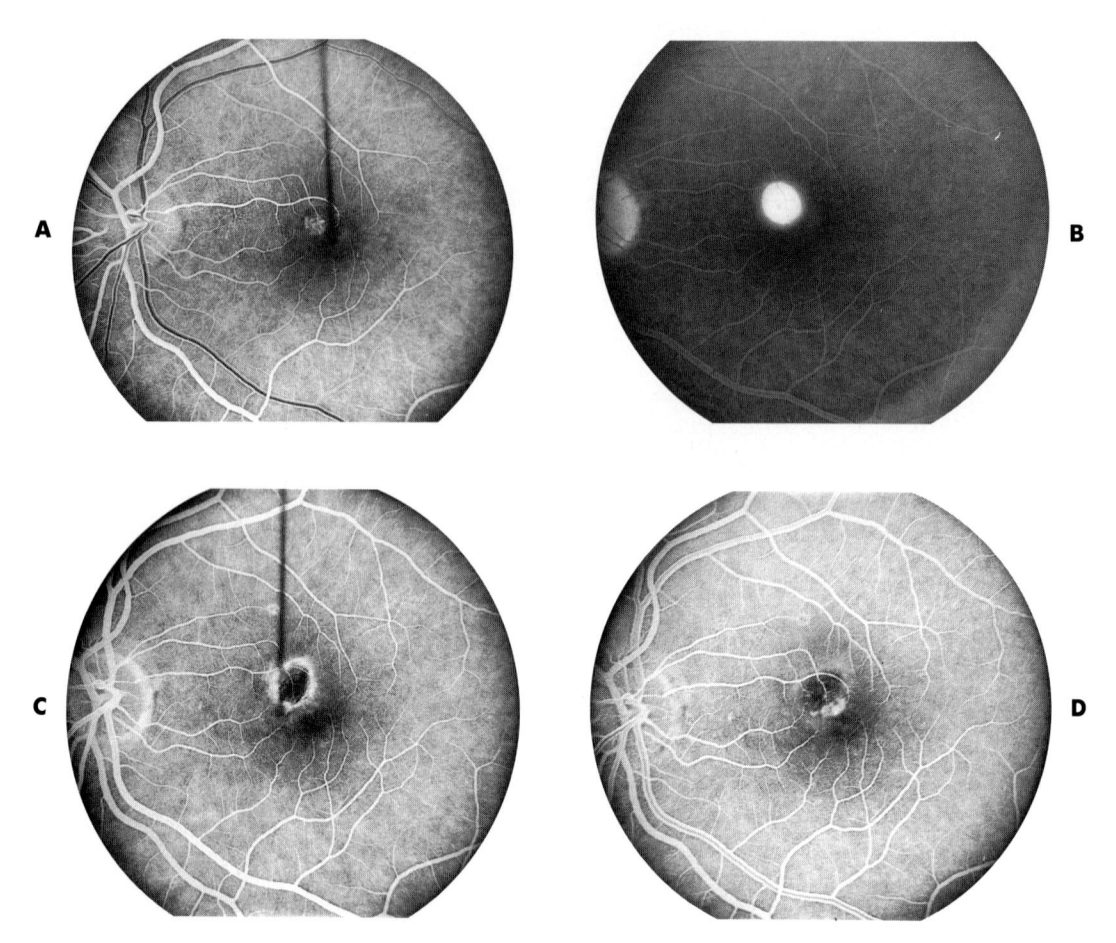

Figure 3-11 Choroidal neovascular membrane. **A,** A fluorescein angiogram reveals lacy initial hyperfluorescence. **B,** Note that it often increases as the study progresses. Several weeks after laser photocoagulation a chorioretinal scar develops. **C,** Another fluorescein angiogram shows hypofluorescence representing closure of the treated CNVM. In over 50% of patients with age-related macular degeneration who have been successfully treated and followed for more than 3 years there is a recurrence, **D,** most commonly seen along the foveal edge of the previous treatment scar.

Well-Defined Membranes. Well-defined or discrete CNVMs appear as progressive focal areas of subretinal hyperfluorescence that are frequently noted during or before the arteriovenous phase of fluorescein angiography. Their borders are initially well defined but become more irregular as fluorescein leaks from their incompetent vasculature and diffuses into the subretinal space (Fig. 3-11, *A* and *B*). Initial frames may reveal a fine vascular network with a cartwheel appearance if a central feeding vessel is noted.[25,44,64a] Areas of hypofluorescence in the surrounding area frequently represent blockage caused by hemorrhage and, less commonly, dense hard exudate. Ophthalmoscopically, discrete CNVMs have a slate gray to green color at the level of the pigment epithelium. They may be elevated compared to the surrounding RPE and have evidence of associated hard exudate, hemorrhage, pigmentation, and subretinal fluid. Involvement of the fovea may give the appearance of cystoid macular edema.

Untreated discrete CNVMs have been documented[41,68] to grow at an average rate of between 10 and 18 μm per day. Most will eventually progress within the foveal avascular zone, ultimately leading to significant loss of vision and disciform scar formation.[5,20,25,44-47,50a]

Occult Membranes. Occult choroidal neovascularization is defined as areas of presumed CNVM formation on the basis of subretinal fluid without discrete areas of fluorescein accumulation at angiography. Multiple areas of punctate hyperfluorescence typically are present and increase in intensity throughout the angiography but are unassociated with atrophy or the formation of drusen. The exact borders of involvement cannot be reasonably determined.[10] Alternatively, areas of elevated RPE may be noted clinically that stain but have a loculated appearance and do not leak aggressively in the late phases of the angiogram. Yannuzzi et al.[73] have classified these as vascularized RPE. Approximately half of all patients presenting with signs of choroidal neovascularization will have evidence of occult changes.[9,10] The significance of this is readily apparent when one recognizes that the benefits of laser photocoagulation for exudative ARMD are predicated on the ability to define the location of the treated lesion. The possible benefits of indocyanine green dye and advances in digital angiography have led to increasing interest in indocyanine green angiography's ability to reveal the position of these vessels.[55,73]

Because available studies often already have evidence of subfoveal involvement, the natural course of occult changes is difficult to determine. Bressler et al.[9] found a statistically significant difference in the number of eyes that developed moderate to severe visual loss depending on whether they proceeded on to disciform scar or continued to show poorly defined leakage.

TREATMENT OF THE COMPLICATIONS AND SEQUELAE OF ARMD

The treatment of exudative complications of ARMD involves primarily the use of laser photocoagulation to CNVMs. Recent reports,[3,24,30,33,65] however, of parenteral antiangiogenic factors and vitrectomy techniques have broadened the number of therapeutic options now available and may in the future lead to improved visual outcomes.

Laser Photocoagulation

Laser photocoagulation is the proven standard of treatment in exudative ARMD. The Moorfields Macular Study, the Macular Photocoagulation Study (MPS), and several other independent prospective trials[44-47,50a] have highlighted its benefit in the treatment of discrete extrafoveal CNVM formation. An additional report by the MPS[47] has shown a statistical benefit with krypton red wavelengths in juxtafoveal involvement and in subfoveal lesions, although from a practical standpoint overall visual results were poor.

Photocoagulation technique in the MPS for age-related neovascularization was directed to whole ablation of an angiographically demonstrated discrete choroidal neovascular membrane in an extrafoveal position (200 to 2500 μm from the center of the foveal avascular zone). This was achieved by the application of 200 μm diameter burns diffusely over the surface of the CNVM and a surrounding additional border of 100 μm. Durations of at least 0.2 second were used, and laser energy was titrated to give a uniformly white burn.[44-47] Post-treatment follow-up was typically scheduled 2 weeks after treatment and involved repeat fluorescein angiography to determine whether total closure of the CNVM had been achieved (Fig. 3-11, *C*).

Despite adequate closure initially, the MPS demonstrated a recurrence rate of 53% within 3 years of treatment, with most recurrences weighted to the first 6 months.[45] Recurrent neovascularization was found most frequently on the foveal edge of a previously treated lesion and often exhibited a rim configuration[45,46] (Fig. 3-11, *D*). Separate areas of involvement became noticeable in almost 10% of eyes during this same follow-up period.[45,46] This finding underlines the diffuse and progressive nature of age-related macular disease. In addition, individuals with documented choroidal neovascularization in one eye have a 2% to over 25% risk per year of developing exudative disease in the contralateral eye.[45,46,62]

Complications of laser photocoagulation in ARMD include inadvertent foveal burns, retinal hemorrhage, choroidal ischemia, retinal vascular occlusion, retinal pigment epithelial tears, and macular pucker.[27,44-47] Long-term follow-up of even stable photocoagulation scars may show concentric expansion of the scar with involvement of the fovea itself.

Vitrectomy

Pars plana vitrectomy (PPV) can be utilized in the treatment of numerous patients who present with the complications of ARMD: (1) subfoveal CNVM formation, (2) subretinal macular hemorrhage, and (3) breakthrough vitreous hemorrhage.

The presence of CNVM formation near the fovea has few practical treatment options involving the real improvement of vision. Foveal photocoagulation is designed to limit scotoma size and often leads to an initial decline of central acuity.[12,47] Recently reports of CNVM removal in cases of ocular histoplasmosis and ARMD[3,65] have shown some potential benefits to PPV with intentional retinotomy and removal of the CNVM en bloc from the subretinal space. Although reported results are better in patients with histoplasmosis and foveal CNVM formation, the removal of discrete neovascularization anterior to the RPE[65] has been shown to be beneficial in selected patients with ARMD (Fig. 3-12).

Patients experiencing large submacular hemorrhage secondary to ARMD often develop catastrophic visual loss because of extensive subretinal hemorrhage and secondary vitreous hemorrhage. Vitrectomy surgery with removal of vitreous hemorrhage alone often leads to improvement in the peripheral vision. Removal of subretinal macular hemorrhage has the added advantage of improving central field as well and limiting the end stage fibrotic reaction that causes extensive disciform scarring[69] (Fig. 3-13). Subretinal clot removal should be undertaken within 1 week of hemorrhage that is due to the development of subretinal fibrosis and the permanent disruption of photoreceptors.[69] The use of tissue plasmingen activator (t-PA), a clot-specific lysing agent, has increased the ease of removing large macular hemorrhages.

Age-related macular degeneration 91

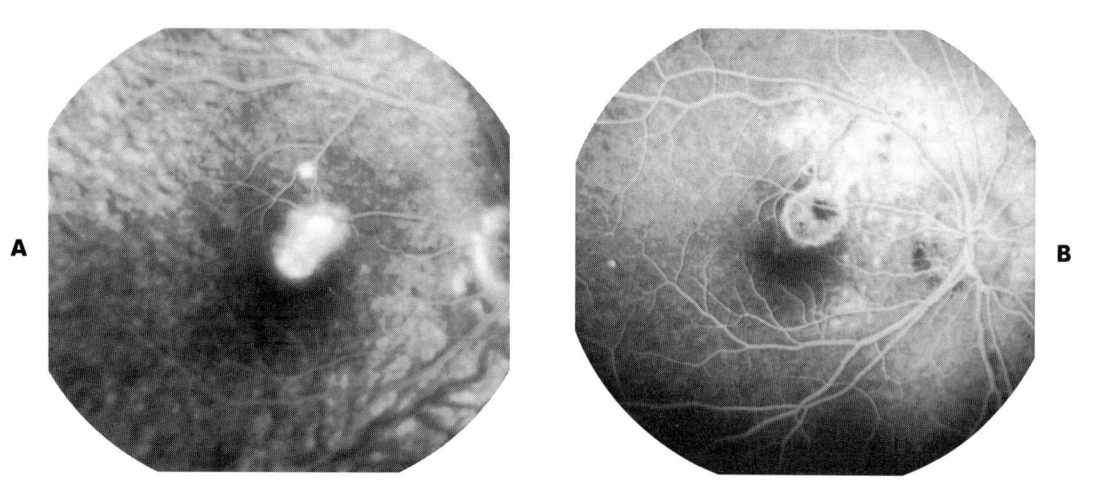

Figure 3-12 Removal of a foveal choroidal neovascular membrane. **A,** There is a discrete CNVM near the fovea. The patient underwent vitrectomy with intentional retinotomy and secondary removal of the membrane. **B,** Postoperatively note that the CNVM is absent.

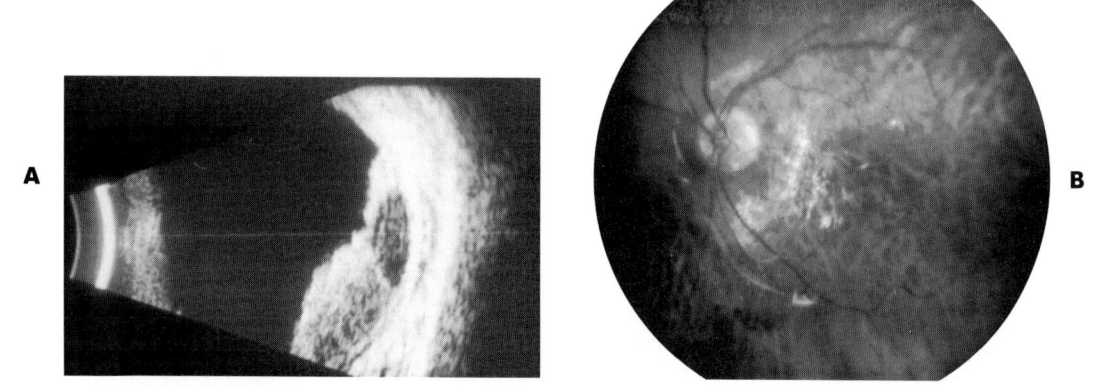

Figure 3-13 Treatment of large subretinal hemorrhages in age-related macular degeneration. **A,** A B-scan ultrasound shows the area of subretinal macular hemorrhage with secondary vitreous hemorrhage. **B,** After pars plana vitrectomy with intentional retinotomy and the use of tissue plasminogen activator to remove a macular clot.

Antiangiogenic Factors

Recent reports by Fung[24] and Guyer et al.[33] have focused attention on the practical application of medical treatment in the control of exudative ARMD. Alpha-interferon is a potent antiangiogenic factor with known abilities in the treatment of some vascular tumors. Its use in patients with CNVMs, however, is controversial and not without systemic and ocular complication.[33] The limited number of patients treatable by laser photocoagulation and the high rate of recurrence in successfully treated patients combine to make the further study of medical treatment protocols an important area of future endeavor.

References

1. Barondes MJ, Pauleikhoff D, Chisholm IH, et al: Bilaterality of drusen.
2. Bastek JV, Siegel EB, Straatsma BR, Foos RY: Chorioretinal juncture: pigmentary patterns of the peripheral fundus, *Ophthalmology* 89:1455, 1982.
3. Berger AS, Kaplan HJ: Clinical experience with the surgical removal of subfoveal neovascular membranes, *Ophthalmology* 99:969, 1992.
4. Boulton M, Marshall J: Effects of increasing numbers of phagocytic inclusions on human retinal pigment epithelial cells in culture: a model for aging, *Br J Ophthalmol* 70:808, 1986.
5. Bressler SB, Bressler NM, Fine SL, et al: Natural course of choroidal neovascular membranes within the foveal avascular zone. *Am J Ophthalmol*
6. Bressler SB, Bressler NM, Maguire MG, et al: Relationship of drusen and abnormalities of the retinal pigment epithelium to the prognosis of neovascular macular degeneration, *Arch Ophthalmol* 108:1442, 1990.
7. Bressler NM, Bressler SB, Seddon JM, et al: Drusen characteristics in patients with exudative versus non-exudative age-related macular degeneration, *Retina* 8:109, 1988.
8. Bressler NM, Bressler SB, West SK, et al: The grading and prevalence of macular degeneration in Chesapeake Bay watermen, *Arch Ophthalmol* 107:847, 1989.
9. Bressler NM, Frost LA, Bressler SB, et al: Natural course of poorly defined choroidal neovascularization associated with macular degeneration, *Arch Ophthalmol* 105:1537, 1988.
10. Bressler SB, Silia JC, Bressler NM, et al: Clinicopathologic correlation of occult choroidal neovascularization in age-related macular degeneration, *Arch Ophthalmol* 110:827, 1992.
11. Burns RP, Feeney-Burns L. Clinico-morphologic correlation of drusen and Bruch's membrane, *Trans Am Ophthalmol Soc* 78:206, 1980.
11a. Casswell AG, Kohen D, Bird AC: The development of neovascularization in the elderly: classification and outcome, *Br J Ophthalmol* 69:397, 1985.
12. Decker WL, Grabowski WM, Annesley WH: Krypton red laser photocoagulation of subretinal neovascular membranes located within the foveal avascular zone, *Ophthalmology* 91:1582, 1984.
13. Duvall J, Tso MOM: Cellular mechanisms of resolution of drusen after laser coagulation, *Arch Ophthalmol* 103:694, 1985.
14. El Baba F, Green WR, Fleishmann J, et al: Clinicopathologic correlation of lipidization and detachment of the retinal pigment epithelium, *Am J Ophthalmol* 101:576, 1986.
14a. Elman MJ, Fine SL, Murphy RP, et al: The natural history of serous retinal pigment epithelium detachment in patients with age-related macular degeneration, *Ophthalmology* 93:224, 1986.
15. Eye Disease Case Control Study Group: Risk factors for neovascular age-related macular degeneration, *Arch Ophthalmol* 110:1701, 1992.
16. Feeney-Burns L, Eldred GE: The fate of the phagosome:conversion to 'age pigment' and impact in human retinal pigment epithelium. Trans Ophthalmol Soc UK 103:416, 1983.
17. Feeney-Burns L, Ellersieck MR: Age-related changes in the ultrastructure of Bruch's membrane, *Am J Ophthalmol* 100:686, 1985.
18. Feeney-Burns L, Hilderbrand ES, Eldridge S: Aging human RPE: morphometric analysis of macular, equatorial, and peripheral cells, *Invest Ophthalmol Vis Sci* 25:195, 1984.
19. Ferris FL: Senile macular degeneration: review of epidemiologic features. *Am J Epidemiol* 118:132, 1983.
20. Ferris FL III, Fine SL, Hyman L: Age-related macular degeneration and blindness due to neovascular maculopathy, *Arch Ophthalmol* 102:1640, 1984.
21. Fisher RF: The influence of age on some ocular basement membranes, *Eye* 1:184, 1987.
22. Fine BS: Lipoidal degeneration of the retinal pigment epithelium, *Am J Ophthalmol* 91:469, 1981.
23. Framingham Eye Study. VI. Macular degeneration, *Surv Ophthalmol* 24:(suppl)428, 1980.
24. Fung WE: Interferon alpha 2a for treatment of age-related macular degeneration, *Am J Ophthalmol* 112:349, 1991.

25. Gass JDM: Drusen and disciform macular detachment and degeneration, *Arch Ophthalmol* 90:206, 1973.
26. Gass JDM, Jallow S, Davis B: Adult vitelliform macular degeneration occurring in patients with basal laminar drusen, *Am J Ophthalmol* 99:445, 1985.
27. Grabowski WM, Decker WL, Annesley WH: Complications of krypton red laser photocoagulation to subretinal neovascular membranes, *Ophthalmology* 91:1587, 1984.
28. Green WR: Senile macular degeneration: a histopathologic study, *Trans Am Ophthalmol Soc* 75:180, 1977.
29. Green WR, McDonnell PJ, Yeo JH: Pathologic features of senile macular degeneration, *Ophthalmology* 92:615, 1985.
30. Gregor Z, Bird AC, Chisholm IH: Senile disciform macular degeneration in the second eye, *Br J Ophthalmol* 61:141, 1977.
31. Gregor Z, Joffe L: Senile macular changes in the black African, *Br J Ophthalmol* 62:547, 1978.
32. Grindle CFJ, Marshall J: Ageing changes in Bruch's membrane and their functional implications, *Trans Ophthalmol Soc UK* 98:172, 1978.
33. Guyer DR, Adamis AP, Gragoudas ES, et al: Systemic antiangiogenic therapy for choroidal neovascularization; what is the role of interferon alfa? *Arch Ophthalmol* 110:1383, 1992.
34. Henkind P, Gartner S: The relationship between retinal pigment epithelium and the choriocapillaris, *Trans Ophthalmol Soc UK* 103:444, 1983.
35. Hogan MJ: Role of the retinal pigment epithelium in macular disease, *Trans Am Acad Ophthalmol Otolaryngol* 76:64, 1972.
35a. Hoskin A, Bird AC, Sehmi K: Tears of detached retinal pigment epithelium, *Br J Ophthalmol* 65:417-422, 1981.
36. Ishibashi T, Patterson R, Ohnishi Y, et al. Formation of drusen in the human eye, *Am J Ophthalmol* 101:342, 1986.
37. Ishibashi T, Sorgente N, Patterson R, Ryan SJ. Pathogenesis of drusen in the primate, *Invest Ophthalmol Vis Sci* 27:184, 1986.
38. Kenyon KR, Maumenee AE, Ryan SJ, et al: Diffuse drusen and associated complication, *Am J Ophthalmol* 100:119, 1985.
39. Killingsworth MC: Age-related components of Bruch's membrane in the human eye, *Graefes Arch Clin Exp Ophthalmol* 225:406, 1987.
40. Klein ML, Jorizzo PA, Watzke RC: Growth features of choroidal neovascular membranes in age-related macular degeneration, *Ophthalmology* 96:1416, 1989.
41. Klein R, Klein BEK, Linton, KLP: Prevalence of age-related maculopathy; the beaver dam eye study, *Ophthalmology* 99:933, 1992.
42. Korte GE, Repucci V, Henkind P: RPE destruction causes choriocapillary atrophy, *Invest Ophthalmol Vis Sci* 25:1135, 1984.
43. Loffler KU, Lee WR: Basal linear deposits in the human macula, *Graefes Arch Clin Exp Ophthalmol* 2324:493, 1986.
44. Macular Photocoagulation Study Group: Argon laser photocoagulation for senile macular degeneration: results of a randomized clinical trial, *Arch Ophthalmol* 100:912, 1982.
45. Macular Photocoagulation Study Group: Argon laser photocoagulation for neovascular maculopathy: three-year results from randomized clinical trials, *Arch Ophthalmol* 104:694, 1986.
46. Macular Photocoagulation Study Group: Argon laser photocoagulation for neovascular maculopathy after five years; results from randomized clinical trials, *Arch Ophthalmol* 109:1109, 1991.
47. Macular Photocoagulation Study Group: Laser photocoagulation of subfoveal neovascular lesions in age-related macular degeneration; results of a randomized clinical trial, *Arch Ophthalmol* 109:1232, 1991.
48. Maguire P, Vine AK: Geographic atrophy of the retinal pigment epithelium, *Am J Ophthalmol* 102:621, 1986.
49. Marshall J: The aging retina: physiology or pathology, *Eye* 1:282, 1987.
50. Moorfields Macular Study Group: Retinal pigment epithelial detachments in the elderly. A controlled trial of argon laser photocoagulation, *Br J Ophthalmol* 66:1, 1982.

50a. Moorfields Macular Study Group: Treatment of senile disciform macular degeneration: a single-blind randomised trial by argon laser photocoagulation, *Br J Ophthalmol* 66:745, 1982.
51. Newsome DA, Swork M, Leone NC, Elston RC, Miller E: Oral zinc in macular degeneration, *Arch Ophthalmol* 106:192, 1988.
52. Pauleikhoff D, Barondes MJ, Minassian D, et al: Drusen as a risk factor in age-related macular disease, *Am J Ophthalmol* 109:171, 1990.
53. Pauleikhoff D, Chen JC, Chisholm IH, Bird AC: Choroidal perfusion abnormality in age-related Bruch's membrane change, *Am J Ophthalmol* 109:211, 1990.
54. Pauleikhoff D, Harper CA, Marshall J, Bird AC: Aging changes in Bruch's membrane: a histochemical and morphologic study, *Ophthalmology* 97:171, 1990.
54a. Poliner LS, Olk JR, Burgess D, Gordon M: Natural history of retinal pigment epithelium detachment in patients with age-related macular degeneration, *Ophthalmology* 93:543, 1986.
55. Regillo CD, Benson WE, Maguire JI, Annesley WH: Indocyanine green angiography and occult choroidal neovascularization. (Accepted for publication in *Ophthalmology*.)
56. Rungger-Brandle E, Englert U, Leuenberger PM: Exocytic clearing of degraded membrane material from pigment epithelium cells in frog retina, *Invest Ophthalmol Vis Sci* 28:2026, 1987.
57. Sarks SH: Aging and degeneration in the macular region: a clinicopathologic study, *Br J Ophthalmol* 60:324, 1976.
58. Sarks SH: Drusen and their relationship to senile macular degeneration, *Aust J Ophthalmol* 8:117, 1980.
59. Sarks SH: Drusen patterns predisposing to geographic atrophy of the retinal pigment epithelium, *Aust J Ophthalmol* 10:91, 1982.
60. Sarks JP, Sarks SH, Killingsworth M: Evolution of geographic atrophy of the retinal pigment epithelium, *Eye* 2:552, 1988.
61. Sarks SH, Van Driel D, Maxwell L, et al: Softening of drusen and subretinal neovascularization, *Trans Ophthalmol Soc UK* 100:414, 1980.
62. Schoeppner G, Chaung EL, Bird AC: The risk of fellow eye visual loss with unilateral retinal pigment epithelial tears, *Am J Ophthalmol* 108:683, 1989.
63. Sheraidah G, Steinmetz R, Maguire JI, et al: Correlation between lipids extracted from Bruch's membrane and age, *Ophthalmology* 100:47, 1993.
64. Smiddy WE, Fine SL: Prognosis of patients with bilateral macular drusen. *Ophthalmology* 91:271-277, 1984.
64a. Teeters VW, Bird AC: The development of neovascularization in senile disciform macular degeneration, *Am J Ophthalmol* 77:1, 1973.
65. Thomas MA, Grand MG, Williams DF, et al: Surgical management of subfoveal choroidal neovascularization, *Ophthalmology* 99:952, 1992.
66. Tso MOM: Pathogenetic factors of aging macular degeneration. *Ophthalmology* 92:628, 1985.
67. Tso MOM, Woodford BJ: Effects of photic injury on the retinal tissues, *Ophthalmology* 92:952, 1983.
68. Vander JF, Morgan CM, Schatz H: Growth rate of subretinal neovascularization in age-related macular degeneration, *Ophthalmology* 96:1422, 1989.
69. Wade EC, Flynn HW, Olsen KR, et al: Subretinal hemorrhage management by pars plana vitrectomy and internal drainage, *Arch Ophthalmol* 108:973, 1990.
70. Wetzig PC: Treatment of drusen-related aging macular degeneration by photocoagulation, *Trans Am Ophthalmol Soc* 86:276, 1988.
71. Young RW: Pathophysiology of age-related macular degeneration, *Surv Ophthalmol* 31:291, 1987.
72. Young RW, Bok D: Metabolism of the retinal pigment epithelium. In Zinn KM, Marmor MF (eds): *The retinal pigment epithelium*. Cambridge Mass, 1979, Harvard University Press, pp 102-123.
73. Yannuzzi LA, Slakter JS, Sorenson JA, et al: Digital indocyanine green videoangiography and choroidal neovascularization. *Retina* 12:191, 1992.

4

Choroidal Neovascularization Associated with Myopic Macular Degeneration

James F. Vander

Choroidal neovascularization associated with myopic macular degeneration typically presents in the young to middle-aged adult with "high myopia." The distinction between "physiologic" and "high" myopia is not strictly correlated with the degree of refractive error, but the likelihood of pathologic changes in the fundus does increase in eyes with greater than 6 to 8 diopters of myopia.[1] Symptoms usually include blurring of vision with metamorphopsia, micropsia, and occasionally a relative central or paracentral scotoma if significant hemorrhaging has occurred.

FINDINGS

The clinical findings resulting from choroidal neovascularization associated with myopic degeneration are similar to those noted in the myriad other causes of choroidal neovascularization: subretinal fluid, hemorrhage, and lipid (Fig. 4-1). Identification of these findings in the presence of other features of the myopic fundus strongly suggests myopic degeneration and secondary choroidal neovascularization. A brief review of the characteristic features of the myopic fundus is therefore in order. The fundus finding most commonly seen with low to moderate degrees of myopia (<6 diopters) is a scleral or choroidal crescent located adjacent to the optic nerve head.[2] Mottled pigmentation from choroidal elements on the inner aspect of the sclera are often present, but the crescent may have the appearance of bare sclera. This crescent is usually found at the temporal aspect of the disc[3,4] and, in physiologic myopia, its width rarely exceeds one third of a disc diameter. Stenstrom and others[5-8] showed that the presence of a peripapillary crescent correlated with increasing axial length but not with total refractive power (corneal plus lens power) of the eye. Examination of the fundus periphery reveals a higher incidence of white without pressure, lattice degeneration, and pavingstone degeneration than in the normal population.[9]

Figure 4-1 Typical subretinal neovascular membrane in a patient with myopia. Note the subretinal blood and fluid temporal to the fovea.

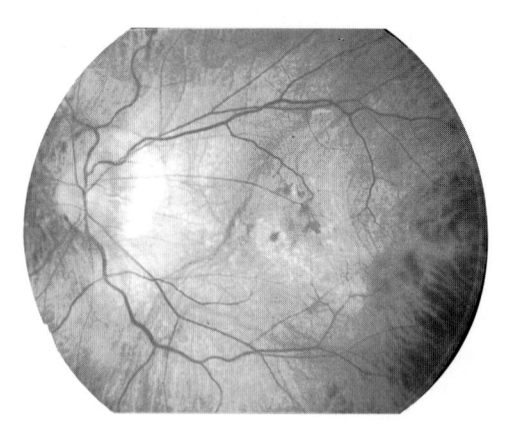

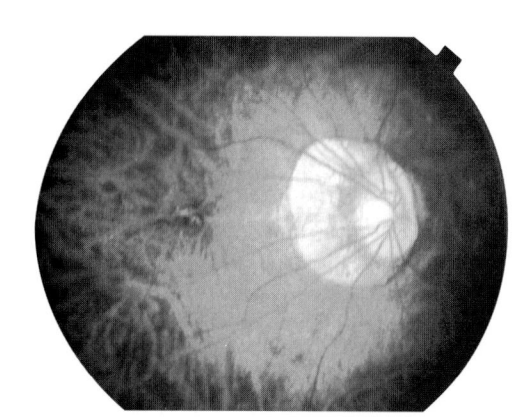

Figure 4-2 Lacquer cracks associated with myopia.

Figure 4-3 Peripapillary crescent associated with myopia. There is also myopic degeneration involving the posterior pole.

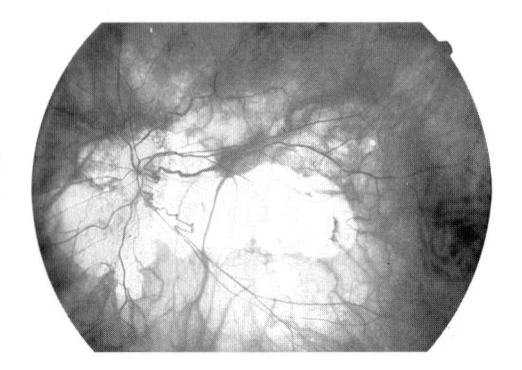

The earliest funduscopic sign of pathologic myopia is diffuse tessellation and pallor of the fundus as a result of retinal pigment epithelial thinning.[1,10,11] Normal development of the choroid and sclera is partially dependent on the presence of normal RPE, and therefore these layers may be thinned secondarily. As a result ectasia often develops in the areas of most pronounced RPE changes. Marked scleral ectasia, known as a staphyloma, is a common feature of pathologic myopia.[12] Staphyloma formation is most common in the posterior pole. A variety of configurations may be found, with most involving the macula and circumpapillary fundus. The wide field of vision and stereopsis provided by the indirect ophthalmoscope are very helpful in the detection of posterior staphylomas.

Lacquer cracks (Fig. 4-2) are yellow-white lines of variable caliber found deep to the retina, principally in the posterior pole.[13-15] They often first appear in the third or fourth decade of life. They are frequently multiple, and normal large choroidal vessels may be seen traversing them. They have no associated visual field changes and do not leak on fluorescein angiography, but their presence is a poor prognostic sign, with extensive degenerative changes usually occurring in the involved fundus area years later. Lacquer cracks probably are a manifestation of mechanical stretching of the eye, but the role of primary degenerative changes cannot be excluded. On histopathologic examination they correspond to areas of fissuring in the RPE, Bruch's membrane, and choriocapillaris.[16]

The peripapillary crescent in pathologic myopia can enlarge to encompass an area several disc diameters across (Fig. 4-3). The margins of the crescent may become irregular as well. Progressive staphyloma formation produces eversion of the optic nerve with forward movement of the lamina cribrosa. This may expose the central retinal vessels posterior to their bifurcations.[2]

Extensive peripheral retinal changes are invariably present in pathologic myopia.[2] Benign changes include pavingstone degeneration and white without pressure. Posterior vitreous detachment tends to occur at an earlier age, there is a higher incidence of lattice degeneration, and the retina is relatively thin compared to that seen in emmetropes. Not surprisingly, then, the risk of retinal tears and detachment, frequently bilateral, is great.

Development of typical symptoms and/or fundus findings suggestive of choroidal neovascularization warrants performing intravenous fluorescein angiography. This study will characteristically show early hyperfluorescence corresponding to the area of choroidal neovascularization (Fig. 4-4). Stereoscopic viewing reveals the hyperfluorescence to be deep to the retina. The hyperfluorescence usually first appears before or during the retinal arterial filling phase. It may have a lacy vascular pattern or frequently will appear as just a spot. The neovascularization leaks fluorescein into the subretinal or subpigmentary epithelial space, so increasing hyperfluorescence with expansion and blurring of margins will be noted as the angiography progresses. Abnormal hyperfluorescence can persist into the late recirculation phases of the study. Identification of the presence or extent of neovascularization may be impaired by the fluorescein blocking defect that results from the presence of subretinal hemorrhage. Frequently there is also extensive abnormality of the macular retinal pigment epithelium, with areas of both increased and absent pigmentation. The resultant window and blocking defects can sometimes make interpretation of the an-

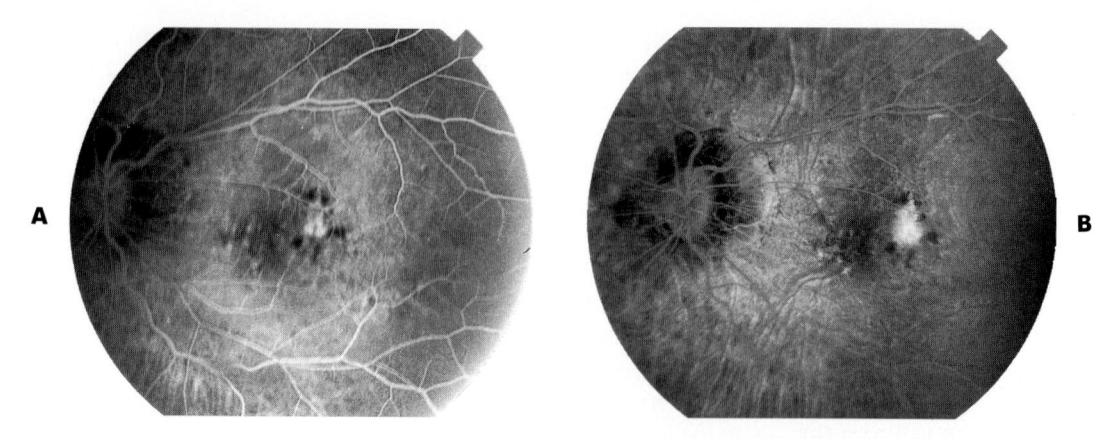

Figure 4-4 Fluorescein angiogram of a patient with subretinal neovascular membrane related to myopia. **A**, Transit phase showing hyperfluorescence of the membrane. **B**, Late recirculation phase showing a leakage of dye into the subretinal space.

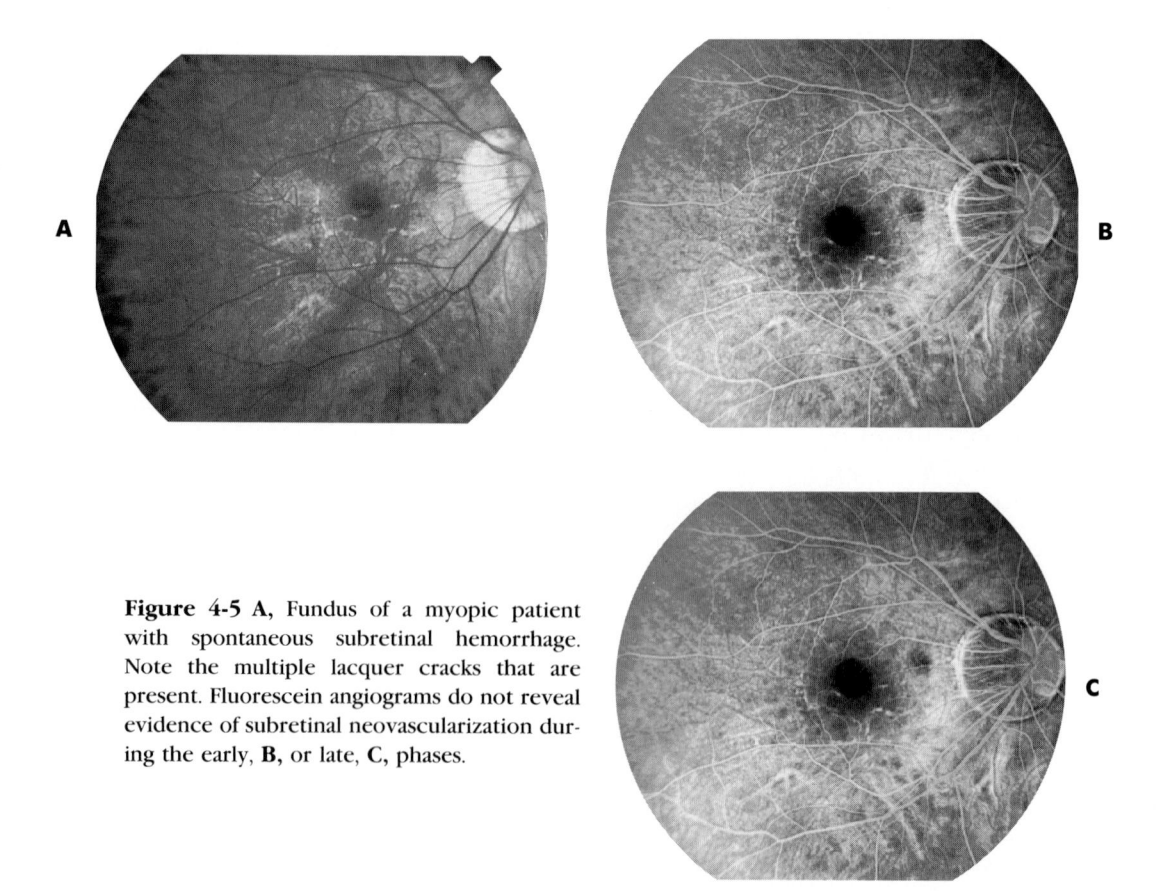

Figure 4-5 A, Fundus of a myopic patient with spontaneous subretinal hemorrhage. Note the multiple lacquer cracks that are present. Fluorescein angiograms do not reveal evidence of subretinal neovascularization during the early, **B**, or late, **C**, phases.

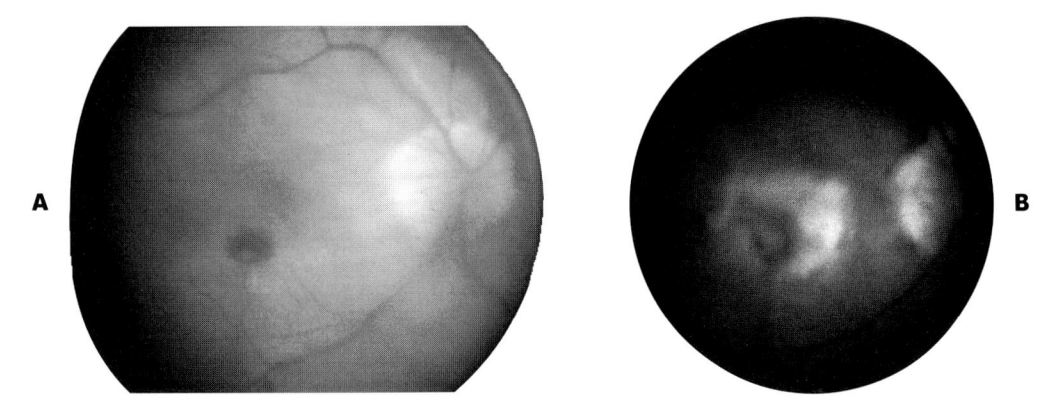

Figure 4-6 A, Typical Fuchs spot associated with myopia. **B,** Five years later a subretinal scar has developed along the foveal edge of the spot, reducing vision to 20/200.

giogram difficult. Careful comparison of the early transit and late recirculation phases, however, should reveal increasing intensity of hyperfluorescence with obscuration of margins if choroidal neovascularization is present.

Spontaneous subretinal hemorrhage can occur in the maculas of high myopes in the absence of identifiable neovascularization (Fig. 4-5). The prognosis for such patients is variable, although many retain excellent visual acuity.

A round or elliptic black lesion known as a Fuchs spot (Fig. 4-6) may occur in pathologic myopia, usually in the macula.[17,18] This lesion is sharply circumscribed, slightly elevated, and of variable size. It usually develops after the age of 35 years and may be found in up to 10% of high myopes. Fuchs' spots are bilateral in 40% of patients, with the second eye becoming affected usually within 5 years. They are often found in an area overlying previous choroidal neovascularization and appear as hyperplasia of the RPE at histopathology. Fibrosis may occur over the Fuchs spot, imparting a gray, yellow, green, or red appearance to the lesion. With time, the spot becomes less distinct and a halo of atrophy develops around it. Similar lesions can develop in the absence of myopia. Like lacquer cracks, Fuchs' spots are a poor prognostic sign, with the development of subsequent widespread chorioretinal degeneration generally the rule.[19]

DIFFERENTIAL DIAGNOSIS

Although verifying the presence of choroidal neovascularization can sometimes be problematic, identifying myopic macular degeneration as the underlying cause of choroidal neovascularization is generally not difficult. Many of the reports in the literature concerning choroidal neovascularization have used arbitrary levels of refractive error to categorize patients in terms of the etiology of their neovascularization. Occasionally, however, patients with a moderate or high degree of myopia will present with the typical funduscopic and angiographic signs of choroidal neovascularization in the absence of other features of a myopic fundus. These cases might be more properly categorized as idiopathic choroidal neovascularization. Although the distinction in terms of management techniques is probably not critical, the long-term prognosis is generally more favorable in this latter condition.

Central serous choroidopathy causes visual symptoms similar to those seen in myopic choroidal neovascularization. Funduscopic examination will typically show a serous detachment of the retina. Recurrent cases may have associated macular pigmentary disturbance that can be bilateral and mimic the pigmentary changes seen in myopia. Fluorescein angiography often shows a spot of deep early hyperfluorescence with expanding blurred margins in the recirculation phases. The other funduscopic and angiographic features of myopic degeneration, however, will not be present. Furthermore, if hemorrhage is present, this strongly suggests the diagnosis of choroidal neovascularization. It is important to bear in mind that some patients with central serous choroidopathy will have myopia. In these cases distinguishing between a myopic refractive error and myopic degeneration is very important, since the recommended treatments for central serous choroidopathy and choroidal neovascularization secondary to myopia are quite different.

TREATMENT

The presence of choroidal neovascularization associated with myopia does not necessarily have quite the ominous implications found with other conditions.[19-22] Overall, up to 50% of patients with choroidal neovascularization can expect spontaneous improvement or stabilization of vision. Although one fourth of extrafoveal neovascular membranes will grow to involve the fovea, as many as a fourth of subfoveal membranes will spontaneously regress and vision improve. The long-term prognosis for these patients, however, is guarded. Recurrent subretinal hemorrhage or marked leakage of fluorescein dye in the presence of a neovascular membrane is a poor prognostic sign.

The role for laser photocoagulation in choroidal neovascularization associated with myopia is unclear. The Macular Photocoagulation Study[23] demonstrated a clear benefit of treatment for patients with well-defined extrafoveal choroidal neovascularization associated with age-related macular degeneration and ocular histoplasmosis syndrome along with idiopathic membranes. Also a beneficial effect of neovascularization extending into the foveal avascular zone was shown,[24] especially for patients with ocular histoplasmosis. Choroidal neovascularization associated with myopia, however, was not assessed in this study, and extrapolation of these results to patients with myopia may not be appropriate. In fact, evidence exists that suggests that photocoagulation of neovascularization with only mild to moderate leakage at fluorescein angiography may worsen the visual prognosis compared to the outcome in untreated patients.[20] Photocoagulation of extrafoveal lesions, with subsequent enlargement of the scar through the foveola resulting in significant visual loss, has been reported in up to 68% of patients.

In the absence of well-defined criteria for treatment and effective parameters of treatment with proven efficacy, the following approach to these patients is proposed: For patients with well-defined extrafoveal neovascularization photocoagulation is probably indicated. Symptomatic patients with extrafoveal membranes that at fluorescein angiography are slowly leaking or poorly defined may benefit from treatment as well. The benefits of treating this type of mem-

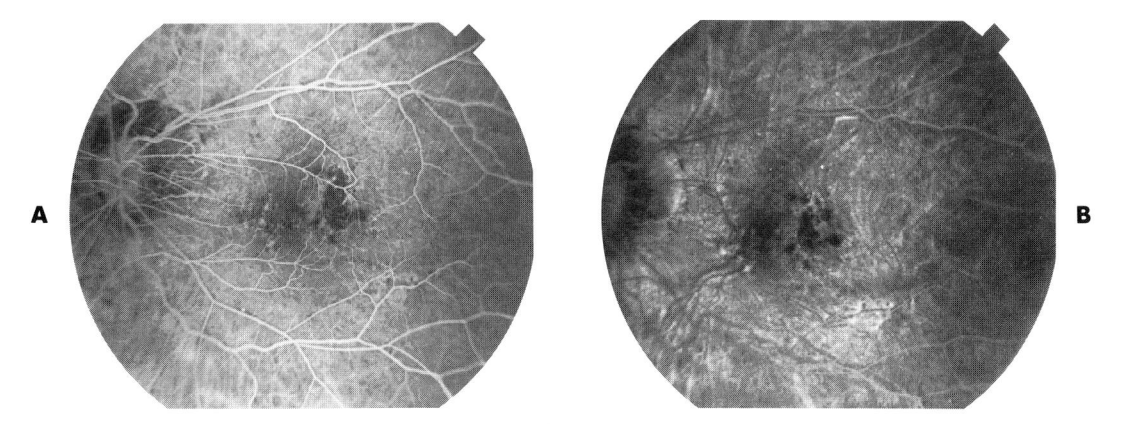

Figure 4-7 A, Three-week posttreatment angiographic appearance of the neovascular membrane in Figure 4-1 showing a hypofluorescent spot in the area of treatment during the transit phase. **B,** No significant leakage is present during the late recirculation phase.

brane, however, are not as clear. Consequently, in the absence of symptoms, observation of these less well-defined membranes is appropriate. Since photocoagulation scars in myopic patients seem particularly prone to progressive enlargement, treatment of choroidal neovascularization that extends up to the edge of or into the foveal avascular zone should be undertaken with extreme caution.

Treatment parameters are similar to those used for other causes of choroidal neovascularization. A gray-white confluent burn completely covering the neovascularization with a margin beyond the edge of about 100 μm is a reasonable end point. A longer-duration burn with relatively lower energy may be advantageous, although this is unproven. The ideal laser wavelength is also uncertain. The argon green laser is effective; but if treatment is undertaken near the fovea, then longer wavelengths such as krypton red may reduce retinal damage from uptake by macular xanthophyll. Fluorescein angiography to assess the adequacy of treatment is usually performed 2 to 3 weeks after photocoagulation (Fig. 4-7). Areas of persistent or recurrent neovascularization that are extrafoveal should probably be treated as soon as recognized.

Development of angiography using indocyanine green as an alternative or a complement to fluorescein may be helpful in managing certain cases of myopic choroidal neovascularization. This technique could prove particularly helpful in outlining the less well-defined or slowly leaking membranes and subsequently assessing the adequacy of treatment.

References

1. Harman NB: An analysis of 300 cases of high myopia in children with a scheme for the grading of the fundus changes, *Trans Ophthalmol Soc UK* 33:202, 1913.
2. Curtin BJ: *The myopias: basic science and clinical management,* Hagerstown Md, 1985, Harper & Row.
3. Fuchs A: Myopia inversa, *Arch Ophthalmol* 37:722, 1947.
4. Hertel E: Über Myopie, *Albrecht von Graefes Arch Ophthalmol* 56:326, 1903.
5. Stenstrom S: Untersuchungen über die Variation and Kovariation der optischen Elemente des menschlichen Auges, 1946 (translated by Woolf D), *Am J Optom* 25:218, 1948.

6. Curtin BJ, Karlin DB: Axial length measurements and fundus changes of the myopic eye, *Am J Ophthalmol* 71:42, 1971.
7. Bulach EK: Correlation between the degree of changes in the ocular fundus and the length of the anteroposterior axis of the eye in myopia, *Vestn Oftalmol* 3:45, 1971.
8. Tokoro T, Kabe S: The relationship between changes in ocular refraction and refraction components and the development of myopia, *Acta Soc Ophthalmol Jpn* 68:1240, 1964.
9. Karlin DB, Curtin BJ: Peripheral chorioretinal lesions and axial length of the myopic eye, *Am J Ophthalmol* 81:625, 1976.
10. Noble KG, Carr RE: Pathologic myopia, *Ophthalmology* 89:1099, 1982.
11. Blach RK: Degenerative myopia. In Krill AE (ed): *Hereditary retinal and choroidal diseases,* vol 2, Hagerstown Md, 1977, Harper & Row.
12. Curtin BJ: The posterior staphyloma of pathologic myopia, *Trans Am Ophthalmol Soc* 75:67, 1977.
13. Klein RM, Curtin BJ: Lacquer crack lesions in pathologic myopia. I, *J Ophthalmol* 79:386, 1975.
14. Shapiro M, Chandra SR: Evolution of lacquer cracks in high myopia, *Ann Ophthalmol* 17:231, 1985.
15. Hogan MJ, Zimmerman LE: *Ophthalmic pathology,* ed 2, Philadelphia, 1962, WB Saunders, pp 257-263.
16. Pruett RC, Weiter JJ, Goldstein RG: Myopic cracks, angioid streaks, and traumatic tears in Bruch's membrane, *Am J Ophthalmol* 103:537, 1987.
17. Donders FC: *On the anomalies of accommodation and refraction of the eye* (translated by Moore WD), London, 1864, New Sydenham Society.
18. Fuchs E: Der centrale schwarze Fleck bei Myopie, *Z Augenheilkd* 5:171, 1901.
19. Hampton GR, Kohen D, Bird AC: Visual prognosis of disciform degeneration in myopia, *Ophthalmology* 90:923, 1983.
20. Avila MP, Weiter JJ, Jalkj AE: Natural history of choroidal neovascularization in degenerative myopia, *Ophthalmology* 91:1573, 1984.
21. Fried M, Siebert A, Meyer-Schwickerath G: Natural history of Fuchs' spot: a long-term follow-up study, *Doc Ophthalmol* 28:215, 1981.
22. Hotchkiss ML, Fine SL: Pathologic myopia and choroidal neovascularization, *Am J Ophthalmol* 91:177, 1981.
23. Macular Photocoagulation Study Group: Argon laser photocoagulation for senile macular degeneration: results of a randomized clinical trial, *Arch Ophthalmol* 100:912, 1982.
24. Macular Photocoagulation Study Group: Krypton laser photocoagulation for neovascular lesions of ocular histoplasmosis, *Arch Ophthalmol* 105:1499, 1987.

5

Central Serous Chorioretinopathy

Joseph I. Maguire

Central serous chorioretinopathy (CSCR) is a common idiopathic dysfunction of the posterior pole affecting the sensory retina, retinal pigment epithelium (RPE), and choroid. Although its exact pathogenesis is unknown, clinical and experimental evidence suggests that the RPE is the fundamental arbitor of CSCR's clinical appearance, if not the primary source of dysfunction.

Hallmarks of this condition include (1) mild to moderate central visual loss not related to optic nerve dysfunction, (2) a discrete temporal course with resolution and possible recurrence, (3) a typical clinical and fluorescein angiographic appearance with rarer variants, and (4) an idiopathic etiology.

In this chapter we will review the clinical appearance of CSCR, its fluorescein angiographic features, demographics, symptoms, systemic associations, variants, pathogenesis, natural course, and long-term prognosis, and its differential diagnosis and treatment.

CLINICAL FEATURES

Ophthalmoscopy

Central serous chorioretinopathy is characterized by a well-demarcated round to oval sensory retinal detachment and/or low serous elevation of the RPE involving the macular region but without associated evidence of choroidal neovascular membrane formation (CNVM) such as hemorrhage or hard exudate. An increased light reflex at the edge of the elevated retina is frequently present with an associated loss of the foveal reflex if fixation is involved. Fine yellow to white deposits on the undersurface of the sensory retina—retinitic precipitates—are sometimes present and may imply chronicity (Fig. 5-1). Abnormalities of the RPE are frequently found within the area of sensory retinal detachment and may include subtle areas of mottled pigmentation, discrete yellow to orange foci resembling small isolated drusen, or frank retinal pigment elevations. These alterations, which may be single or multiple, are usually less than one quarter of a disc diameter.[12,25,29,57,59] Gass[12] points out the frequent presence of pigment epithelial detachment in CSCR, although Wessing[56,57] notes that more than 90% of his patients had sensory retinal elevations alone and less than 10% of cases were observed to have either pigment epithelial eleva-

Figure 5-1 Central serous chorioretinopathy in a 28-year-old man. A well-demarcated area of subretinal fluid is present within the fovea. Retinitic precipitates in the papillomacular bundle appear as yellow foci similar to drusen.

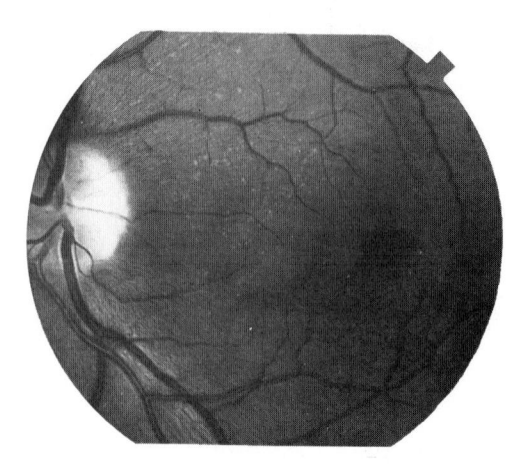

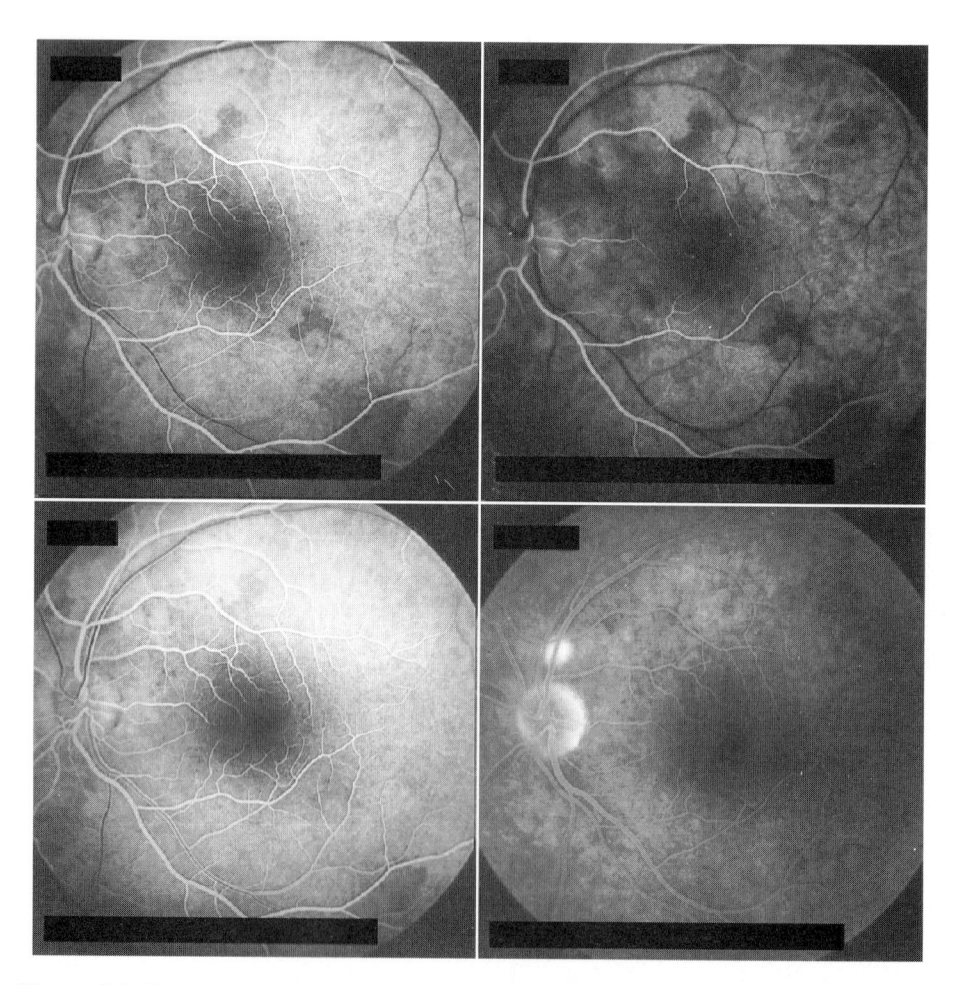

Figure 5-2 Fluorescein transit in a patient with central serous chorioretinopathy. Areas of patchy delayed choroidal fluorescence (DCF) are still visible in the laminar venous phase *(lower left)*. Note the discrete area of hyperfluorescence at the level of the retinal pigment epithelium after the completion of venous transit in an area of initial DCF just above the optic nerve *(lower right)*.

Central serous chorioretinopathy 105

tions alone or in conjunction with subretinal fluid. Limited histopathologic reports of CSCR[17,22] have thus far failed to characterize RPE detachments.

The remaining clinical appearance of the posterior pole and anterior segment is normal. Retinal abnormalities in CSCR are unassociated with other ocular findings; the optic nerve is free of anomalies, the vitreous is clear of cellular reaction, and there are usually no retinal vascular alterations.

Fluorescein Angiography

Although the diagnosis of CSCR is frequently made on the basis of history and ophthalmoscopic findings, fluorescein angiography often serves as a useful adjunct.

The fluorescein angiographic pattern characteristically involves a focus of discrete hyperfluorescence at the level of the RPE that expands circumferentially, resulting in eventual diffusion of fluorescein into the subsensory retinal space (Fig. 5-2). Unlike choroidal neovascular membrane formation, these foci of hyperfluorescence are often delayed until the conclusion of arterial-venous transit.[35,37] Nearly 30% of eyes may have more than one area of evolving hyperfluorescence, with as many as seven spots having been reported.[9,50,56] These "leakage" sites are typically grouped in a perifoveal location, with most being present in a 1 mm band 0.5 mm from the foveal avascular zone center.[50,56] A

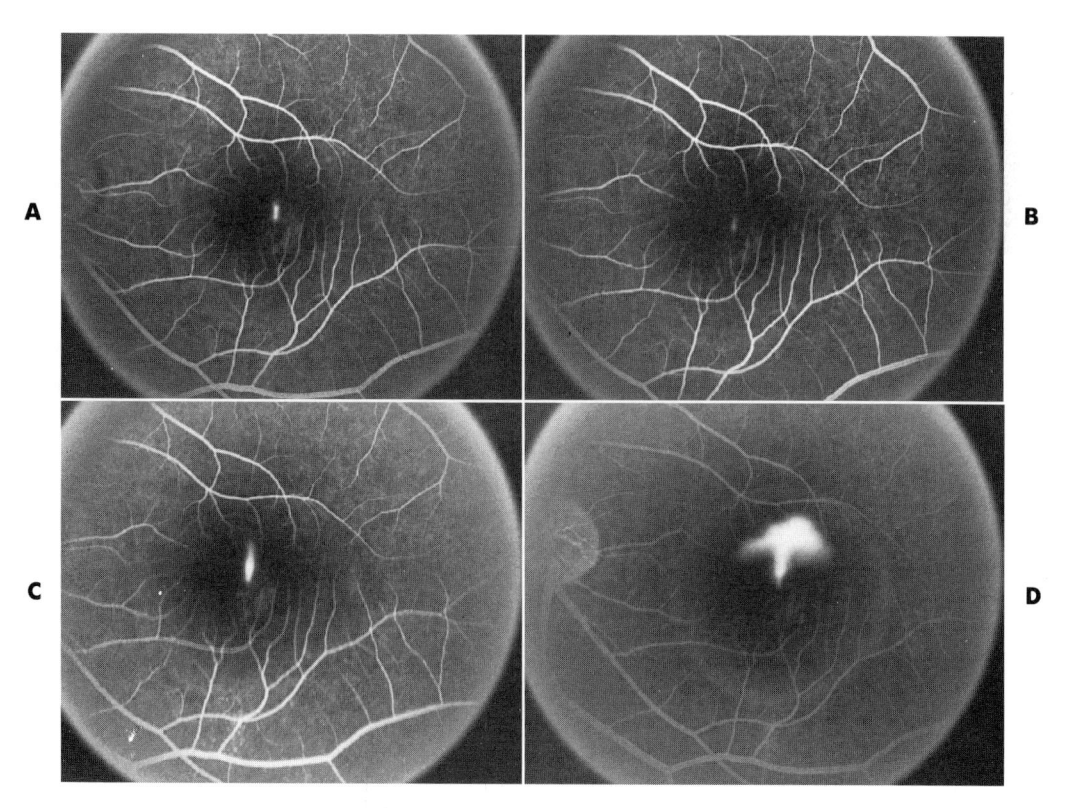

Figure 5-3 Fluorescein angiogram of a patient with the "smokestack" presentation of central serous chorioretinopathy. An initial discrete focus of hyperfluorescence, **A**, expands upward, **B** and **C**, and forms a mushroom configuration in the late frames of the study, **D**.

predilection for the area superonasal to the fovea has been described in several studies.[9,50,56] Many of these eyes have patchy choroidal filling patterns similar to those described in some age-related macular degeneration patients[41] (Fig. 5-2). Sites of RPE abnormality are frequently noted in these areas of delayed fluorescence and may imply either a delayed choroidal perfusion or an increased barrier to fluorescein transmittance.[5,30,41]

Alternatively, the classic "smokestack" pattern of hyperfluorescence has been reported[9,48,50,56,59] in 7% to 20% of affected eyes. This appearance is characterized by progressive upward expansion of fluorescein dye within the exudative detachment. It assumes a mushroom configuration as dye comes into contact with the upper limit of the sensory retinal detachment during the recirculation and late frames of the angiogram. The phenomenon has been attributed to the entry of low-density fluid into the serous retinal detachment cavity, which then rises by convection (Fig. 5-3).

Evidence of previous involvement appears angiographically as RPE transmission defects in both the involved and the contralateral eye, even in the absence of symptoms. Areas of new CSCR involvement are often near these stippled zones of fluorescence.[28]

Symptoms

Central serous chorioretinopathy produces symptoms if fixation is involved. These include mild central blurring of vision to the 20/40 range, which may be corrected with hyperopic overrefraction. Metamorphopsia—usually micropsia—with Amsler grid abnormalities, a relative central scotoma, and prolonged retinal recovery after photic exposure are frequently reported complaints. Such symptoms need to be differentiated from optic nerve disease, and this can be done by evaluation of pupillary function, Ishiara plates, photostress testing, and formal visual fields if necessary. The patient is usually without systemic complaints and has an unremarkable past medical history and general physical examination.

Etiology

Central serous chorioretinopathy is predominantly found in young healthy adults between the ages of 20 and 45 years, with a 10:1 male preponderance.[12,59] Associations with trauma, pregnancy, allergy, migraine, and certain medications such as antibiotics and steroids have all been noted.[3,18,21,53] Gelber and Schatz[15] and Yannuzzi[58] have described a significant proportion of their patients to have Type A personality behavior patterns. Increased catecholamine release in such individuals was postulated as a contributor in the pathogenesis of CSCR. Yoshioka[61] and Yoshioka et al.[62] have experimentally reproduced CSCR in monkeys after repeated intravenous injections of epinephrine. Histologic findings in these eyes included endothelial cell alteration in the choriocapillaris with platelet-fibrin clots and overlying RPE alterations.

NATURAL COURSE

An episode of CSCR ordinarily has a defined course of several weeks to months with resultant resolution of the initial clinical findings and return to normal visual acuity.[7,16,27] Some patients, however, may experience persistent visual blur, reduced retinal sensitivity and color perception, along with distortion that may last months or become permanent despite clinical resolution.[4,11,52] Chaung et al.[4] have noted persistent psychophysical abnormalities in areas of previous CSCR involvement despite normal acuities.

Recurrences in the same or contralateral eye are not unusual in up to 50% of patients.[7,12,28,57,59] These additional episodes are usually noted within 1 year of previous occurrences but may be separated by several years. New occurrences may be located anywhere within the macula, many close to previous episodes.

A subset of eyes will develop clinical and angiographic evidence of progressive diffuse retinal pigment epithelial decompression with inferior tracking of subretinal fluid leading to progressive macular dysfunction and visual loss. The reasons for this progression are unclear but may support theories of more diffuse, rather than focal, RPE abnormalities in CSCR.[28,46]

DIFFERENTIAL DIAGNOSIS

The differential diagnosis of CSCR should include all macular exudative or pseudoexudative processes resulting in pigment epithelial and/or sensory retinal elevation. Accurate historical, systemic, ophthalmoscopic, and angiographic evaluation helps shorten the list of likely alternate diagnoses.

Age-Related Macular Degeneration (ARMD)

Since CSCR is a condition found mainly in young to middle-aged adults, patients over the age of 50 years should be viewed with some caution prior to the establishment of a diagnosis based solely on ophthalmoscopic grounds. Clearly, CSCR shares common clinical features with ARMD, and these distinctions become more difficult as patient age progresses past 50.[8,28,60] Evidence of extensive drusen or choroidal neovascularization, including retinal hemorrhage or hard exudate, is not consistent with a diagnosis of CSCR. Fluorescein angiography may be useful in these situations, although cases of chronic CSCR may be difficult to differentiate from occult neovascularization or diffuse RPE alterations found in nonexudative ARMD (Fig. 5-4).

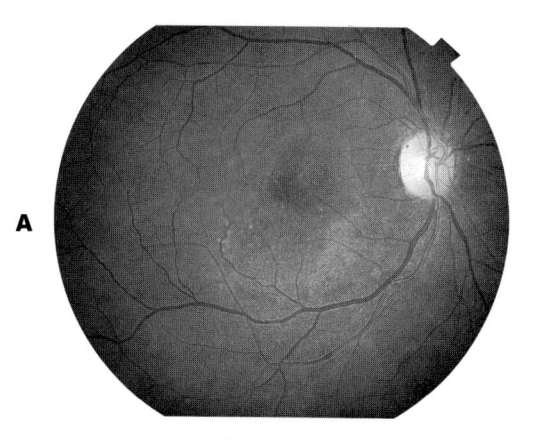

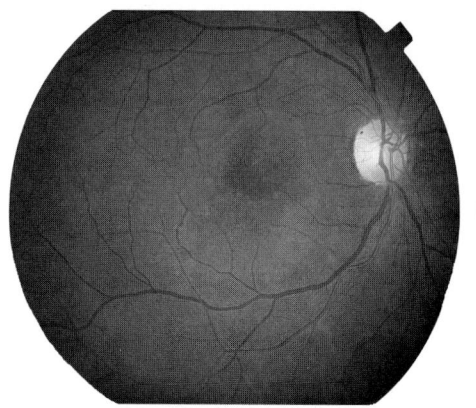

Figure 5-4 Chronic central serous chorioretinopathy. Fluorescein angiography reveals extensive areas of mottled hyperfluorescence present at the level of the retinal pigment epithelium, **A.** This eye also evidenced inferior tracking with dependent subretinal fluid. Clinical findings are often subtle when compared to the extensive angiographic changes **B.**

Congenital Optic Nerve Pits

Pits of the optic nerve are frequently associated with macular detachment because of sensory retinal elevation or, as more recently suggested, retinoschis. These are congenital abnormalities and believed to be abnormal vestiges of the embryonic epithelial papilla.[26,31] Symptoms of central visual loss in young adults with associated well-demarcated macular fluid, loss of the foveal reflex, pigment epithelial alterations, and retinitic precipitates all closely mimic in clinical features CSCR.[26] Ophthalmoscopic evaluation of the optic nerve usually reveals an oval to round well-demarcated depression in the temporal optic nerve tissue that may vary from white to black and be easily overlooked in cursory macular examinations.

Choroidal Tumors

Many choroidal tumors may involve the posterior pole, resulting in elevation of the macula and possible accumulation of intra- or subretinal fluid. Choroidal melanomas, choroidal hemangiomas, and metastatic carcinomas can all mimic CSCR.[10] Close biomicroscopic evaluation is usually sufficient to eliminate these entities.

Choroidal Inflammatory Disease

Many primary and secondary ocular inflammatory conditions may lead to the development of overlying RPE dysfunction with the resultant accumulation of fluid in the subretinal space and hyperfluorescent foci at fluorescein angiography (Fig. 5-5). These findings may be unassociated with overlying retinal vascular abnormalities, making their diagnosis difficult. Posterior scleritis, sympathetic ophthalmia, Harada's disease, and secondary involvement from systemic conditions (e.g., systemic lupus erythematosus, polyarteritis nodosa, and other related collagen vascular disorders) may all mimic CSCR[25,57]; however, the presence of associated inflammatory signs, including anterior segment or vitreous cells, disc edema, scleral injection, and ocular discomfort—along with systemic abnormalities and pertinent historical information—will help eliminate these conditions.

Choroidal Vascular Disease

Accelerated or malignant hypertension, toxemia, coagulopathies, and the abovementioned inflammatory conditions may all lead to sensory retinal detachment and RPE abnormalities. Segmental closure of choroidal vessels with secondary pigment epithelial disruption is thought to be the mode of action.[6,14]

Retinal Detachment

Rhegmatogenous retinal detachment may be responsible for subtle subretinal fluid within the macula, but the association of retinal tears and extension of fluid to the retinal periphery (i.e., the ora serrata) are sufficient to make this diagnosis.

Exudative retinal detachment can be associated with many vascular and inflammatory conditions as well as with idiopathic entities like the uveal effusion syndrome.

Macular Hole

Full-thickness and lamellar macular hole formation, impending macular hole, and pseudomacular hole associated with surface wrinkling all demonstrate a well-demarcated orange foveal pattern that may resemble a focal RPE elevation or abnormality similar to that found in CSCR.

Optic Neuropathies

Optic nerve disease often involves young to middle-aged adults and produces a central field deficit. Optic neuritis may even follow a several-week time course of visual improvement similar to that with CSCR. The presence of an afferent pupillary defect, color plate changes, and optic nerve abnormalities, along with the absence of macular findings, will differentiate these conditions.

PATHOGENESIS

The etiology of CSCR is unknown, although clinical and experimental data suggest a primary or secondary dysfunction of the RPE as the principal determiner of the clinical and angiographic appearance in this condition. Early speculation was based on fluorescein angiographic findings of dye "leakage" into the subsensory retinal compartment. This led to the hypothesis that a focal RPE defect was allowing free fluid movement in a choroidal-to-vitreal direction. Increasing information, however, regarding RPE physiology and fluid dynamics in the eye makes this less certain.* Recent theories[5,30,32,44,49] have focused on alterations in choroidal perfusion and changes in the relative polarity of RPE cells—with resultant changes in ion flux and bulk fluid flow. Our understanding of CSCR development requires the application of general physical principles, ophthalmoscopic and angiographic observations, ocular fluid dynamics, and retina/retinal pigment epithelial/choroidal pathophysiology. An important physical point to keep in mind regards the process of *diffusion* (i.e., unrestricted movement of free particles down a concentration gradient, such as with fluorescein, does not require fluid movement).

Important clinical points in CSCR include
1. Movement of fluorescein dye in the normal eye is restricted by the zonulae occludentes—tight junctions—of the RPE cells. This normally prevents fluorescein from entering the subretinal space.
2. Serous fluid accumulates in a discrete subretinal location without progressive expansion.
3. Focal laser treatment to the RPE focus of increasing hyperfluorescence shortens the natural course of individual episodes.

Important experimental observations include the following:
1. Intraocular fluid normally moves in a vitreal-to-choroidal direction, with prime contributors to this flow being
   a. Hydrostatic pressure
   b. High oncotic pressure of the choroid
   c. Retinal pigment epithelial cell polarity, which creates fluid flow in an apical (retinal side) to basal (choroidal side) direction

---

*References 32-34, 40, 42, 51, 62.

2. The sensory retina offers greater resistance to fluorescein and water movement than the RPE does. This differential resistance is also likely to contribute to retinal adhesion.[40,42,51]
3. Destruction of RPE cells leads initially to greater fluid outflow in the direction of the choroid in experimentally produced serous retinal detachments.

Piccolino[44] and Spitznas[49] first challenged conventional views of CSCR pathogenesis by emphasizing that the direction of fluorescein dye did not necessarily correspond to fluid movement. Spitznas[49] theorized that fluid accumulation beneath the retina was due to a change in RPE cell polarity. Under these conditions pigment epithelial cells would reverse the normal direction of their cell membrane ion pumps, leading to secondary fluid movement in a retinal direction. This fluid flow would initially be transcellular but would later cause disruption of the RPE tight junctions with resultant fluorescein "leakage" into the subretinal space. Eventually a steady state would be achieved wherein the reversal of flow created by localized abnormal RPE cells would be checked by surrounding normal functioning RPE cells.[49]

Marmor[32] elaborated on these thoughts by suggesting that damaged metabolic transport across the retinal pigment epithelium occurs in the presence of an intact blood-retina barrier. In this scenario an alteration of ion flux across the RPE results not in a reversal but in slowed movement of water across the pigment epithelium. This decreased flow is then overwhelmed by a focal RPE "leak" that allows fluid to pass from the choroid to the subretinal space. Choroidal vasculature pulsations or vitreoscleral movement during saccades are postulated as the driving force in propelling choroidal fluid through this leakage site.[32]

All present working hypotheses of fluid dynamics in CSCR assume a choroidal source for the subretinal fluid. It would seem logical, however, to consider the source to be from the vitreal side of the retina. Normal fluid flow within the eye is known to occur in a vitreal-to-choroidal direction. Choroidal oncotic pressure, ocular hydrostatic pressure, and active pigment epithelial transport all contribute to this unidirectional flow. Resistance to normal fluid movement is known to be greater in the sensory retina than the RPE.[40,42,51] This relative difference in fluid conductivity helps maintain retinal apposition. If a primary event, such as segmental choroidal hypoperfusion, were to slow RPE transport and increase resistance to solute flow across the pigment epithelium to a point where it superseded retinal resistance, then the development of a sensory retinal detachment would become possible. This would not require a reversal of the normal fluid flow across the pigment epithelium as suggested by Spitznas.[49] Disruption of the blood-retinal barrier could also be secondary to the same primary event that led to RPE transport dysfunction (e.g., hypoperfusion). The movement of fluorescein from the choroid could then be viewed simply as a molecule flowing down its concentration gradient.

A recent review of fluorescein angiographic data[30] has shown a delayed choroidal fluorescence (DCF) in over 50% of CSCR patients. Of this group, a significant number had their focus of RPE leakage at a confluence of these hypofluorescent areas, which appeared as watershed zones between individual short posterior ciliary arteries. Delayed choroidal filling has also been noted with indocyanine green angiography, and similar fluorescein angiographic findings have been reported in patients with ARMD.[19,20,41,47] Since vascular watershed zones are known to be more susceptible to hypoperfusion, areas of pigment epithelium overlying them should be more at risk for metabolic dysfunction.

Treatment

Conventional therapy for CSCR involves either (1) reassurance with conservative observation until spontaneous resolution or (2) focal laser photocoagulation.* Laser photocoagulation has been shown to shorten the duration of an individual episode of CSCR and lead to resolution within 2 to 4 weeks. Some authors[27,45] have suggested that laser also decreases the frequency of recurrences while lessening the possible development of a chronic form of the disease, and therefore improving the long-term visual prognosis; however, other prospective data have failed to show a long-term benefit in these treated eyes and question the need for intervention in a usually self-limited and benign macular condition.

Guidelines for laser therapy have been suggested by several authors.† These approaches require an individualized approach with special attention given to the patient's personal needs and the eye's clinical and fluorescein angiographic findings. Treatment of foveal and near parafoveal foci of hyperfluorescence should be avoided. Recommendations for treatment include

1. Occupational demands (patients whose employment requires fine binocular vision and stereopsis)
2. Progressive visual loss to less than 20/40
3. Prolonged course (eyes in which symptoms and clinical findings have been present without evidence of resolution for greater than 4 months)
4. Previous episodes (patients who have experienced previous episodes that resulted in visual loss in the affected or contralateral eye; these individuals should be considered for earlier intervention with photocoagulation)
5. Biomicroscopic evidence of permanent changes in retinal, RPE, or choroidal morphology

Although both direct treatment of RPE leakage sites and indirect applications to removed areas within the sensory detachment have been advocated, more recent studies seem to favor direct treatment alone.[7,46,55] It is important to emphasize that these studies have small numbers of patients. The mechanism of laser effect in direct treatment is thought to involve debridement of abnormal RPE cells, allowing subsequent occupation of these treated areas by normal pigment epithelium, which reestablishes the blood-retina barrier.[37,46] In addition, focal elimination of the RPE barrier is known to speed the resorption of subretinal fluid in experimentally produced retinal detachments.[36-38]

Since focal elimination of the pigment epithelium alone is the goal of treatment, care should be taken to avoid excessive energies, which might produce unwanted retinal or choroidal injury. Complications of exuberant laser therapy are well documented and include permanent paracentral scotomas and the development of choroidal neovascular membrane formation.[23,45,55] The incidence of CNVM development has been reported to vary between 0% and 5% and may be explained in at least some cases by misdiagnosis of ophthalmoscopic and fluorescein angiographic features.[23]

---

*References 7, 24, 27, 39, 45, 46, 54, 55.
†References 27, 39, 45, 46, 54, 55.

Treatment strategy involves the application of subconfluent light gray laser burns to the area of focal angiographic hyperfluorescence. A larger spot size, with longer duration and low energy levels, will give the desired effect while minimizing the risk of damage to Bruch's membrane and subsequent CNVM formation.[7,27,45,46]

VARIANTS

Chronic CSCR

Although the majority of eyes with CSCR will have self-limited episodes with return to near normal vision, some will develop chronic or recurrent areas of dependent subretinal fluid accumulation and RPE alteration that extend inferiorly from the macula to the peripheral fundus.[8,23,60] These pigment epithelial tracts assume a teardrop shape and originate in the macula, often in a peripapillary location.[23a,60] They are best seen with fluorescein angiography and may be easily missed on biomicroscopic evaluation (Fig. 5-5). Associated retinal abnormalities, including retinal capillary telangiectasia, cystoid macular edema, hard exudate formation, disciform scarring, and bone spicule formation, have all been described as well as atrophy of the choriocapillaris.[23a,60]

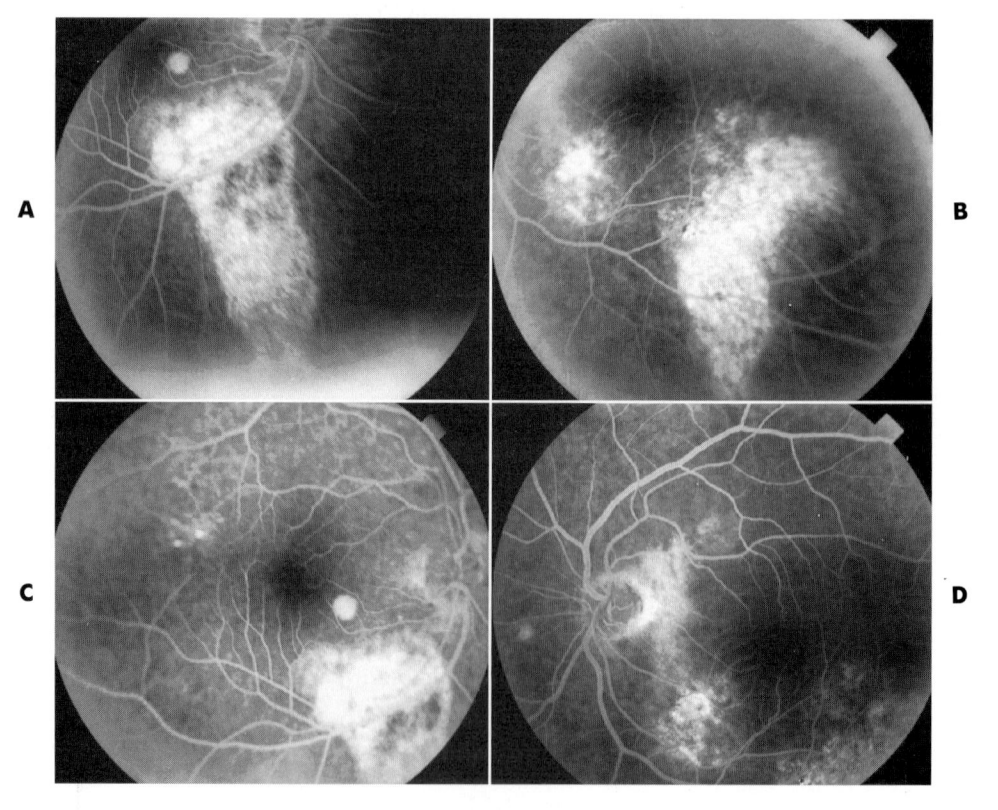

Figure 5-5 Chronic central serous chorioretinopathy. Inferior tracking of subretinal fluid causes extensive pigment epithelial alterations well visualized on fluorescein angiography, **A** and **B.** This patient had bilateral involvement. Note the well-circumscribed pigment epithelial elevation in the nasal parafovea of the right eye, **C.**

Patients with these findings tend to be older than those with typical CSCR. Vision loss is dependent on the location of the RPE defects, but 25% of patients will have a visual acuity of 20/200 or less.[60] The possibility of occult choroidal neovascularization should always be considered.

Bullous CSCR

Bullous CSCR presents an unusual clinical picture, a more extreme variant of the spectrum associated with this disorder. Patients tend to be male (over 90% of the cases) and often have bilateral involvement with multiple areas of RPE elevation larger than in the more typical cases. These lead to bullous sensory retinal detachments with shifting fluid and the presence of a grayish yellow subretinal fibrinous exudate[1,11] (Fig. 5-6). As in other cases of CSCR, the patients are in generally good health, although Gass[13] has reported two individuals who also had renal failure. The differential diagnosis includes vascular, inflammatory, and idiopathic conditions associated with pigment epithelial alteration and exudative retinal detachment.

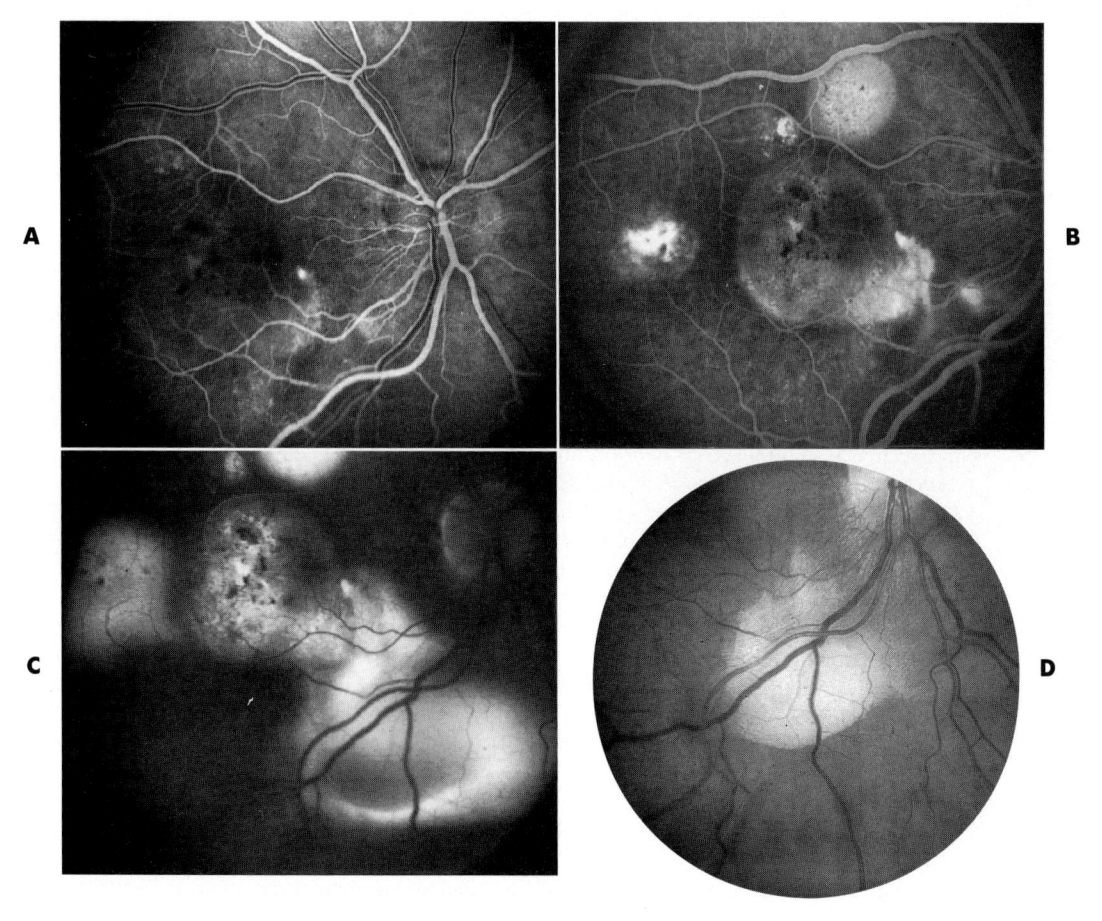

Figure 5-6 Bullous central serous chorioretinopathy. Note the focus of hyperfluorescence at the level of the retinal pigment epithelium in the laminar venous phase, **A.** Fluorescein is later found to cascade inferiorly into a larger area of exudative retinal detachment, **B** and **C.** A yellow subretinal fibrinous exudate is well seen in the area of serous elevation, **D.**

References

1. Benson WE, Shields JA, Annesley WH, Tasman W: Central serous chorioretinopathy with bullous retinal detachment, *Ann Ophthalmol* 12:920-924, 1980.
2. Brown GC, Shields JA, Goldberg RE: Congenital pits of the optic nerve head. II. Clinical studies in humans, *Ophthalmology* 87:51-65, 1980.
3. Cassel GH, Brown GC, Annesley WH: Central serous chorioretinopathy: a seasonal variation? *Br J Ophthalmol* 68:724-726, 1984.
4. Chaung EL, Sharp DM, Fitzke FW, et al: Retinal dysfunction in central serous retinopathy, *Eye* 1:120-125, 1987.
5. Cotallo JL, Salvador R, Andres M, et al: Pathogenesis of idiopathic central serous chorioretinopathy: vascular choroidal hypothesis, *Arch Soc Esp Oftalmol* 53:491-500, 1987.
6. de Venecia G, Jampol LM: The eye in accelerated hypertension. II. Localized serous detachments of the retina in patients, *Arch Ophthalmol* 102:68-73, 1984.
7. Ficker L, Vafadis G, While A, Leaver P: Long-term follow-up of a prospective trial of argon laser photocoagulation in the treatment of central serous retinopathy, *Br J Ophthalmol* 72:829-834, 1988.
8. Frederick AR: Multifocal and recurrent (serous) choroidopathy (MARC) syndrome: a new variety of idiopathic central serous choroidopathy, *Doc Ophthalmol* 56:203-235, 1984.
9. Friberg TR, Campagna J: Central serous chorioretinopathy: an analysis of the clinical morphology using image-processing techniques, *Graefes Arch Clin Exp Ophthalmol* 227:201-205, 1989.
10. Fry WE, Spaeth EB: Subacute circumscribed macular retinochoroiditis simulating intraocular tumor, *Trans Am Acad Ophthalmol* 59:346-355, 1955.
11. Fuhrmeister H: A long-term study of morphological and functional developments after central serous chorioretinitis, *Klin Monatsbl Augenheilkd* 182:549-551, 1983.
12. Gass JDM: Pathogenesis of disciform detachment of the neuro-epithelium. II. Idiopathic central serous choroidopathy, *Am J Ophthalmol* 63:587-615, 1967.
13. Gass JDM: Bullous retinal detachment: an unusual manifestation of idiopathic central serous choroidopathy, *Am J Ophthalmol* 75:810-821, 1973.
14. Gaudric A, Sterkers M, Coscas G: Retinal detachment after choroidal ischemia, *Am J Ophthalmol* 104:364-372, 1987.
15. Gelber GS, Schatz H: Loss of vision due to central serous chorioretinopathy following psychological stress, *Am J Psychiatry* 144:46-50, 1987.
16. Gilbert CM, Owens SL, Smith PD, Fine SL: Long-term follow-up of central serous chorioretinopathy, *Br J Ophthalmol* 68:815-820, 1984.
17. Green WR: Central serous chorioretinopathy. In Spencer WH (ed): *Ophthalmic pathology: an atlas and textbook,* Philadelphia, 1985, WB Saunders, pp 1017-1018.
18. Harada T, Harada K: Six cases of central serous choroidopathy induced by systemic corticosteroid therapy, *Doc Ophthalmol* 60:37-44, 1985.
19. Hayashi K, Hasegawa Y, Tokoro T: Indocyanine green angiography of central serous chorioretinopathy, *Int Ophthalmol* 9:37-41, 1986.
20. Hayashi K, Laey JJ: Indocyanine green angiography of choroidal neovascular membranes, *Ophthalmologica* 190:30, 1985.
21. Hurault De Ligny B, Sirbat D, Kessler M, et al: Ocular side effects of flumequine: 3 cases of central serous retinopathy, *Therapie* 39:595-600, 1984.
22. Ikui H: Histological examination of central serous retinopathy, *Folia Ophthalmol Jpn* 20:1035-1043, 1969.
23. Ishibashi R, Yoshioka H: Relationship between idiopathic central serous choroidopathy and idiopathic macular choroidal neovascularization, *Folia Ophthalmol Jpn* 40:316-320, 1989.
23a. Jalkh AE, Jabbour N, Avila MP, et al: Retinal pigment epithelium decompression. I. Clinical features and natural course, *Ophthalmology* 91:1544-1548, 1984.
24. Klein ML, Van Buskirk FM, Friedman E, et al: Experience with nontreatment of central serous chorioretinopathy, *Arch Ophthalmol* 91:247-250, 1974.
25. Klien BA: Macular and extramacular serous chorioretinopathy: with remarks upon the role of an extrabulbar mechanism in its pathogenesis, *Am J Ophthalmol* 64:3-23, 1961.

26. Kranenbrug EW: Crater-like holes in the optic disc and central serous retinopathy, *Arch Ophthalmol* 64:912-928, 1960.
27. Leaver P, Williams C: Argon laser photocoagulation in the treatment of central serous retinopathy, *Br J Ophthalmol* 63:674-677, 1979.
28. Levine R, Brucker AJ, Fane R: Long-term follow-up of idiopathic central serous chorioretinopathy by fluorescein angiography, *Ophthalmology* 96:854-859, 1989.
29. Lu JG, Friberg TR: Idiopathic central serous retinopathy in China: a report of 600 cases (624 eyes) treated by acupuncture, *Ophthalmic Surg* 18:608-611, 1987.
30. Maguire JI, Annesley WH, Fischer DH: Delayed choroidal fluorescence in central serous chorioretinopathy. (Submitted for publication.)
31. Mann I: *Developmental abnormalities of the eye,* ed 2, Philadelphia, 1957, JB Lippincott, pp 113-116.
32. Marmor MF: New hypothesis on the pathogenesis and treatment of serous retinal detachment. *Graefes Arch Clin Exp Ophthalmol* 226:548-552, 1988.
33. Marmor MF, Maack T: Enhancement of retinal adhesion and subretinal fluid resorption by acetazolamide, *Invest Ophthalmol Vis Sci* 23:121-124, 1982.
34. Moseley M, Johnson NF, Foulds WS: Vitreo-scleral fluid transfer in the rabbit, *Acta Ophthalmol* 56:769-776, 1978.
35. Mutlak JA, Dutton GN: Fluorescein angiographic features of acute central serous retinopathy: a retrospective study, *Acta Ophthalmol* 67:467-469, 1989.
36. Negi A, Marmor MF: Experimental serous retinal detachment and focal pigment epithelial damage, *Arch Ophthalmol* 102:445-449, 1984.
37. Negi A, Marmor MF: Healing of photocoagulation lesions affects the rate of subretinal fluid resorption, *Ophthalmology* 91:1678-1683, 1984.
38. Negi A, Marmor MF: Quantitative estimation of metabolic transport of subretinal fluid, *Invest Ophthalmol Vis Sci* 27:1564-1568, 1986.
39. Novak MA, Singerman LJ, Rice TA: Krypton and argon laser photocoagulation for central serous chorioretinopathy, *Retina* 7:162-169, 1987.
40. Orr G, Goodnight R, Lean JS: Relative permeability of retina and retinal pigment epithelium to the diffusion of tritiated water from vitreous to choroid, *Arch Ophthalmol* 104:1678-1680, 1986.
41. Pauleikhoff D, Chen JC, Chisholm IH, Bird AC: Choroidal perfusion abnormality in age related macular disease, *Am J Ophthalmol* 109:171, 1991.
42. Pederson JE, Cantrill HL: Experimental retinal detachment. V. Fluid movement through the retinal hole, *Arch Ophthalmol* 102:136-139, 1984.
43. Peyman GA, Bok D: Peroxidase diffusion in the normal and laser-coagulated primate retina, *Invest Ophthalmol* 11:35-45, 1972.
44. Piccolino FC: Central serous chorioretinopathy some considerations on the pathogenesis, *Ophthalmologica* 182:204-210, 1982.
45. Robertson DM: Argon laser photocoagulation treatment in central serous chorioretinopathy, *Ophthalmology* 93:972-974, 1986.
46. Robertson DM, Ilstrup D: Direct, indirect, and sham laser photocoagulation in the management of central serous chorioretinopathy, *Am J Ophthalmol* 95:457-466, 1983.
47. Scheider A, Nasemann JE, Lund OE: Fluorescein and indocyanine green angiographies of central serous choroidopathy by scanning laser ophthalmoscopy, *Am J Ophthalmol* 115:50-56, 1993.
48. Shimizu K, Tobari I: Central serous retinopathy dynamics of subretinal fluid, *Mod Probl Ophthalmol* 9:152-157, 1971.
49. Spitznas M: Pathogenesis of central serous retinopathy: a new working hypothesis, *Graefes Arch Clin Exp Ophthalmol* 224:321-324, 1986.
50. Spitznas M, Huke J: Number, shape, and topography of leakage points in acute type I central serous retinopathy, *Graefes Arch Clin Exp Ophthalmol* 225:437-440, 1987.
51. Tsuboi S, Fujimoto T, Uchihori Y, et al: Measurement of retinal permeability to sodium fluorescein in vitro, *Invest Ophthalmol Vis Sci* 25:1146-1150, 1984.
52. van Meel GJ, Smith VC, Pokorny J, van Norren D: Foveal densitometry in central serous choroidopathy, *Am J Ophthalmol* 98:359-368, 1984.

53. Wakakura M, Ishikawa S: Central serous chorioretinopathy complicating systemic corticosteroid treatment, *Br J Ophthalmol* 68:329-331, 1984.
54. Watzke RC, Burton TC, Leaverton PE: Ruby laser photocoagulation therapy of central serous retinopathy. Part I: a controlled clinical study. II. Factors affecting prognosis, *Trans Am Acad Ophthalmol Otolaryngol* 78:205-211, 1974.
55. Watzke RC, Burton YC, Woolsen RF: Direct and indirect laser photocoagulation of central serous choroidopathy, *Am J Ophthalmol* 88:914-918, 1979.
56. Wessing A: Grundsatzliches zum diagnostischen fortschritt durch die fluoreszenzanangiographie, *Ber Dtsch Ophthalmol Gesundhdt* 73:566-568, 1975.
57. Wessing A: Central serous retinopathy and related lesions, *Mod Probl Ophthalmol* 9:148-151, 1971.
58. Yannuzzi LA: Type-A behavior and central serous chorioretinopathy, *Retina* 7:111-131, 1987.
59. Yannuzzi LA, Gitter KA, Schatz H: Central serous chorioretinopathy. In *The macula: a comprehensive text and atlas,* Baltimore, 1979, Williams & Wilkins, pp 145-165.
60. Yannuzzi LA, Shakin JL, Fisher YL, Altomonte MA: Peripheral retinal detachments and retinal pigment epithelial atrophic tracts secondary to central serous pigment epitheliopathy, *Ophthalmology* 91:1554-1572, 1984.
61. Yoshioka H: Some new findings in central serous choroidopathy, *Folia Ophthalmol Jpn* 38:42-56, 1987.
62. Yoshioka H, Katsume Y, Akune H: Experimental central serous chorioretinopathy. I. Clinical findings, *Jpn J Ophthalmol* 25:112-118, 1981.
63. Zauberman H: Adhesive forces between the retinal pigment epithelium and sensory retina. In Zinn K, Marmor MF (eds): *The retinal pigment epithelium,* Cambridge Mass, 1979, Harvard University Press, p 226.

6

Idiopathic Macular Holes

James F. Vander

Idiopathic macular holes generally occur in older patients, affecting women more often than men, and typically reduce visual acuity to the 20/100-20/400 range.[1] Bilateral holes occur in less than 10% to 20% of cases.[2] Once a full-thickness macular hole has formed, the visual loss is usually stationary although, rarely, spontaneous improvement or deterioration can occur. Painless blurring of vision with a central scotoma is the usual presenting symptom. Metamorphopsia may also be present. While some patients may be symptomatic during the process of macular hole formation (a process which may occur over several days or weeks, as discussed below), many cases are discovered only after incidental closure of the fellow eye or at the time of routine ophthalmological evaluation.

FINDINGS

Examination of a patient with an idiopathic macular hole will reveal diminished visual acuity with preservation of the peripheral field. The Amsler grid will show a central scotoma or, frequently, just central distortion. The anterior segment is normal. Fundoscopic examination will reveal an absence of retinal tissue, usually fairly well centered on the fovea. The hole is generally circular and of variable size, measuring between 200 and 1000 μm in most cases (Fig. 6-1). The absence of foveal tissue enhances visualization of the choroid and RPE, producing a relative cherry-red spot. Yellow flecks resembling drusen may be seen at the level of the RPE within the hole (Fig. 6-2) and may represent localized proliferation of the RPE similar to those seen in patients with chronic retinal detachment.[3]

A hallmark of idiopathic macular holes is the presence of an associated halo of serous retinal detachment.[1] The size of this halo is variable, although generally at least a small amount of fluid is present. Progressive enlargement characteristic of most typical *rhegmatogenous* retinal detachments is uncommon. There is often secondary intraretinal edema present overlying the subretinal fluid as well. Spontaneous resolution of the subretinal fluid, with resultant visual improvement, has been reported.[4] After the edges of the retina flatten, the holes have been noted ophthalmoscopically to "disappear."

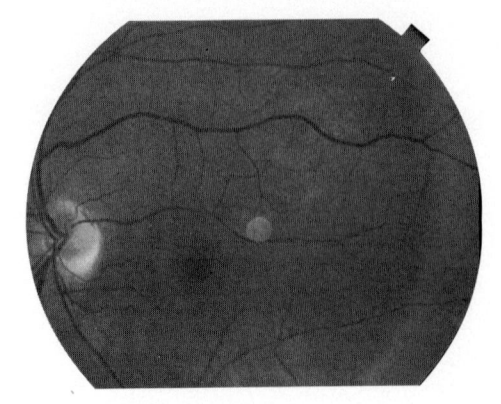

Figure 6-1 Typical appearance of an idiopathic macular hole.

Figure 6-2 Flecks within the base of a macular hole at the level of the retinal pigment epithelium.

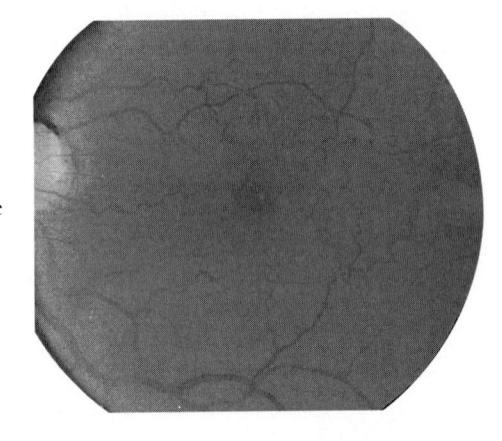

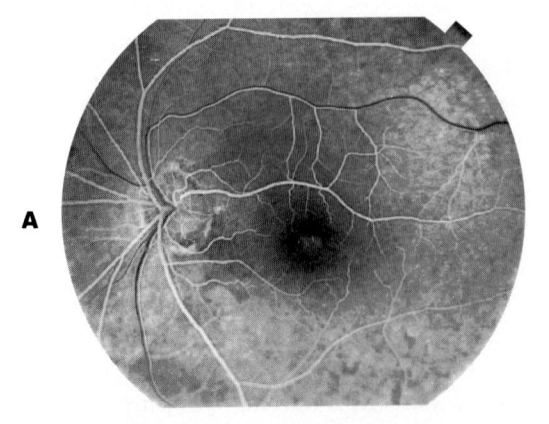

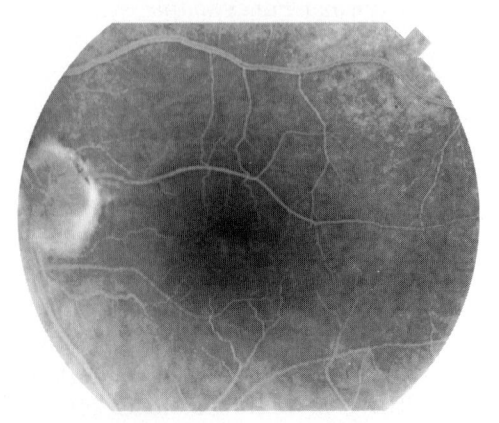

Figure 6-3 Fluorescein angiogram of a patient with a macular hole. **A,** The transit phase shows hyperfluorescence at the level of the retinal pigment epithelium corresponding to the size of the hole. **B,** The late recirculation phase shows staining of the same area.

Fluorescein angiography is occasionally helpful in the diagnosis of macular hole. There is usually a circular area of early hyperfluorescence comparable in size to the hole seen clinically[3] (Fig. 6-3). This transmission defect will usually fade as the background choroidal blush fades. Proposed etiologies for it include thinning of the RPE and loss of the macular xanthophyll. Heavily pigmented fundi may not show it well.

PATHOGENESIS

The etiology and natural history of full-thickness macular holes have been a matter of considerable controversy, producing numerous theories.[5-6] Much of the confusion relates to widely varying interpretations of the status of the posterior vitreous and the central fovea in patients with idiopathic macular hole. For example, the prevalence of complete posterior vitreous detachment (PVD) at the time of macular hole diagnosis has ranged from 12% to 100%![5-10] One hypothesis, favored by those who noted a high incidence of PVD,[5-7] is that abnormal vitreoretinal adhesion at the fovea in combination with anteroposterior traction occurring at the time of the PVD leads to hole formation. Morgan and Schatz[9] proposed the concept of "involutional macular thinning," in which relative choroidal vascular insufficiency in the fovea produces atrophic retinal changes that, along with vitreoretinal traction, leads to hole formation.

More recently Gass[10] has suggested that contraction of prefoveal cortical vitreous produces tangential traction on the retina leading to hole formation. In addition, he has proposed a staging system outlining the evolution of idiopathic macular holes (Fig. 6-4). Given the confusion and inconsistencies that have characterized our understanding of macular holes, development of such a classification is a critical advancement. Although Gass' hypothesis and classification are unproven, they are consistent with most observations related to macular holes and are currently held in wide favor.

- A Stage 1 macular hole is defined as a yellow spot or ring in the fovea with a loss of the normal foveal depression (Fig. 6-5). It results when tangential traction of cortical vitreous causes a foveolar detachment. Mild visual loss with metamorphopsia at distance or near is frequently present. Fluorescein angiography shows minimal or no central hyperfluorescence without late staining. Spontaneous release of the vitreous from the fovea, with resolution of symptoms and reformation of the foveal reflex, may occur. Others will progress to development of a full-thickness hole. The exact incidence of this progression is unknown, although the risk seems to be highest in patients with an idiopathic macular hole in the fellow eye.
- A Stage 2 hole is a full-thickness defect, usually measuring less than 200 μm in diameter, that may show yellow RPE precipitates and well-defined hyperfluorescence on fluorescein angiography. The vision may drop further at this stage depending on whether the small hole is central or eccentric. This hole will typically progress over several days or weeks to a typical Stage 3 or Stage 4 macular hole measuring ≥500 μm with associated subretinal fluid at the edges and diminished vision.

    Gass categorizes holes as Stage 3 if there is vitreofoveal separation but the remainder of the premacular vitreous remains adherent and Stage 4 if there is posterior vitreous separation.

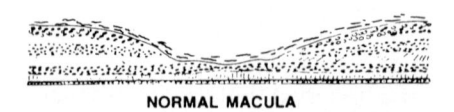

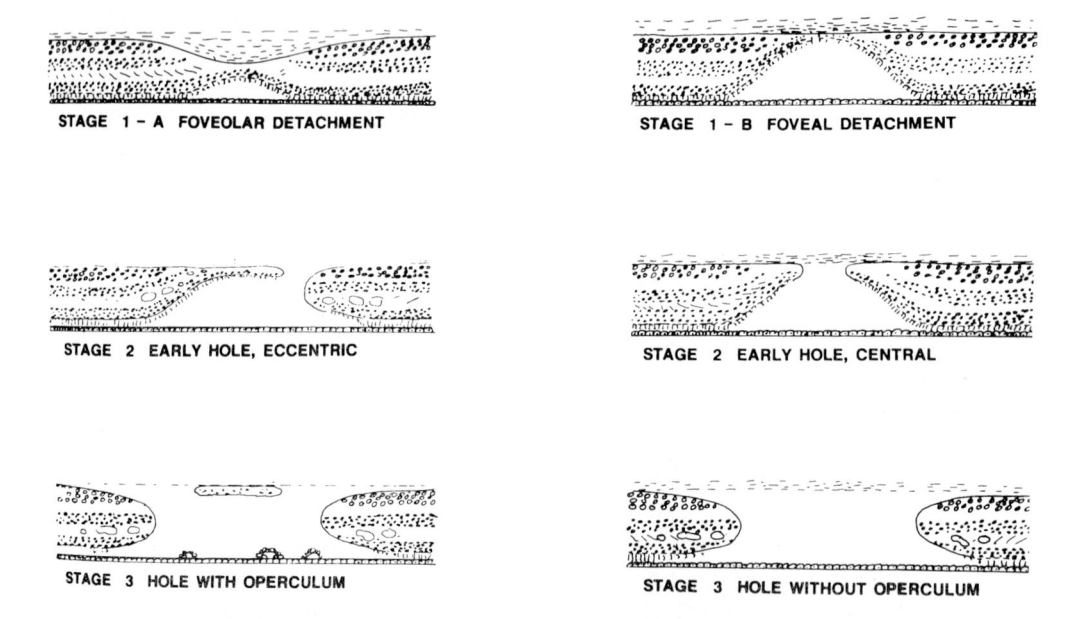

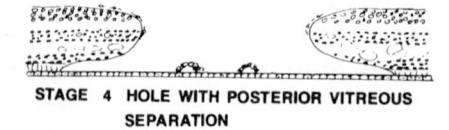

Figure 6-4 Stages of idiopathic macular hole development according to the Gass classification.

From Johnson RN, Gass JD: *Ophthalmology* 95:917, 1988.

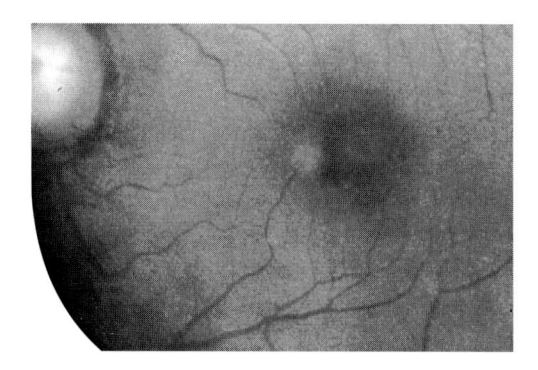

Figure 6-5 Stage 1B impending macular hole.

DIFFERENTIAL DIAGNOSIS
Pseudomacular Hole

Distinguishing between a true and a pseudomacular hole can sometimes be problematic, especially since these patients tend to be older and frequently have some degree of cataract that may impair optimum visualization of the macular detail. Longstanding cystoid macular edema may lead to rupture of the inner wall of the foveolar cyst. This inner lamellar hole may appear similar to a full-thickness idiopathic macular hole with its associated halo of fluid. These patients will not have the yellow deposits at the RPE seen within a full-thickness hole, however. Also, fluorescein angiography will show late leakage within the intact cystic cavities, but the ruptured cyst does not retain fluorescein dye and so should appear hypofluorescent, in contrast to an idiopathic macular hole.[3]

Epiretinal membranes and vitreoretinal traction syndrome are two abnormalities of the vitreoretinal interface that might be confused with idiopathic macular hole.[3] Occasionally holes within an epiretinal membrane will occur over the fovea and produce an excavated foveal appearance. Again, yellow deposits will not be noted within the "hole." A halo of subretinal fluid is not present with the epiretinal membrane. Careful contact lens biomicroscopy in such cases will usually reveal a bright light reflex within the hole, indicating preservation of a thin layer of retinal tissue in the foveola. Aiming a thin slit beam focused on the central macula may be helpful. If the patient notes a definite gap in the line of light, this strongly suggests a full-thickness hole. Frequently, however, patients will note a *bend* or *waviness* in the line, a response that is less helpful since it may occur in patients with a true hole or a pseudohole. Fluorescein angiography will generally show minimal (if any) hyperfluorescence in the macula as opposed to the discrete changes seen with a full-thickness macular hole. Epiretinal membranes may occasionally be associated with a full-thickness macular hole, but it is seldom known whether the membrane preceded the hole or vice versa.

Vitreoretinal traction syndrome is an unusual condition that occurs as the result of an abnormally strong adhesion between the vitreous and macula during the development of a posterior vitreous detachment. This anterior retinal traction will produce a tenting of the retina and definite anteroposterior vitreomacular traction, which should be apparent ophthalmoscopically.[11] Vitreoretinal traction syndrome is thought to progress to development of a full thickness macular hole only rarely.

Macular Hole from Known Causes

As noted above, true full-thickness macular holes may develop in association with other well-defined entities. In addition to vitreoretinal interface abnormalities, holes may be related to myopia, trauma, rhegmatogenous retinal detachment with a peripheral retinal tear, and photic retinopathy. Although the appearance of the hole itself may be identical to that of an idiopathic macular hole, the patient's history or other funduscopic features makes distinguishing these entities a simple task in most cases.[3]

TREATMENT

Traditionally, macular holes have been thought to be untreatable. Attempts with juxtafoveal laser photocoagulation met with very minimal success.[12] Recently, however, renewed interest has developed in the treatment of macular hole and prehole conditions using vitrectomy techniques.

When considering treatment, it is important to distinguish between treatment for impending macular hole and that for preexisting idiopathic macular hole. Impending macular hole patients would be those meeting the description of Stage 1 described by Gass. If untreated, this condition results in full-thickness hole formation and visual loss in some *but not all* patients. Theoretically, vitrectomy with release of the premacular cortical vitreous could result in release of foveal traction and prevent progression to a full-thickness hole.[13] Smiddy et al.[15] and Jost et al.,[14] in uncontrolled pilot studies, reported on the technical feasibility of this technique. Both had favorable results. The rate of progression to a full-thickness hole was 20% in each study, and relatively few complications were noted. Symptomatic relief with recovery of vision occurred in the majority of cases. Since the natural rate of progression is unknown, however, it is uncertain whether prophylactic vitrectomy should be recommended at this time for all patients with Stage 1 holes. Most investigators believe that the risk of progression is substantially higher for patients with a hole in the fellow eye. It seems reasonable therefore, to offer surgery for patients with a Stage 1 hole in one eye and a full-thickness hole in the fellow eye. Since progression to a full-thickness hole can occur fairly quickly, patients with a full-thickness hole in one eye should be advised to monitor the fellow eye regularly and instructed to report any changes that occur.

The effectiveness of treatment for full-thickness holes is also uncertain. Although a large prospective long-term natural history study has not been published, it is widely accepted that the vast majority of eyes with an idiopathic macular hole will remain stable. As noted previously, though, well-documented cases of spontaneous "closure" of a hole, with resorption of subretinal fluid and visual improvement, have been reported. It has been postulated[13] that adherent cortical vitreous at the edges of a macular hole causes persistence of the subretinal fluid around the hole. Release of this tangential traction might then allow the RPE to "pump" this fluid and reattach the retina. Spontaneous release of the cortical vitreous could account for the sporadic cases of improvement that have been noted.

Based on this theory, considerable interest has been generated during the last few years in the possible surgical management of idiopathic macular hole. Pars plana vitrectomy with careful attention to pealing the cortical vitreous from the retinal surface and then fluid-air exchange has been tried by several inves-

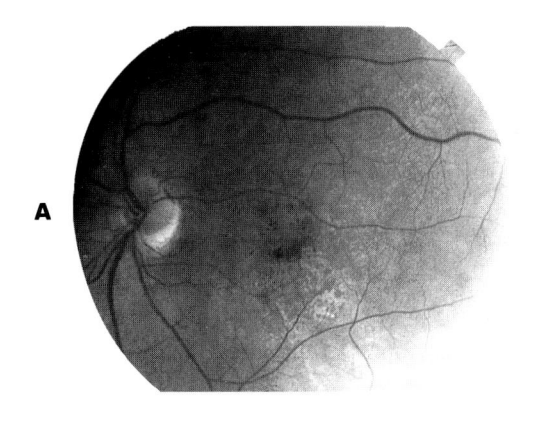

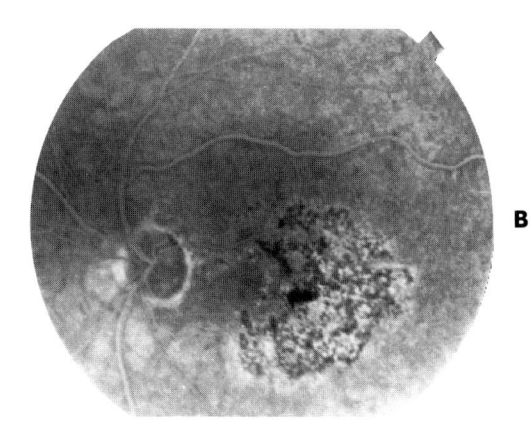

Figure 6-6 A, Full thickness macular hole in the patient in Figure 6-3, *B*, several weeks after vitrectomy with cortical vitreous delamination. The hole is closed, but extensive pigmentary mottling is present clinically, **B.** Vision after surgery initially was counting fingers but gradually improved to 20/50.

tigators. Kelly and Wendel[16] have reported in a pilot study that in nearly 60% of cases the retina could be reattached around the hole. Additional reports by Poliner[17] and Glaser[18] have also shown a high rate of retinal reattachment. Kelly and Wendel[16] reported visual improvement in about 40% of eyes, with some eyes improving to 20/40 or better. Although no type of retinopexy was performed in their study, other investigators have advocated additional techniques, such as application of growth factors, to enhance retinal adhesion to the underlying RPE.

Not surprisingly, complications can occur with this procedure: retinal detachment, cataract, and intraoperative enlargement of the hole. Poliner[17] described an unusual macular pigmentary response in a large percentage of cases in which the retina was successfully reattached (Fig. 6-6). Whether this is a mechanical or a photic process and what the long-term visual significance of the response is remain uncertain.

Factors that might be expected to affect the likelihood of visual recovery after surgical repair include the duration of the hole prior to surgery and the relative sizes of the hole and surrounding halo of subretinal fluid. Although there is no clear evidence that these are critical factors, it seems reasonable to predict that small holes with a relatively large amount of fluid and holes of recent onset would have the most favorable prognosis.

As with prophylactic surgery in cases of impending macular holes, there are no clearcut recommendations concerning treatment for patients with full-thickness holes. As with any elective procedure, the patient's visual needs, status of the fellow eye, and general health are critical factors to be considered.

References

1. Aaberg TM, Blair CJ, Gass JDM: Macular holes, *Am J Ophthalmol* 69:555-562, 1970.
2. Bronstein MA, Trempe CL, Freeman HM: Fellow eyes of eyes with macular holes, *Am J Ophthalmol* 92:757-761, 1981.
3. Gass JDM: *Stereoscopic atlas of macular diseases: diagnosis and treatment,* ed 3, St Louis, 1987, Mosby, vol 2, pp 684-693.
4. Lewis H, Cowan GM, Straatsma BR: Apparent disappearance of a macular hole with development of an epiretinal membrane, *Am J Ophthalmol* 102:172-175, 1986.

5. Avila MP, Jalkh AE, Murakami K, et al: Biomicroscopic study of the vitreous in macular breaks, *Ophthalmology* 90:1277-1283, 1983.
6. Trempe CL, Weiter JJ, Furukawa H: Fellow eyes in cases of macular hole: biomicroscopic study of the vitreous, *Arch Ophthalmol* 104:93-95, 1986.
7. McDonnell PJ, Fine SL, Hillis AI: Clinical features of idiopathic macular cysts and holes, *Am J Ophthalmol* 93:777-786, 1982.
8. Morgan CM, Schatz H: Idiopathic macular holes, *Am J Ophthalmol* 99:437-444, 1985.
9. Morgan CM, Schatz H: Involutional macular thinning: a pre-macular hole condition, *Ophthalmology* 93:153-161, 1986.
10. Gass JDM: Idiopathic senile macular hole: its early stages and pathogenesis, *Arch Ophthalmol* 106:629-639, 1988.
11. Smiddy WE, Michels RG, Glaser BM, et al: Vitrectomy for macular traction caused by incomplete vitreous separation, *Arch Ophthalmol* 106:624-628, 1988.
12. Schocket SS, Lakhanpal V, Xiaoping M, et al: Laser treatment of macular holes, *Ophthalmology* 95:574-582, 1988.
13. Johnson RN, Gass JDM: Idiopathic macular holes: observations, stages of formation, and implications for surgical intervention, *Ophthalmology* 95:917-924, 1988.
14. Jost BF, Hutton WL, Fuller DG, et al: Vitrectomy in eyes at risk for macular hole formation, *Ophthalmology* 97:843-847, 1990.
15. Smiddy WE, Michels RG, Glaser BM, et al: Vitrectomy for impending idiopathic macular holes. *Am J Ophthalmol* 105:371-376, 1988.
16. Kelly NE, Wendel RT. Vitreous surgery for idiopathic macular holes: results of a pilot study, *Arch Ophthalmol* 109:654-659, 1991.
17. Poliner LS, Tornambe PE: Retinal pigment epitheliopathy after macular hole surgery, *Ophthalmology* 99:1671-1677, 1992.
18. Glaser BM, Michels RG, Kupperman BD, et al: Transforming growth factor–β_2 for the treatment of full-thickness macular holes: a prospective randomized study, *Ophthalmology* 99:1162-1173, 1992.

7

Macular Dystrophies

Eric P. Shakin

The macular dystrophies include a heterogeneous group of hereditary conditions that are either confined to the fovea alone or associated with other ocular and systemic manifestations. These conditions are best classified by the anatomic localization of the disease to the level of the choroid, Bruch's membrane, retinal pigment epithelium, outer retina, or vitreoretinal interface. Some dystrophies are further subclassified by visual physiology evaluation. Since the literature abounds with a plethora of macular dystrophies, this chapter will deal only with the more common and recently described dystrophies that affect primarily the macula.

CLINICAL PRESENTATIONS

Patients with macular dystrophies present, in the first or second decade of life, with a variety of visual symptoms—diminished acuity, dyschromatopsia, nyctalopia, central and paracentral scotomas, and metamorphopsia. They may have strabismus or nystagmus associated with a congenital or an acquired defect within the first few years (e.g., juvenile retinoschisis or stationary monochromatism). Whereas hemeralopia is a common symptom in patients with cone deficits, photophobia is more typical in patients with albinism or Leber's congenital amaurosis. Nyctalopia usually indicates a concomitant abnormality of the rod system and/or myopia. These visual symptoms can be evaluated by specific visual physiology examination.

DIAGNOSTIC APPROACH

The clinical history is valuable in assessing patients with dystrophies. The history should include age, onset of symptoms, pedigree analysis, review of systems, and medications being taken. Prior clinical diagnostic tests and fundus photographs of the patient and relatives may also be helpful. Clinical examination is essential in determining the extent of pathology. Biomicroscopy of the posterior pole with a white, red, and red-free lights accentuates abnormalities such as pigment accumulation.

```
Stationary           ┌─ Anomalous
cone defects ────────┤  trichromatism
                     │
                     ├─ Dichromatism              ┌─ Rod
                     │                            ├─ Cone
                     └─ Monochromatism ───────────┤
                                                  ├─ Blue cone
                                                  └─ Central cone


                     ┌─ Cone dystrophy
                     │                            ┌─ Retinitis pigmentosa
Acquired             │                            │  and allied disorders
cone defects ────────┼─ Cone-rod dystrophy ───────┤
                     │                            └─ Enhanced S cone
                     │                               syndrome
                     │
                     └─ Dominant macular dystrophy
                        (S-cone dysfunction)
```

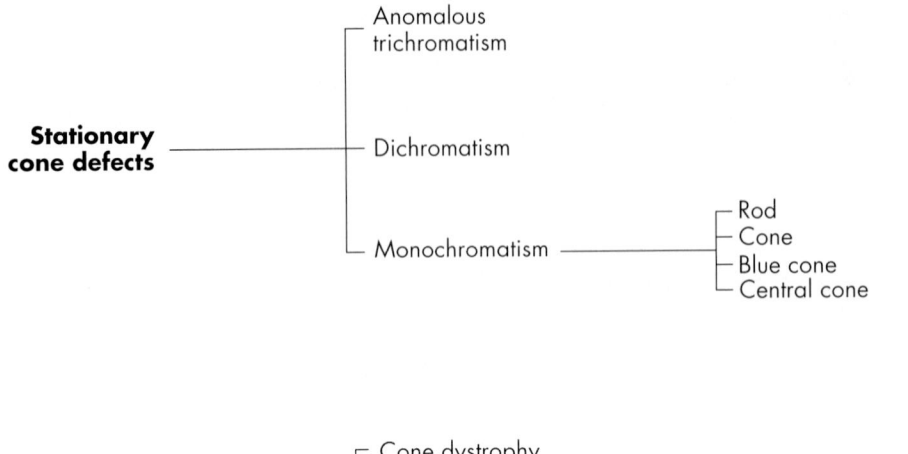

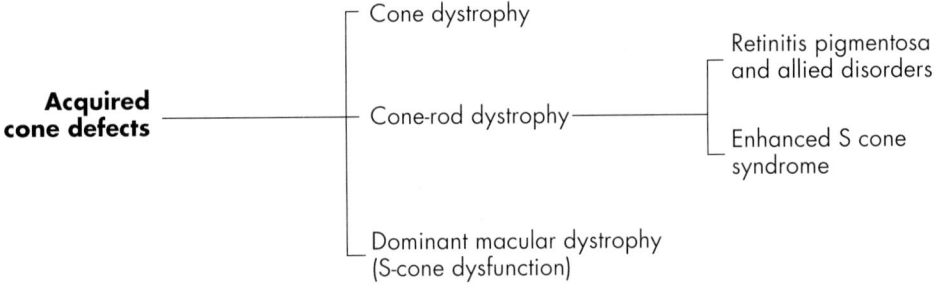

Figure 7-1 Congenital color vision defects versus progressive cone dystrophies.

Visual physiology testing may be of some limited value. Specialized psychophysical tests for macular function include the Amsler grid, modulation transfer function (contrast sensitivity and flicker fusion frequency), automated perimetry with a white and red test object, and macular photostress test. Color vision testing includes pseudoisochromatic plates and arrangement tests. Congenital defects may sometimes be distinguished from acquired defects. Retinal diseases (Fig. 7-1) that cause primarily a photoreceptor degeneration are associated with Type I (red-green) defects.* Most retinal diseases causing visual loss are associated with a Type III (blue-yellow) defect, which may progress to a Type I defect in advanced stages.[1] These tests are helpful to the extent that they better quantify the degree of visual loss and sometimes help differentiate macular pathology from an optic neuropathy.

Dark adaptometry is utilized in the investigation of nyctalopia. The test target is between 10 and 15 degrees temporal to fixation. On occasion, a patient with a macular dystrophy who either fixates on the test target or has abnormal retinal function temporal to fixation will have an abnormal dark adaptation curve.

Electrodiagnostic testing also plays a role in the diagnosis of macular dystrophies.[2] The electroretinogram reflects a mass retinal response that is not usually affected by pathology confined to the fovea. Certain conditions with ophthalmoscopic manifestations confined to the macula, however, such as cone dys-

---

*Verriest classification.

trophies, juvenile retinoschisis, or the enhanced S cone syndrome, have distinct electroretinographic abnormalities. The electrooculogram may be subnormal in many macular dystrophies because of diffuse involvement of the retinal pigment epithelium (RPE). The Arden ratio (light peak/dark trough) is considered normal if above 1.8 and distinctly abnormal if below 1.5.

The focal electroretinogram, which utilizes a flashing 3- to 4-degree stimulus, may be useful for differentiating optic nerve disease from macular disease and has been loosely correlated with visual acuity. The pattern electroretinogram utilizes a pattern of constant luminance, which is reduced by disease affecting the inner retina and optic nerve. Pattern visual evoked cortical potentials represent mostly foveal activity; consequently, they are of reduced amplitude and sometimes increased latency with macular disease.

Fluorescein angiography, likewise, plays a role in the diagnosis of some of these disorders. There may be delayed filling of the choriocapillaris or abnormalities of choroidal perfusion in disorders involving Bruch's membrane or the choriocapillaris.[3] Hypofluorescence may also be associated with blockage from pigment accumulation in addition to nonperfusion and may be helpful, for example, in distinguishing an accumulation of lipofuscin in vitelliform dystrophy from a pigment epithelial detachment. Hyperfluorescence occurs with transmission window defects, neovascularization, and leakage. Since many of the macular dystrophies are potentially associated with the development of choroidal neovascular membranes, fluorescein angiography and indocyananine green videoangiography may be helpful in detecting the neovascular membrane in an area of degeneration.

DYSTROPHIES OF THE NEUROSENSORY RETINA

Macular dystrophies that involve primarily the retina include vitreoretinal dystrophies, disorders of photoreceptor function, and dominant cystoid macular dystrophy. Also a dystrophy of the inner retina may be one of the manifestations of metabolic storage disease. For example, patients with generalized gangliosidosis have enzyme deficiencies associated with a macular halo (cherry-red spot) and optic atrophy in certain cases.[4] Other metabolic storage diseases[4] or various syndromes of unknown etiology (e.g., Alport's syndrome[5]) may be associated primarily with a macular dystrophy. However, such syndromes will not be discussed in this chapter.

Vitreoretinal Dystrophies

Juvenile (X linked) retinoschisis presents with a stellate maculopathy (Fig. 7-2) in all patients and peripheral retinoschisis with visible inner-wall holes in nearly half the patients.[6] The foveal schisis or cysts coalesce, and subsequently atrophy of the macula associated with pigmentary changes and further visual loss develops over an interval of 3 to 4 decades. The foveal schisis characteristically does not hyperfluoresce during fluorescein angiography. Vitreous hemorrhage, retinal detachment, and progressive macular degeneration are causes of visual loss.[7] These children may also have associated nystagmus and strabismus. Electroretinography typically demonstrates a reduced b-wave under photopic and scotopic conditions.[8] Carriers are clinically normal, although some psychophysical aberrations with regard to abnormal rod-cone interactions have been de-

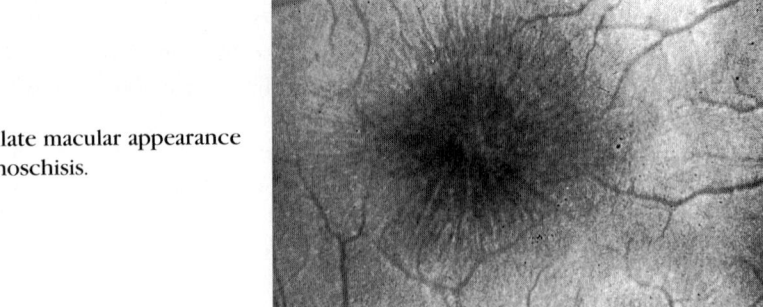

Figure 7-2 Stellate macular appearance in X-linked retinoschisis.

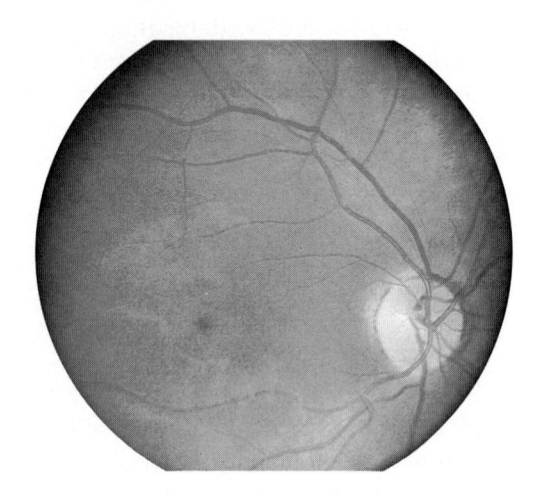

Figure 7-3 Cone dystrophy demonstrating a bull's-eye macula.

scribed.[9] The genetic defect has been identified[10] in one pedigree (Xp22 locus). It should be distinguished from Goldmann-Favre syndrome and Wagner's syndrome.

Photoreceptor Dystrophies

Cone Disorders. The symptoms of a progressive cone dystrophy (Fig. 7-3), which start between the second and fourth decades of life, include decreasing vision, acquired dyschromatopsia (tritan- and protanlike defects), hemeralopia, and occasionally nystagmus. It is inherited most commonly as an autosomal recessive or dominant disorder.[11,12] The clinical findings include macular degeneration, sometimes in an annular distribution, a golden tapetal sheen, temporal pallor of the optic disc, and rarely the Mizuo-Nakamura phenomenon with X-linked cone dystrophy.[13]

There is an absent cone response on the electroretinogram under both photopic conditions (flicker and single flash) and scotopic conditions (x-wave, or a_p component). There is also an abnormal cone adaptation curve with dark adaptometry. This psychophysical response distinguishes a cone dystrophy from a Type II cone-rod dystrophy.[14] Recently, a 6.5 kilobase deletion on the gene for red cone pigment has been identified in a subset of X-linked cone dystrophy.[15]

Some patients with a cone-rod dystrophy (inverse or central retinitis pigmentosa) present initially with a cone dysfunction. There is pigment clumping within the vascular arcades with diffuse mottling of the retinal pigment epithelium and choroidal atrophy. There may also be other stigmas of retinitis pigmentosa, such as waxy pallor of the optic disc and attenuated retinal vessels. The visual field defects are limited to the area of retinal involvement. Both the cone response and the rod response of the ERG are diminished.[16,17] In addition, fundus albipunctatus has been reported[18] in association with a cone dystrophy.

The congenital color vision defects should be distinguished from the progressive cone dystrophies (Fig. 7-1). Clinically, congenital monochromatism may have similarities with visual physiology testing and there may be either pigmentary alterations in the macula (blue cone monochromatism) or foveal hypoplasia (achromatopsia).[12]

Dominant macular dystrophy (S cone system dysfunction) was described by Bresnick et al.[19] as an autosomal dominant–inherited condition, manifested by pigmentary alterations in the fovea, that affects central visual acuity. There is an inherent defect in the S-cone system encoding short wavelengths. There is also an increased b-wave implicit time of the electroretinogram under photopic conditions with a 30-hertz stimulus. The patients have a typical tritanlike defect with abnormal spectral sensitivity in the short-wavelength range. This contrasts with the cone dystrophies, which affect the longer-wavelength cones (red/green defects). Advanced cone dystrophies and autosomal dominant optic atrophy should be distinguished from this condition.

Rod-Cone Disorders. The enhanced S cone syndrome[20,21] represents a probable hereditary disorder of photoreceptor function. Patients may have variably decreased vision in the second and third decades of life with nyctalopia, midperipheral scotomas, and normal color vision. They have cystoid architectural changes in their maculars, which do not leak during fluorescein angiography. In addition, there are associated yellow flecks and pigmentary alterations near the vascular arcades.

The electroretinogram is peculiar to this disorder. The rod response is markedly reduced with attenuated stimuli, but there is a maximum response with increased latency under scotopic conditions when a brighter stimulus is used. The cone response under photopic conditions is similar to the response under scotopic conditions because of the larger amplitudes and increased latency with bright stimuli.

There is a mismatch under photopic conditions, with increased sensitivity and increased amplitude when short wavelengths are utilized compared to longer-wavelength stimuli.

Inner Retinal Dystrophy. Cystoid macular edema is an autosomal dominant condition that presents with hyperopia and visual loss in the first or second decade of life. It includes cystoid macular edema associated with macular depigmentation, peripheral corpuscular pigment clumping, and accumulation of vitreous cells.[22] The ERG is normal, and the EOG may be subnormal with decreased vision. Fluorescein angiography demonstrates hyperfluorescent leakage from both the retinal pigment epithelium and the perifoveal capillaries. Recently, oral acetazolamide and grid laser photocoagulation have been described[23] in the treatment of this disorder or cystoid macular edema associated with other retinal dystrophies.[23]

DYSTROPHIES OF THE RETINAL PIGMENT EPITHELIUM

Fundus flavimaculatus (Stargardt's disease[24]) (Fig. 7-4) is an autosomal recessive or, less commonly, autosomal dominant condition (dominant progressive foveal dystrophy,[25] progressive atrophic macular dystrophy[26]) that frequently presents in the first or second decade of life. Often these children will have visual complaints preceding the onset of ophthalmoscopic changes. Visual acuity may progressively deteriorate to the 6/60 level, with red-green dyschromatopsia. Approximately 70% of patients have 6/30 vision or better by the age of 19 years, and 39% have 6/30 vision or better by age 39. When visual acuity has decreased to the 20/40 level, about 48% patients will progress to the 6/30 level or worse over an interval of 2 years.[27] The autosomal dominant variant of Stargardt's disease progresses more slowly than the recessive variant.

The four types of fundus flavimaculatus[28] include (1) atrophic maculopathy with parafoveal flecks, (2) atrophic maculopathy with a cone dystrophy, (3) atrophic maculopathy with advanced rod-cone dystrophy, and (4) flecks without an associated maculopathy.

The macular appearance may initially be normal. Patients then develop mottling of the RPE with perifoveal yellow-white flecks, and finally atrophy of the RPE associated with a beaten bronze reflex in over half the cases. The yellow-white flecks are linear or pisciform and may extend from the macula to the equator of the fundus.

Fluorescein angiography demonstrates attenuation of the background choroidal fluorescence ("silent choroid") in 83% of cases.[27] There may be hyperfluorescent transmission window defects corresponding to atrophy of the RPE.

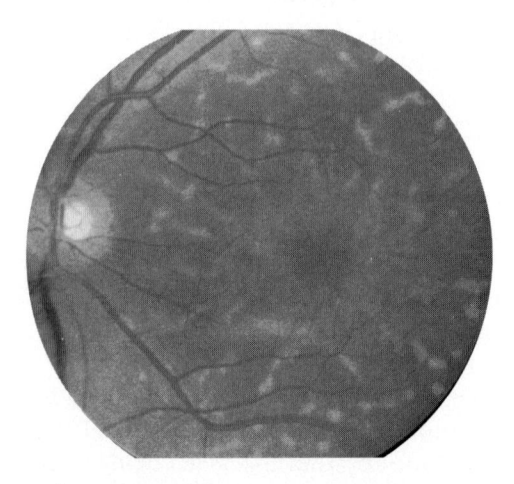

Figure 7-4 Fundus flavimaculatus demonstrating parafoveal flecks.

Macular dystrophies

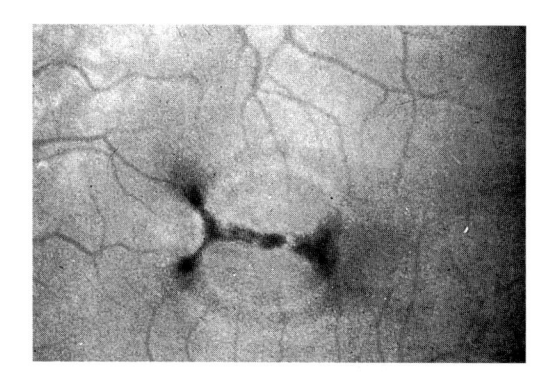

Figure 7-6 Butterfly pattern dystrophy.

Figure 7-7 Reticular pattern dystrophy.

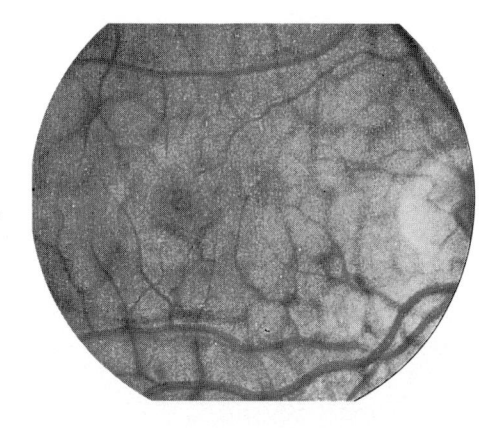

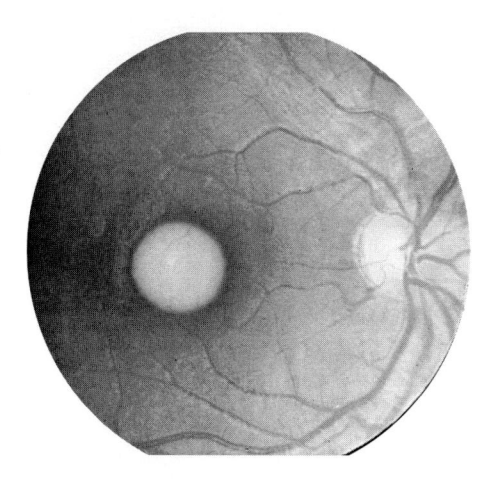

Figure 7-8 Vitelliform dystrophy demonstrating the vitelliform stage.

Figure 7-9 Vitelliform dystrophy demonstrating a pseudohypopyon.

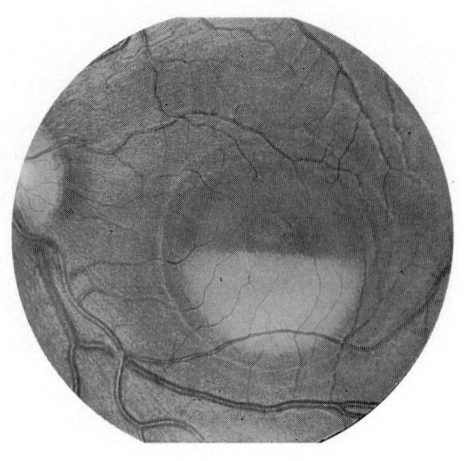

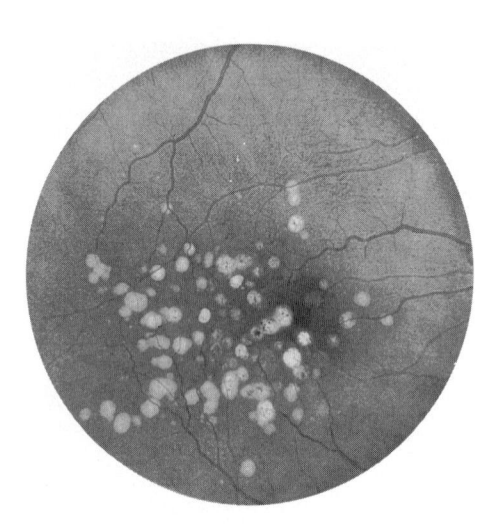

Figure 7-10 Dominant drusen.

Figure 7-11 Central areolar choroidal dystrophy.

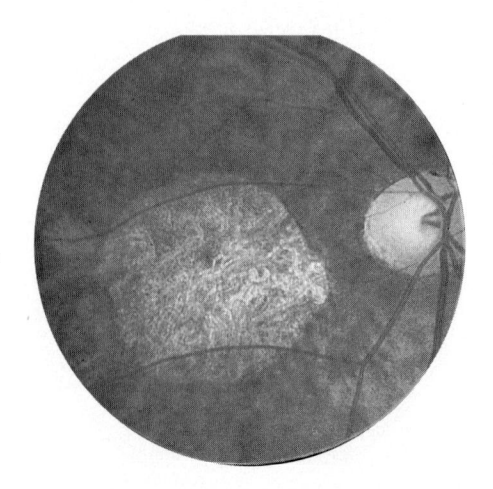

does not necessarily worsen even in the more advanced stages.[54] Fluorescein angiography usually reveals areas of blocked hypofluorescence corresponding to the pigment deposits. The pigment deposits may possibly be accumulations of lipofuscin.[53] Although the electroretinogram is usually normal (except for the c-wave), the electrooculogram is consistently reduced with a subnormal Arden ratio (light peak/dark trough) in affected patients and carriers.

Dominant (familial) drusen[55,56] (Fig. 7-10) are not uncommonly observed in clinical practice. They may be first noted in the third decade of life, and they accumulate and become more confluent with advancing years. There may be a combination of hard and soft drusen, sometimes arranged in a mosaic ("honeycomb") pattern associated with atrophy of the retinal pigment epithelium in later stages. Fluorescein angiography typically reveals discrete hyperfluorescence of the drusen that wanes in the recirculation phase of the study. There is associated mottled hyperfluorescence from loss of the RPE.

Although the visual prognosis is not predictable, visual acuity usually remains stable until the age of 40 to 50 years. The electrooculogram is subnormal in advanced cases. Familial drusen should, of course, be distinguished from secondary drusen associated with age-related macular disease, overlying choroidal lesions, prior damage to the retinal pigment epithelium, and other conditions occurring with macular degeneration. The type of drusen and location are not specific for this condition.

DYSTROPHIES OF BRUCH'S MEMBRANE

Various disorders such as Sorsby's pseudoinflammatory macular dystrophy, angioid streaks, age-related macular degeneration, and myopic degeneration can be hereditary. Sorsby's pseudoinflammatory macular dystrophy[57-59] (hereditary hemorrhagic macular dystrophy[60]) is a rare familial condition that may have an autosomal dominant inheritance. The patient presents around the age of 40 with diminished vision and bilateral retinal edema, hemorrhages, exudates, and discrete drusenoid yellow-white spots. This all evolves into a cicatricial phase followed by atrophy of the pigment epithelium and choriocapillaris. Fluorescein angiography reveals delayed perfusion of the choriocapillaris and mottled hyperfluorescence corresponding to the pigmentary changes. The electroretinogram or electrooculogram may be reduced in advanced cases. Laser photocoagulation can play a role in the treatment of choroidal neovascular membrane associated with the condition.[61]

DYSTROPHIES OF THE CHOROID

Choroidal dystrophies involve atrophy of the choroid with secondary retinal atrophy. They may be classified as diffuse or regional choroidal vascular atrophy. Disorders associated with diffuse choroidal vascular atrophy include choroideremia, gyrate atrophy, and diffuse choriocapillaris atrophy.

Central areolar choroidal dystrophy[62] (Fig. 7-11) is usually an autosomal dominant disorder that initially presents in the third decade of life. There is a localized progressive loss of the RPE and choriocapillaris in the macula. The larger choroidal vessels are preserved. Pigment clumping may be seen in some of the atrophic areas. Variations of this condition include choroidal atrophy limited to a peripapillary or paramacular (circinate) distribution that may enlarge to involve the fovea. Visual acuity slowly deteriorates to the 6/30 level or worse. Electrophysiologic testing is usually normal. Fluorescein angiography reveals a well-circumscribed transmission defect with a silhouette of the larger choroidal vessels and leakage along the edge of the atrophy.

Central areolar pigment epithelial dystrophy (CAPE) is an autosomal dominant condition[63,64] associated with atrophy of the RPE in the first decade of life. Vision and the prognosis are good for these patients, in contrast to those for patients with central areolar choroidal dystrophy. It is possible that certain macular dystrophies represent a spectrum of the same disease. Some authors[65] have proposed that North Carolina macular dystrophy, central areolar pigment epithelial dystrophy, and central areolar choroidal dystrophies are different phenotypes of the same macular dystrophy.

References

1. Hart WM: Acquired dyschromatopsias, *Surv Ophthalmol* 32:10, 1987.
2. Carr RE, Siegel IM; *Electrodiagnostic testing of the visual system: a clinical guide,* Philadelphia 1990, FA Davis.
3. Piguet B, Palmvang IB, Chisholm IH, et al: Evolution of age-related macular degeneration with choroidal perfusion abnormality, *Am J Ophthalmol* 113:657, 1992.
4. Gass JDM: *Stereoscopic atlas of macular diseases: diagnosis and treatment,* ed 3, St Louis, 1977, Mosby, p 312.
5. Setala K, Ruusuvaara P: Alport syndrome with hereditary macular degeneration, *Acta Ophthalmol* 67:409, 1989.
6. Harris GS, Yeung JWS: Maculopathy of sex-linked juvenile retinoschisis, *Can J Ophthalmol* 11:1, 1976.
7. Deutman AF: Vitreoretinal dystrophies. In Krill AE (ed): *Krill's Hereditary retinal and choroidal diseases,* Hagerstown Md, 1977, Harper & Row.
8. Peachey NS, Fishman GA, Derlacki DJ, Brigell MG: Psychophysical and electroretinographic findings in X-linked juvenile retinoschisis, *Arch Ophthalmol* 105:513, 1987.
9. Arden GB, Gorin MB, Polkinghorne PJ, et al: Detection of the carrier state of X-linked retinoschisis, *Am J Ophthalmol* 105:590, 1988.
10. Dahl N, Goonewardena P, Chotai J, et al: DNA linkage analysis of X-linked retinoschisis, *Hum Genet* 78:228, 1988.
11. Krill AE, Deutman AF, Fishmann M: The cone degenerations, *Doc Ophthalmol* 35:1, 1973.
12. Goodman G, Ripps H, Siegel IM: Cone dysfunction syndromes, *Arch Ophthalmol* 70:214, 1963.
13. Heckinlively JR, Weleber RG: X-linked recessive cone dystrophy with tapetal-like sheen: a newly recognized entity with Mizuo-Nakamura phenomenon, *Arch Ophthalmol* 104:1322, 1986.
14. Massof RW, Finkelstein D: Subclassifications of retinitis pigmentosa from two-color scotopic static perimetry, *Doc Ophthalmol Proc Ser* 26:219, 1981.
15. Reichel E, Bruce AM, Sandberg MA, Berson EL: An electroretinographic and molecular genetic study of X-linked cone degeneration, *Am J Ophthalmol* 108:540, 1989.
16. Gass JDM: *Stereoscopic atlas of macular diseases,* ed 3, St Louis, 1987, Mosby, vol 1, p 288.
17. Francois J, DeRouck A, Cambie E, DeLaey JJ: Visual functions in pericentral and central pigmentary retinopathy, *Ophthalmologica* 165:38, 1972.
18. Miyake Y, Shiroyama N, Sugita S, et al: Fundus albipunctatus associated with cone dystrophy, *Br J Ophthalmol* 76:375, 1992.
19. Bresnick GH, Smith VC, Pokorny J: Autosomal dominantly inherited macular dystrophy with preferential short-wavelength sensitive cone involvement, *Am J Ophthalmol* 108:265, 1989.

20. Marmor MF, Jacobson SG, Foerster MH, et al: Diagnostic clinical findings of a new syndrome with night blindness, maculopathy, and enhanced S-cone sensitivity, *Am J Ophthalmol* 110:124, 1990.
21. Fishman GA, Peachey NS: Rod-cone dystrophy associated with rod system electroretinogram obtained under photopic conditions, *Ophthalmology* 96:913, 1989.
22. Deutman AF, Pinckers AJLG, Aan de Kerk AL: Dominantly inherited cystoid macular edema, *Am J Ophthalmol* 82:540, 1976.
23. Cox SN, Hay E, Bird AC: Treatment of chronic macular edema with acetazolamide, *Arch Ophthalmol* 106:1190, 1988.
24. Stargardt K: Über familiare progressive Degeneration in der Maculgegend des Auges, *Albrecht von Graefes Arch Klin Ophthalmol* 71:534, 1909.
25. Cibis GW, Morey M, Harris DJ: Dominantly inherited macular dystrophy with flecks (Stargardt), *Arch Ophthalmol* 98:1785, 1980.
26. Deutman AF: Macular dystrophies. In Ryan SJ (ed): *Retina* St Louis, 1989, Mosby, Chapter 69, pp 263-264.
27. Fishman GA, Farber M, Patel BS, Derlacki DJ: Visual acuity loss in patients with Stargardt's macular dystrophy, *Ophthalmology* 94:809, 1987.
28. Noble KG, Carr RE: Stargardt's disease and fundus flavimaculatus, *Arch Ophthalmol* 97:1281, 1979.
29. Fishman GA, Farban JS, Alexander KR: Delayed rod dark adaptation in patients with Stargardt's disease, *Ophthalmology* 98:957, 1991.
30. Noble KG, Carr RE, Siegel IM: Pigment epithelial dystrophy, *Am J Ophthalmol* 83:751, 1977.
31. O'Donnell FE, Welch RB: Fenestrated sheen macular dystrophy: A new autosomal dominant maculopathy, *Arch Ophthalmol* 97:1292, 1979.
32. Daily MJ, Mets MB: Fenestrated sheen macular dystrophy. *Arch Ophthalmol* 102:855, 1984.
33. Sneed SR, Sieving PA: Fenestrated sheen maculopathy, *Am J Ophthalmol* 112:1, 1991.
34. Deutman AF: Benign concentric macular dystrophy, *Am J Ophthalmol* 78:384, 1974.
35. Van den Biesen PR, Deutman AF, Pinckers AJLG: Evolution of benign concentric annular macular dystrophy, *Am J Ophthalmol* 100:73, 1985.
36. Lefler WH, Wadsworth JAC, Sidbury JB: Hereditary macular degeneration and aminoaciduria, *Am J Ophthalmol* 71:224, 1971.
37. Small KW, Killian J, McLean WC: North Carolina's dominant progressive foveal dystrophy: how progressive is it? *Br J Ophthalmol* 75:401, 1991.
38. Gass DJM: A clinicopathologic study of a peculiar foveamacular dystrophy, *Trans Am Ophthalmol* 72:139, 1974.
39. Epstein GA, Rabb MF: Adult vitelliform macular degeneration: diagnosis and natural history, *Br J Ophthalmol* 64:733, 1980.
40. Deutman AF, Van Blommestein JDA, Henkes HE, et al: Butterfly-shaped pigment dystrophy of the fovea, *Arch Ophthalmol* 83:558, 1970.
41. Prensky JG, Bresnick GH: Butterfly-shaped macular dystrophy in four generations, *Arch Ophthalmol* 101:1198, 1983.
42. Sjögren H: Dystrophia reticularis laminae pigmentosa retinae, *Acta Ophthalmol* 28:279, 1950.
43. Kingham JD, Fenzl RE, Willerson D, Aaberg TA: Reticular dystrophy of the retinal pigment epithelium, *Arch Ophthalmol* 96:1177, 1978.
44. Benedikt O, Werner W: Kleine Mitteilungen aus der Praxis: für die Praxis, *Klin Monatsbl Augenheilkd* 159:794, 1971.
45. Jimenez-Sierra JM, Ogden TE, Van Boemel GB: *Inherited retinal diseases* St Louis, 1989, Mosby, pp 59-81.
46. Slezak H, Hommer K: Fundus pulverulentus, *Albrecht von Graefes Arch Klin Exp Ophthalmol* 178:177, 1969.
47. Hsieh RC, Fine BS and Lyons JS: Pattern dystrophies of the retinal pigment epithelium. *Arch Ophthalmol* 95:429, 1977.

48. Cortin P, Archer D, Maumenee IH, et al: A patterned macular dystrophy with yellow plaques and atrophic changes, *Br J Ophthalmol* 64:127, 1980.
49. Marmor MF, Byers B: Pattern dystrophy of the pigment epithelium, *Am J Ophthalmol* 84:32, 1979.
50. Singerman LJ, Berkow JW, Patz A: Dominant slowly progressive macular dystrophy, *Am J Ophthalmol* 83:680, 1977.
51. De Jong PTVM, Delleman W: Pigment epithelial pattern dystrophy, *Arch Ophthalmol* 100:1416, 1982.
52. O'Donnell FE, Schatz H, Reid P, Green WR: Autosomal dominant dystrophy of the retinal pigment epithelium, *Arch Ophthalmol* 97:680, 1979.
53. Blodi CF, Stone EM: Best's vitelliform dystrophy, *Ophthalmic Ped Genet* 2:49, 1990.
54. Mohler CW, Fine SL: Long-term evaluation of patients with Best's vitelliform dystrophy, *Ophthalmology* 88:688, 1981.
55. Deutman AF, Jansen LMAA: Dominantly inherited drusen of Bruch's membrane, *Br J Ophthalmol* 54:373, 1970.
56. Marmor MF: Dominant drusen. In Heckenlively JR, Arden GB (eds): *Principles and practice of clinical electrophysiology of vision,* St Louis, 1991, Mosby, Chapter 87, pp 664-668.
57. Sorsby A, Joll-Mason ME and Gardener N: A fundus dystrophy with unusual features, *Br J Ophthalmol* 33:67, 1949.
58. Forsius HR, Eriksson AW, Suvanto EA, Alanko HI: Pseudoinflammatory fundus dystrophy with autosomal recessive inheritance, *Am J Ophthalmol* 94:634, 1982.
59. Hamilton WK, Ewing CC, Ives EJ, Carruthers JD: Sorsby's fundus dystrophy, *Ophthalmology* 96:1755, 1989.
60. Wu G, Pruett RC, Baldinger J, Hirose T: Hereditary hemorrhagic macular dystrophy, *Am J Ophthalmol* 111:294, 1991.
61. Polkinghorne PJ, Capon MRC, Berninger T, et al: Sorsby's fundus dystrophy, *Ophthalmology* 96:1763, 1989.
62. Noble KG: Central areolar choroidal dystrophy, *Am J Ophthalmol* 84:310, 1977.
63. Fetkenhour CL, Gurney N, Dobbie JG, Choromokos E: Central areolar pigment epithelial dystrophy, *Am J Ophthalmol* 81:745, 1976.
64. Leveille AS, Morse PH, Kiernan JP: Autosomal dominant central pigment epithelial and choroidal degeneration, *Ophthalmology* 89:1407, 1982.
65. Small KW, Hermsen V, Gurney N, et al: North Carolina macular dystrophy and central areolar pigment epithelial dystrophy, *Arch Ophthalmol* 110:515, 1992.

PART III

Retinal Vascular Disease

8

Treatment of Nonproliferative Diabetic Retinopathy

William E. Benson

PATIENT PRESENTATION

Case 1. A 42-year-old diabetic man presents with a visual acuity of 20/20 in the right eye and 20/70 in the left eye. Examination is within normal limits except for nonproliferative diabetic retinopathy in both eyes. There is no macular edema in the right eye. The left eye has a circinate ring of hard exudates that is mostly inferior to the foveal avascular zone (FAZ) but there are definite hard exudates in the FAZ.

CLINICAL FINDINGS AND SYMPTOMS

Macular edema (retinal thickening), an important manifestation of nonproliferative diabetic retinopathy (NPDR), is the leading cause of legal blindness in diabetics. The intercellular fluid comes from leaking microaneurysms or from diffuse capillary leakage. Microaneurysms are the first ophthalmoscopically detectable manifestation of background retinopathy. Beginning as dilations in the capillary wall where pericytes are absent, microaneurysms are initially thin walled. Later, endothelial cells proliferate and lay down layers of basement membrane material around themselves. Despite the multiple layers of basement membrane, they are permeable to water and large molecules, allowing the accumulation of water and lipid in the retina. Since fluorescein passes easily across their walls, we usually see many more microaneurysms at fluorescein angiography than are apparent at ophthalmoscopy.

When the wall of a capillary or microaneurysm is weakened enough, it may rupture, giving rise to an intraretinal hemorrhage. If the hemorrhage is deep (i.e., in the inner nuclear layer or outer plexiform layer), it usually is round or oval ("dot or blot"). If it is in the nerve fiber layer, it takes a flame or splinter shape indistinguishable from that seen in hypertensive retinopathy.

If the leakage of fluid is severe enough, lipid may accumulate in the retina. The outer plexiform layer is first to be affected. In some cases lipid is scattered through the macular; in others it accumulates in a ring around a group of leaking microaneurysms, or around microaneurysms surrounding an area of capillary nonperfusion (Fig. 8-1). This patterns is called circinate retinopathy.

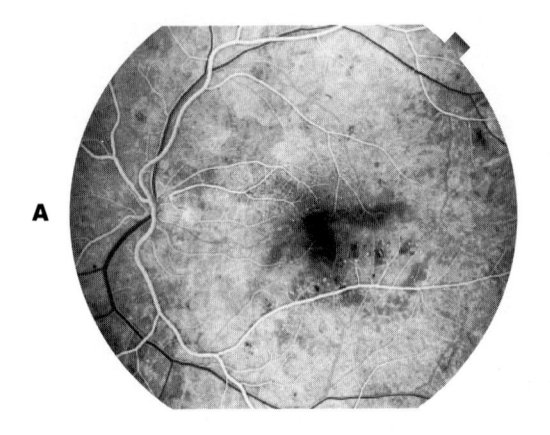

Figure 8-1 Fluorescein angiogram of an eye with diabetic retinopathy. **A,** The arteriovenous transit phase shows microaneurysms scattered throughout the macula. There is some blockage of the background fluorescence by the dense hard exudates. **B,** At 27 seconds small areas of capillary nonperfusion are surrounded by clusters of microaneurysms along the inferotemporal artery. **C,** The late phase shows considerable leakage from the microaneurysms. Laser treatment will be concentrated in this area. The leaking microaneurysms superiorly do not contribute to the macular edema and do not require treatment.

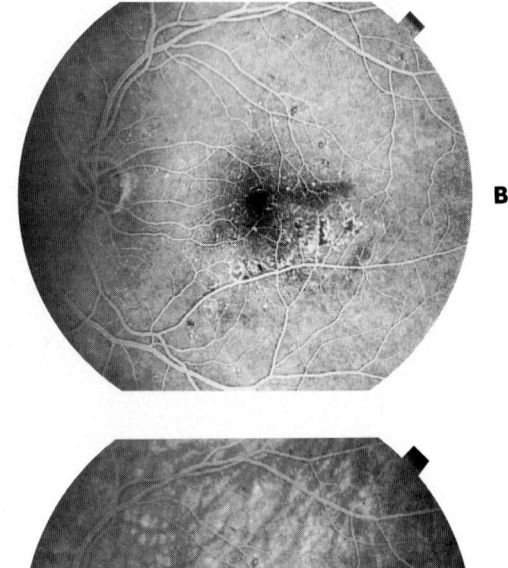

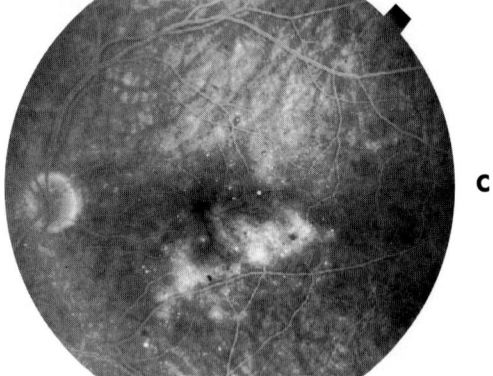

The decreased visual acuity in patients with diabetic macular edema (ME) is worse at near than at distance. Difficulty in reading is usually the most bitter complaint. Patients also complain of decreased color vision, decreased dark adaptation, micropsia, and sometimes metamorphopsia.

DIFFERENTIAL DIAGNOSIS

The entity that most closely mimics diabetic retinopathy is radiation retinopathy, which may also have microaneurysms, soft and hard exudates, intraretinal hemorrhages, macular edema, and neovascularization of the disc and retina. Radiation retinopathy should be suspected in patients who have had radiotherapy of orbital, sinus, nasopharyngeal or intracranial lesions. Fluorescein angiography also helps in the differentiation. In radiation retinopathy there are many fewer microaneurysms than there are in diabetic retinopathy.

Malignant hypertension, which may have intraretinal hemorrhages, soft exudates, hard exudates, and macular edema, also mimics diabetic retinopathy. Microaneurysms, however, are generally not a feature of hypertensive retinopathy. Furthermore, most diabetic hemorrhages are of the dot and blot variety because they are in the middle retinal layers whereas most hypertensive hemorrhages have a splinter shape because they are in the nerve fiber layer. Although splinter hemorrhages and soft exudates are common in diabetic retinopathy, if their number is out of proportion to the other findings or if disc edema is present the patient's blood pressure must be taken.

Central retinal vein obstruction usually has dilated veins and retinal hemorrhages, and frequently has macular edema. It is generally distinguished from diabetic retinopathy by its rapidity of onset and its unilaterality. The dilation of retinal veins is often more severe than in diabetic retinopathy, and the hemorrhages are mostly superficial and not deep. Microaneurysms may be present, but are few in acute obstructions. The same findings help differentiate branch retinal vein obstruction from diabetic retinopathy. In addition, the findings are nearly all confined to either the superior or the inferior half of the retina.

The ocular ischemic syndrome commonly has intraretinal hemorrhages and microaneurysms, but they are located predominantly in the periphery or midperiphery. Macular edema is common. Fluorescein angiography shows delayed choroidal and retinal filling, increased arteriovenous transit time, and late staining of the retinal arteries. Electroretinography shows a reduced b-wave because of inner retinal ischemia as well as a reduced a-wave because of outer retinal ischemia from poor choroidal perfusion. In diabetic retinopathy the a-wave is less affected.

DIAGNOSTIC APPROACH

Macular edema should be suspected in any diabetic patient with decreased vision. Clinically, retinal thickening is best detected by stereoscopic biomicroscopy with a contact, 60 diopter, or 90 diopter lens. If the center of the macula is involved, there is loss of the foveal reflex. Another clue is blurring of the normal retinal pigment epithelial and choroidal background pattern caused by scattering of light from the multiple interfaces the edema creates. They decrease the retina's translucency. Finally, the pockets of fluid in the outer plexiform layer, if large enough, can be seen as cystoid spaces. Usually cystoid macular edema is seen in eyes with other signs of severe background diabetic retinopathy such as numerous hemorrhages or exudates. In rare cases, however, cystoid macular edema caused by generalized diffuse leakage from the entire capillary network can be seen in eyes with very few other signs of diabetic retinopathy.

The examiner should look for clinically significant macular edema (CSME), which has been defined by the Early Treatment Diabetic Retinopathy Study (ETDRS) as edema that has reduced or is threatening to reduce vision. Affected eyes have one of the following characteristics:
1. Retinal thickening (edema) at or within 500 μm of the center of the foveal avascular zone (FAZ)
2. Hard exudates at or within 500 μm of the center of the FAZ, *if* associated with thickening of the adjacent retina
3. Retinal thickening (edema) 1 diopter or larger within 1 diopter of the center of the FAZ.

It will be noted that the ETDRS made no statement regarding whether visual acuity had to be decreased before treatment was given. In fact, eyes with 20/20 or better were treated. Nevertheless, with the exception of eyes with hard exudates threatening the FAZ, I almost never treat unless vision is actually decreased. I also do not obtain fluorescein angiography until treatment is contemplated. The diagnosis of CSME is made on the basis of the fundus examination, not the fluorescein angiogram; there is no benefit in obtaining a "baseline angiogram." Fluorescein angiography is performed for the following reasons: (1) to prove that decreased vision is caused by macular edema and not by central macular ischemia, (2) to identify leaking microaneurysms, (3) to locate areas of diffuse capillary leakage, and (4) to establish areas of capillary nonperfusion.

MANAGEMENT

Arnall Patz[1] pioneered the treatment of diabetic macular edema. Several other studies, using the argon laser[2-9] or the xenon arc,[9-13] have also been reported, but the benefits of treatment were controversial until the results of the largest clinical trial on the subject, the ETDRS[14] appeared.

The prognosis is affected by the pattern of leakage. Patients in whom most of the retinal capillaries are normal or nearly normal, but who have macular edema caused by focal areas of leakage surrounded by a ring of hard exudate (circinate retinopathy), have the best prognosis. Patients with widespread diffuse leakage from a myriad of microaneurysms or from multiple capillaries do less well, especially if they have cystoid macular edema. Patients who have occlusion of capillaries surrounding the foveal avascular zone or who have a large accumulation of lipid in the FAZ may respond to treatment, but the prognosis is poor.

The most commonly accepted treatment strategy ("focal treatment") was published by the ETDRS. It calls for identification (by fluorescein angiography) and photocoagulation (with the argon green laser) of "treatable lesions":

1. Focal leaks (e.g., microaneurysms) 500 or more μm from the center of the macula thought to be causing retinal thickening and/or hard exudates
2. Areas of diffuse capillary leakage
3. Areas of capillary nonperfusion

The treating ophthalmologist attempts to close all leaking microaneurysms. The endpoint is whitening or blackening. Areas of diffuse leakage and capillary nonperfusion are treated with a "grid" pattern of 100 or 200 μm burns of moderate intensity placed one burn width apart. In some cases there are so many microaneurysms that treating them all would destroy extensive confluent areas of retina. Grid treatment is then used.[3,5,15,16]

The treatment often causes an initial worsening of visual acuity, so the patients should be forewarned. Frequently it takes 3 to 4 months before the benefits of treatment are seen. Retreatment should be considered if there is persistent macular edema and treatable lesions can be identified. In subsequent treatment(s) the ophthalmologist can consider treatment of focal leaks 300 to 500 μm from the center of the macula thought to be causing retinal thickening and/or hard exudates if (1) visual acuity is 20/40 or worse and (2) such treatment is not likely to destroy the remaining perifoveal capillary network.

The exact mechanism of the beneficial effect of grid treatment is not known. One possibility is that destruction of the outer retinal layers and the retinal pigment epithelium (RPE) permits better diffusion of oxygen from the choriocapillaris into the inner retinal layers. Another possibility was suggested by Marshall et al.[17] In pig eyes they demonstrated evidence of mitotic activity in retinal capillaries following both argon and krypton laser treatment. They thought that alterations in the outer blood-retina barrier might allow the diffusion of substances capable of stimulating retinal endothelial cell division and repair, which in turn might reestablish the inner blood-retina barrier.

Most authors agree that the prognosis is best in cases with localized leakage with or without circinate rings of hard exudate. In my experience the prognosis is not good, but treatment should still be considered, in cases with

1. Significant central capillary nonperfusion
2. Severe cystoid macular edema
3. Hard exudates in the FAZ
4. Visual acuity 20/200 or less

OTHER EXAMPLES OF TREATMENT

Case 2. A 52-year-old man presents with nonproliferative diabetic retinopathy in both eyes. Visual acuity in the right eye is 20/50. This eye has a few circinate rings of hard exudates that do not impinge on the FAZ, but there is thickening of the center (Fig. 8-2).

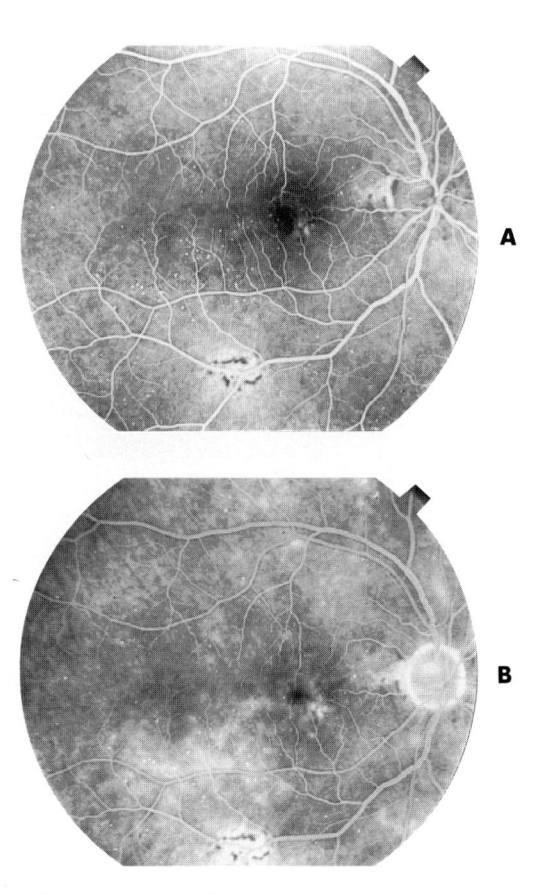

Figure 8-2 Case 2. At 34 seconds multiple leaking microaneurysms can be seen inferotemporal to the FAZ. There is no capillary nonperfusion. An old chorioretinal scar exists along the inferotemporal vein. **B,** The late phase shows that most of the leakage is coming from inferotemporal microaneusyrms. This area will be treated by focal applications in an attempt to occlude them. In addition, microaneurysms inferonasal to the FAZ will be treated.

Case 3. A 23-year-old woman presents with preproliferative diabetic retinopathy in both eyes. There is diffuse macular edema in the right eye, along with several soft exudates (Fig. 8-3).

Case 4. A 33-year-old woman who had undergone panretinal photocoagulation and a vitrectomy for nonclearing vitreous hemorrhage presents with a visual acuity of 20/60. She has diffuse macular edema with some hard exudates just superotemporal to the FAZ. A venous loop is present along the superotemporal retinal vein and the superotemporal artery is sheathed (Fig. 8-4).

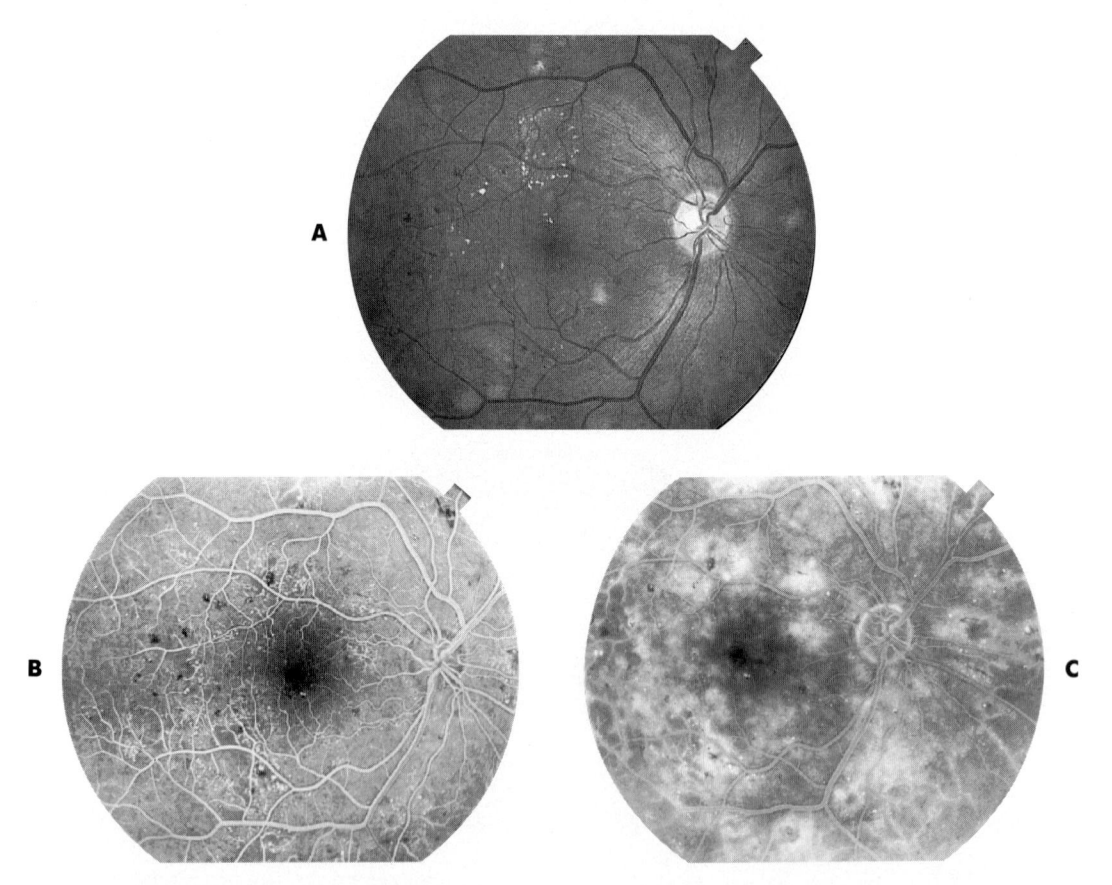

Figure 8-3 Case 3. **A,** Preproliferative diabetic retinopathy. There is diffuse macular edema with soft exudates. **B,** At 22 seconds into the fluorescein angiogram multiple microaneurysms can be seen. **C,** Diffuse late leakage.

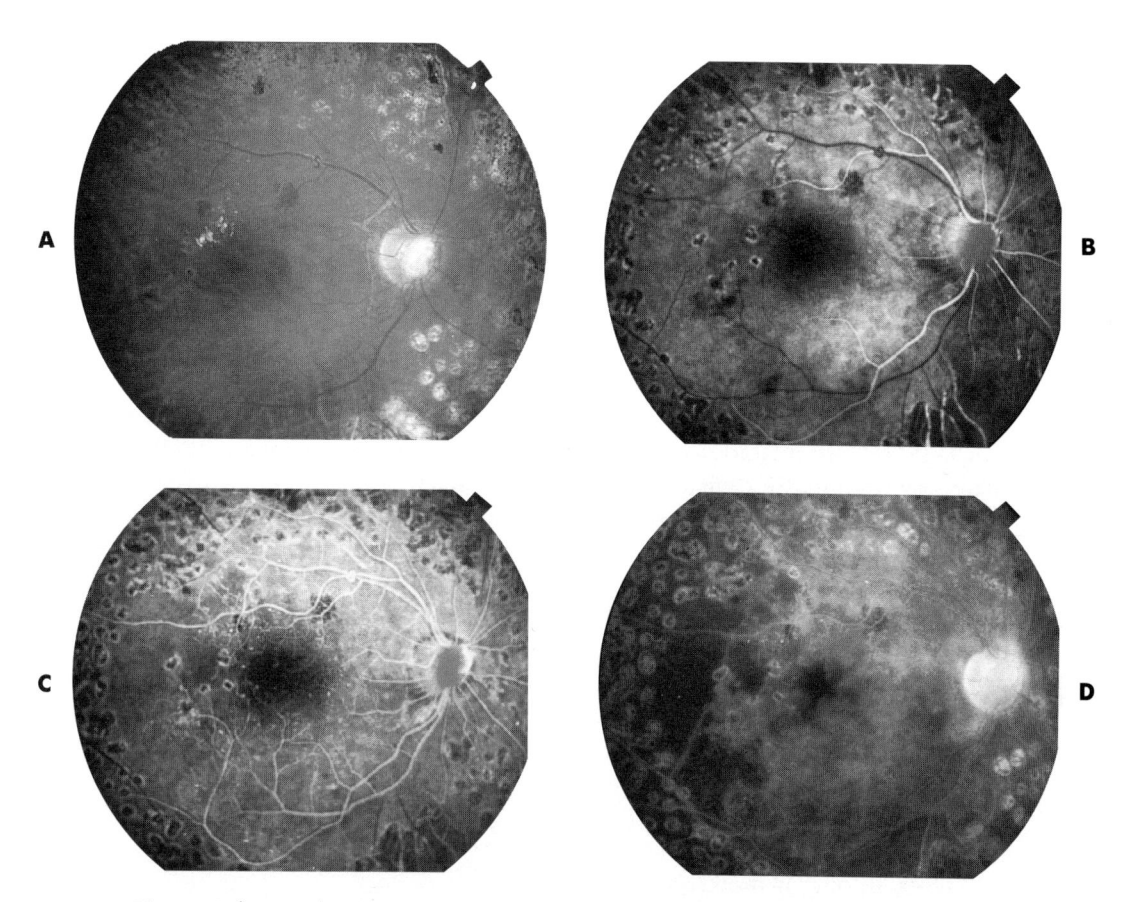

Figure 8-4 Case 4. **A,** Following panretinal photocoagulation and vitrectomy for a nonclearing vitreous hemorrhage, visual acuity is 20/60. There is diffuse macular edema with some hard exudates just superotemporal to the FAZ. A venous loop is present along the retinal vein, and the retinal artery is sheathed. **B,** At 22 seconds into the fluorescein angiogram incomplete filling of the superotemporal and inferotemporal arteries can be seen. There are five old laser burns just temporal to the FAZ. **C,** At 28 seconds very few microaneurysms are evident. Note the extensive capillary nonperfusion temporal to the macula. The hard exudates seen in **A** are at the edge of the area of capillary nonperfusion. **D,** The late phase shows diffuse leakage from the macular capillaries. The treatment strategy is to place a grid of 200 μm spots 500 μm from the center of the FAZ to the area previously treated by panretinal photocoagulation.

RESULTS OF THE ETDRS

The Early Treatment Diabetic Retinopathy Study was designed to help evaluate the results of focal treatment for macular edema. In addition, many eyes received panretinal photocoagulation if they had severe NPDR or early neovascularization because there was, and is, some controversy regarding the management of such eyes. To be able to interpret the ETDRS results, one must understand the terms "severe NPDR" and "neovascularization less than HRC."

Intermediate between NPDR and proliferative diabetic retinopathy (PDR) is a stage known as preproliferative diabetic retinopathy (PPDR) characterized by signs of increasing retinal hypoxia such as soft exudates, capillary nonperfusion at fluorescein angiography, numerous intraretinal hemorrhages, venous beading and loops, and intraretinal microvascular abnormalities (IRMA). Soft exudates, also called cotton wool spots or nerve fiber layer infarctions, are white fluffy lesions in the nerve fiber layer caused by occlusion of the precapillary arterioles. Fluorescein angiography shows no capillary perfusion in the area of the soft exudate. Microaneurysms frequently surround the hypoxic area. Venous beading is an important sign of sluggish retinal circulation. Venous loops are nearly always adjacent to large areas of capillary nonperfusion. Focal vitreous traction may contribute to their formation. Intraretinal microvascular abnormalities (IRMA) are dilated capillaries that seem to function as collateral channels. They are frequently difficult to differentiate from surface retinal neovascularization. Fluorescein, however, does not leak from intraretinal microvascular abnormalities but leaks profusely from neovascularization. Surrounding IRMA are large patches of capillary hypoperfusion. Although soft exudates are often thought to be the hallmark of PPDR, the Early Treatment Diabetic Retinopathy Study found that IRMA, venous abnormalities, and numerous hemorrhages are all much more predictive of the imminence of PDR. From their data, these investigators defined severe NPDR as

Hemorrhages in four quadrants
or
Venous abnormalities in two or more quadrants
or
IRMA in one or more quadrants

The Diabetic Retinopathy Study found that not all eyes with PDR require panretinal photocoagulation. Those that do are said to have high-risk characteristics (HRC), which are defined as (1) neovascularization of the disc (NVD) larger than half a disk area, (2) any NVD with vitreous or preretinal hemorrhage, and/or (3) neovascularization elsewhere (NVE) larger than half a disk area with vitreous or preretinal hemorrhage. Therefore an eye may have neovascularization, but may not require PRP, because a treatment benefit has not been proven. Such eyes are said to have "neovascularization less than HRC."

The end point for "moderate visual loss" in the ETDRS was doubling of the visual angle. For an eye that started the study with 20/20, doubling would be 20/40. For an eye starting with 20/50, doubling would be 20/100. After 5 years of follow-up, the following results were reported for eyes with macular edema and mild (nonproliferative) diabetic retinopathy, which were divided into three groups[18]: The *first* group (controls) did not receive any macular focal treatment. However, if they developed high-risk characteristics (HRC), panretinal photocoagulation (PRP) was given. The *second* group received immediate focal treatment but did not receive PRP unless severe NPDR developed. The *third* group received focal treatment and PRP within 4 months of each other. Table 8-1 shows that eyes receiving only focal treatment were much more likely to maintain good visual acuity than eyes receiving only focal treatment were much more likely to maintain good visual acuity than eyes receiving no focal treatment; however, the eyes that received PRP as part of their initial treatment did worse than both these groups. Clearly, panretinal photocoagulation is *not* part of the treatment of macular edema because it causes early visual loss!

Table 8-1 Doubling of the Visual Angle in Eyes With Macular Edema and Mild NPDR

	4 months (%)	1 year (%)	3 years (%)	5 years (%)
Controls (no treatment unless HRC)	4	9	21	30
Immediate focal and PRP if severe NPDR develops	3	5	11*	22
Immediate PRP, focal 4 months later	10*	16*	23	30

*Statistically significant.

Table 8-2 Doubling of the Visual Angle in Eyes With Macular Edema and Severe NPDR

	4 months (%)	1 year (%)	3 years (%)	5 years (%)
No treatment unless HRC	7	16	24	32
Immediate focal and PRP	12	16	23	26

Unfortunately, the ETDRS could not answer the question as to how effective is focal treatment alone in patients with macular edema and *severe* NPDR, because all such eyes were randomized to either no treatment unless HRC developed (controls) or immediate focal macular treatment *and* PRP. Table 8-2 shows the risk of moderate visual loss (doubling of the visual angle) in eyes with severe NPDR.

From these results, since the eyes receiving immediate focal macular treatment and PRP were twice as likely to have a decrease in visual acuity as were eyes receiving no treatment at all, we can conclude that eyes with ME and severe NPDR should not be treated with PRP.[20] The recommended course is to treat with focal applications only and monitor the patient closely for HRC.

Thus, as far as preservation of visual acuity goes, the ETDRS established that PRP should not be given to eyes without HRC. We also need to look, however, at the results in preventing severe visual loss that can result from PDR. In other words, can PRP be justified in eyes with severe NPDR if it retards the onset of HRC (and, therefore, of PDR) and prevents severe visual loss? The data in Table 8-3 show that if preventing HRC is a major goal early PRP should be given.

In other words, early PRP reduces the rate at which eyes with not only severe but also mild NPDR progress to HRC by approximately 50%, however, we must remember that the goal of performing a PRP is not to prevent HRC but to preserve visual function. As discussed above, PRP has a deleterious effect on visual acuity in eyes with macular edema. To better understand why, we must be cautious. We must look also at the effect on visual acuity in eyes with either severe NPDR or neovascularization less than HRC and no macular edema. The results are given in Table 8-4.

Table 8-3 Five-Year Incidence of High-Risk Characteristics

	Controls (%)	Immediate PRP (%)
No ME* (all eyes)	38	19
ME and mild NPDR	27	14
ME and severe NPDR	61	29

*ME, Macular edema; NPDR, nonproliferative diabetic retinopathy.

Table 8-4 Effect of PRP on Eyes With Severe NPDR and No Macular Edema

	Doubling of the visual angle			
	4 months (%)	1 year (%)	3 years (%)	5 years (%)
Deferred PRP	0.6	3.6	9.8	17.6
Immediate PRP	3.8*	7.5*	13.6	15.5

*Statistically significant.

Table 8-5 Very Bad Outcomes in Eyes With Severe NPDR and Macular Edema

	<5/200 alone (%)	<5/200 or vitrectomy (%)
Focal and immediate PRP	4.7	6.9
No laser unless HRC	6.5	10.3

Clearly, there is a heavy price to be paid for an immediate PRP. Eyes with no treatment at all were less likely to suffer a moderate loss of vision than the treated eyes were. At 1 year eyes with severe NPDR and no ME were twice as likely to have doubling of the visual angle as were eyes that had not been treated. By this criterion, they did better in the long run but the difference did not appear until 5 years. Finally, we could make the case that it might be worth the price to be paid in mild loss of visual acuity caused by early PRP if the PRP prevented severe visual loss (defined as a visual acuity of less than 5/200) or the need for a vitrectomy later. Table 8-5 shows these data.

As regards severe visual loss, eyes receiving an immediate PRP did slightly better in the long run than eyes not receiving PRP until HRC developed. In my opinion, with the exceptions listed below, the difference between 4.5% and 6.5% is not sufficient to justify an early PRP. I recommend treating the macular edema and monitoring closely for the development of HRC. Nevertheless, there are certain patients who are known to be at high risk for whom PRP can be considered. These patients

1. Have severe bilateral NPDR
2. Have rapidly progressing NPDR
3. Have had a poor outcome in one eye
4. Cannot be relied upon to return for follow-up
5. Are pregnant

References

1. Patz A, Schatz H, Berkow JW, et al: Macular edema: an overlooked complication of diabetic retinopathy, *Trans Am Acad Ophthalmol Otolaryngol* 77:34-42, 1973.
2. Wiznia RA: Photocoagulation of non-proliferative exudative diabetic retinopathy, *Am J Ophthalmol* 88:22-27, 1979.
3. Blankenship GW: Diabetic macular edema and argon laser photocoagulation. A prospective randomized study, *Ophthalmology* 86:69, 1979.
4. Ticho U, Patz A: The role of capillary perfusion in the management of diabetic macular edema, *Am J Ophthalmol* 76:880-886, 1973.
5. Whitelocke RAE, Kearns M, Blach RK, Hamilton AM: The diabetic maculopathies, *Trans Ophthalmol Soc UK* 99:314-320, 1979.
6. Reeser R, Fleischman J, Williams GA, Goldman A: Efficacy of argon laser photocoagulation in the treatment of circinate diabetic retinopathy, *Am J Ophthalmol* 92:762, 1981.
7. Schatz H, Patz A: Cystoid maculopathy in diabetics, *Arch Ophthalmol* 94:761-768, 1976.
8. Murphy RP: Current status of treatment of nonproliferative and proliferative diabetic retinopathy. In Friedman EA, L'Esperance FA (eds): *Diabetic renal-retinal syndrome,* New York, 1982, Grune & Stratton, vol 2, pp 217-242.
9. Spalter HF: Photocoagulation of circinate maculopathy in diabetic retinopathy, *Am J Ophthalmol* 71:242-250, 1971.
10. Spalter HF: Diabetic maculopathy, *Metab Pediatr System Ophthalmol* 1984;7:211-215, 1984.
11. Rubenstein K, Myoka U: Treatment of diabetic maculopathy, *Br J Ophthalmol* 56:1-5, 1972.
12. Cheng H, Kohner EM, Keen H, et al: Photocoagulation in the treatment of diabetic maculopathy: interim report of a multicentre controlled study, *Lancet* 2:1110-1113, 1975.
13. Townsend C, Bailey J, Kohner EM: Xenon are photocoagulation in the treatment of diabetic maculopathy, *Trans Ophthalmol Soc UK* 99:13-16, 1979.
14. The Early Treatment Diabetic Retinopathy Research Study Group: Photocoagulation for diabetic macular edema: ETDRS report no. 1, *Arch Ophthalmol* 103:1796-1806, 1985.
15. McDonald HR, Schatz H: Grid photocoagulation for diffuse macular edema, *Retina* 5:65-71, 1985.
16. Olk RJ: Modified grid argon laser photocoagulation for diffuse diabetic macular edema, *Ophthalmology* 93:938-948, 1986.
17. Marshall J, Clover G, Rothery S: Some new findings on retinal irradiation by krypton and argon lasers, *Doc Ophthalmol Proc Ser* 36:21-37, 1984.
18. The Early Treatment Diabetic Retinopathy Study Group: Early photocoagulation for diabetic retinopathy: ETDRS report no. 9, *Ophthalmology* 98:766-785, 1991.
19. Benson WE, Brown GC, Tasman W: *Diabetes and its ocular complications,* Philadelphia, 1988, WB Saunders, Chapter 17, pp 154-162.
20. Early Treatment Diabetic Retinopathy Study Research Group: Early photocoagulation for diabetic retinopathy: ETDRS report no. 9, *Ophthalmology* 98:766-785, 1991.

9

Treatment of Proliferative Diabetic Retinopathy

William E. Benson

PATIENT PRESENTATION

Case 1. A 35-year-old diabetic woman presented with a 1-day history of decreased vision. Visual acuity was 20/20 in the right eye and counting fingers in the left. Ocular examination was normal except for the fundus findings. In the right eye she had neovascularization of the optic disc three disc areas in extent, scattered microaneurysms, and dot and blot hemorrhages. In the left eye she had a central vitreous hemorrhage (Fig. 9-1). The diagnosis of proliferative diabetic retinopathy in both eyes and vitreous hemorrhage in the left eye was made.

CLINICAL FINDINGS AND SYMPTOMS OF PROLIFERATIVE RETINOPATHY

Although the macular edema, exudates, and capillary occlusions seen in background diabetic retinopathy often cause legal blindness, afflicted patients usually maintain ambulatory or better vision. Proliferative diabetic retinopathy (PDR), however, may result in severe vitreous hemorrhage or retinal detachment with hand-movements vision or worse. When the edema, exudates, and occlusions occur on or within one disc diameter of the optic disc, they are referred to as NVD (neovascularization of the disc). When they arise further than one disc diameter away, they are called NVE (neovascularization elsewhere).

Proliferative vessels usually arise from veins and often begin as a collection of fine naked vessels. When the stimulus for growth of new vessels is present, the path taken by vessels is along the route of least resistance. For example, the absence of a true internal limiting membrane on the disc could explain the prevalence of new vessels at that location. Also neovascularization seems to grow more easily on a performed connective tissue framework. Thus the detached posterior vitreous face is a frequent site of new vessel growth. The new vessels, initially naked, usually progress through a stage of further proliferation with connective tissue formation. As PDR progresses, the fibrous component becomes more prominent. Vitreous traction is transmitted to the retina along these proliferations and may lead to traction retinal detachment.

Treatment of proliferative diabetic retinopathy 153

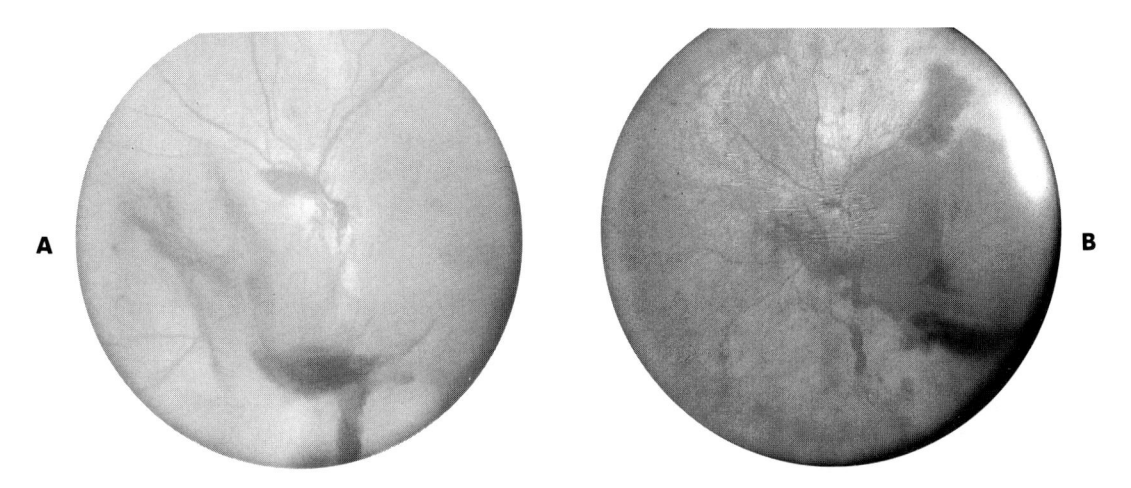

Figure 9-1 Left eye of Case 1. **A,** Probable neovascularization of the optic disc and vitreous hemorrhage. **B,** Despite the large hemorrhage, there is room for peripheral panretinal photocoagulation.

NVE nearly always initially grows toward zones of retinal ischemia until posterior vitreous detachment occurs. Posterior vitreous detachment in diabetics is characterized by a slow overall shrinkage of the entire formed vitreous rather than by the formation of cavities resulting from vitreous destruction.[1] Davis[2] and Davis et al.[3] have stressed the role of the contracting vitreous in the production of vitreous hemorrhage, retinal breaks, and retinal detachment. Neovascular vessels do not "grow" forward into the vitreous cavity; they are pulled into it by the contracting vitreous to which they are adherent. Confirmation of the importance of the vitreous in the development and progression of proliferative retinopathy comes from long-term follow-up of eyes that have undergone successful vitrectomy. The existent neovascularization regresses and leaks less fluorescein, and new areas of neovascularization rarely arise.

It has long been assumed that sudden vitreous contractions tear the fragile new vessels, causing vitreous hemorrhage, however, 62% to 83% of diabetic vitreous hemorrhages occur during sleep,[4,5] possibly because of an increase in blood pressure secondary to early morning hypoglycemia or to rapid eye movement (REM) sleep. Since so few hemorrhages occur during exercise, we do not restrict the activity of patients with proliferative retinopathy.

DIFFERENTIAL DIAGNOSIS

The correct diagnosis is usually made easily because nearly all patients with PDR have had a long history of diabetes mellitus. Furthermore, most patients with PDR have bilateral retinopathy, although it may not always be symmetric. In patients who are not diabetic, radiation retinopathy, branch retinal vein obstruction, sarcoidosis, and sickle cell hemoglobinopathy must be considered. Radiation retinopathy and branch retinal vein obstruction were discussed in Chapter 8. Sarcoidosis is usually associated with other signs of uveitis and retinal periphlebitis. Sickle cell hemoglobinopathy should be suspected in black patients whose neovascularization is mostly anterior to the vortex veins and in whom there are no posterior signs of diabetic retinopathy.

TECHNIQUE OF PANRETINAL PHOTOCOAGULATION

I generally do not obtain fluorescein angiography before performing panretinal photocoagulation (PRP), although some retinal specialists do so they can document known NVD and NVE and identify small areas of NVE. If there is no significant cataract, I use the argon green laser. The Rodenstock panfunduscope is good for the first burns because its wide field of vision enables one to avoid the macula.[6,7] It provides an excellent view of the fundus from the disc to the equator and sometimes even anterior to the equator. This lens is especially helpful if a retrobulbar anesthetic injection is required for analgesia since, with the associated akinesia, complete treatment with the Goldmann three-mirror lens is difficult. The patient cannot move his eye to help the physician treat hard-to-reach areas between the various viewing zones of the lens. Typical initial settings are a 200 μm spot size, a 0.1-second exposure time, and 200 mW of power. The power is increased until a whitish lesion is obtained. The first step is to make a ring of coagulations around the macula to help avoid unintentional macular burns (Fig. 9-2). Lesions are spaced about half a burn width apart. Areas of NVE are treated with confluent burns and surrounded with a 500 μm zone of confluent burns. NVE, especially when it is not elevated into the vitreous, can often be obliterated by such treatment. Burns of wide diameter and long duration are most effective, because they deliver the maximum heat to the inner retina. After the row delimiting the macula has been placed, treatment is continued out to the far periphery. For treatment of the periphery the Goldmann three-mirror lens and 500 μm spots are used. Generally a total of 1600 to 2000 burns are placed.

Burns along the long ciliary nerves are often painful, but most patients will have little or no discomfort until the treatment approaches the equator. If the patient cannot tolerate the required intensity of burns, the physician can suspend treatment, give the patient a mild tranquilizer, and resume treatment 30 to 45 minutes later. An alternative is to use 200 μm burns. If this option is selected, 6.25 times more burns are required to coagulate the same area of retina, because the formula for the area of a circle is pi times the radius squared (πr^2). A third alternative is to use a 0.5-second exposure time. A final alternative is to give retrobulbar anesthesia.

Doft and Blankenship[8] have shown that treatment in a single session has no more long-term complications than treatment in divided sessions. Nevertheless, we usually divide the treatment into three sessions because this strategy is less likely to cause transient myopia, angle closure, and cystoid macular edema. Furthermore, many patients who cannot tolerate 1600 to 2000 burns in one session unless retrobulbar anesthesia is given can tolerate 550 to 700 burns.

For many years, the efficacy of PRP was controversial. Many authors reported good results,[9-24] but occasionally the untreated eyes did as well as the treated eyes.[25] For many reasons none of these reports was able to prove statistically that treatment was beneficial. Some of these reports were discussed by Ederer and Hiller[26] in their classic paper on clinical trials. They stressed that to achieve statistical validity, a study had to have (1) proper controls, (2) randomization, (3) masking of both the treater and the patient, (4) easily defined criteria for determining the outcome of treatment or of nontreatment, (5) adequate number of patients, and (6) proper statistical analysis. Their paper must be read by anyone who wants to interpret scientific literature properly. The controversy

Treatment of proliferative diabetic retinopathy 155

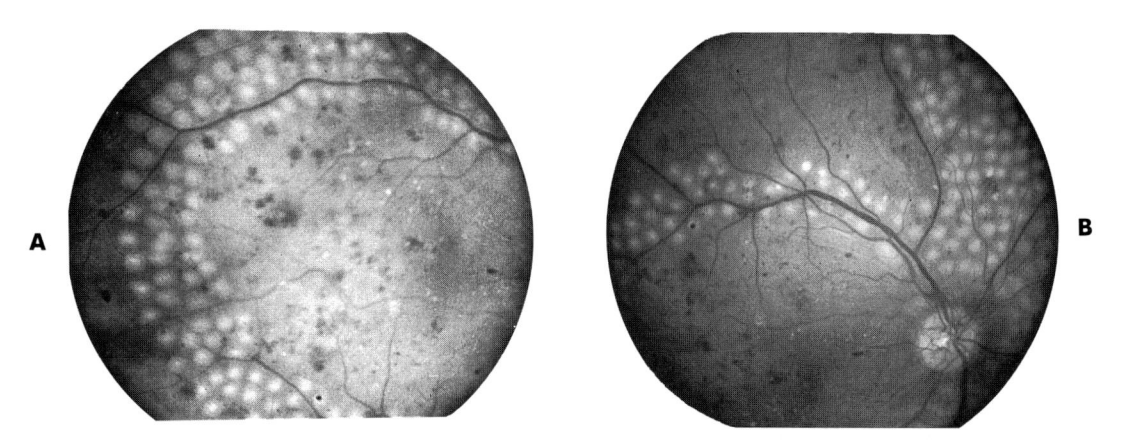

Figure 9-2 The first step in a panretinal photocoagulation is to outline the macula.

was finally resolved when Dr. Matthew Davis initiated and led one of the best clinical trials ever done, the Diabetic Retinopathy Study (DRS).[27]

The DRS enrolled 1758 patients, all of whom had a visual acuity of 20/100 or better, had received no previous photocoagulation, and had PDR in one eye or severe nonproliferative retinopathy in both eyes. One eye was treated with either argon blue-green laser or xenon arc PRP. In addition, NVE was treated with confluent burns. The end point was a visual acuity of 5/200 or worse on two consecutive visits 4 months apart. The DRS conclusively proved that either treatment modality was better than nontreatment. After 3 years of follow-up the 5/200 end point was reached by 26.4% of controls, as opposed to only 8% of eyes treated with xenon arc PRP and 13% of those treated with argon laser PRP. The difference between the results for argon versus xenon was not statistically significant.[28,29] In eyes receiving argon laser the DRS initially treated NVD with direct burns until it was found that the results were just as good in eyes that received indirect treatment alone.

Further analysis of the data enabled the investigators to determine which eyes benefited most from treatment. Any eye with (1) NVD less than half a disc diameter in area with associated vitreous hemorrhage, (2) NVD greater than half a disc diameter in area with or without associated vitreous hemorrhage, or (3) NVE with associated vitreous hemorrhage was found to be at particularly high risk of visual loss. Such eyes were said to have high-risk characteristics (HRC). At the end of 3 years of follow-up many fewer treated eyes had severe loss of vision (defined as less than 5/200) than did the untreated control eyes. The results of treatment versus no treatment are shown in the Table 9-1.

These results prove that PRP is clearly beneficial for all eyes with HRC. Furthermore, the greatest treatment benefit was in eyes with early NVD. PRP as soon as HRC have developed is much more likely to preserve visual acuity than it is after they have advanced. A similar conclusion was reached by Yassur et al.,[30] who noted that eyes with early NVD are much less likely to progress to fibrovascular proliferation after PRP than are eyes with moderate or advanced NVD. This is important because eyes with fibrovascular proliferation are more likely to go on to develop traction retinal detachment or dragging of the macular than are eyes without it.

Table 9-1 Effect of Panretinal Photocoagulation in Preventing Severe Visual Loss (<5/200) in Eyes with High-Risk Characteristics (3 Years After Treatment)

	Treated eyes (%)	Control eyes (%)
NVE greater than half a disc area and vitreous hemorrhage	7	30
NCD less than half a disc area and vitreous hemorrhage	4	26
NVD greater than half a disc area and no hemorrhage	9	26
NVD greater than half a disc area and vitreous hemorrhage	20	37

It should be stressed that PRP usually does not cause total regression of neovascularization.[28] Overall, in only 30% of treated eyes was there total regression of NVD. In eyes with mild NVD (less than half a disc diameter in area) 41% had total regression. Partial regression was seen in another 27%. By comparison, only 13% of the untreated eyes with mild NVD had partial regression and another 13% had total regression.

OTHER STUDIES ON PANRETINAL PHOTOCOAGULATION

Other large randomized clinical trials[31-33] have also found that PRP is beneficial to the treated eyes. Blankenship and Doft[34] reported that the prognosis is best if some regression occurs within 3 weeks. They studied eyes that had NVD greater than half a disc diameter in area before treatment. Of those that regressed to less than half a disc diameter by 3 weeks after treatment, 50% had total regression by 6 months and another 28% remained stable. Conversely, if little or no regression was seen by 3 weeks after PRP, only 36% later regressed to either mild or no NVD by 6 months. Furthermore, eyes with prompt regression of the neovascularization have an excellent visual prognosis.[35]

Case 1. (Continued) This patient clearly has high-risk characteristics and requires PRP in both eyes. The left eye (see Fig. 9-1) should be treated immediately, before the vitreous hemorrhage spreads and prevents any treatment at all. The ophthalmologist should treat, as a semiemergency, all of the retina that is not obscured by the hemorrhage. In many cases this necessitates retrobulbar anesthesia. On the next visit PRP will be begun in the right eye.

Case 2. A 24-year-old man has received 2000 500 μm burns, but his neovascularization of the disc has not regressed.

Case 3. A 28-year-old woman received 2000 500 μm burns 4 months ago. She presents with "floaters" and is found to have a small vitreous hemorrhage (Fig. 9-3).

Should additional treatment be given to Cases 2 and 3? Some experts[36-39] have recommended supplementing the treatment in both cases, even if this requires as many as 7985 burns. There is no proof, however, that the visual prognosis of eyes treated with this strategy is any better than that of eyes treated with a standard PRP and no supplements. Furthermore, the additional supplements can be expected to increase the unavoidable complications of PRP (e.g., loss of peripheral visual field and poor dark adaptation). Finally, it must be re-

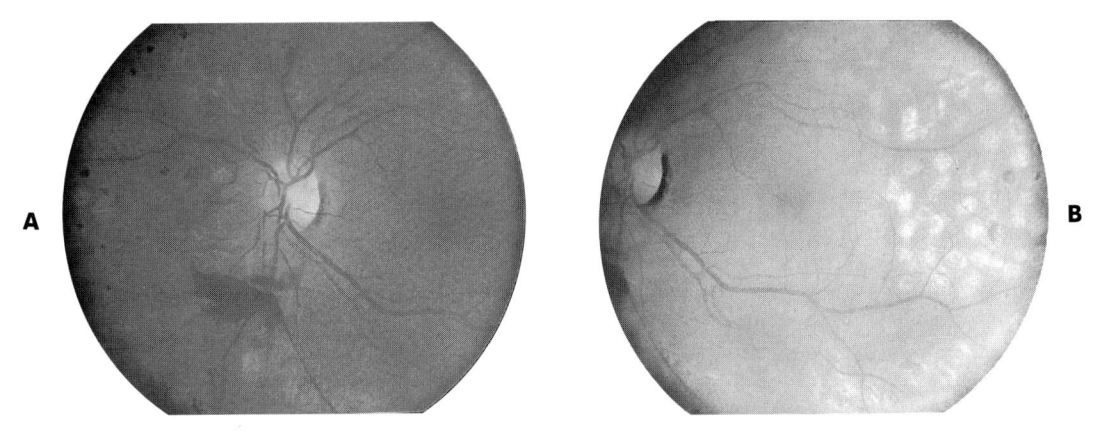

Figure 9-3 Case 3. Vitreous hemorrhage 3 months after panretinal photocoagulation.

membered that the results of the DRS were obtained before the widespread use of modern vitrectomy techniques. Many of the eyes that had a poor visual result in the DRS would today have a vitrectomy and a good visual outcome. In summary, whether supplementary treatment should be given is not known. Most retinal specialists would attempt to close areas of NVE directly, except for highly elevated ones. Whether supplements should be given for NVD remains controversial.

The krypton laser (wavelength 647 nm) causes less damage to the inner retinal layers than does either the argon blue-green laser (wavelengths 488 and 514 nm), the argon green laser, or the xenon arc photocoagulator. Therefore, since the krypton laser damages the nerve fiber layer least, when used for PRP it might be expected to cause less visual field loss than the other instruments. Schulenburg et al.[40] randomized 12 eyes with NVD to either argon blue-green PRP or krypton PRP. Both lasers caused equal resolution of the NVD. The krypton-treated eyes had slightly less visual field loss, but the difference was not striking (average of only 2 degrees less than in eyes treated with the argon blue-green laser).

COMPLICATIONS OF PRP

There are numerous complications of PRP.[41,42] Many patients develop a syndrome similar to Adie's with chronic dilation, hypersensitivity to 0.125% pilocarpine, light-near dissociation, and sector iris sphincter palsy.[43,44] Young patients frequently complain of asthenopia because of decreased accommodation.[45] Common retinal complications include decreased visual acuity.[46,47] from cystoid macular edema or macular pucker, decreased color vision,[48,49] decreased visual field,[40,47] and decreased dark adaptation.[50] Rarer, but devastating, complications are inadvertent foveolar burns, choriovitreal proliferation, choroidal neovascular membranes, and transient closed angle glaucoma.[41]

MECHANISM OF THE EFFICACY OF PRP

The mechanism by which panretinal photocoagulation causes regression of NVD and of NVE not directly treated is unknown. There are several theories.

The first[51] assumes that the diseased retinal vessels can deliver only a limited quantity of oxygen to the retina. Treatment eliminates enough retina to allow the retinal circulation to supply the remaining retina better. In other words, the rationale for treatment is analogous to that for thinning out a new forest of saplings: those remaining achieve maximum growth.

A second theory,[52-57] similar to the first, stresses the fact that the maximum damage caused by photocoagulation is in the outer retinal layers. The photoreceptors use approximately two thirds of the oxygen supply to the retina.[58] Therefore eliminating them facilitates diffusion of oxygen from the richly oxygenated choriocapillaris to the adjacent photoreceptors and inner retina. Although the choriocapillaris is initially occluded by laser burns, in most cases it regenerates to supply the needed oxygen.[59] Strong support for this theory is that in experimental animals, if the retinal circulation is occluded by a probe, the oxygen tension over a laser burn is actually higher than it is over adjacent retina.[52-54] Further evidence of improved oxygenation of the retina is constriction of dilated retinal arteries and veins and decreased blood flow, both of which can be observed clinically[60-62] and in experimental animals.[63] Also, in diabetics, the retinal blood volume is decreased[64] and the retina's autoregulatory capacity is improved.[61,62] With the choriocapillaris now supplementing the retinal circulation, there is less need for a high retinal blood flow. The principal proponents of this second theory[56,57] believe that the main stimulus for neovascularization is vasodilation. When the veins constrict, the stimulus for neovascularization is decreased.

A third theory[65-70] recognizes the improvement in retinal oxygenation following PRP but postulates that the main effect is to decrease the production of a vasoproliferative factor by the hypoxic retina. Since less of this factor would be available to diffuse from hypoxic areas to adjacent retina and to the optic disc, the stimulus for NVE and NVD would be decreased.

PANRETINAL CRYOTHERAPY

Haut, Lempert, and Schimek were pioneers in the use of peripheral retinal cryotherapy.[71-73] Some 8 to 12 cryotherapy lesions are placed in each quadrant, just posterior to the ora serrata and under direct visualization if possible. If retinal freezing cannot be seen ophthalmoscopically, the freeze is held for 10 to 15 seconds. The main indications for this treatment[71-80] are media too hazy to allow either argon or krypton laser PRP and repeated vitreous hemorrhages despite a complete PRP. Reported benefits include accelerated resorption of longstanding vitreous hemorrhages[73,74,77,78,80] and regression of neovascularization.[71-80] The main complication is development or acceleration of a traction retinal detachment. In some series[74,76-80] this followed treatment in as many as 25% to 33% of the eyes.

We believe that peripheral retinal cryotherapy is a treatment modality that should be considered before vitrectomy but that should be avoided in patients with traction retinal detachment or areas of strong vitreoretinal adhesion. A careful ultrasound examination is mandatory before this treatment can be considered in eyes with opaque media.

References

1. Foos RY, Kreiger AE, Forsythe AB, et al: Posterior vitreous detachment in diabetic subjects, *Ophthalmology* 87:122, 1980.
2. Davis MD: Vitreous contraction in proliferative diabetic retinopathy. Arch Ophthalmol 74:741, 1965.
3. Davis MD, et al: Clinical observations concerning pathogenesis of diabetic retinopathy. In Goldberg MD, Fine SL (eds): *Symposium on the treatment of diabetic retinopathy* (publication no. 1890), Washington DC, 1969, U.S. Public Health Service.
4. Anderson B Jr: Activity and diabetic vitreous hemorrhage, *Ophthalmology* 87:137, 1980.
5. Tasman W: Diabetic vitreous hemorrhage and its relationship to hypoglycemia, *Mod Probl Ophthalmol* 20:413, 1979.
6. Lobes LA Jr, Benson WE, Grand MG: Panfunduscope contact lens for argon laser therapy, *Ann Ophthalmol* 13:713, 1981.
7. Blankenship GW: Panretinal laser photocoagulation with a wide-angle fundus contact lens, *Ann Ophthalmol* 14:362, 1982.
8. Doft BG, Blankenship GW: Single versus multiple treatment sessions of argon laser panretinal photocoagulation for proliferative diabetic retinopathy, *Ophthalmology* 89:772, 1982.
9. Okun E, Cibis P: The role of photocoagulation in the treatment of proliferative diabetic retinopathy, *Arch Ophthalmol* 75:337, 1966.
10. Wetzig PC, Jepson CN: Treatment of diabetic retinopathy by light coagulation, *Am J Ophthalmol* 62:459, 1966.
11. Meyer-Schwickerath G, Schott K: Diabetic retinopathy and photocoagulation, *Am J Ophthalmol* 66:597, 1968.
12. Okun E, Johnston GP: The role of photocoagulation in the treatment of proliferative diabetic retinopathy: continuation and follow-up studies. In Goldberg MF, Fine SC (eds): *Symposium on the treatment of diabetic retinopathy,* Washington DC, 1968, U.S. Department of Health, Education, and Welfare, pp 523-535.
13. Okun E: The effectiveness of photocoagulation in the treatment of proliferative diabetic retinopathy, *Trans Am Acad Ophthalmol Otolaryngol* 72:246, 1968.
14. Dobree JH, Taylor E: Treatment of proliferative diabetic retinopathy by light coagulation, *Trans Ophthalmol Soc UK* 88:313, 1968.
15. Dobree JH, Taylor E: Treatment of proliferative diabetic retinopathy by repeated light coagulation: a seven year review, *Br J Ophthalmol* 57:73, 1973.
16. Aiello LM, Beetham WP, Balodimos MC, et al: Ruby laser photocoagulation in the treatment of diabetic proliferating retinopathy: preliminary report. In Goldberg MF, Fine SL (eds): *Symposium on the treatment of diabetic retinopathy,* Washington DC, 1968, U.S. Department of Health, Education, and Welfare, pp 437-463.
17. Beetham WP, Aiello LM, Balodimos MC, Koncz L: Ruby laser photocoagulation of early diabetic neovascular retinopathy, *Arch Ophthalmol* 83:261, 1970.
18. L'Esperance FA: An ophthalmic argon laser photocoagulation system; design, construction and laboratory investigations, *Trans Am Ophthalmol Soc* 66:827, 1968.
19. Little HL, Zweing HC, Peabody RR: Argon laser slit lamp retinal photocoagulation, *Trans Am Acad Ophthalmol Otolaryngol* 74:85, 1970.
20. Krill AE, Archer DB, Newell FW, Chishti ML: Photocoagulation in diabetic retinopathy, *Am J Ophthalmol* 72:299, 1971.
21. Geltzer AI: Laser photocoagulation and diabetic retinopathy, *Rhode Island Med J* 55:275, 1972.
22. Zetterstrom B: The value of photocoagulation in diabetic retinopathy, *Acta Ophthalmol (Kbh)* 50:351, 1972.
23. L'Esperance FA: The treatment of ophthalmic vascular disease by argon laser photocoagulation, *Trans Am Acad Ophthalmol Otolaryngol* 73:1077, 1969.
24. L'Esperance FA: Argon laser photocoagulation of diabetic retinal neovascularization: a five year appraisal, *Trans Am Acad Ophthalmol Otolaryngol* 77:6, 1973.

25. Irvine AR, Norton EWD: Photocoagulation in diabetic retinopathy, *Am J Ophthalmol* 71:437, 1971.
26. Ederer F, Hiller R: Clinical trials, diabetic retinopathy and photocoagulation. A reanalysis of five studies, *Surv Ophthalmol* 19:267, 1975.
27. Diabetic Retinopathy Study Research Group: Preliminary report on effects of photocoagulation therapy, *Am J Ophthalmol* 81:383, 1976.
28. Diabetic Retinopathy Study Research Group: Photocoagulation treatment of proliferative diabetic retinopathy: the second report of diabetic retinopathy study findings, *Ophthamology* 85:82, 1978.
29. Diabetic Retinopathy Study Research Group: Four risk factors for severe visual loss in diabetic retinopathy: third report, *Arch Ophthalmol* 97:654, 1979.
30. Yassur Y, Pickle LW, Fine SL, et al: Optic disc neovascularization in diabetic retinopathy. II. Natural history and results of photocoagulation treatment, *Br J Ophthalmol* 64:77, 1980.
31. Hercules BL, Gayed II, Lucas SB, Jeacock J: Peripheral retinal ablation in the treatment of proliferative diabetic retinopathy: a three-year interim report of a randomized, controlled study using the argon laser, *Br J Ophthalmol* 61:555, 1977.
32. British Multicentre Study Group: Photocoagulation for proliferative diabetic retinopathy: a randomized controlled clinical trial using the xenon-arc, *Diabetologia* 26.109, 1984.
33. Oosterhuis JA, Beintema MR, Lemkes HHLM, et al: Photocoagulation treatment in diabetic retinopathy: a two-year pre- and five-year post-treatment study, *Doc Ophthalmol* 48:101, 1979.
34. Doft BH, Blankenship G: Retinopathy risk factor regression after laser panretinal photocoagulation for proliferative diabetic retinopathy, *Ophthalmology* 91:1453, 1984.
35. Vander JF, Duker JS, Benson WE, et al: Long-term stability and visual outcome after favorable initial response of proliferative diabetic retinopathy to panretinal photocoagulation, *Ophthalmology* 98:1575, 1991.
36. Rogell GD: Incremental panretinal photocoagulation; results in treating proliferative diabetic retinopathy, *Retina* 3:308, 1983.
37. Vine AK: The efficacy of additional argon laser photocoagulation for persistent, severe proliferative diabetic retinopathy, *Ophthalmology* 92:1532, 1985.
38. Aylward GW, Pearson RV, Jagger JD, et al: Extensive argon laser photocoagulation in the treatment of proliferative diabetic retinopathy, *Br J Ophthalmol* 73:197, 1989.
39. Singerman LJ: PDR in juvenile-onset diabetics: high-risk proliferative diabetic retinopathy in juvenile-onset diabetics, *Retina* 1:18, 1981.
40. Schulenberg WE, Hamilton AM, Blach RK: A comparative study of argon laser and krypton laser in the treatment of diabetic optic disc neovascularisation, *Br J Ophthalmol* 63:412, 1979.
41. Benson WE, Brown GC, Tasman W: *Diabetes and its ocular complications,* Philadelphia, 1988, WB Saunders, Chapter 16, pp 144-153.
42. Schiodte N: Ocular effects of panretinal photocoagulation, *Acta Ophthalmol* 66:(suppl 186):9, 1988.
43. Lobes LA, Bourgnon P: Pupillary abnormalities following argon laser ablation for proliferative diabetic retinopathy, *Ophthalmology* 92:234, 1985.
44. Rogell GD: Internal ophthalmoplegia after argon laser panretinal photocoagulation, *Arch Ophthalmol* 97:904, 1979.
45. Lerner BC, Lakhanpal V, Schocket SS: Transient myopia and accommodative paresis following cryotherapy and panretinal photocoagulation, *Am J Ophthalmol* 97:704, 1984.
46. Ferris FL, Podgor MJ, Davis MD: The Diabetic Retinopathy Research Group: Macular edema in diabetic retinopathy study patients, *Ophthalmology* 94:754, 1987.
47. Hamilton AM, Townsend C, Khoury D, et al: Xenon arc and argon laser photocoagulation in the treatment of diabetic disc neovascularization. I. Effect on disc vessels, visual fields, and visual acuity, *Trans Ophthalmol Soc UK* 101:87, 1981.

48. Birch J, Hamilton AM: Xenon arc and argon laser photocoagulation in the treatment of diabetic disc neovascularization. II. Effect on color vision, *Trans Ophthalmol Soc UK* 101:93, 1981.
49. Birch-Cox J: Defective colour vision in diabetic retinopathy before and after laser photocoagulation, *Mod Probl Ophthalmol* 19:326, 1978.
50. Pender PM, Benson WE, Compton H, et al: The effects of panretinal photocoagulation on dark adaptation in diabetics with proliferative retinopathy, *Ophthalmology* 88:635, 1981.
51. Blach R, Hamilton AM: The technique and indications for photocoagulation in diabetic retinopathy. I. Principles of photocoagulation, *Int Ophthalmol* 1:19, 1978.
52. Wolbarsht ML, Landers MB III: The rationale of photocoagulation therapy for proliferative diabetic retinopathy: a review and a model, *Ophthalmic Surg* 11:235, 1980.
53. Stefansson E, Landers MB III, Wolbarsht ML: Increased retinal oxygen supply following pan-retinal photocoagulation and vitrectomy in lensectomy, *Trans Am Ophthalmol Soc* 79:307, 1981.
54. Stefansson E, Machemer R, deJuan E, et al: Retinal oxygenation and laser treatment in patients with diabetic retinopathy, *Am J Ophthalmol* 113:36, 1992.
55. Stefansson E, Hatchell DL, Fisher BL, et al: Panretinal photocoagulation and retinal oxygenation in normal and diabetic cats, *Am J Ophthalmol* 101:657, 1986.
56. Wolbarsht ML, Landers MB III, Stefansson E: Vasodilation and the etiology of diabetic retinopathy: a new model, *Ophthalmic Surg* 1981;12:104-107.
57. Stefansson E, Landers MB III, Wolbarsht ML: Oxygenation and vasodilation in relation to diabetic and other proliferative retinopathies, *Ophthalmic Surg* 17:209, 1983.
58. Weiter JJ, Zuckerman R: The influence of the photoreceptor-RPE complex on the inner retina, *Opthahlmology* 87:1133, 1980.
59. Perry DD, Risco JM: Choroidal microvascular repair after argon laser photocoagulation, *Am J Ophthalmol* 93:787, 1982.
60. Feke GT, Green GJ, Goger DG, McMeel JW: Laser doppler measurements of the effects of panretinal photocoagulation on retinal blood flow, *Ophthalmology* 89:757, 1982.
61. Grunwald JE, Riva CE, Brucker AJ, et al: Effect of panretinal photocoagulation on retinal blood flow in proliferative diabetic retinopathy, *Ophthalmology* 93:590, 1986.
62. Grunwald JE, Brucker AJ, Petrig BL, et al: Retinal blood flow regulation and the clinical response to panretinal photocoagulation in proliferative diabetic retinopathy, *Ophthalmology* 96:1518, 1989.
63. Hill DW, Young S: Diversion of retinal blood flow by photocoagulation, *Br J Ophthalmol* 62:251, 1978.
64. Koerner F, Fries F, Niesel P, Dubied P: Zur Interpretation der retinalen Kreislaufzeiten bei der diabetischen Retinopathie vor und nach Photokoagulation, *Klin Monatsbl Augenheilkd* 172:440, 1978.
65. Michaelson IC: The mode of development of the vascular system of the retina with some observations on its significance for certain retinal diseases, *Trans Ophthalmol Soc UK* 78:137, 1948.
66. Glaser BM, D'Amore PA, Michels RG, et al: The demonstration of angiogenic activity from ocular tissues, *Ophthalmology* 87:440, 1980.
67. Glaser B: Extracellular modulating factors and the control of intraocular neovascularization, *Arch Ophthalmol* 106:603, 1988.
68. Imre G: Studies on the metabolism of retinal neovascularisation: role of lactic acid, *Br J Ophthalmol* 48:75, 1965.
69. Zauberman H, Michaelson IC, Bergman F, et al: Stimulation of neovascularization of the cornea by biogenic amines, *Exp Eye Res* 8:77, 1969.
70. Ben Ezra D: Neovasculogenesis: Triggering factors and possible mechanisms, *Surv Ophthalmol* 24:167, 1979.
71. Haut J, Robert P, Chatellier PH, Leon MC: Place de la cryothérapie dans le traitement de la rétinopathie diabétique, *Bull Mem Soc Fr Ophtalmol* 90:124, 1978.

72. Lempert P: Cryoablation for diabetic retinopathy, *Am Ophthalmol* 11:740, 1979.
73. Schimek RA, Spencer R: Cryopexy treatment of proliferative diabetic retinopathy, *Arch Ophthalmol* 97:1276, 1979.
74. Oosterhuis JA, Bijlmer-Gortner H: Cryotreatment in proliferative diabetic retinopathy: long-term results, *Ophthalmologica (Basel)* 181:81, 1980.
75. Bergen RL, Mignone B: Cryocoagulation for proliferative diabetic retinopathy, *Ann Ophthalmol* 12:1209, 1980.
76. Ramsey RC, Cantrill HL, Knobloch WH: Cryoretinopexy for proliferative diabetic retinopathy, *Can J Ophthalmol* 17:17, 1982.
77. Daily MJ, Gieser RG: Treatment of proliferative diabetic retinopathy with panretinal cryotherapy, *Ophthalmic Surg* 9:741, 1984.
78. Buettner H, Johnson RO: Retinal cryoablation for complications of proliferative diabetic retinopathy (PDR). Presented at the annual meeting of the Retina Society, September 1981.
79. Lim ASM, Ang BC: Cryoapplication in diabetic retinopathy, *Int Ophthalmol* 9:139, 1986.
80. Mosier MA, DelPiero E, Gheewala SM: Anterior retinal cryotherapy in diabetic vitreous hemorrhage, *Am J Ophthalmol* 100:440, 1985.

10

Retinal Arterial Obstructive Disease

Gary C. Brown

HISTORICAL BACKGROUND

In 1859 von Graefe[1] described the appearance of a central retinal artery obstruction in a patient with endocarditis and multiple systemic emboli. Fifteen years later, in 1874, Loring[2] implicated focal obstructive disease within the central retinal artery as a cause of central retinal artery obstruction. By the turn of the twentieth century, over two dozen reports of central retinal artery obstruction were present in the literature.

CLINICAL CHARACTERISTICS

Symptoms[3]

Patients with acute central retinal artery obstruction usually have a history of painless unilateral loss of vision that occurs over a period of several seconds or less. In some patients a history of episodes of amaurosis fugax (periods of unilateral visual loss lasting for seconds to minutes) can be elicited as a precursor to the obstructive event.

Background Features[4]

The mean age of patients with central retinal artery obstruction is in the sixties, although the entity has also been seen in children.[5] Men are afected more than women, and there appears to be no predilection for one eye over the other. Bilateral involvement is seen in approximately 1% to 2% of cases. In these instances the possibilities of giant cell arteritis and cardiac abnormalities that predispose to the formation of emboli should be considered.

Included among the pathophysiologic mechanisms responsible for retinal arterial obstruction are emboli,[6] hemorrhage under an atherosclerotic plaque,[7] intraluminal thrombosis,[8] spasm,[9] vasculitis,[10] dissecting aneurysm,[11] and hypertensive necrosis.[12]

Clinical Findings

Visual acuity in eyes with central retinal artery obstruction is usually in the counting fingers to hand movements range. In eyes in which the acuity is no light perception, the possibilities of concomitant choroidal obstruction (ophthalmic artery obstruction) or damage to the optic nerve should be considered.[13] An afferent pupillary response is often present at the outset of the obstruction and thus precedes the retinal whitening observed ophthalmoscopically.

The anterior segment is usually normal in eyes with acute central retinal artery obstruction. In approximately 17% to 18% of cases iris neovascularization can occur.[14] The new vessels develop at a mean time of 4 weeks after the obstruction, with a range of 1 to 12 weeks. When iris neovascularization is already present at the time of visual loss, the possibility of underlying carotid artery obstructive disease as the cause of the new vessels should be considered.[15]

Posterior segment signs include narrowing of the retinal arteries, in severe cases associated with segmentation ("boxcarring") of the blood column. Superficial whitening of the retina usually develops within minutes to hours, and a cherry-red spot can be seen in the foveola, where the macular retina is the thin-

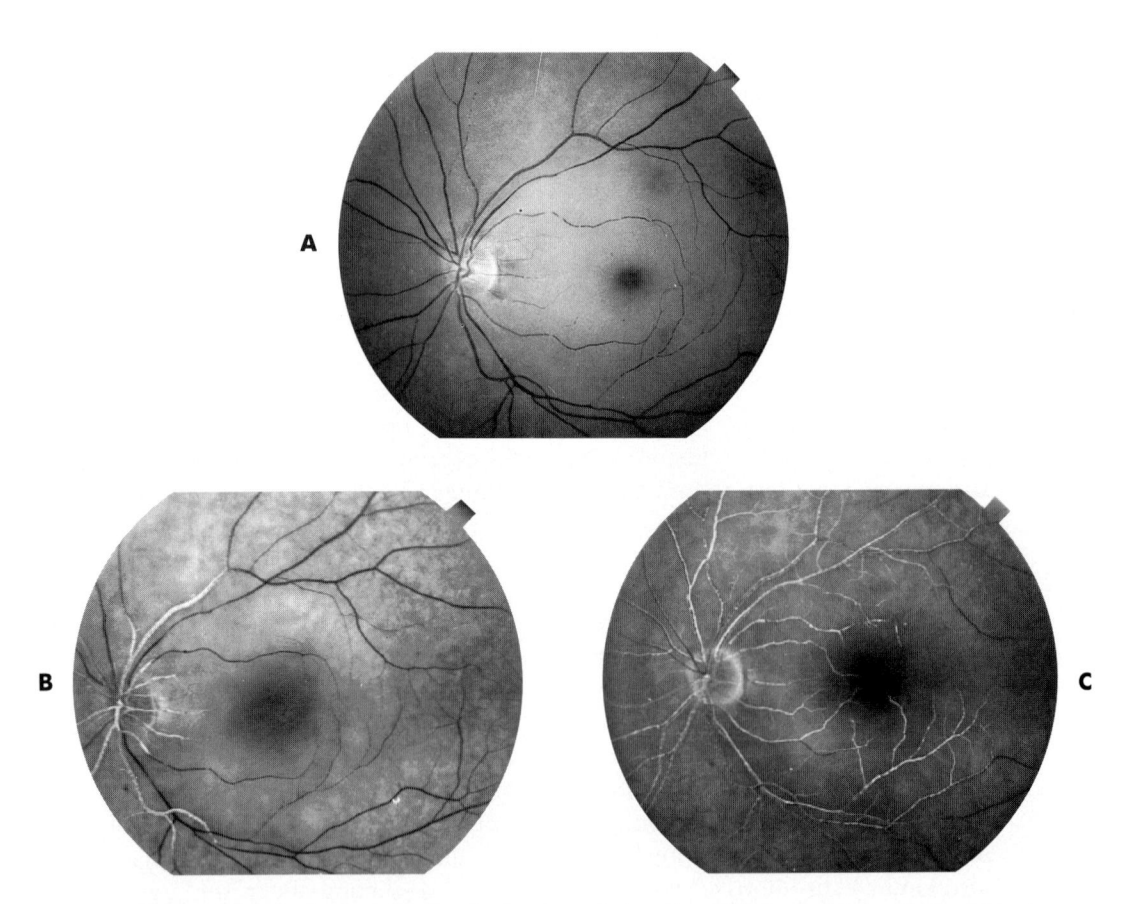

Figure 10-1 A, Acute central retinal artery obstruction with superficial retinal whittening and a cherry red spot in the foveola. Segmentation of the blood column ("boxcarring") can be seen in some of the retinal arteries and veins. **B,** Intravenous fluorescein angiogram corresponding to **A** at approximately 56 seconds after injection. There is delayed filling of the retinal arterial system. **C,** At greater than 10 minutes after injection, some of the retinal vessels are still not filled. Segmentation of the blood column is evident in most of the vessels.

nest and the underlying retinal pigment epithelium and choroid can still be seen (Fig. 10-1). Resolution of the retinal whitening generally occurs over a period of 2 to 6 weeks. In about 10% of cases a patient cilioretinal artery spares the foveolar retina (Fig. 10-2). In this situation, the visual acuity improves to 20/20 to 20/50 in 80% eyes.[16]

Emboli are seen with the retinal arterial system in about 20% of eyes with central retinal artery obstruction.[6] The most common are *cholesterol* emboli ("Hollenhorst plaques") (Fig. 10-3), which have a glistening yellow appearance and usually arise from the carotid arteries, *calcific* emboli (Fig. 10-4), which tend to be larger and whiter and arise from the aortic valve, and *fibrin-platelet* emboli (Fig. 10-5), yellow plugs that tend to be transient and can arise from the carotid system or the cardiac valves. It is the fibrin-platelet emboli that cause some cases of amaurosis fugax. The observation of a retinal arterial embolus, whether associated with a retinal arterial obstruction or not, implies a poorer prognosis for longevity compared to an age-matched population.[17]

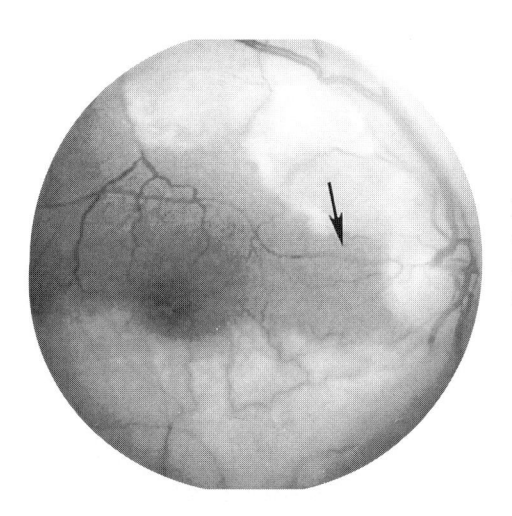

Figure 10-2 Acute central retinal artery obstruction with sparing of the central macula by a patent cilioretinal artery *(arrow)*. The visual acuity returned to 20/20.

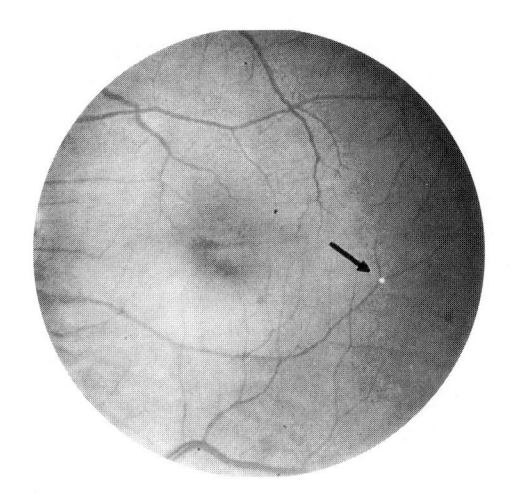

Figure 10-3 Cholesterol embolus ("Hollenhorst plaque") *(arrow)* lodged at a bifurcation within the superior retinal artery.

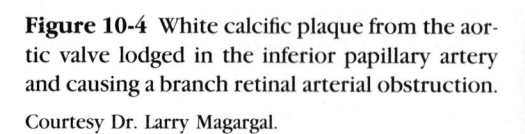

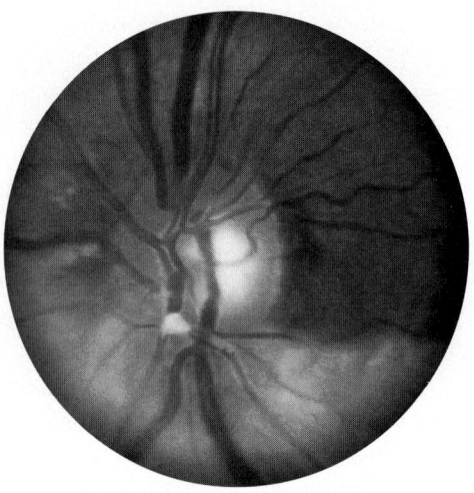

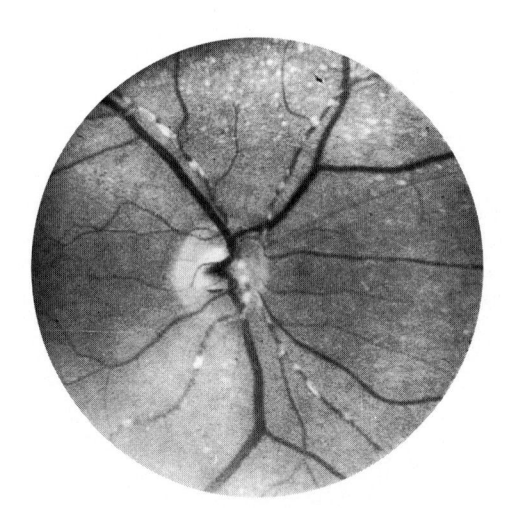

Figure 10-4 White calcific plaque from the aortic valve lodged in the inferior papillary artery and causing a branch retinal arterial obstruction.

Courtesy Dr. Larry Magargal.

Figure 10-5 Platelet-fibrin emboli within the retinal arterial system.

Figure 10-6 Electroretinogram from an eye with a central retinal artery obstruction *(top)*. There is diminution of the b-wave amplitude. The contralateral normal eye is shown in the *bottom* tracing.

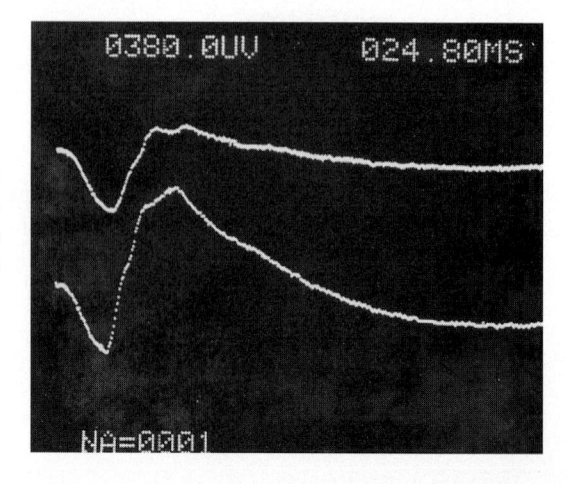

Table 10-1 Disease Entities Associated with Retinal Arterial Obstruction

I. ABNORMALITIES CONTRIBUTING TO EMBOLUS FORMATION

Systemic arterial hypertension (via atherosclerotic plaque formation; can also cause hypertensive necrosis)
Carotid artery atherosclerosis
Cardiac valvular disease
  Rheumatic
  Mitral valve prolapse
Thrombus after myocardial infarction
Cardiac myxoma
Tumors
Intravenous drug abuse
Lipid emboli
  Pancreatitis
  Purtscher's retinopathy (trauma)
Loiasis
Radiologic studies
  Carotid angiography
  Lymphangiography
  Hysterosalpingography
Head and neck corticosteroid injection
Retrobulbar corticosteroids
Deep vein thrombosis (via paradoxical embolus)

II. TRAUMA (VIA COMPRESSION, SPASM, OR DIRECT VESSEL DAMAGE)

Retrobulbar injection
Orbital fracture
Anesthesia
Penetrating injury
Drug- and/or alcohol-induced stupor
Nasal surgery

III. COAGULOPATHIES

Sickle cell disease
Homocystinuria
Oral contraceptives
Pregnancy
Platelet and factor abnormalities
Lupus anticoagulants
Protein S deficiency
Protein C deficiency
Antithrombin III deficiency

IV. OCULAR CONDITIONS ASSOCIATED WITH RETINAL ARTERIAL OBSTRUCTION

Prepapillary arterial loops
Optic disc drusen
Increased intraocular pressure (with sickling hemoglobinopathy)
Toxoplasmosis
Optic neuritis

V. COLLAGEN VASCULAR DISEASES

Systemic lupus erythematosis
Polyarteritis nodosa
Giant cell arteritis
Wegener's granulomatosis
Liebow's lymphogranulomatosis

VI. OTHER VASCULITIDES

Orbital mucormycosis
Radiation retinopathy
Behçet's disease

VII. MISCELLANEOUS ASSOCIATIONS

Ventriculography
Fabry's disease
Sydenham's chorea
Migraine
Hypotension
Fibromuscular hyperplasia
Nasal oxymethazolone
Lyme disease

Ancillary Studies[4]

Intravenous fluorescein angiography (Fig. 10-1) often reveals delayed retinal arterial filling. Nevertheless, the most common angiographic sign is delayed retinal arteriovenous transit time (the time from first appearance of the eye within the retinal arteries of the temporal vascular arcade until the corresponding retinal veins are completely filled; normal ≤ 11 seconds). Staining of the retinal vessels is generally not seen.

Electroretinography (Fig. 10-6) typically discloses a diminution of the b-wave amplitude due to ischemia of the inner retinal layers.

Systemic Associations

Systemic arterial hypertension is encountered in about 65% of patients with central retinal artery obstruction, and diabetes mellitus is found in a third.[3] A fourth of the patients have cardiac valvular disease, and 20% have a carotid stenosis greater than 50%.

A systemic workup is indicated in most cases of central retinal artery obstruction. The most common related abnormalities are listed in the above paragraph, but consideration should also be given to the other abnormalities listed in Table 10-1.

DIFFERENTIAL DIAGNOSIS

An acute ophthalmic artery obstruction (Fig. 10-7) is the abnormality most likely to be confused with an acute central retinal artery obstruction. The features that differentiate the two entities are shown in Table 10-2.

Central retinal artery/vein obstruction (Fig. 10-8) has the fundus appearance of superficial retinal whitening and a cherry-red spot seen with central retinal artery obstruction but, in addition, demonstrates the dilated tortuous retinal veins and retinal hemorhages usually seen with central retinal vein obstruction. Eyes with central retinal artery/vein obstruction have an 80% chance of developing iris neovascularization, with the growth of new blood vessels occurring at a mean of 6 weeks after the obstructive event.[18]

Aminoglycoside toxicity to the retina after an inadvertent intravitreal injection of the drug produces retinal whitening and a cherry-red spot similar to that seen with a central retinal artery obstruction within minutes of the injection.[19] Unlike a typical central retinal artery obstruction, it generally leads to a hemorrhagic retinal necrosis within days and can also cause a serous detachment of the retina.

Metabolic storage diseases (e.g., Tay Sachs) may cause superficial retinal whitening but occur in a completely different setting from that usually encountered with central retinal artery obstruction. They are most often present in young children and are associated with longstanding serious neurologic and systemic sequelae.

MANAGEMENT

Unfortunately, a consistently effective treatment is lacking for reversal of the visual loss associated with central retinal artery obstruction. Digital massage of the globe and massage via an in-and-out movement with the Goldmann contact lens have been advocated in an attempt to dislodge an obstructing embolus.

Retinal arterial obstructive disease 169

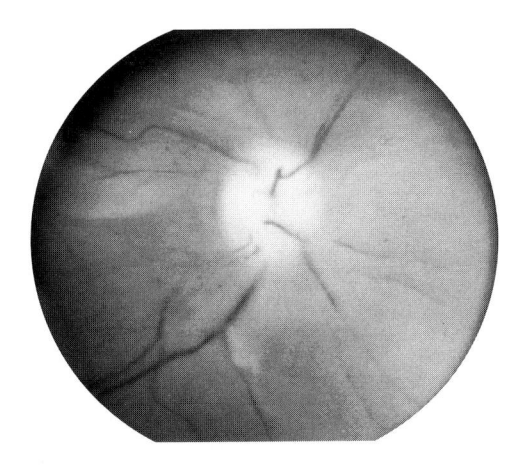

Figure 10-7 Acute ophthalmic artery obstruction secondary to mucormycosis of the orbit. Intense retinal whitening is present but there is no cherry-red spot. Visual acuity was no light perception.

Figure 10-8 Combined central retinal artery and vein obstructions.

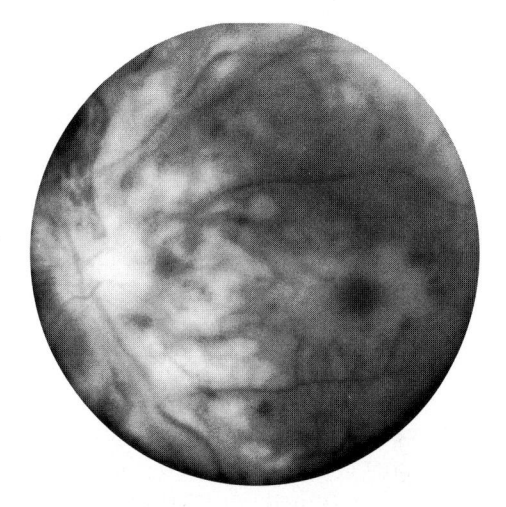

Table 10-2 Differentiating Features Between Acute Central Retinal Artery and Acute Ophthalmic Artery Obstructions

Features	Central retinal artery	Ophthalmic artery
Visual acuity	Typically CF-HM	Usually NLP
Fundus appearance		
Acute		
Cherry-red spot	Present	± Present
Whitening	Mild to moderate	Severe
Late		
RPE changes	Absent	Present
Optic atrophy	Mild to moderate	Severe
Fluorescein angiography		
Abnormal choroidal flow	Usually absent	Present
Abnormal retinal flow	Present	Present
Late deep staining	Absent	± Present
Electroretinography	Reduced b-wave amplitude	Reduced or absent a- and b-wave amplitudes

CF, counting fingers; HM, hand movements; NLP, no light perception; Abn, abnormal; Obstr, obstruction.
From Brown GC, Magargal LE, Sergott R: *Ophthalmology* 93:1371, 1986.

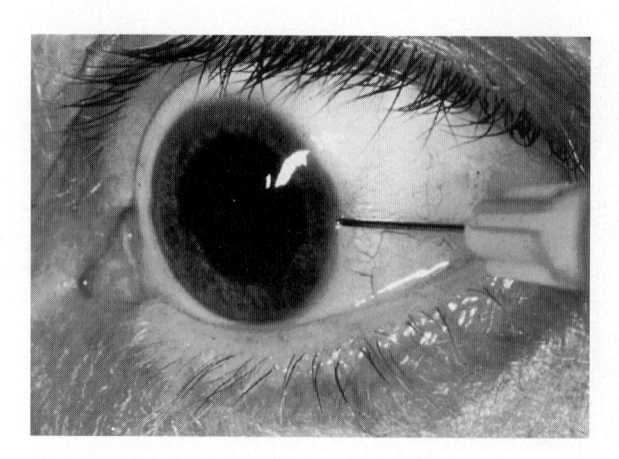

Figure 10-9 Anterior chamber paracentesis at the limbus.

Anterior chamber paracentesis has been advocated if the obstruction is caught within 24 hours after onset. A 27- to 30-gauge needle is inserted into the anterior chamber at the limbus and 0.15 to 0.30 ml of aqueous is removed (Fig. 10-9). Breathing a mixture of 95% oxygen and 5% carbon dioxide has also been attempted.[4]

It has been shown[20] that 35% of eyes with acute central retinal artery obstruction improve at least three Snellen gradations after anterior paracentesis. Uncertainty exists, however, whether the improvement observed with this treatment modality is any better than that with the natural course of the disease.

Anecdotal reports of improvement in vision after the administration of sublingual nitroglycerin[21] and the systemic administration of anticoagulants[22] also exist.

Panretinal photocoagulation has been effective in eradicating the iris neovascularization that can occur after central retinal artery obstruction; in approximately 65% of cases there is regression of the new vessels.[23] Since the visual acuity does not improve in these instances, the goal is to prevent the development of neovascular glaucoma and maintain a pain-free, cosmetically acceptable eye with a limited amount of vision.

BRANCH RETINAL ARTERY OBSTRUCTION

Patients with branch retinal artery obstruction typically relate a history of sudden and painless visual loss in a portion of the visual field of one eye. Visual acuity is usually 20/40 or better, since part of the foveola is usually spared.[24]

Fundus examination reveals sectoral superficial retinal whitening in the distribution of the obstructed vessel. The borders of the ischemic area are often whiter than other parts since there is axoplasmic damming at the juncture of the normal and abnormal areas (Fig. 10-10). Posterior segment neovascularization can rarely develop after branch retina vein obstruction.[25,26]

The systemic workup for branch retinal artery obstruction is similar to that for central retinal artery obstruction; the diseases that cause both are essentially the same (Table 10-1). Ocular treatment is generally not administered since the visual prognosis is good.

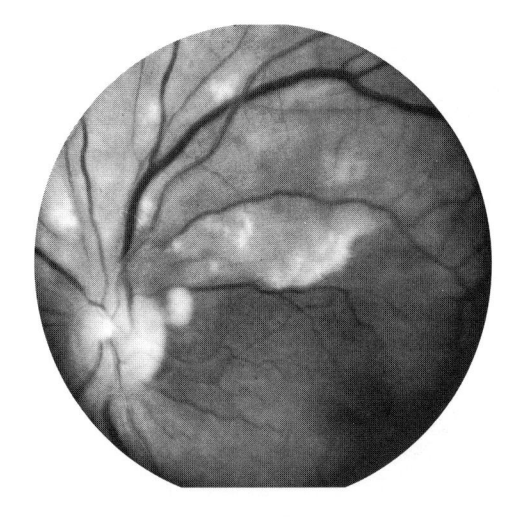

Figure 10-10 Branch retinal artery obstruction secondary to an embolus on the optic disc. The whitening is more pronounced at the border of the ischemic area because axoplasmic flow is blocked in this region.

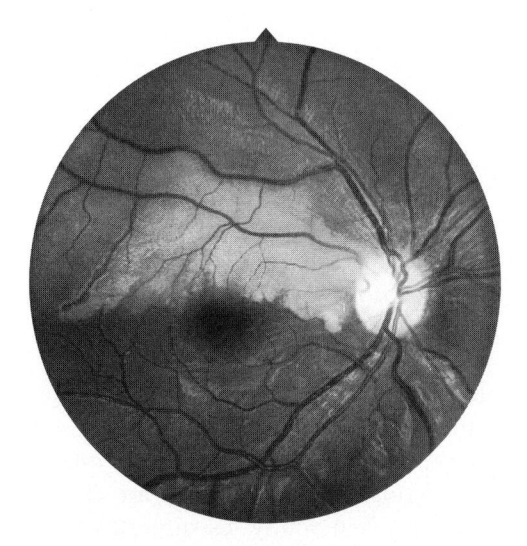

Figure 10-11 Acute isolated cilioretinal artery obstruction.

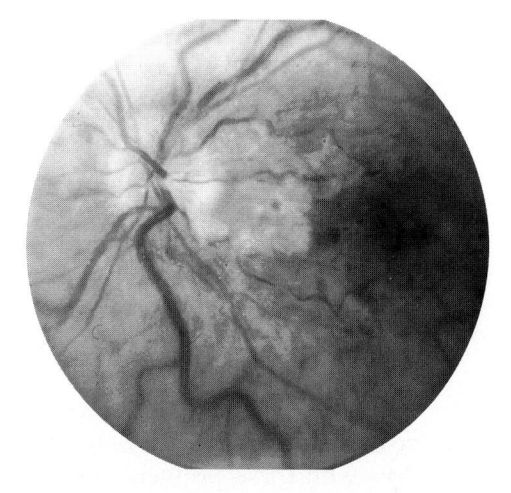

Figure 10-12 Cilioretinal artery obstruction in an eye with concomitant central retinal vein obstruction.

CILIORETINAL ARTERY OBSTRUCTION[27]

Obstruction of the cilioretinal artery occurs in three forms: (1) isolated, (2) with central retinal vein obstruction, and (3) with anterior ischemic optic neuropathy.

Isolated cilioretinal artery obstruction (Fig. 10-11) accounts for about 40% of the cases. Its clinical appearance is retinal whitening along the course of the obstructed vessel, usually in the macula. Approximately 90% of eyes with an isolated cilioretinal artery obstruction will achieve a visual acuity of ≥ g20/40 without treatment.

Cilioretinal artery obstruction associated with central retinal vein obstruction (Fig. 10-12) also accounts for about 40% of the cases. There is retinal whit-

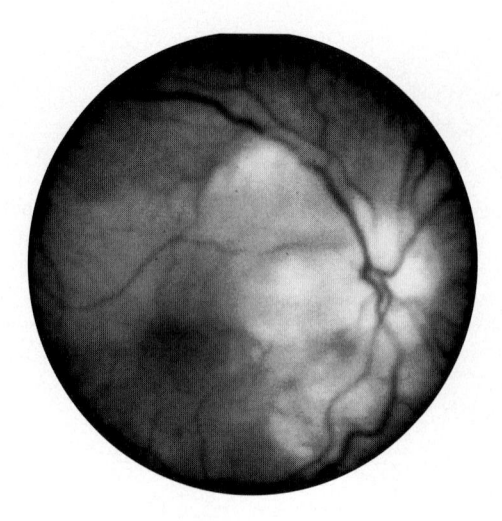

Figure 10-13 Cilioretinal artery obstruction in an eye with anterior ischemic optic neuropathy secondary to giant cell arteritis. Visual acuity was no light perception, primarily because of the optic neuropathy.

ening along the course of the cilioretinal artery in association with retinal venous dilation and retinal hemorrhages. The optic disc is often swollen, and it is believed that the swelling may contribute to external pressure on the artery and, in part, contribute to the arterial obstruction. Seventy percent of the eyes with a cilioretinal artery obstruction in association with a central retinal vein obstruction will eventually reach an acuity of 20/40 or better without treatment.

In eyes with cilioretinal artery obstruction associated with anterior ischemic optic neuropathy there is whitening of the retina along the course of the obstructed artery as well as swelling of the optic disc (Fig. 10-13). The dilated veins and hemorrhages found with central retinal vein obstruction are absent. Eyes with these problems tend to have poor visual acuity, usually 20/400 or worse. It is not surprising that cilioretinal artery obstruction and anterior ischemic optic neuropathy can be seen together, since both are manifestations of the obstruction of branches derived from the posterior ciliary arteries.

The workup for eyes with cilioretinal artery obstruction is similar to that for central retinal artery obstruction. In particular, the possibility of giant cell arteritis as an underlying cause should be considered when cilioretinal artery obstruction and anterior ischemic optic neuropathy are seen together.

COTTON-WOOL SPOTS

Cotton-wool spots are superficial foci of retinal whitening that are are usually a quarter disc area or less in size (Fig. 10-14). They are located in the posterior pole and have been shown to develop following axoplasmic damming in the retinal nerve fiber layer in regions of focal ischemia. The ischemia is believed to develop secondary to the obstruction of a terminal retinal arteriole.

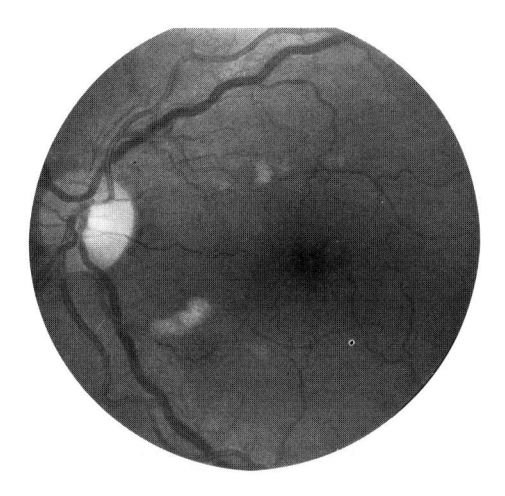

Figure 10-14 Multiple cotton-wool spots.

Patients with cotton-wool spots may notice small scotomas corresponding to the lesions, but central visual acuity is generally unaffected. Specific treatment for the eye is therefore not routinely administered. The cotton-wool spots usually disappear over a period of 5 to 7 weeks, although they can remain longer in patients with diabetic retinopathy.

Diabetic retinopathy is the most common cause of cotton-wool spots. When known diabetics are excluded, however, 95% of patients with a fundus appearance characterized by the presence of a single cotton-wool spot or a predominance of cotton-wool spots can be found to have an underlying cause.[28] A systemic workup is therefore indicated. Approximately one fifth of these patients have been shown to have diabetes mellitus that is discovered only by an abnormal glucose tolerance test. Another fifth have systemic arterial hypertension that is poorly controlled, usually with a diastolic blood pressure of $\geq$ 110 mm Hg. Other underlying causes include collagen vascular diseases, human immunodeficiency virus retinopathy, cardiac emboli, carotid artery obstructive disease, and essentially those entities that can also cause central retinal artery obstruction (Table 10-1).

References

1. von Graefe A: Ueber Embolie der arteria centralis retinae als Urscahe plotzlicher Erblingdung, *Arch Ophthalmol* 5:136-157, 1859.
2. Duke-Elder S, Dobree H: *System of ophthalmology,* St Louis 1967, Mosby, vol 10, pp 66-97.
3. Brown GC: Arterial obstructive disease and the eye, *Ophthalmol Clin North Am* 3:373-392, 1990.
4. Brown GC: Retinal arterial obstructive disease. In Ryan SJ (ed): *Retina,* St Louis, 1989, Mosby, vol 2, Chapter 73,pp 403-419.
5. Brown GC, Magargal LE, Shields JA, et al: Retinal arterial obstruction in children and young adults, *Ophthalmology* 88:18-25, 1981.
6. Brown GC, Magargal LE: Central retinal artery obstruction and visual acuity, *Ophthalmology* 82:14-19, 1982.
7. Dahrling BE: The histopathology of early central retinal artery occlusion, *Arch Ophthalmol* 73:506-510, 1965.

8. Perraut LE, Zimmerman LE: The occurrence of glaucoma following occlusion of the central retinal artery: a clinicopathologic report of six cases with a review of the literature, *Arch Ophthalmol* 61:845-865, 1959.
9. Graveson GS: Retinal arterial occlusion in migraine, *Br Med J* 2:838-840, 1949.
10. Appen RE, Wray SH, Cogan DG: Central retinal artery occlusion. *Am J Ophthalmol* 79:374-381, 1975.
11. Wolter JR, Hansen RD: Intimo-intimal intussusception of the central retinal artery, *Am J Ophthalmol* 92:486-491, 1981.
12. Leishman R: The eye in general vascular disease: hypertension and arteriosclerosis, *Br J Ophthalmol* 41:641-701, 1957.
13. Brown GC, Magargal LE, Sergott R: Acute obstruction of the retinal and choroidal circulations, *Ophthalmology* 93:1371-1382, 1986.
14. Duker JS, Brown GC: Iris neovascularization associated with obstruction of the central retinal artery, *Ophthalmology* 95:1244-1249, 1988.
15. Brown GC: The ocular ischemic syndrome. In Ryan SJ (ed), *Retina*, St Louis, 1989, Mosby, vol 2, Chapter 88, pp 547-559.
16. Brown GC, Shields JA: Cilioretinal arteries and retinal arterial occlusion, *Arch Ophthalmol* 97:84-92, 1979.
17. Savino PJ, Glaser JS, Cassady J: Retinal strike. Is the patient at risk? *Arch Ophthalmol* 95:1185-1189, 1977.
18. Brown GC, Duker J, Lehman R, et al: Combined central retinal artery/central retinal vein obstruction, *Int Ophthalmol* 17:9-17, 1993.
19. Brown GC, Eagle RC, Shakin EP, et al: Retinal toxicity of intravitreal gentamicin, *Arch Ophthalmol* 108:1740-1744, 1990.
20. Augsburger JJ, Magargal LE: Visual prognosis following treatment of acute central retinal artery obstruction, *Br J Ophthalmol* 64:913-917, 1980.
21. Kuritzky S: Nitroglycerin to treat acute loss of vision, *N Engl J Med* 323:1428, 1990.
22. Schmidt D, Schumacher M, Wakhloo AK: Microcatheter urokinase infusion in central retinal artery obstruction. *Am J Ophthalmol* 113:429-434, 1992.
23. Duker JS, Brown GC: The efficacy of panretinal photocoagulation for neovascularization of the iris after central retinal artery obstruction, *Ophthalmology* 96:92-95, 1989.
24. Karjalainen K: Occlusion of the central retinal artery and retinal branch arterioles, *Acta Ophthalmol* 109:5-96, 1971.
25. Brown GC, Reber R: An unusual presentation of branch retinal artery obstruction in association with ocular neovascularization, *Can J Ophthalmol* 21:103-106, 1986.
26. Kraushar MF, Brown GC: Retinal neovascularization after branch retinal arterial obstruction, *Am J Ophthalmol* 104:294-296, 1987.
27. Brown GC, Moffat K, Cruess A, et al: Cilioretinal artery obstruction, *Retina* 3:182-187, 1983.
28. Brown GC, Brown MM, Hiller T, et al: Cotton wool spots, *Retina* 5:206-214, 1985.

11

Central Retinal Vein Obstruction

Arunan Sivalingam

CLINICAL PRESENTATION

Central retinal vein obstruction (CRVO) is diagnosed when a patient presents with hemorrhage in all four quadrants of the retina. In addition, the retinal veins are usually found to be dilated and tortuous. The clinical appearance varies from a few scattered hemorrhages to diffuse and marked hemorrhages within the superficial and deep retina. Cotton-wool spots are also, at times, associated with CRVO. Two major complications that have occurred are reduced central vision secondary to cystoid macular edema and neovascular glaucoma secondary to iris neovascularization.

Most patients who develop central retinal vein obstruction are over 50 years of age. Between 50% and 70% have associated hypertension, cardiovascular disease, and/or diabetes mellitus.[1] Other risk factors for CRVO include glaucoma and hypercoagulable states such as multiple myeloma and Waldenstrom's macroglobulinemia.[2]

The symptoms of CRVO range from a mild and/or transient episode of visual blurring to severe visual loss to the level of 20/200 or less. In addition, patients presenting with severe, end stage CRVO usually have ocular pain secondary to neovascular glaucoma.

HISTOPATHOLOGY AND PATHOPHYSIOLOGY

Green et al.[3] demonstrated thrombosis of the central retinal vein in the area of the lamina cribrosa as a constant histopathologic finding in 29 consecutive eyes with central retinal vein obstruction. The visual damage produced by venous obstruction depends primarily on the rapidity of its development and the availability of collateral pathways for the venous outflow. The resolution of central retinal vein occlusion depends on the rate of venous recanalization as well as the establishment of the optociliary shunt vessels. Some investigators also believe there is a component of retinal arterial insufficiency enhancing the severity of central retinal vein obstruction. Little clinical or experimental evidence support this view, however.

Two types of CRVO, ischemic and nonischemic, have been described. The differing clinical and pathologic manifestations are believed to influence visual prognosis.

Nonischemic Central Retinal Vein Obstruction

In the nonischemic type of CRVO the retinal veins may be dilated and tortuous. Usually there are dot and blot hemorrhages in all four quadrants, but, in contrast to the ischemic variety of central retinal vein obstruction, the amount of intraretinal hemorrhage is minimal (Fig. 11-1). There may be a few or no cotton-wool spots associated with this type of CRVO. In the acute phase of the obstruction, central vision may be diminished secondary to cystoid macular edema. Characteristically visual acuity in nonischemic CRVO is better than that in ischemic CRVO (i.e., better than 20/200). This variant comprises the majority of vein obstructions and it can vary in frequency from 50% to 78% depending on the study.[4,5]

Tools that may help differentiate ischemic from nonischemic CRVO are the fluorescein angiogram and the electroretinogram. A wide-angle fluorescein angiogram using a 60-degree fundus camera is helpful in evaluating and documenting the degree of retinal nonperfusion. According to Magargal et al.,[6] when the ischemic index (nonperfused area/total area) was less than 10%, only 1% of eyes developed neovascular glaucoma. In the indeterminate group (ischemic index 11% to 50%), 7% progressed to neovascular glaucoma. Thus an eye with minimal or total capillary nonperfusion has a very small risk of neovascular glaucoma (Fig. 11-2). Some eyes, however, have too much retinal hemorrhage for adequate quantitation of capillary nonperfusion by fluorescein angiography.

The electroretinogram may also be helpful in categorizing central retinal vein obstruction. The average b/a-wave amplitude ratio in a single light flash ERG was greater than 1 for a nonischemic central retinal vein occlusion compared to less than 1 for the ischemic variety.[7,8] The b/a amplitude ratio reflected the degree of retinal ischemia and had value in predicting which cases were at risk for developing neovascular glaucoma.

Ischemic Central Vein Occlusion

Some 22% to 31% of all eyes presenting with central vein obstruction have the ischemic variant of CRVO[5,6,9] and 67% of these patients will develop some form of ocular neovascularization.[5] Whereas 60% of these patients develop iris neovascularization, two thirds will progress to develop neovascular glaucoma.[5,10] In comparison, less than 10% develop retinal neovascularization. Hence, determination of the ischemic versus nonischemic variant is important in management.

Many clinical and ophthalmologic findings accompany ischemic central retinal vein obstruction. Patients usually present with severe visual loss, usually vision worse than 20/200. In addition, it has been shown[11] that an afferent pupillary defect is often present with ischemic central retinal vein obstruction. Ophthalmoscopic examination usually reveals confluent intraretinal hemorrhage with multiple cotton-wool spots (Fig. 11-3 and 11-4).

May et al.[12] were the first to suggest that ischemic CRVO is diagnosed when greater than 10 disc diameters of capillary nonperfusion is seen. Although no investigator has defined the critical amount of capillary nonperfusion necessary

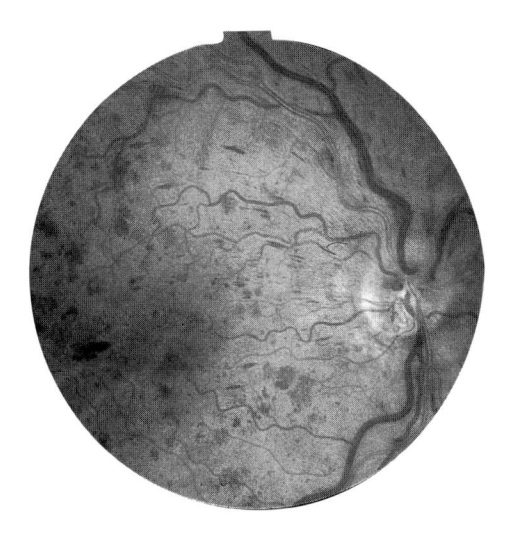

Figure 11-1 Fundus photograph of the right eye of a patient with nonischemic central retinal vein obstruction. There are dilated and tortuous veins and a few dot-blot hemorrhages in the posterior pole.

Figure 11-2 Fluorescein angiogram of the patient in Figure 11-1 showing good capillary perfusion consistent with a nonischemic central retinal vein obstruction.

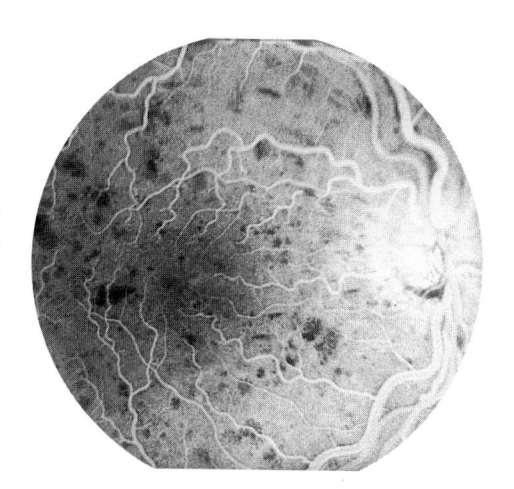

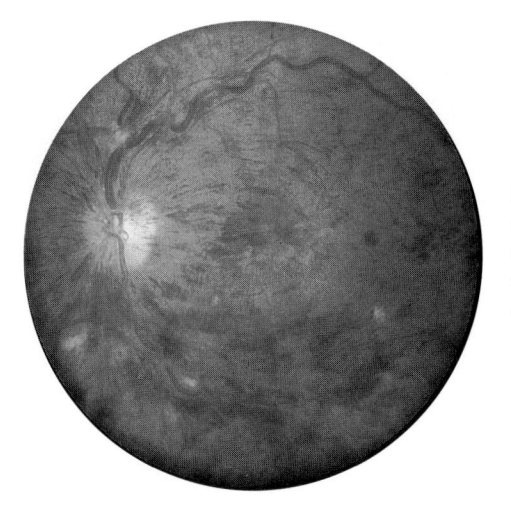

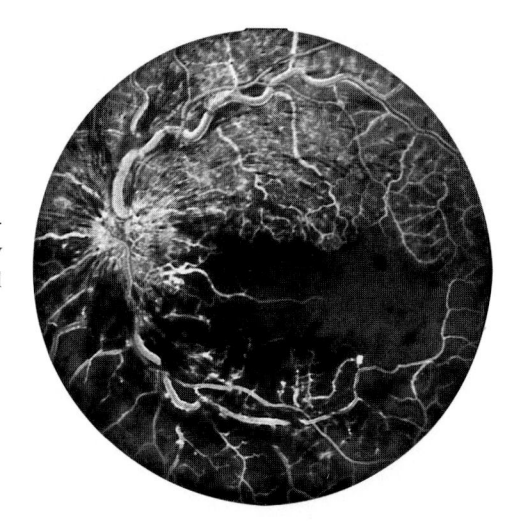

Figure 11-3 Fundus photograph of the left eye of a patient with ischemic central retinal vein obstruction. There are dilated and tortuous veins with extensive intraretinal hemorrhage and cotton-wool spots.

Figure 11-4 Fluorescein angiogram of the patient in Figure 11-3 showing extensive capillary nonperfusion consistent with an ischemic central retinal vein obstruction.

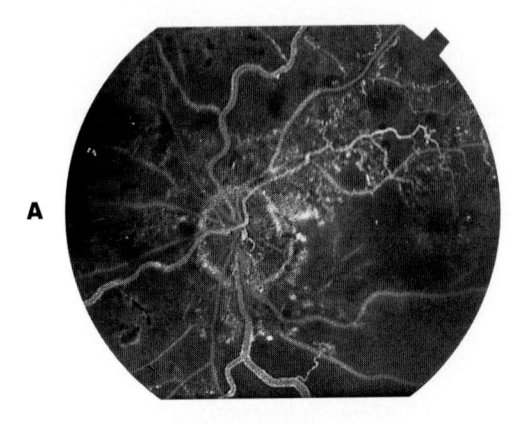

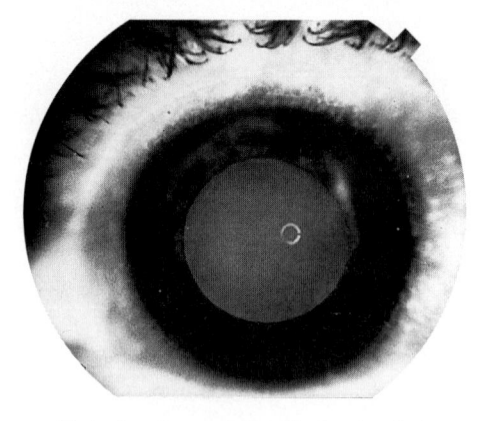

Figure 11-5 A, Fluorescein angiogram of an eye with ischemic central retinal vein obstruction showing marked capillary dropout. **B,** Iris angiogram of the eye showing neovascularization of the iris.

Figure 11-6 Fundus photograph of a left eye showing confluent retinal hemorrhages without cotton-wool spots.

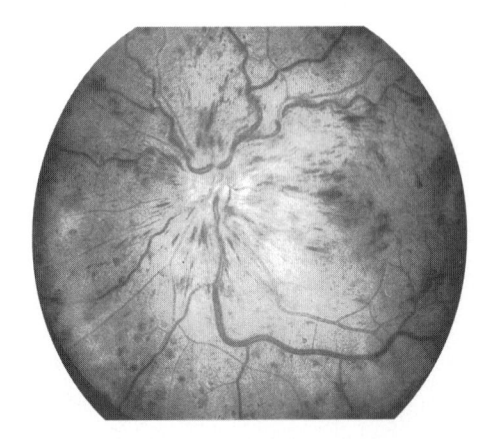

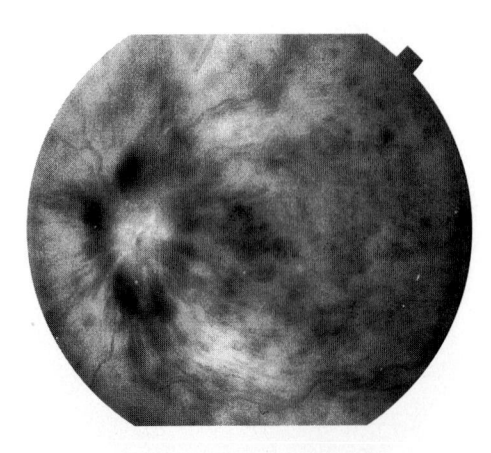

Figure 11-7 One month later, same patient as in Figure 11-6 presenting with neovascular glaucoma. Now however, there are worsening intraretinal hemorrhages, poor visual acuity, and cystoid macular edema consistent with ischemic central retinal vein obstruction.

for development of neovascularization of iris, subsequently Magargal et al.[6] used an ischemic index of greater than 50% (10 disc diameters of nonperfusion) as the critical number in determining whether the central vein occlusion was ischemic or not. Forty-five percent of patients with an ischemic index of 50% or greater developed neovascular glaucoma. Thus an eye with extensive capillary nonperfusion has a significant risk of developing neovascular glaucoma (Fig. 11-5).

The electroretinogram may be helpful in diagnosis of the ischemic CRVO. It has been shown[7,8] that a b/a-wave amplitude ratio of less than 1 can be classified as ischemic central retinal vein obstruction. They showed that no patients with b-wave to a-wave ratio greater than 1 developed neovascularization of the iris. Recently Kay et al.[13] have shown that, in addition to the b/a-wave amplitude ratio, the prolonged b-wave implicit time is important as a predictor of eyes that are at risk for development of iris neovascularization.

One must also realize that some 5% to 20% of patients presenting with nonischemic central retinal vein obstruction will progress to an ischemic variety of central retinal vein occlusion.[14,15] The transition may occur from 2 weeks to 26 months after initial diagnosis. Eyes that progress have features of both

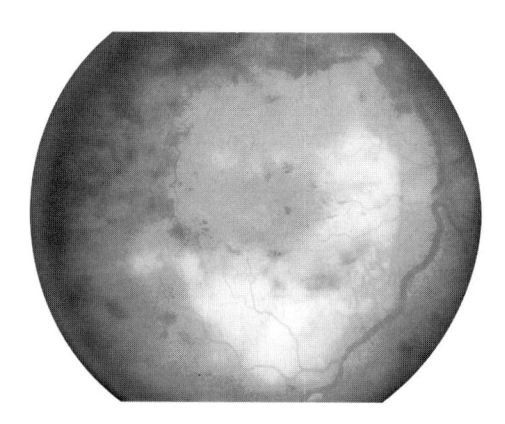

Figure 11-8 Fundus photograph of a right eye showing intraretinal hemorrhages with yellow lipid exudates.

Figure 11-9 Fluorescein angiogram of the patient in Figure 11-8 demonstrating the extensive capillary dropout.

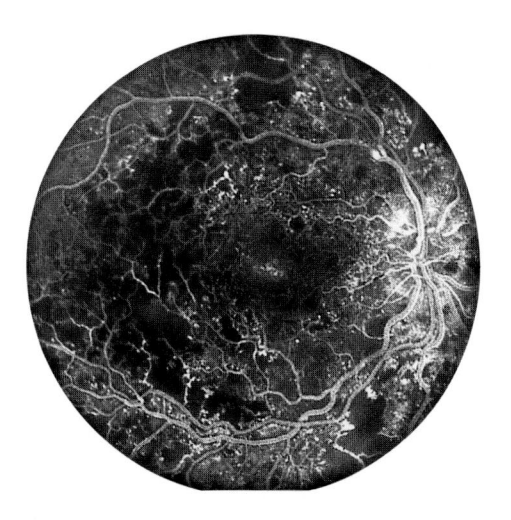

nonischemic and ischemic CRVO. For example, poor initial visual acuity, severe macular edema, and an increase in the amount of intraretinal hemorrhage typical of ischemic CRVO are usually seen in these cases. On the other hand, eyes in this group usually lack the capillary nonperfusion and cotton-wool spots seen with the nonischemic variety. Thus, if a patient with CRVO has minimal or no capillary nonperfusion at fluorescein angiography, poor visual acuity, and marked macular edema with increasing retinal hemorrhage, that individual is at high risk to progress to ischemic CRVO[15] (Figs. 11-6 and 11-7).

Approximately 2% of patients with CRVO have marked accumulation of exudates in the fundi.[16] This is usually associated with hypertriglyceridemia. All the patients with exudates described by Brown[16] had poor visual acuity, evidence of retinal ischemia on fluorescein angiograms, and neovascularization of the iris. Thus progressive worsening of the lipid exudation may also be an indicator of ischemic central retinal vein obstruction (Figs. 11-8 and 11-9).

TREATMENT

Several studies[11,17] have indicated that panretinal photocoagulation before the development of neovascularization iris may prevent neovascular glaucoma in eyes with ischemic central retinal vein obstruction. There have been studies demonstrating a beneficial effect of treatment in CRVO patients, but the number of eyes studied was small and randomization did not always include retinal perfusion characteristics. Although most retrospective and prospective studies showed benefit with panretinal photocoagulation for the prevention of neovascular glaucoma, Hayreh[18] recently reported no statistically significant difference between treated and nontreated eyes with regard to the development of ocular neovascularization or visual acuity.

No treatment for macular edema resulting from central retinal vein occlusion has been shown to be effective. There have been some studies showing improvement in macular edema after grid pattern photocoagulation.[19,20] Although these studies have shown some improvement in the macular edema, visual acuity did not always improve after treatment.

References

1. Gutman FA: Evaluation of a patient with central retinal vein occlusion, *Ophthalmology* 90:481-483, 1983.
2. Gass JDM: Stereoscopic atlas of macular diseases: diagnosis and treatment, ed 3, St Louis, 1987, Mosby, p 426.
3. Green WR, Chan CC, Hutchins GM, Terry JM: Central retinal vein occlusion: a prospective histopathologic study of 29 eyes in 28 cases, *Retina* 1:27-55, 1981.
4. Magargal LE, Brown GC, Augsburger JJ, Parrish RK II: Neovascular glaucoma following central retinal vein obstruction, *Ophthalmology* 88:1095-1101, 1981.
5. Hayreh SS, Rojas P, Podhajsky P, et al: Ocular neovascularization with retinal vascular occlusion. III. Incidence of ocular neovascularization with retinal vein occlusion, *Ophthalmology* 90:488-506, 1983.
6. Magargal LE, Donoso LA, Sanborn GE: Retinal ischemia and risk of neovascularization following central retinal vein obstruction, *Ophthalmology* 89:1241-1245, 1982.
7. Barber C, Galloway NR, Reacher M, Salem H: The role of the electroretinogram in the management of central retinal vein occlusion, *Doc Ophthalmol Proc Ser* 40:149-159, 1984.

8. Sabates R, Hirose T, McMeel JW: Electroretinography in the prognosis and classification of central retinal vein occlusion, *Arch Ophthalmol* 101:232-235, 1983.
9. Sinclair SH, Gragoudas ES: Prognosis for rubeosis iridis following central retinal vein occlusion, *Br J Ophthalmol* 63:735-743, 1979.
10. Zegarra H, Gutman FA, Conforto J: The natural course of central retinal vein occlusion, *Ophthalmology* 86:1931-1939, 1979.
11. Servais GE, Thompson S, Hayreh SS: Relative afferent pupillary defect in central retinal vein occlusion, *Ophthalmology* 93:301-303, 1986.
12. May DR, Klein ML, Peyman GA, Raichland M: Xenon arc panretinal photocoagulation for central retinal vein occlusion: a randomized prospective study, *Br J Ophthalmol* 63:725-734, 1979.
13. Kaye SB, Harding SP: Early electroretinography in unilateral central retinal vein occlusion as a predictor of rubeosis iridis, *Arch Ophthalmol* 106:353-356, 1988.
14. Hayreh SS: Classification of central retinal vein occlusion, *Ophthalmology* 90:458-474, 1983.
15. Minturn J, Brown GC: Progression of nonischemic central retinal vein obstruction to the ischemic variant, *Ophthalmology* 93:1158-1162, 1986.
16. Brown GC: Central retinal vein obstruction with lipid exudates, *Arch Ophthalmol* 107:1001-1005, 1991.
17. Laaitikainen L, Kohner EM, Khoury D, Blach, RK: Panretinal photocoagulation in central retinal vein occlusion: a randomized controlled clinical study, *Br J Ophthalmol* 61:741-753, 1977.
18. Hayreh SS: Ocular neovascularization in central retinal vein occlusion. Presented at the symposium on central vein occlusion, 10th Annual Macula Society Meeting, Paris, June 1987.
19. Gutman FA, Zegarra H, Nothnagel A: Laser treatment of macular edema secondary to central retinal vein occlusion, *Int Ophthalmol* 10:100, 1987.
20. Klein ML, Finkelstein D: Laser photocoagulation of macular edema in central retinal vein occlusion. Presented at the symposium on central vein occlusion, 10th Annual Macula Society Meeting, Paris, June 1987.

12

Retinal Branch Vein Occlusion

J. Arch McNamara

Retinal venous occlusive disease is second only to diabetic retinopathy as a cause of retinal vascular disease.[1] The exact pathogenesis of branch retinal vein occlusion (BRVO) is not known, but arteriosclerosis has been implicated. It is postulated[2] that pressure on the vein by the thick wall of an arteriosclerotic artery may cause turbulence of blood flow, endothelial cell damage, and thrombosis, as proposed for central retinal vein occlusion.

BRVO occurs with equal frequency in men and women. The typical age range is between 50 and 70 years. Hypertension is a well-recognized association with BRVO,[3,4] as has been borne out in recent case-controlled studies.[5,6] Both those studies also recognized male gender as a significant risk factor for BRVO. Rath et al.[6] found open-angle glaucoma to be a significant risk factor whereas Johnson et al.[5] did not. Both studies did not find diabetes mellitus to be a risk factor whereas previous noncontrolled studies have suggested that possibility.

Branch retinal vein occlusion typically presents with sudden onset of decreased vision. Patients may complain of a sectoral visual field defect. The superotemporal quadrant is most often affected with the inferotemporal quadrant affected in almost all of the remainder of cases. Inferonasal BRVO is rare, but this may be related to the fact that patients so affected would be minimally, if at all, symptomatic and are therefore unlikely to present. The fundus appearance is pathognomonic; there is a segmental distribution of intraretinal hemorrhages that typically fan out towards the retinal periphery from the site of the occlusion. With greater degrees of ischemia, nerve fiber layer infarcts may be present. The occlusion usually occurs at the site of an artery overcrossing a vein. In their series of 25 cases of BRVO, Duker and Brown[7] found all occlusions to be at the site of an artery overcrossing a vein. Weinberg et al.[8] found 97.6% of 84 cases to be so affected. Venous overcrossings occur at 30% of all crossings in normal retinas.[9] The location and extent of branch retinal vein obstruction determines the degree to which vision will be affected. The closer to the optic nerve, the greater the likelihood of visual impairment. If only macular tributaries are involved, the findings may be subtle, but vision will usually be decreased.[10]

The clinical course of BRVO is variable. Approximately 50% of patients with decreased vision due to macular edema of less than 1 year's duration will re-

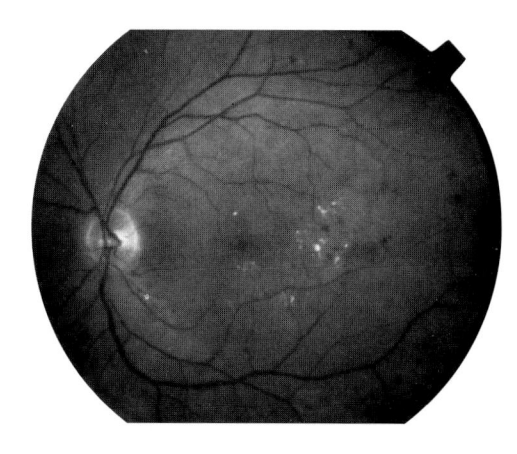

Figure 12-1 Nonproliferative diabetic retinopathy with scattered hemorrhages and hard exudates inferiorly mimicking branch retinal vein occlusion.

gain vision of 20/40 or better. Approximately 50% of eyes with extensive BRVO have large areas of retinal capillary nonperfusion, and 40% of these eyes develop neovascularization. The neovascularization usually appears between 3 and 6 months. Approximately 60% of patients with neovascularization will have hemorrhage into the vitreous.

Bilateral branch retinal vein occlusion is rare, less frequent than bilateral central retinal vein occlusion (which occurs in 6%[11] to 14%[12] of cases). The incidence of bilateral BRVO is 2.3% according to Pollack et al.[13]

DIFFERENTIAL DIAGNOSIS

Branch retinal vein occlusion has such a pathognomonic clinical appearance in its early stages that it is difficult to be mistaken in the diagnosis. The segmental hemorrhages extending away from an arteriovenous crossing site are highly characteristic. Diabetic retinopathy (Fig. 12-1) and radiation retinopathy have similar clinical findings (intraretinal hemorrhages, nerve fiber layer infarcts, macular edema, and intraretinal hard exudates), but the distribution of these lesions is more diffuse.

Macular branch retinal vein occlusion may present more of a diagnostic dilemma.[10] Although the retinal findings fan out from an arteriovenous crossing site, the limited area of involvement may be mistaken for mild nonproliferative diabetic retinopathy, radiation retinopathy, or parafoveal retinal telangiectasis. Diabetic retinopathy can usually be correctly diagnosed by obtaining a history of diabetes mellitus and noting bilateral findings. Radiation retinopathy will most often be associated with a history of radiation treatment. Parafoveal retinal telangiectasis does not occur along the distribution of retinal veins and frequently crosses the horizontal meridian. Fluorescein angiography may be helpful in further clarifying the diagnosis.

DIAGNOSTIC APPROACH

Clinical Examination

In the acute presentation of BRVO, visual acuity may range from normal to counting fingers depending on the location and severity of the occlusion. The final vision, however, is often improved over that at presentation. Orth and Patz[1] tabulated the final visual acuity results from several studies and found that a final vision of 20/40 or better occurred in 53% of cases.

Iris neovascularization is a distinctly rare occurrence in association with BRVO. Orth and Patz[1] observed only two cases in their review article.

The fundus examination in BRVO differs depending on the phase of the disease. In the acute phase (0 to 6 months) there is often extensive intraretinal hemorrhage throughout the distribution of the occluded vessel. If the occlusion is proximal, hemorrhages may be seen in the fovea. The vein beyond the occlusion site is usually dilated. With greater degrees of obstruction and hence ischemia, nerve fiber layer infarcts may be seen. Vision may be decreased because of foveal hemorrhage, macular edema, macular ischemia, or a combination of these factors. When the reason for decreased vision is not immediately apparent, ischemia is suspected. Fluorescein angiography frequently aids in determining the cause of decreased visual acuity.

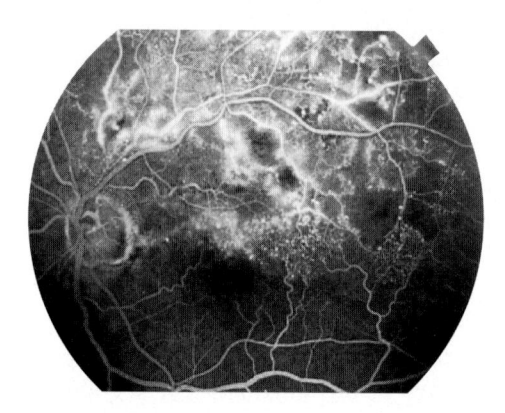

Figure 12-2 Venous phase of a fluorescein angiogram showing superotemporal branch retinal vein occlusion. Note the retinal capillary microaneurysms (pinpoint spots of hyperfluorescence)

Figure 12-3 Branch retinal vein occlusion with macular edema. Note the loss of a foveal reflex.

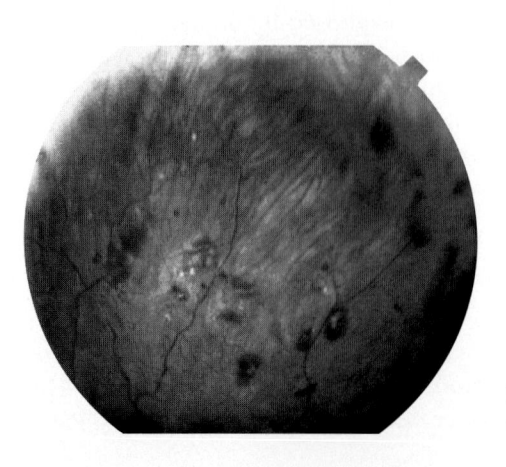

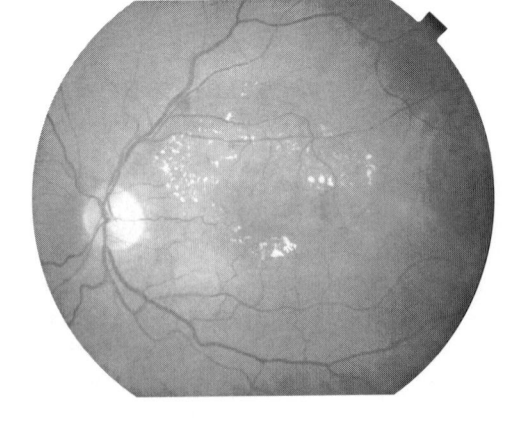

Figure 12-4 Peripheral retinal neovascularization secondary to branch retinal vein occlusion.

In the chronic phase (after 3 to 6 months) the majority of intraretinal hemorrhages may have resorbed. Nerve fiber layer infarcts have usually disappeared by this time as well. Other microvascular abnormalities are frequently present, however. When the vein occlusion has been extensive, collateral vessel formation across the horizontal raphe is usually seen. Intraretinal microvascular abnormalities (IRMA), similar to those seen in nonproliferative diabetic retinopathy, and retinal capillary microaneurysms (Fig. 12-2) may be present in chronic BRVO. Macular edema as evidenced by retinal thickening is a frequent cause of persistent decreased vision in chronic BRVO (Fig. 12-3). Cystoid macular edema may develop from chronic macular edema. If there is significant retinal capillary ischemia, neovascularization of the disc or retina may also occur (Fig. 12-4).

Rare late complications of BRVO include macular retinal pigment epithelial atrophy, macular hole, traction retinal detachment, and combined traction/rhegmatogenous retinal detachment.

Fluorescein Angiography

Fluorescein angiography (FA) is useful in the evaluation of branch retinal vein occlusion. It aids in the prognosis and helps guide laser photocoagulation. In the acute phase of the disease FA provides little information since hemorrhage usually blocks the underlying retinal microvasculature. Additionally, it is recommended to wait at least 3 months before considering laser photocoagulation for macular edema, obviating the need for FA until then.

When the acute phase has ended (3 to 6 months), FA is useful in detecting macular pathology, retinal capillary nonperfusion, and neovascularization. As

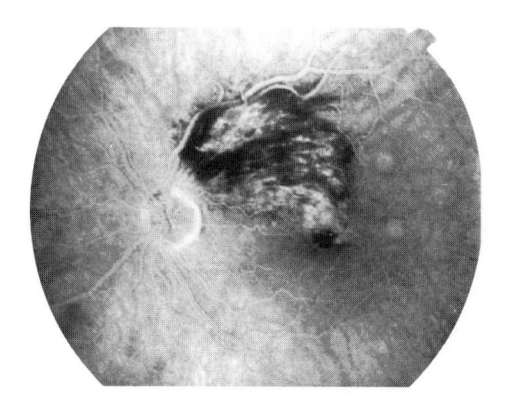

Figure 12-5 Fluorescein angiogram of a recent branch retinal vein occlusion with intraretinal hemorrhage appearing as hypofluorescence.

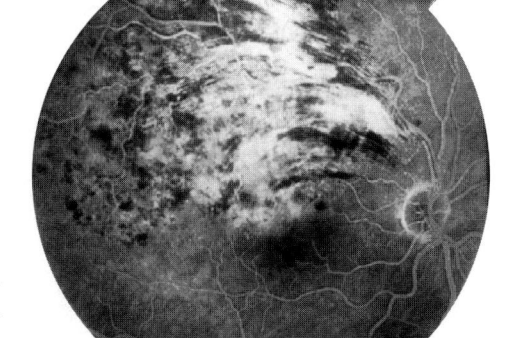

Figure 12-6 Hyperfluorescence in the superior foveal area caused by macular edema secondary to branch retinal vein occlusion.

previously mentioned, vision may be decreased because of macular hemorrhage, macular edema, macular ischemia, or a combination thereof. Hemorrhage can usually be seen clinically and appears as blocked fluorescence at FA (Fig. 12-5). Macular edema is manifested by increasing hyperfluorescence with late leakage of dye into the surrounding retina (Fig. 12-6). Cystic spaces may fill with dye if cystoid macular edema is present. Nonperfusion in the macula and retinal periphery appears as relative hypofluorescence adjacent to areas of normal fluorescence (Fig. 12-7). Collateral vessels may be seen to fill and are usually located in the temporal macula (Fig. 12-8).

Neovascularization is a particularly worrisome finding since it may lead to vitreous hemorrhage. It appears as early intense hyperfluorescence with late leakage. Neovascularization elsewhere (NVE) (i.e., other than of the disc) typically appears at the border of perfused and nonperfused retinal capillaries (Fig. 12-9). Neovascularization of the disc (NVD) is less frequently seen, being present usually when there is extensive retinal capillary nonperfusion.

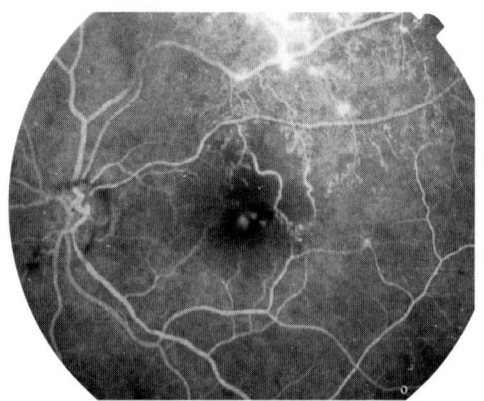

Figure 12-7 Hypofluorescence caused by retinal capillary nonperfusion in the macula.

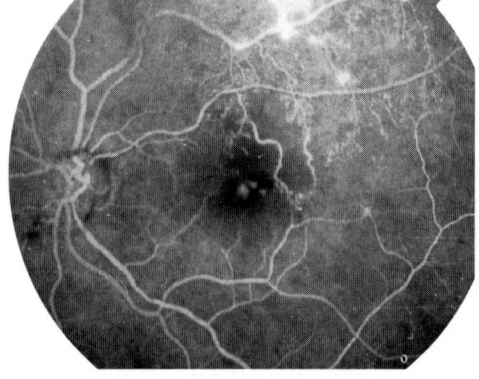

Figure 12-8 Filling of collateral vessels temporal and nasal to the fovea.

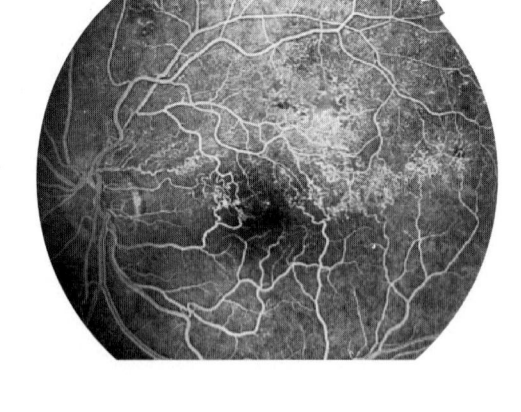

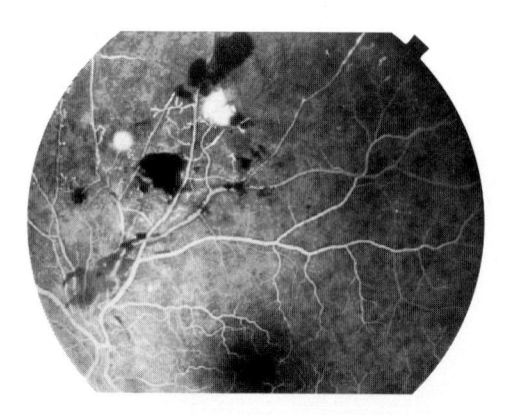

Figure 12-9 Hyperfluorescence at the border between a perfused and a nonperfused retinal capillary bed caused by neovascularization.

MANAGEMENT

Medical Therapy

Despite histopathologic evidence that the branch retinal vein becomes thrombosed in BRVO,[14] anticoagulant therapy has not been shown to be of any benefit in preventing or managing this disease. Anticoagulant therapy has systemic risks and may even increase the amount of hemorrhage in the acute phase of BRVO.

Arterial hypertension is a known association of BRVO.[3-6] Although lowering elevated blood pressure may have no effect on the progression of BRVO, it seems prudent for other health reasons to attempt better control of the hypertension.

Open-angle glaucoma has been recognized[6] as a risk factor for BRVO. Similar to elevated blood pressure, it is not known whether lowering the intraocular pressure (IOP) would have any beneficial effect on BRVO. It would also be prudent to reduce elevated IOP in patients with glaucoma and BRVO.

Laser Therapy

Photocoagulation has been studied for the management of the complications of branch retinal vein occlusion since Meyer-Schwickerath[15] first introduced this form of therapy in 1960. The Branch Vein Occlusion Study,[16,17] a prospective, randomized, and controlled clinical trial sponsored by the National Eye Institute, established laser photocoagulation as an appropriate treatment for both macular edema and neovascularization secondary to BRVO.

The first report of the Branch Vein Occlusion Study[16] concerned treatment for macular edema. Patients with branch retinal vein occlusion and vision of 20/40 or worse because of macular edema were randomized to treatment or no treatment. (Treatment is not recommended if macular nonperfusion explains the visual loss.) Of treated eyes, 65% gained two or more lines of vision from baseline compared to only 37% of controls. Treatment was recommended for such eyes.

Laser treatment is delivered in a grid pattern over the area of retinal capillary leakage involving the fovea. A 100 µm spot size at 0.1 second with sufficient power to cause a dull white burn should be used. In the Branch Vein Occlusion Study an argon blue-green laser was used. Although there has been no clinical trial specifically to address the best wavelength for treating macular edema, yellow, red, and green wavelengths have been used with success. Yellow has the advantage of not being absorbed by the macular xanthophyll pigment. A high-quality angiogram of less than 1 month's duration should be used to diagnose the macular edema. Treatment may be brought up to the edge of the foveal avascular zone but should not go beyond. Treatment over intraretinal hemorrhage should be avoided since damage to the nerve fiber layer may occur. In addition, direct treatment of collateral vessels should be avoided.

The second report of the Branch Vein Occlusion Study[17] addressed laser photocoagulation for the prevention of neovascularization and vitreous hemorrhage in branch retinal vein occlusions five or more disc areas in size. There was a decreased incidence in the development of neovascularization in the group treated with scatter laser before neovascularization occurred. In the group that already had neovascularization before treatment, 29% of lasered eyes developed vitreous hemorrhage compared to 61% of control eyes. The study

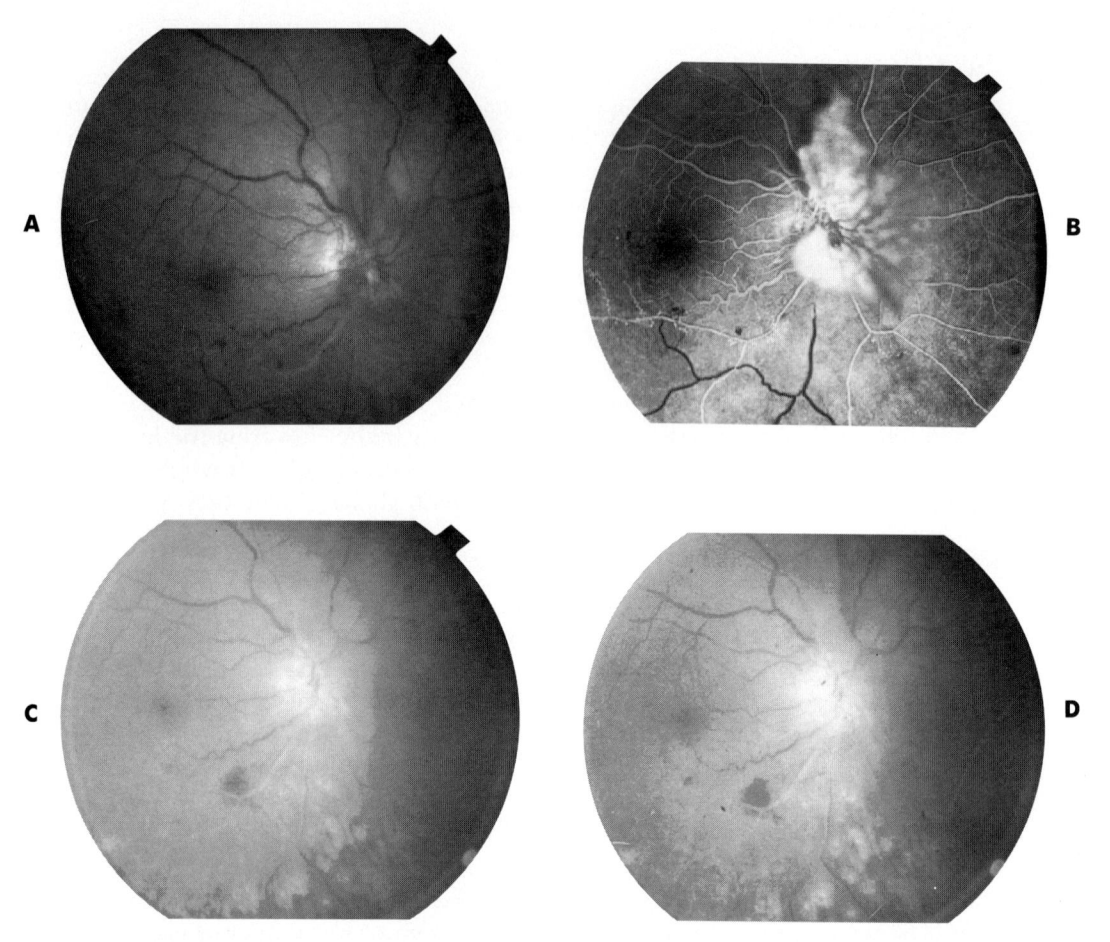

Figure 12-10 A, Before treatment. Note the extensive neovascularization of the disc (NVD) secondary to a branch retinal vein occlusion. **B,** Transit phase of a fluorescein angiogram demonstrating leakage of dye from the NVD. **C,** After laser. Note the regressing NVD. **D,** Postoperative fluorescein angiogram demonstrating decreased leakage of the dye.

was not designed to determine whether treatment should be applied before or after the development of neovascularization; but, from the data, 12% of nonperfused eyes treated before the neovascularization appeared could be expected to develop vitreous hemorrhage compared to 9% of eyes treated after the neovascularization occurred. This suggests that there may be no advantage to treating before the development of neovascularization. It was therefore recommended that eyes with BRVO and neovascularization should have scatter laser photocoagulation to the involved quadrant.

The Branch Vein Occlusion Study used an argon blue-green laser, but argon green, which is commonly available, may be more desirable for scatter treatment. Applications of 200 to 500 µm spot size at 0.1-second intervals were scattered throughout the involved quadrant spaced approximately one burn with apart. Areas of intraretinal hemorrhage should be avoided. A dull white burn is also desirable for scatter treatment (Fig. 12-10).

Vitrectomy

Occasionally, vitreous hemorrhage will be so severe and persistent that vitrectomy is indicated. Rarely traction or combined traction/rhegmatogenous retinal detachments may occur as a result of cicatricial complications from branch retinal vein occlusion. Vitreous surgery techniques may be beneficial in these complicated retinal detachment.[18]

CONCLUSION

Branch retinal vein occlusion is not a benign disease. Fortunately, however, it is rarely bilateral, and significant clearing often occurs within the first few months after onset. In patients with persistently decreased vision (less than 20/50) grid laser photocoagulation offers hope for some visual recovery. Careful follow-up of patients with BRVO is necessary in monitoring for the development of neovascularization.

References

1. Orth DH, Patz A: Retinal branch vein occlusion, *Surv Ophthalmol* 22:357-376, 1978.
2. Green WR, Chan CC, Hutchins GM, et al: Central retinal vein occlusion: a prospective histopathologic study of 29 eyes of 28 cases, *Retina* 1:27-55, 1981.
3. Gutman FA, Zegarra H: The natural course of temporal retinal branch vein occlusion, *Trans Am Acad Ophthalmol Otolaryngol* 78:178-192, 1974.
4. Blankenship GW, Okun E: Retinal tributary vein occlusion. Histology and management by photocoagulation, *Arch Ophthalmol* 89:363-368, 1973.
5. Johnson RL, Brucker AJ, Steinmann W, et al: Risk factors of branch retinal vein occlusion, *Arch Ophthalmol* 103:1831-1832, 1985.
6. Rath EZ, Frank RN, Shin DH, et al: Risk factors for retinal vein occlusions: A case-control study, *Ophthalmology* 99:509-514, 1992.
7. Duker JS, Brown GC: Anterior location of the crossing artery in branch retinal vein occlusion, *Arch Ophthalmol* 107:998-1000, 1989.
8. Weinberg, D, Dodwell DG, Fern SA: Anatomy of arteriovenous crossings in branch retinal vein occlusion, *Am J Ophthalmol* 109:298-302, 1990.
9. Jensen VA: Clinical studies of tributary thrombosis in the central retinal vein, *Acta Ophthalmol* 1(suppl. 10):1, 1936.
10. Joffe L, Goldberg RE, Magargal LE, et al: Macular branch retinal vein occlusion, *Ophthalmology* 87:91-97, 1980.
11. Magargal LE Brown GC, Augsburger JJ, et al: Neovascular glaucoma following central retinal vein obstruction, *Ophthalmology* 88:1095-1101, 1981.
12. Hayreh SS, Rojas P, Podhajsky, et al: Ocular neovascularization with retinal vascular occlusion. III. Incidence of ocular neovascularization with retinal vein occlusion, *Ophthalmology* 90:488-506, 1983.
13. Pollack A, Dottan S, Oliver M: The fellow eye in retinal vein occlusive disease, *Ophthalmology* 96:842-845, 1989.
14. Frangieh GT, Green WR, Barraquer-Somers E, et al: Histopathologic study of nine branch retinal vein occlusions. *Arch Ophthalmol* 100:1132-1140, 1982.
15. Meyer-Schwickerath G: *Light coagulation* (translated and edited by Drance SM), St Louis, 1960, Mosby.
16. Branch Vein Occlusion Study Group: Argon laser photocoagulation for macular edema in branch vein occlusion, *Am J Ophthalmol* 98:271-282, 1984.
17. Branch Vein Occlusion Study Group: Argon laser scatter photocoagulation for prevention of neovascularization and vitreous hemorrhage in branch retinal vein occlusion, *Arch Ophthalmol* 104:34-41, 1986.
18. Russell SR, Blodi CF, Folk JC: Vitrectomy for complicated retinal detachments secondary to branch retinal vein occlusions, *Am J Ophthalmol* 108:6-9, 1989.

13

Hypertension

Eric P. Shakin
Alfred C. Lucier

Hypertension affects about 20% of all individuals in the United States. Adult hypertension is defined as a blood pressure greater than or equal to 140/95 torr in men over 45 years of age (or greater than 160/95 in women of any age).[1]

Arterial hypertension is primary (essential hypertension) in the vast majority of the patients (over 90%).[1] The etiology of secondary hypertension includes renal disease, endocrine, metabolic, or toxic disorders, neurogenic disorders, pregnancy-induced hypertension and hemodynamic disorders. The systemic manifestations vary with the severity (mild to malignant) and chronicity of the hypertension. The morbidity and prognosis of patients with hypertension are multifactorial and depend on age, race, gender, smoking, obesity, lipid profile, presence of diabetes mellitus, and evidence of end organ damage. Hypertensive changes in the eye have been correlated with prognosis and morbidity.[1-3]

ARTERIOSCLEROSIS

Arteriosclerosis is integrally related to hypertension at the clinical and pathological level. The term "arteriosclerosis" refers to fibrosis and hyalinization of the arterial intima; "atherosclerosis" refers to arteriosclerosis and fatty infiltration of the larger arteries (greater than 300 μm in diameter). Hypertension causes smooth muscle hypertrophy of the media and focal arteriolar necrosis. Arteriosclerotic and hypertensive histopathologic changes occur concomitantly in many patients.[4] The larger arteriosclerotic retinal arteries are not responsive to autoregulation and narrow in response to lower blood pressure, in contrast to vasoconstriction with hypertension in normal retinal arteries.[5] Although hyperlipidemia is associated with atherosclerosis (of larger blood vessels), it is not a risk factor for arteriosclerosis of retinal arterioles.[6]

The ocular manifestations of hypertension are usually observed in an asymptomatic individual or occasionally before the discovery of systemic hypertension. There is a wide spectrum of ocular manifestations of hypertension (Fig. 13-1). It behooves the examining physician to measure the patient's blood pressure in the office when confronted with these various fundus manifestations.

Hypertension

```
Arteriolar  ──►  Focal arteriolar  ──►  Retinal hemorrhage, exudate,  ──►  Papilledema
narrowing         constriction              nerve fiber layer infarct
                      │                              ▲
                 Arteriosclerosis ─────────────────────┘
```

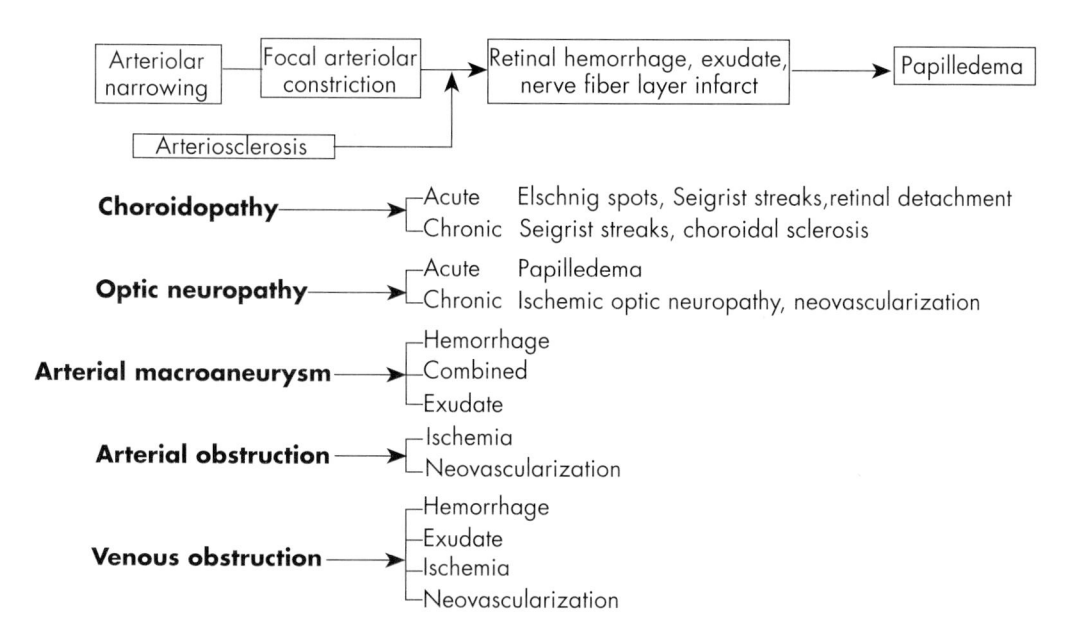

Choroidopathy ──► ┬─ Acute   Elschnig spots, Seigrist streaks, retinal detachment
                     └─ Chronic Seigrist streaks, choroidal sclerosis

Optic neuropathy ──► ┬─ Acute   Papilledema
                         └─ Chronic Ischemic optic neuropathy, neovascularization

Arterial macroaneurysm ──► ┬─ Hemorrhage
                               ├─ Combined
                               └─ Exudate

Arterial obstruction ──► ┬─ Ischemia
                             └─ Neovascularization

Venous obstruction ──► ┬─ Hemorrhage
                           ├─ Exudate
                           ├─ Ischemia
                           └─ Neovascularization

Figure 13-1 Ocular manifestations of hypertension.

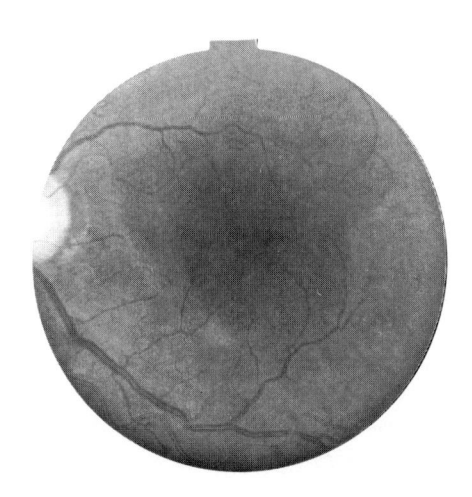

Figure 13-2 Hypertensive retinopathy demonstrating arteriosclerosis and arteriovenous crossing changes.

RETINAL VASCULAR CHANGES

Hypertensive retinopathy was probably first described by Marcus Gunn[7] in 1898. In essential or subacute hypertension the ophthalmoscopic appearance of the retinal blood vessels is characterized by changes in caliber and the light reflex. The normal arteriole to venule ratio (2:3) is reduced because of the attenuation of arteriole caliber. The degree of arteriosclerosis is described by the light reflex and arteriovenous crossing changes. The presence of venous compression and sclerotic changes along the wall of the artery and vein causes apparent loss of visualization and attenuation of venous blood flow (Gunn's sign)[8] (Fig. 13-2).

Usually the artery crosses anterior to the vein (in about two thirds of patients), although the anterior location of the artery is seen almost exclusively in patients with venous obstructions.[9]

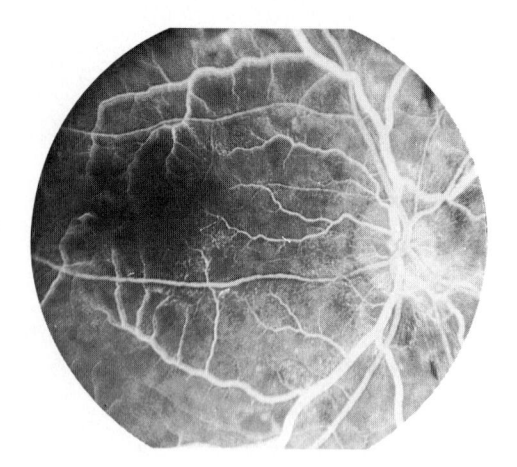

Figure 13-3 Fluorescein angiogram of hypertensive retinopathy.

There is loss of the acute angle of crossing between the artery and vein with arteriovenous nicking. The lateral deviation of the vein as well as the arcuate displacement of the vein toward the outer retina is described as Salus' sign (arc of Salus).[10,11] The arteriovenous crossing changes are caused by sclerosis of the venous wall and a change in the length of arterioles from arteriosclerosis.

The retinal vascular changes are not specific for or predictive of hypertension. Crossing changes have been described in only one third of men with a blood pressure over 151/90 mm Hg.[12] Retinal artery attenuation is not a reliable indicator of hypertension. Only one third of patients with hypertension have narrowed retinal arteries.[13] Often arteriosclerotic retinal arteries appear narrow and become more prevalent with increasing age. Retinal artery attenuation is a more sensitive indicator of hypertension in younger patients than in older patients.[14] Focal arteriolar narrowing can be seen with vasospasm in acute or chronic hypertension. The focal constriction may be reversible with control of blood pressure or it may persist. The caliber of the retinal arteries varies with treatment. Usually the smaller retinal arteries are dilated after control of blood pressure, but the larger retinal arteries can have a variable response.[13]

Other associated manifestations of hypertensive retinopathy include microaneuryms, retinal, capillary telangiectasias, vascular incompetence, and retinal capillary nonperfusion. These may develop in the vicinity of the nerve fiber layer infarcts. Retinal exudates and intraretinal hemorrhages subsequently develop from changes at the capillary level. The presence of hemorrhages and exudates indicates more advanced retinopathy. Intravenous fluorescein angiography confirms the presence of the various manifestations of hypertensive retinopathy, including ischemic maculopathy in some patients with decreased vision. (Fig. 13-3). In patients with secondary hypertension from hemodynamic disorders such as coarctation of the aorta, there may also be associated retinal arteriolar tortuosity.[15]

Several classifications have evolved since the clinical description of hypertensive retinopathy by Keith, Wagener, and Barker.[16] Most are based on morphologic changes in the retinal vasculature, the light reflex of retinal arterioles, and the presence of cotton-wool spots, hemorrhages, hard exudates, and disc edema. A pathophysiologic classification includes a vasoconstrictive phase, an exudative phase, a sclerotic phase, and complications of the sclerotic phase.[17]

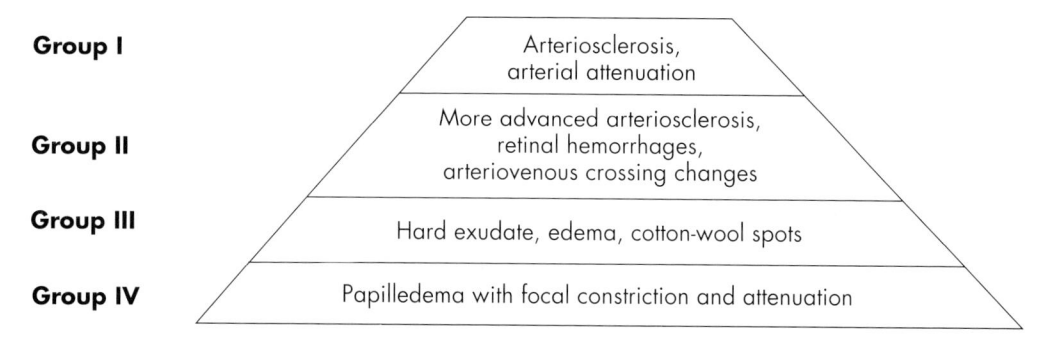

Group I	Arteriosclerosis, arterial attenuation
Group II	More advanced arteriosclerosis, retinal hemorrhages, arteriovenous crossing changes
Group III	Hard exudate, edema, cotton-wool spots
Group IV	Papilledema with focal constriction and attenuation

Figure 13-4 Modified Keith-Wagener-Barker classification of hypertensive retinopathy.

The Scheie[18] classification separates hypertensive changes from arteriolar sclerotic light reflexes. In particular, the light reflex is graded on a scale of 0 to 4, such that copper and silver wiring designate grades 3 and 4 respectively. The Keith-Wagener-Barker classification combines arteriosclerosis with other retinal changes. Each successive group includes characteristics of the preceding group. Group I to IV range from mild to malignant hypertensive retinopathy, respectively (Fig. 13-4). Prognosis has been correlated with the stage of retinopathy, ranging from a 71% 10-year survival for group I to about a 21% 10-year survival (or median survival of about 3.5 years) for group IV hypertensive retinopathy.

Other retinal conditions associated with essential hypertension include retinal arterial macroaneurysms, retinal capillary occlusions, ischemic maculopathy, macular edema, ocular ischemia, ischemic optic neuropathy, arterial and venous obstructive disease, and retinal neovascularization.[20] The clinical course and response to treatment of age-related macular disease,[21] branch retinal vein obstruction,[22] and diabetic retinopathy[23] are influenced by the presence of essential hypertension. Some of these disorders will be discussed in other chapters.

ACUTE HYPERTENSION

Acute hypertension may accelerate or enter a malignant phase characterized by fibrinoid necrosis of the choroidal vessels and disc edema.[24] (Fig. 13-5). Accelerated hypertension usually refers to a recent increase in blood pressure with fundus changes without papilledema.[25] Initially hemorrhages and nerve fiber layer infarcts develop in the distribution of radial peripapillary capillaries. There is diffuse and focal arteriolar narrowing. The hard exudates, typically manifested as a circinate ring in the fovea, follow within several weeks. There have also been a small number of cases of acute macular neuroretinopathy reported[26] after an acute elevation of blood pressure induced by intravenous sympathomimetics. The optic disc and choroid were normal in these patients.

Papilledema develops in the malignant phase of acute hypertension (Fig. 13-6). Patients have associated manifestations of hypertensive encephalopathy, including headache, vomiting, transient paresis, convulsions, stupor, and visual disturbances as well as possible cardiac decompensation and renal failure. Ma-

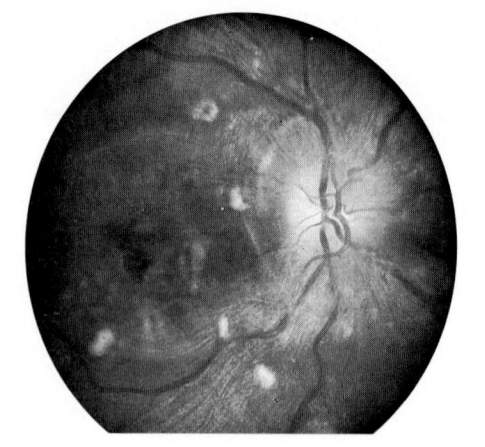

Figure 13-5 Malignant hypertension.

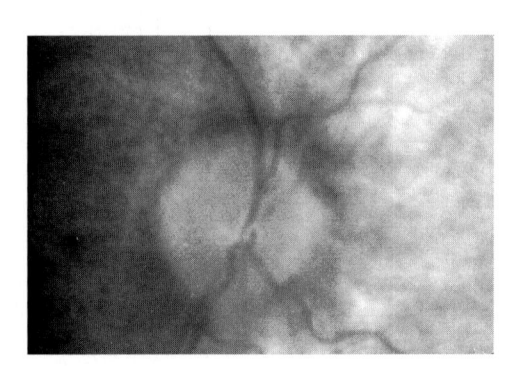

Figure 13-6 Papilledema in malignant hypertension.

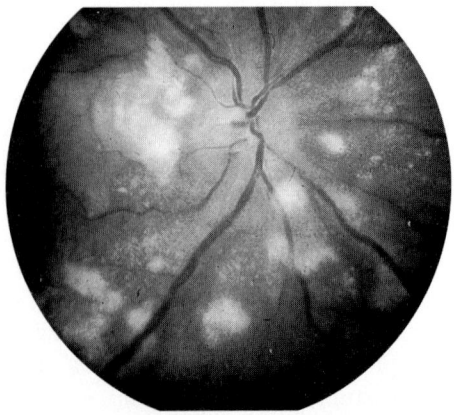

Figure 13-7 Malignant hypertension demonstrating acute Elchnig spots.

lignant hypertension is a medical emergency in which the diastolic blood pressure should be reduced toward 90 torr. An abrupt reduction in blood pressure has been associated with permanent visual loss.[27]

Choroid

Hypertensive choroidopathy is a common manifestation of acute hypertension.[25] Focal infarcts develop in the choriocapillaris or small choroidal arterioles appearing as yellow spots at the level of the retinal pigment epithelium and leaking on fluorescein angiography (Fig. 13-7). Rarely, localized serous retinal detachments may occur with the leakage. These focal infarcts heal as hyperpigmented centers surrounded by a halo of depigmentation (Elschnig spot). Siegrist's streaks are hyperpigmented areas along the course of sclerotic choroidal arteries in acute or chronic hypertension.

Optic Disc

In the early stages of accelerated hypertension the optic disc appears hyperemic, the disc capillaries dilate, and the retinal veins become engorged associated with retinal edema; then papilledema develops. The mechanisms for optic disc edema in malignant hypertension include increased intracranial pressure, venous stasis, axoplasmic swelling, and possibly ischemia.[28]

In patients with chronic hypertension there may be optic disc involvement manifested by peripapillary hemorrhages and optic disc edema. Subsequently optic atrophy occurs with an ischemic optic neuropathy.

PREGNANCY-INDUCED HYPERTENSION

Pregnancy-induced hypertension (5% of pregnancies) is characterized by the presence of hypertension, edema, and proteinuria (preeclampsia). Preeclampsia may progress to eclampsia if seizures develop. Pregnancy-induced hypertension usually commences in the second half of gestation. Certain coagulation disorders—such as disseminated intravascular coagulation and thrombocytopenia—may develop concomitantly with preeclampsia/eclampsia. Pregnancy-induced hypertension resolves within 1 to 5 months post-partum. Some patients develop an underlying chronic hypertension or continue to have hypertension. Visual complaints (e.g., diplopia or blurred vision) are present in up to 50% of the patients with pregnancy-induced hypertension. Retinal vascular changes are commonly identified.[29]

The earliest fundus manifestations include reversible focal arteriolar spasm. Arteriolar narrowing and focal arteriolar constrictions have been loosely correlated with the diastolic blood pressure.[30] Sometimes there are associated intraretinal hemorrhages, exudates, and nerve fiber layer infarcts. Disc edema evolves with the onset of malignant hypertension. Serous retinal and retinal pigment epithelial detachments rarely occur.

The serous retinal detachments are usually not associated with significant retinopathy. They are believed to arise from a disturbance in the choroidal circulation. There may be residual pigmentary alterations and Elschnig spots after the subretinal fluid resorbs. The vascular changes improve after medical management or delivery. The visual prognosis is good in most patients unless optic atrophy, an arterial occlusion, or cortical blindness occurs.

The severity of the retinopathy has in the past been correlated with both maternal and fetal prognoses[29] however, the use of ophthalmoscopy in terms of diagnosis and management of preeclampsia is limited. The presence of retinopathy alone in a patient with pregnancy-induced hypertension is not an indication to terminate a pregnancy.[30]

References

1. Williams GH, Jagger PI, Braunwald E: Hypertensive vascular disease. In Isselbacher KJ, Adams RD, Braunwald E, et al (eds): *Harrison's Principles of internal medicine,* ed 9, New York 1980, McGraw-Hill, Chapter 251.
2. Walsh JB: Hypertensive retinopathy: description, classification, and prognosis, *Ophthalmology* 89:1127, 1982.
3. Breslin DJ, Gifford Rw Jr, Fairbairn JF, Kearns TP: Prognostic importance of ophthalmoscopic finding in essential hypertension, *JAMA* 195:335, 1966.
4. Wise GN, Dollery CT, Henkind P: *The retinal circulation,* New York, 1971, Harper & Row, Chapter 13.
5. Ibid, Chapter 6.
6. Orlin C, Lee K, Jampol LM, Farber M: Retinal arteriolar changes in patients with hyperlipidemias, *Retina* 8:6, 1988.
7. Gunn M: On ophthalmoscopic evidence of general arterial disease, *Trans Ophthalmol Soc UK* 18:356, 1898.
8. Gunn M: Ophthalmoscopic appearance of arterial changes associated with chronic renal disease, of increased arterial tension, *Trans Ophthalmol Soc UK* 12:124, 1892.
9. Duker J, Brown GC: Anterior Location of crossing artery in branch retinal vein obstruction, *Arch Ophthalmol* 107:998, 1989.
10. Salus R: Veränderungen der Netzhautvenen bei allg. Blutdrucksteigerung, *Klin Monatsbl Augenheilkd* 82:471, 1929.
11. Seitz R: The retinal vessels (translated by Blodi FC), St Louis, 1964, Mosby.
12. Bechgaard P, Kopp H, Nielsen JH: One thousand hypertensive patients followed from 16 to 22 years, *Acta Med Scand* 154(suppl 312):175, 1956.
13. Ramalho PS, Dollery CT: Hypertensive retinopathy: caliber changes in retinal blood vessels following blood pressure reduction and inhalation of oxygen, *Circulation* 37:580, 1968.
14. Daniels SR, Lipman MJ, Burke MJ, Loggie JMH: The prevalence of retinal vascular abnormalities in children and adolescents with essential hypertension, *Am J Ophthalmol* 111:205, 1991.
15. Johns KJ, Johns JA, Fenman SS: Retinal vascular abnormalities in patients with coarctation of the aorta, *Arch Ophthalmol* 109:1266, 1991.
16. Keith NM, Wagener HP, Barker NW: Some different types of essential hypertension: their course and prognosis, *Am J Med Sci* 197:332, 1939.
17. TSO M, Jampol LM: Pathophysiology of hypertensive retinopathy, *Ophthalmology* 89:1132, 1982.
18. Scheie HG: Evaluation of ophthalmoscopic changes of hypertension and arteriolar sclerosis, *Arch Ophthalmol* 49:117, 1953.
19. Breckenridge A, Dollery CT, Parry EH: Prognosis of treated hypertension: changes in life expectancy and causes of death between 1952 and 1967, *Q J Med* 39:411, 1970.
20. Becker RA: Hypertension and arteriolsclerosis. In Duane TD, Jaeger EA (eds): *Clinical ophthalmology,* Hagerstown Md, 1989, Harper & Row.
21. Macula Photocoagulation Study Group: Argon laser photocoagulation for senile macula degeneration, *Arch Ophthalmol* 100:912, 1982.
22. Branch Vein Occlusion Study Group: Argon laser for macular edema in branch vein occlusion, *Am J Ophthalmol* 98:271, 1984.
23. Klein R, Klein BEK, Moss SE, et al: The Wisconsin epidemiologic study of diabetic retinopathy. III. Prevalence and risk of diabetic retinopathy when age at diagnosis is 30 or more years, *Arch Ophthalmol* 102:527, 1984.

24. Spencer WH, *Ophthalmic pathology,* Philadelphia, 1985, WB Saunders, p 1037.
25. Murphy RP, Chew EY: Hypertension. In Ryan SJ, Ogden TE, Schachat AP, et al (eds): *Retina,* St Louis, 1989, Mosby, Chapter 78.
26. O'Brien DM, Farmer SG, Kalina RE, Leon JA: Acute macular neuroretinopathy following intravenous sympathomimetics, *Retina* 9:281, 1989.
27. Hayreh SS: Hypertension. In Gold GH, Weingeist TA (eds): *The eye in systemic disease.* Philadelphia, 1990, JB Lippincott, Chapter 226, p 664.
28. Hayreh SS, Servais, Verdi PS: Fundus lesions in malignant hypertension. V. Hypertensive optic neuropathy, *Ophthalmology* 93:74, 1986.
29. Sunness JS: The pregnant woman's eye, *Survey Ophthalmol* 32:219, 1988.
30. Jaffe G, Schatz H: Ocular manifestations of preeclampsia, *Am J Ophthalmol* 103:309, 1987.

14

Idiopathic Parafoveal Telangiectasis

Robert C. Kleiner

In 1952 Reese[1] proposed the term "retinal telangiectasis" to describe a presumed developmental vascular anomaly that typically was uniocular, occurred mainly in adolescent males, and included the lesions of Coats' disease and Leber's miliary aneurysms. The vascular anomaly consists of coarse dilation of the retinal capillaries with microaneurysms and saccular dilation of the adjacent venules and arterioles and shows a propensity for the superotemporal quadrant and perimacular area, although all regions of the retina can be affected.

In 1968 Gass[2] described several patients who differed notably from the typical patients with retinal telangiectasis in that they had discrete patches of telangiectatic capillaries adjacent to the fovea. Similar cases were subsequently reported by Hutton et al.[3,4] and Chopdar.[5] Finally, in 1982, Gass and Oyakawa[6] proposed the term "idiopathic juxtafoveal retinal telangiectasis" to separate this group of patients from those with typical retinal telangiectasis or Coats' disease. The condition is now more commonly referred to as idiopathic parafoveal telangiectasis.

CLINICAL DESCRIPTION

Patients with idiopathic parafoveal telangiectasis may complain of blurred vision, metamorphopsia, or a central scotoma, although the disease is occasionally found on routine examination of an otherwise asymptomatic patient.[5] Most patients are between 40 and 70 years of age.[4,6,7] Although both sexes can be affected, there is some predilection for men.[6,7,8]

Clinical signs are confined to the macular region (Fig. 14-1). Careful examination may reveal visible telangiectasis of the parafoveal capillaries. Gass[6] described the presence of "right-angle venules," or venules dipping into the deep retinal plexis at right angles to the retinal surface.[6] In some patients the vascular findings may be subtle and detected only by fluorescein angiography. Blunting of the foveal reflex, macular edema, or cystic macular changes may be present. In some patients tiny yellow refractile opacities may be present in the superficial retina adjacent to the fovea.[9] Patients with bilateral disease may have

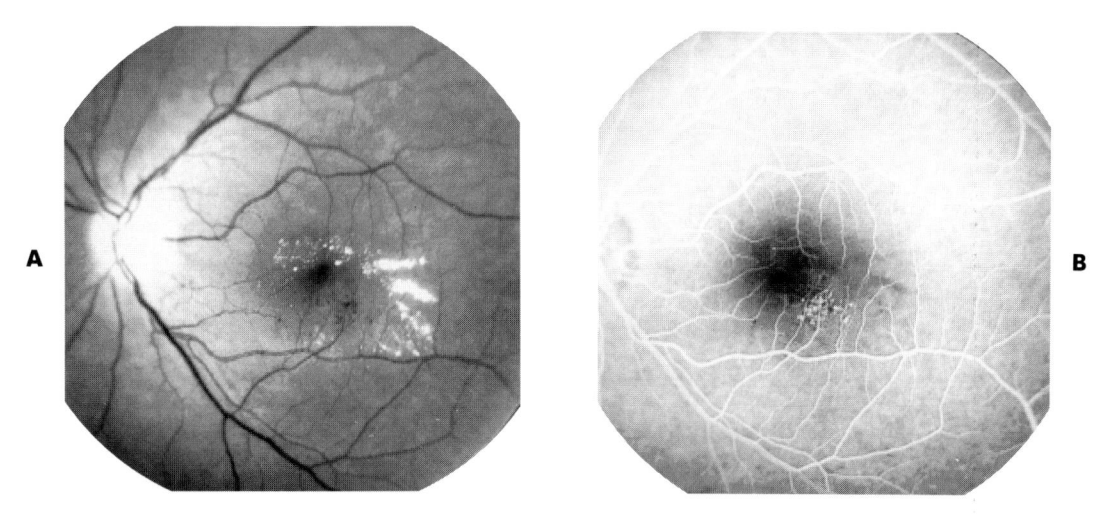

Figure 14-1 Red-free photograph, **A,** and fluorescein angiogram, **B,** of a patient with parafoveal telangiectasis showing lipid exudate from the telangiectatic capillaries and microaneurysms adjacent to the fovea.

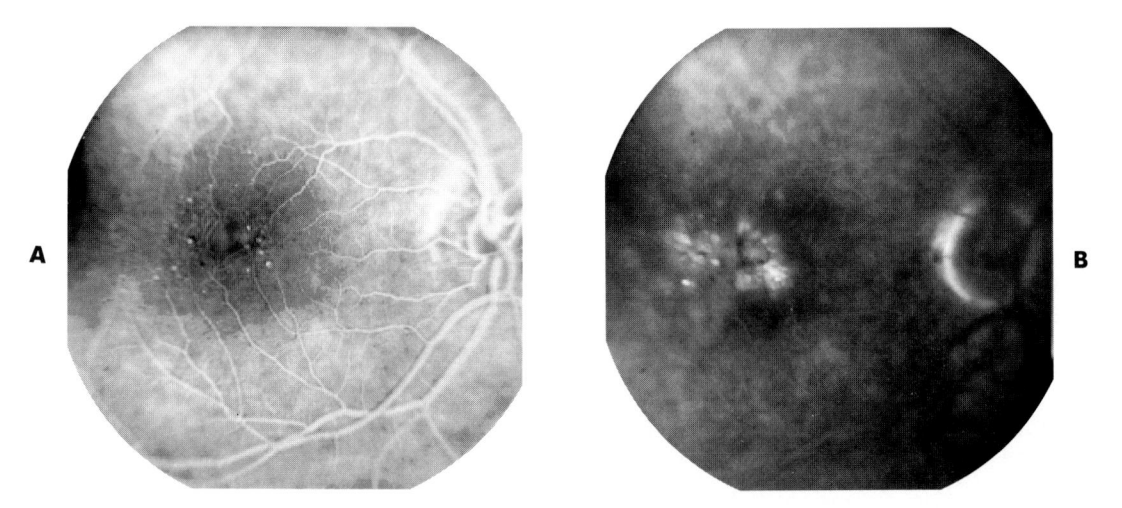

Figure 14-2 Early, **A,** and late, **B,** fluorescein angiogram frames of a patient with parafoveal telangiectasis showing the parafoveal capillaries with aneurysm formation, widening of the foveal avascular zone, and late cyst formation.

asymmetric involvement with changes in the fellow eye evident only by fluorescein angiography.

Late complications include changes at the macular consisting of pigment epithelial clumping and subretinal scarring that resemble disciform lesions. Subretinal neovascularization and chorioretinal anastomoses may occur.[6,7] Chronic cystoid macular edema can lead to formation of a macular hole.[6,10]

Fluorescein angiography reveals telangiectasis of the parafoveal capillaries with microaneurysm formation and late leakage (Fig. 14-2). In many cases the area of telangiectasis is drained by medium-sized retinal venules that cross similar-sized retinal arterioles superior and inferior to the involved region. In

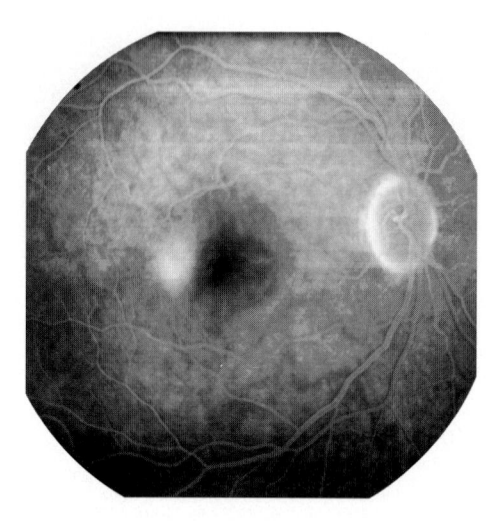

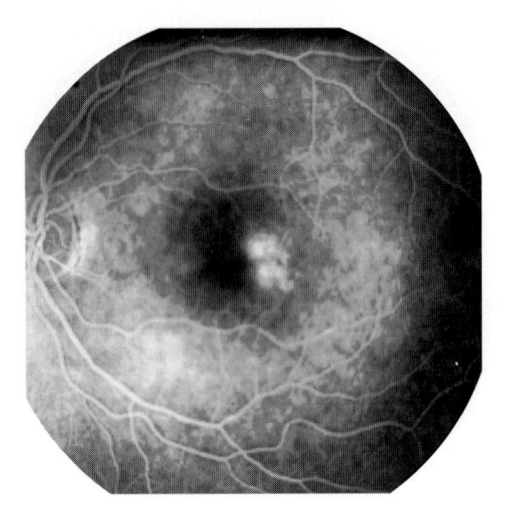

Figure 14-3 Late fluorescein leakage temporal to the fovea in both eyes of a patient with Gass Type II parafoveal telangiectasis.

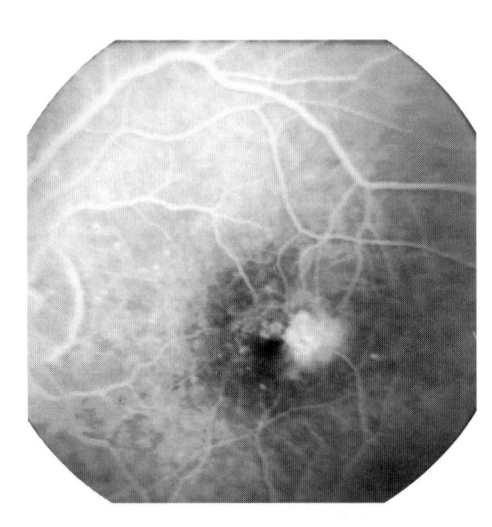

Figure 14-4 Subretinal neovascular membrane present temporal to the fovea in a patient with bilateral parafoveal telangiectasis.

contrast to branch vein occlusion, telangiectatic vessels do not respect the horizontal raphe; they do not affect the entire capillary bed distal to the arteriovenous crossing, only the portion in the juxtafoveal region.[6]

Gass[6] subdivided his patients with idiopathic parafoveal telangiectasis into four groups: group I comprising men with telangiectasis largely confined to the temporal half of the juxtafoveal area, group II comprising mostly men with symmetric involvement of the temporal half of both juxtafoveal areas (Fig. 14-3), group III consisting of patients of both sexes with involvement of all the parafoveal capillary bed in both eyes, and group IV consisting of one patient who had telangiectasis associated with optic disc pallor. Other authors[7] prefer to make a distinction only between unilateral and bilateral disease.

Visual prognosis is usually good, with most patients retaining visual acuity of 20/40 or better.[6,7] The visual prognosis is somewhat better for patients with unilateral disease than for those with bilateral disease. Retinal pigment epithelial changes and subretinal neovascularization resulting in severe loss of vision are more likely to occur in patients with bilateral disease (Fig. 14-4). Severe visual loss can also occur from chronic cystic changes and macular hole formation.

ETIOLOGY AND PATHOLOGY

The etiology of idiopathic parafoveal telangiectasis is unknown. One histopathologic study[11] failed to find any telangiectatic retinal vessels. Rather, there was thickening of the walls of the retinal capillaries caused by marked proliferation of the basement membrane that resulted in narrowing of the capillary lumina. Extensive degeneration of pericytes was also observed with occasional areas of degenerated endothelial cells. These changes were seen, to some extent, throughout the retina and not just in the parafoveal area. The authors postulated that the fluorescein angiographic appearance of telangiectasis is due to rapid diffusion of the dye into the thickened walls of the capillaries at sites of endothelial degeneration with subsequent leakage into the surrounding tissues.

In some cases there may be a hereditary component to the disease. Ehlers and Jensen[12] reported central retinal angiopathy with retinal capillary obliteration in three family members of two successive generations. Deutman et al.[13] described a family with autosomal dominantly inherited cystoid macular edema caused by leaking parafoveal capillaries. The angiographic features of these cases are identical to those seen in parafoveal telangiectasis. Hutton et al.[4] reported two sisters with parafoveal telangiectasis, and Chew et al.[14] reported two brothers with the same disease.

Rarely, systemic abnormalities may be associated with parafoveal telangiectasis. Campo and Reeser[15] discussed a patient with occlusions of both common carotid arteries who had bilateral retinovascular changes suggestive of parafoveal telangiectasis. Parafoveal telangiectasis has been shown[15] to be relatively common in patients with fascioscapulohumeral muscular dystrophy. Grand et al.[17] have described a hereditary syndrome characterized by frontoparietal lobe pseudotumor and parafoveal capillary obliteration, telangiectasis, and microaneurysm formation.

One patient in Gass' series[6] had an abnormal glucose tolerance test. Chew et al.[14] reported five patients with Type II diabetes mellitis who had bilateral parafoveal telangiectasis as the primary retinovascular finding. They commented that the histopathologic features described by Green et al.[11] were similar to those observed in diabetic patients. The finding of primary telangiectasis in five diabetics may have been coincidental and secondary to population bias.[18] Millay et al.,[19] however, examined 25 patients with parafoveal telangiectasis and normal fasting blood glucose levels. Abnormal glucose tolerance test results were found in 5 of 8 with bilateral disease and 6 of 17 with unilateral disease.

Casswell et al.[7] speculated that in bilateral cases the site of primary involvement might be the retinal pigment epithelium. They thought that this would explain the prevalence of subretinal neovascularization in bilateral disease and its absence in uniocular disease. In one of their patients the retinal edema was

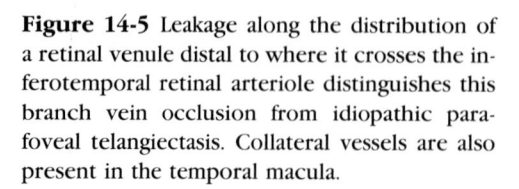

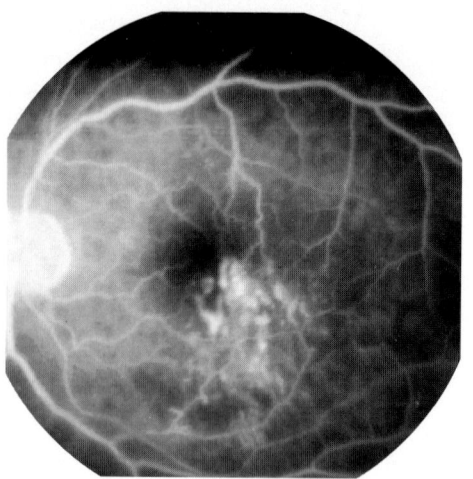

Figure 14-5 Leakage along the distribution of a retinal venule distal to where it crosses the inferotemporal retinal arteriole distinguishes this branch vein occlusion from idiopathic parafoveal telangiectasis. Collateral vessels are also present in the temporal macula.

derived almost totally from the retinal pigment epithelium. In Deutman's series of dominantly inherited cystoid macular edema[13] most patients had a subnormal EOG an a normal ERG, again suggesting widespread dysfunction of the retinal pigment epithelium as a possible cause of leaking retinal capillaries.

DIFFERENTIAL DIAGNOSIS

Other conditions that produce telangiectatic capillaries in the macula with secondary edema include diabetic retinopathy, branch vein occlusion, and radiation retinopathy. A history of any prior radiation treatment should always be obtained and a blood glucose or glucose tolerance test should be considered. The fluorescein angiogram should be carefully examined for signs of branch vein occlusion, including blockage at an arteriovenous crossing, delayed venous filling, areas of nonperfusion, and collateral vessel formation (Fig. 14-5).

The distinction between idiopathic parafoveal telangiectasis and Coats' disease has already been discussed. Coats' disease is most often uniocular in men and can occur anywhere in the retina whereas idiopathic parafoveal telangiectasis is limited to the parafoveal area. Unlike idiopathic parafoveal telangiectasis, Coats' disease is associated with lipid deposition, capillary nonperfusion, microaneurysms, fusiform and saccular dilation of retinal venules and arterioles, and exudative retinal detachment.[20]

In early stages idiopathic parafoveal telangiectasis can be confused clinically with central serous retinopathy although the distinction can easily be made with fluorescein angiography. The small refractile deposits associated with idiopathic parafoveal telangiectasis may resemble those seen in crystalline retinopathies.[20] Other causes of macular edema associated with leaking retinal capillaries should be considered—including vitritis, pars planitis, the Irvine Gass syndrome, retinitis pigmentosa, hypogammaglobulinemia,[21] and muscular dystrophy.[22] The subretinal neovascularization and subsequent subretinal scarring that may accompany bilateral idiopathic parafoveal telangiectasis are sometimes confused with age-related macular degeneration.

TREATMENT

Photocoagulation applied to the areas of leakage in a grid fashion has been reported[6,7] and seems to be successful in some cases. Early workers employed xenon and argon photocoagulation, but use of krypton red can be considered when treating close to the fovea.

Since the visual prognosis is usually good, treatment should be considered only for patients whose vision drops progressively below the 20/40 level. Laser treatment may also be indicated for neovascular complications.

References

1. Reese AB: Telangiectasis of the retina and Coats' disease, *Am J Ophthalmol* 42:1-8, 1952.
2. Gass JDM: A fluorescein angiographic study of macular dysfunction secondary to retinal vascular disease. V. Retinal telangiectasis, *Arch Ophthalmol* 80:592-605, 1968.
3. Hutton WI, Snyder WB, Vaiser A, Siperstein MD: Retinal microangiopathy without associated glucose intolerance, *Trans Am Acad Ophthalmol Otolaryngol* 76:968-980, 1971.
4. Hutton WI, Snyder WB, Fuller D, Vaiser A: Focal parafoveal retinal telangiectasis, *Arch Ophthalmol* 96:1362-1367, 1978.
5. Chopdar A: Retinal telangiectasis in adults: fluorescein angiographic findings and treatment by argon laser, *Br J Ophthalmol* 62:243-250, 1978.
6. Gass JDM, Oyakawa RT: Idiopathic juxtafoveolar retinal telangectasis, *Arch Ophthalmol* 100:769-780, 1982.
7. Casswell AG, Chaine G, Rush P, Bird AC: Paramacular telangiectasis, *Trans Ophthalmol Soc UK* 100:769-780, 1986.
8. Terasvirta M, Tuovinen E: Idiopathic uniocular juxtafoveolar retinal telangiectasis in a female patient, *Acta Ophthalmol* 63(suppl):60-61, 1985.
9. Moisseiev J, Lewis H, Bartov E, et al: Superficial retinal refractile deposits in juxtafoveal telangiectasis, *Am J Ophthalmol* 1:604-605, May 1990.
10. Patel B, Duvall J, Tullo AB: Lamellar macular hole associated with idiopathic juxtafoveolar telangiectasis, *Br J Ophthalmol* 72:550-551, 1988.
11. Green WR, Quigley HA, DeLa Cruz Z, Cohen B: Parafoveal retinal telangiectasis: light and electron microscopy studies, *Trans Ophthalmol Soc UK* 100:162-168, 1980.
12. Ehlers N, Jensen VA: Hereditary central retinal angiopathy, *Acta Ophthalmol* 51:171-178, 1973.
13. Deutman AF, Pinckers AJLG, Aan De Kerk AL: Dominantly inherited cystoid macular edema, *Am J Opthalmol* 82:540, 1976.
14. Chew EY, Murphy RP, Newsome DA, Fine SL: Parafoveal telangiectasis and diabetic retinopathy, *Arch Ophthalmol* 104:71-75, 1986.
15. Campo RV, Reeser FH: Retinal telangiectasia secondary to bilateral carotid artery occlusion, *Arch Ophthalmol* 101:1211-1213, 1983.
16. Gurwin EB, Fitzsimons RB, Sehmi KS, Bird AC: Retinal telangiectasis in facioscapulohumeral muscular dystrophy with deafness, *Arch Ophthalmol* 103:1695-1700, 1985.
17. Grand MG, Kaine J, Fulling K, et al: Cerebroretinal vasculopathy: a new hereditary syndrome, *Ophthalmology* 95(5):649-659, 1988.
18. Mansour A: Parafoveal telangiectasis and diabetic retinopathy, *Arch Ophthalmol* 104:972, 1986.
19. Millay RH, Klein ML, Handelman IL, Watzke RC: Abnormal glucose metabolism and parafoveal telangiectasis, *Am J Ophthalmol* 102:363-370, September 1986.
20. Brucker A, Robinson F: Primary retinal vascular abnormalities. In Yanuzzi L (ed): *Laser photocoagulation of the macula*, Philadelphia, 1989, JB Lippincott.
21. Frenkel M, Russe HP: Retinal telangiectasis associated with hypogammaglobulinemia, *Am J Ophthalmol* 63:215, 1967.
22. Small RG: Coats' disease and muscular dystrophy, *Trans Am Acad Ophthalmol Otolaryngol* 72:225-231, 1968.

15

Coats' Disease

William S. Tasman

In 1908 Coats[1] published the first of two articles in which he described a condition characterized by retinal vascular changes and exudates. In the second article,[2] in 1912, angiomatosis retinae was differentiated from the entity that he had described in 1908. Also in 1912, Leber[3] wrote an article in which he described what has now become known as Leber's multiple miliary aneurysms with retinal degeneration.

PRESENTING SIGNS AND SYMPTOMS

Coats' disease is usually diagnosed between the ages of 2 and 16 years. In most cases when the diagnosis is made it is the result of failing an eye test in school or, in infants, the appearance of a yellowish rather than a red reflex. The disease occurs most often in males, although females may be affected.[4] Unilaterality is the rule, but bilateral involvement occurs in about 8% of patients.

CLINICAL FINDINGS

Coats' disease is characterized by vascular abnormalities that appear as small red "light bulbs" in the retinal periphery with subretinal exudation[1,2] (Figs. 15-1 and 15-2). The vascular changes include aneurysmal alterations, and at fluorescein angiography there is evidence of capillary nonperfusion in the affected area of the retina (Fig. 15-3). These aneurysmal changes show a marked predilection for the temporal area of the retina, especially the superotemporal quadrant. The exudate, on the other hand, tends to accumulate in the posterior pole as well as in the area of vascular abnormality.

The disease may vary in children younger than 4 years as compared to those over 4.[5] In the older age group most of the patients, if verbal, complain of blurred vision. Many, however, are asymptomatic and are picked up only on routine school examinations. Occasionally the exudate in the posterior pole is discovered by a referring ophthalmologist.

Children under the age of 4 often present with leukokoria or strabismus and may be referred to rule out retinoblastoma. If the exudate is in the macular

Coats' disease 205

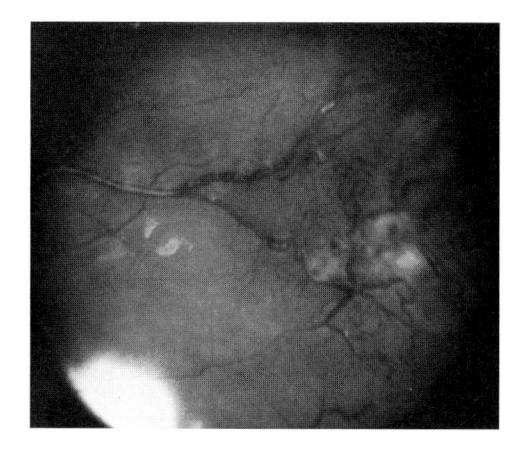

Figure 15-1 Peripheral retinal telangiectasias.

Figure 15-2 Exudation in the posterior pole secondary to the abnormal vasculature seen in Figure 15-1.

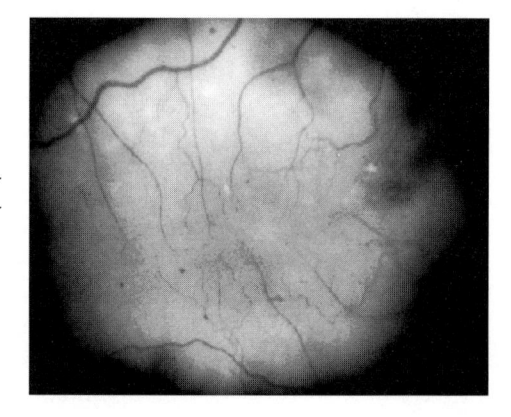

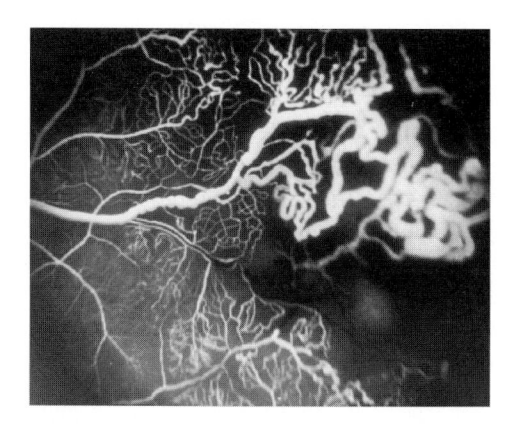

Figure 15-3 Fluorescein angiogram showing nonperfusion in the area of a retinal vascular abnormality.

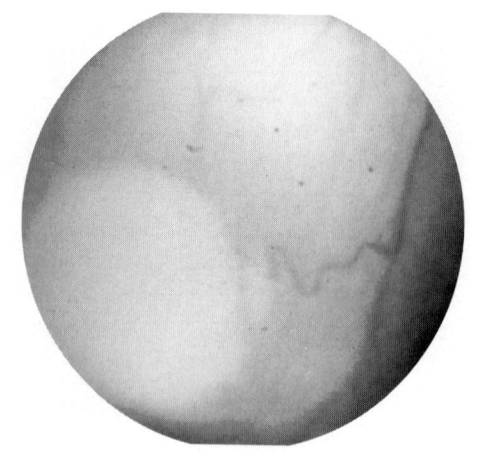

Figure 15-4 Endophytic retinoblastoma.

area, there is generally poor fixation in the affected eye. Although many eyes do not have associated serous retinal detachment, occasional patients may present with a total retinal detachment and the retina ballooned up just behind the lens. In far advanced cases in which there is no resolution of the disease following treatment, neovascularization of the iris may occur and this may lead to neovascular glaucoma.

DIFFERENTIAL DIAGNOSIS

Clearly, the disorder that first must be differentiated from Coats' disease is the malignant intraocular tumor of infancy and childhood, retinoblastoma. In a report by Howard and Ellsworth[6] 254 cases (3.9%) initially diagnosed as retinoblastoma were subsequently discovered to be Coats' disease. Retinoblastoma, the most common primary ocular malignant tumor of childhood and infancy, is diagnosed at an average age of 18 months. There is no sexual predilection as is the case with Coats' disease. In addition, approximately one third of retinoblastoma patients may have bilateral involvement. There may also be a family history that will help in making the determination as to the correct diagnosis since retinoblastoma is inherited as an autosomal dominant disorder when the germinal mutation is present. Generally, a white intraocular mass can be viewed ophthalmoscopically (Fig. 15-4). The most difficult diagnostic problem is when the retinoblastoma occurs as an exophytic presentation. In these situations a tumor is frequently beneath detached retina (Fig. 15-5).

Some patients with exophytic retinoblastoma and overlying nonrhegmatogenous retinal detachment may have telangiectatic-like vessels, which makes the differential diagnosis from Coats' disease more difficult. In such cases ultrasonography can be extremely helpful, since it may reveal the presence or absence of subretinal calcifications. It does not prove to be a major benefit, however, in detecting optic nerve extraocular extension and heavily calcified retinoblastoma.

Haik[7] has recommended that CT scanning is the single most valuable test because of its ability to delineate intraocular morphology, calcified subretinal densities, vascularities within the subretinal space (through the use of contrast enhancement), and finally associated orbital intracranial abnormalities. On the

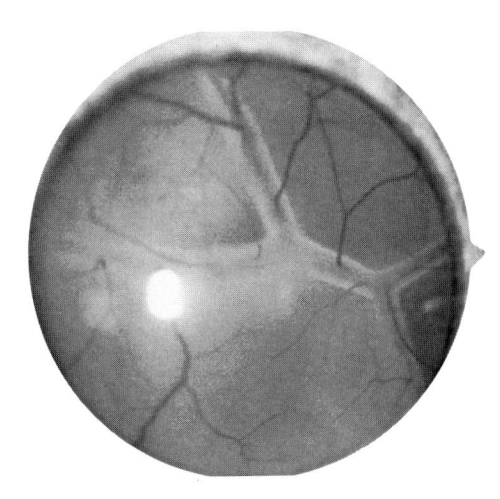

Figure 15-5 Nonrhegmatogenous retinal detachment overlying an exophytic retinoblastoma.

negative side, computed studies require multiple thin slices both before and after contrast introduction and expose the patient to low levels of radiation if repeated studies are performed.

Haik[7] also points out that MRI is valuable for providing insights into the structure and composition of tissues but is limited in its ability to detect calcium, which may be fairly easily seen by ultrasound and CT.

Aqueous lactic dehydrogenase and isoenzyme levels are not particularly helpful in distinguishing between Coats' disease and retinoblastoma. When a diagnosis of Coats' disease rather than retinoblastoma has been established, subretinal fluid will reveal cholesterol crystals in patients with Coats' disease.

Another condition that must be differentiated from Coats' disease is angiomatosis retinae. This was first included in the description of the disorder by Coats in 1908.[1] Angiomatosis is one of the phakomatoses and is inherited as an autosomal dominant trait. It is associated with visceral and central nervous system hemangioblastomas, the latter occurring in about 18% of patients. Visceral cysts and tumors, including renal cell carcinoma and pheochromocytomas, have also been noted in patients with von Hippel–Lindau angiomatosis retinae. Generally this can be differentiated from Coats' disease because of an afferent feeder arteriole and an afferent draining venule that enter and leave the tumor mass (Fig. 15-6). Advanced cases of angiomatosis retinae make the differential diagnosis more difficult, but angiomatosis tends to be bilateral in 30% to 50% of patients and affects both sexes equally. Whereas patients under the age of 10 years with Coats' disease have a negative family history, patients in the second or third decade of life with angiomatosis retinae tend to become symptomatic and may have a family history of the disorder. This is certainly not an absolute rule, however; we have seen patients with capillary angiomas on the optic nerve head as young as 6 years old.

Cavernous hemangioma of the retina occurs in both sexes equally, is usually localized, has no associated exudation, and at fluorescein angiography shows the dye within saccular vascular channels (Fig. 15-7).

Other conditions to be differentiated from Coats' disease include *Toxocara* endophthalmitis, persistent hyperplastic vitreous, familial exudative vitreoretinopathy, and retinopathy of prematurity. The diagnosis of these latter conditions can usually be made on the basis of history, clinical examination, and family

Figure 15-6 Fluorescein angiogram revealing afferent and efferent vessels servicing a capillary angioma.

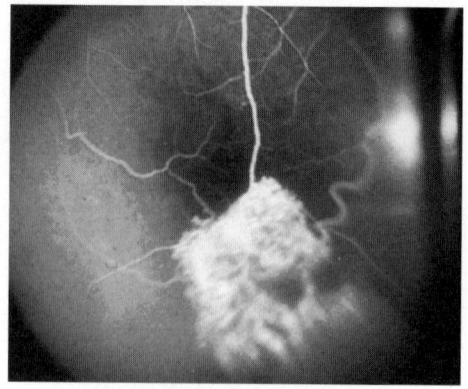

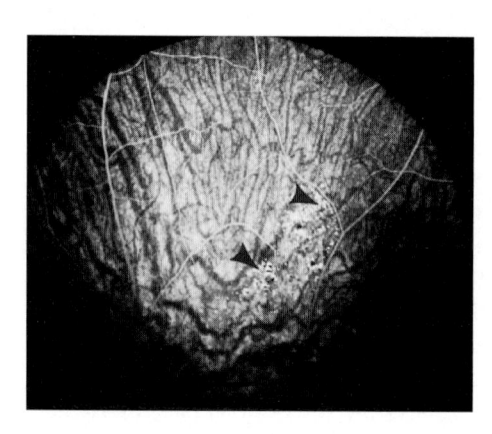

Figure 15-7 Cavernous hemangioma of the retina. Fluorescein has pooled in the vascular saccules *(arrows)*.

Figure 15-8 Residual proliferative band in a patient with Coats' disease 6 years after treatment. The patient had developed a traction retinal detachment that required vitrectomy.

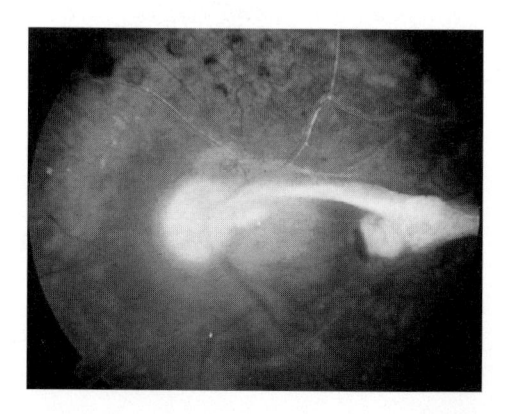

history. Haik,[7] however, has reported that in about 20% of cases presenting with leukokoria the diagnosis could not be established using standard clinical techniques. It was in these instances that the auxiliary diagnostic techniques of ultrasonography, computed tomography, and magnetic resonance imaging were employed to achieve greater diagnostic accuracy.

TREATMENT

Many treatments have been tried over the years, including even the use of antibiotics, vitamins, and steroids. Diathermy coagulation was utilized before the development of lasers and cryotherapy. In 1960 Meyer-Schwickerath[8] first reported the use of photocoagulation in the treatment of retinal telangiectasias with secondary subretinal exudate. Several other series using photocoagulation or cryotherapy[5,9] were reported in the 1970s and were encouraging; but the failure to restore normal vision in many cases, the high likelihood of recurrence, and the apparently dismal course of children with more than two quadrants of the retina involved with telangiectasia proved discouraging.

In our experience cryotherapy has been more effective than laser applications to the telangiectatic vessels. This may well be due to a poor reaction to laser photocoagulation because of the subretinal exudation. Furthermore, eyes with more than two quadrants of abnormal telangiectatic vessels appear to have a poorer prognosis for eventual resolution of the disease. New treatment may be necessary after 2 months if the initial treatment does not lead to resolution of the vascular abnormalities.

In cases with an associated retinal detachment, some authors favor cryotherapy without drainage of fluid. Our preference is for a scleral buckling procedure (to bring the retina into apposition with the pigment epithelium) and then drainage of subretinal fluid with cryotherapy to the abnormal vessels.

We have seen two patients who showed resolution of exudates and elimination of the abnormal vasculature following treatment with cryotherapy and in one case of scleral buckling. In the first patient, treated by cryotherapy alone, proliferative vitreoretinopathy developed 6 years later and required vitrectomy to reattach the retina (Fig. 15-8).

Haik[7] has advocated the use of vitreoretinal surgery in patients with Coats' disease and retinal detachment, including subretinal drainage and simultaneous intravitreal infusion followed by photocoagulation cryotherapy.

Undoubtedly, the successful treatment of advanced Coats' disease depends on reattachment of the retina and elimination of the abnormal retinal vessels. The goal, of course, is to maintain the integrity of the eye and to prevent neovascular glaucoma. One must be prepared, however, for the fact that visual acuity is probably going to be permanently compromised.

References

1. Coats G: Forms of retinal disease with massive exudation, *R Lond Ophthalmol Hosp Rep* 17:440-525, 1908.
2. Coats G: Über Retinitis exsudative (Retinitis haemorrhagica externa), *Albrecht von Graefes Arch Klin Exp Ophthalmol* 81:275-327, 1912.
3. Leber T: Über eine durch Vorkommen multipler Miliaraneurysmen charakterisierte Form von Retinaldegeneration, *Arch Ophthalmol* 81:1-14, 1912.

4. Tasman W: Coats' disease. In Tasman W (ed): *Retinal diseases in children,* Hagerstown Md, 1971, Harper & Row, pp 59-69.
5. Ridley ME, Shields JA, Brown GC, Tasman W: Coats' disease, *Ophthalmology* 89:1381-1387, 1982.
6. Howard GM, Ellsworth RM: Differential diagnosis of retinoblastoma: a statistical survey of 500 children. I. Relative frequency of the lesions which stimulate retinoblastoma, *Am J Ophthalmol* 60:610-617, 1965.
7. Haik BG: Advanced Coats' disease, *Trans Am Ophthalmol Soc* 89:371-476, 1991.
8. Pesch KJ, Meyer-Schwickerath G: Lichtkoagulation bei Morbus Coats und Retinitis Leber, *Klin Monatsbl Augenheilkd* 151:846-853, 1967.
9. Egerer I, Tasman W, Tomer TT: Coats' disease, *Arch Ophthalmol* 92:109-112, 1974.

16

Hemoglobinopathies

Richard E. Goldberg

This chapter emphasizes the vitreoretinal manifestations of sickling hemoglobinopathies and the resultant clinical decisions regarding their management. The sickle cell diseases comprise a hereditary form of hemolytic disease occurring predominantly, but not exclusively, in blacks.[46] It is postulated[46] that the gene that predisposes people to sickle cell disease arose by a natural selection process possibly for protection against malaria in the African black population.

Understanding the sickling hemoglobinopathies integrates both basic science and clinical medicine. Pathologic alterations of this disease process reflect the degree of hematologic abnormality, the coexistent ocular constituents, and the tissues that are affected. Homozygous sickle cell anemia (hemoglobin SS) and heterozygous hemoglobinopathies (sickle cell hemoglobin C disease, hemoglobin S–thalassemia, and sickle cell trait) are discussed in this chapter. The hematologic and systemic features of hemoglobinopathies will not be addressed.

SICKLE CELL ANEMIA

In 1910 James Herrick[25] described the first case of sickle cell anemia. Some 13 years later Taliaferro and Huck[47] recognized an abnormal gene as the cause of this disorder. In 1949 Pauling et al.[35] investigated sickle cell anemia and introduced the concept of a "molecular disease," in which an abnormal gene results in an abnormal protein and leads to a clinical disorder. In that same year Neel[34] subdivided the disease into its appropriate homozygous and heterozygous states.

Hemoglobinopathies are a group of hemolytic disorders caused by the presence of an abnormal hemoglobin. Normal adult hemoglobin is composed of two alpha-peptide and two beta-peptide chains. The alpha-peptide chains contain 141 amino acids, and the beta-peptide chains 146 amino acids. Normal hemoglobin has glutamic acid in position 6 on the beta-peptide chain; sickle hemoglobin has valine in this position,[5] and in hemoglobin C lysine is in the sixth position.[33] Electrophoresis can be used to demonstrate these differences, based on the principle that the hemoglobins migrate differently as charged particles in an electric field.[23,33] These amino acid differences in the hemoglobin molecules alter erythrocyte morphology (resulting in a less flexible sickle shape) increase the viscosity of blood, and induce vasoocclusive as well as hemolytic phenomena.[2] It has been shown[38] that intracellular polymer formation can determine the rheologic properties of erythrocytes as well as the change in shape.[38] Reduced sickle hemoglobin is markedly insoluble. Deoxygenation tends to occur on the venous or capillary side of the network. With the advent of the sickling process, the seminal sequence of erythrostasis may occur.[26]

Homozygotes for the sickle gene (SS) lack HbA and make up approximately 0.4% of blacks in the United States. Heterozygous sickle cell trait (AS) is seen in about 8% of the black population in the United States. Some 25% of children whose parents each have sickle cell trait will have sickle cell disease. Sickle cell HbC (SC) disease is a combination of near-equal or equal concentrations of hemoglobin S and hemoglobin HbC as found in 0.1% to 0.2% of the American black population.[23,48]

The thalassemias are a group of genetically inherited hypochromic microcytic anemias characterized by partial or complete lack of globin synthesis (as opposed to amino acid substitutes) of the two peptide chains (alpha or beta) associated with excessive production of the other peptide chain.[33,46]

Skin and Orbit

Both SS and SC hemoglobinopathies have been reported with orbital swelling.[5]

Anterior Segment

Conjunctiva. The conjunctiva sign (also called comma sign) consists of multiple, short, dark red, comma- or corkscrew-shaped vascular fragments apparently isolated from other vessels. Sausagelike dilations, vascular loops, linear vessel dilations, stasis, telangiectasis, and icterus are described.[33,41] The anomalous segments are best observed in the lower portion of the lower bulbar conjunctiva covered by the lid.[5,33]

The *conjunctiva sign,* diminished by heat of the slit lamp (because of vasodilation), is alternatively enhanced by vasoconstrictors (e.g., phenylephrine).[5,33] Its pathogenesis is unsettled but appears to be related to the percentage of irreversibly sickled cells, which, insoluble, form a gel or "birefringent tactoid."[33,23]

Individuals with SS hemoglobin display more evident conjunctiva signs than patients with SC hemoglobin do. In sickle cell trait the conjunctiva sign is usually absent.[33]

Iris. The manner in which hemoglobinopathies affect the iris (iris atrophy or abnormal sphincter function) may be detected by slit lamp biomicroscopy and/or fluorescein angiography. These may be isolated or part of the syndrome of anterior segment ischemia. The latter sometimes follow scleral buckling or trauma. Self-perpetuating intravascular sickling is the proposed etiology. Hypoxia leads to sickling, followed by vascular occlusions that produce ischemia and further hypoxia.[1,5,33]

Iris neovascularization (rubeosis iridis) also may develop in the presence of severe retinal hypoxia.[5]

Posterior Segment

Optic Nerve. Plugs of sickled erythrocytes can involve the capillary and precapillary arterials on the optic disc *(disc sign)* and segments of blood are noted within the small vessels on the disc surface.[6,23,33] The optic neuropathy reflects a vasoocclusive process. The alterations may be transient and often are not severe enough to alter visual function although both optic atrophy and disc edema can occur.[6,23,33] Ischemic optic neuropathy may be bilateral.

Optociliary shunts and neovascularization of the disc have been documented. The pathophysiology of the optociliary shunts is compromised outflow in the central retinal vein[18] and the ischemic stimulus for disc neovascularization may be accentuated by other diseases (e.g., diabetes).

Neovascularization of the optic disc has been described in SS, SC, and sickle cell trait. The ischemic peripheral retina is treated by peripheral retinal laser photocoagulation to eliminate the release of angiogenic factor(s) and induce regression of disc neovascularization.[6,8,30]

Choroid. Choroidal ischemia is demonstrated as attenuation and/or focal absence of the choriocapillaris in the equatorial and peripheral fundus or chorioretinal degeneration from posterior ciliary artery occlusion.[33,3]

Macular Retina. Sickle cell maculopathy includes infarction of the macula with abnormal perfusion, retinal depressions, macular holes and preretinal fibrosis.[4]

Macular holes may be due to macular ischemia and/or traction from more peripheral fibrovascular tissue. Occlusions can be transient and, as such, sickling hemoglobinopathy should be appreciated as a cause of transient or intermittent visual loss.[14]

Vessel involvement in the posterior pole ranges from perimacular capillary dropout and the appearance of perifoveal avascular zones to minor branch vessel occlusion, major branch vascular occlusion and central retinal and possibly central retinal vein occlusion.[7] Subtle lesions may remain undetected unless they reduce visual acuity or produce visual field defects.[49] Lack of correlation can exist between loss of macular capillaries and macular sensory function. Impairment of vision is generally more significant with involvement of the larger vessels.[14]

Even without evidence of macular retinal vascular involvement, patients with sickle cell anemia can show color vision defects when compared with normal controls.[4]

Fluorescein angiography is most helpful in revealing alterations in the angioarchitecture which may elude conventional methods of clinical evaluation. By this method one can detect microaneurysms, enlarged segments (most likely occluded precapillary arterioles or capillaries), hairpin-shaped loops, broken arcades, and widening and irregularity of the foveal avascular zone[33] (Fig. 16-1).

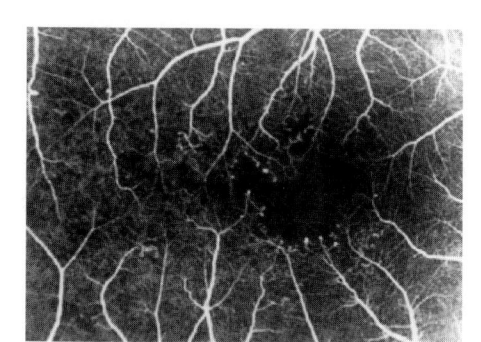

Figure 16-1 Enlargement of the foveal avascular zone in sickling.

Courtesy Morton F. Goldberg, M.D., The Wilmer Eye Institute, Baltimore.

Nagpal et al.[32] reported that angioid streaks occurred in 1% to 2% of the different forms of sickling hemoglobinopathies. Most commonly noted in patients with homozygous sickle cell disease, the streaks have also been reported occasionally in patients with sickle cell SC disease, sickle cell β-thalassemia, and sickle cell trait. Condon and Serjeant[10] found that the prevalence of angioid streaks increases with age in individuals with SS disease and reported an incidence of 22% in patients over the age of 40 years.

The pathogenesis of angioid streaks in hemoglobinopathies is uncertain. The theory of chronic hemolysis and iron deposition is favored by some, but histochemical and light electron microscope studies of two eyes of a patient with homozygous sickle cell disease[27] demonstrated heavy calcification and breaks in Bruch's membrane. Thus calcifications rather than iron deposition may lead to brittleness of Bruch's membrane and angioid streaks.

Peripheral Retina. Retinal vascular abnormalities in sickling hemoglobinopathies may be divided into nonproliferative and proliferative categories.

Nonproliferative changes result directly or indirectly from vascular occlusive phenomena. Intravascular sickling, subsequent ischemic necrosis of an arteriolar wall, and bleeding into the surrounding tissue can result in a salmon patch or black sunburst. In the former, initially the inner retinal and/or submembranous hemorrhage is red; but within days to weeks gradations appear related to the thickness of the blood, the slow rate of resolution, the degeneration of erythrocytes, and the desaturation of the initial red color, resulting in an orange-red appearance[2] that may lighten to a yellow or white color. Following resorption of the blood, a retinoschisis cavity may be formed bound anteriorly by the retinal limiting membrane, and within the schisis cavity iron-laden macrophages and deposits of inorganic iron can provide the clinical appearance of refractile iridescent spots.[2] Such salmon patch hemorrhages, usually located at the equator, have been described[20] with their associated sequelae in SS, SC, and S-thal disease.

Located in the peripheral fundus, round (with a somewhat irregular border) black sunbursts (often with a retinal arteriolar vessel leading into the lesion) are residua of full-thickness retinal and deep intraretinal accumulations of blood.[2] Clinicopathologic correlations of these sunbursts show proliferation of retinal pigment epithelium with migration of pigment into the outer retinal layers and varying degrees of overlying retinal degeneration.[2] Mottled brown areas (round or flat lesions one to two disc diameters in size) are intermediates in the progression of a salmon patch to a black sunburst.

Salmon patches, iridescent spots, and black sunbursts occur most frequently with SS and SC diseases, occasionally with S-thal disease, and rarely with the sickle cell trait.[2]

Peripheral retinal whitening is stated[33] to occur in 80% to 90% of SS, SC, and S-thal groups but this phenomenon is similar to white-without-pressure seen in the general population and probably is nonspecific for hemoglobinopathy.

Retinal vein dilation and tortuosity have been reported,[46] and intravascular sludging could lead to central retinal vein occlusion.[2]

Central or branch retinal arterial occlusion can occur with sickling disease and may be precipitated by a sickling crisis, especially with SS disease. Sickle trait alone is unlikely to cause major arterial occlusion but in combination with ocular trauma and increased ocular pressure may do so.[45] Central retinal artery occlusion in proliferative sickle cell retinopathy has been reported after retrobulbar injection for photocoagulation treatment of proliferative sickle cell retinopathy.[36]

Proliferative changes (proliferative sickle cell retinopathy, PSR) have been divided by Goldberg into five stages[33,47]: (I) peripheral arteriolar occlusions, (II) proliferative arteriolar-venular anastomoses, (III) neovascularization and fibrous changes, (IV) vitreous hemorrhage, and (V) retinal detachment.

Arteriolar occlusion of the retinal vessels occurs particularly in the equatorial temporal periphery.[40] Sickling of the red blood cells results in a thrombotic event thought by some to be at the point in the circulation where oxygen saturation is lowest; others relate that there are measurable quantities of intracellular polymerized hemoglobin S inside sickled erythrocytes even at oxygen saturations of 85% to 90%.

The most peripheral arterioles, especially at dichotomous branching sites, are initially involved and closure gradually spreads posteriorly as a centripetal recession.[33] Blood flow may resume after occlusion, however. Occluded vessels initially appear dark red because aggregations of sickled deoxygenated blood occlude the lumina of the arterioles.[33] In time, conversion to yellow or white "ghost" vessels secondary to organization of intraluminal blood or even resumption of normal appearance can occur.[33]

The electroretinogram may be helpful in assessing the consequences of peripheral retinal ischemia and may prove to be of value in monitoring patients with sickling hemoglobinopathy.[36,37]

Arteriolar-venular or arteriovenous anastomoses (Stage II) occur at the junction of perfused and nonperfused retina. Unlike true neovascularization, these vessels are not thought to leak in the early or late stages of fluorescein angiography[33] (Fig. 16-2).

Neovascularization of the disc[15] and temporal macula[17] (Stage III) has been reported, but proliferative retinopathy is essentially a disorder of the peripheral retina.[46] The neovascularizations ("sea fans") resemble the marine inverte-

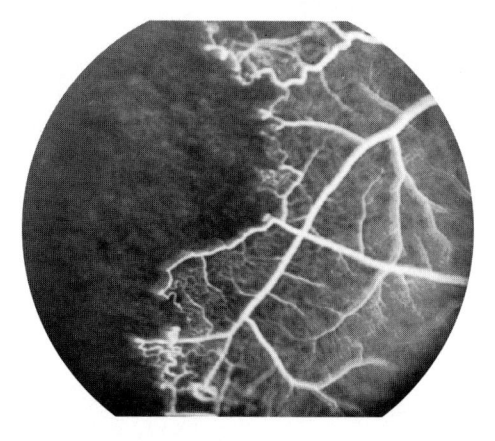

Figure 16-2 Venous phase frame of a fluorescein angiogram in sickle retinopathy showing the confluent gray zone of retinal capillary nonperfusion *(left)* and prominent arteriovenous collaterals along the avascular-vascular interface.

Courtesy James J. Augsburger, M.D., Philadelphia.

Figure 16-3 Early phase fluorescein angiogram of neovascularization ("sea fan") in a patient with proliferative sickle retinopathy.

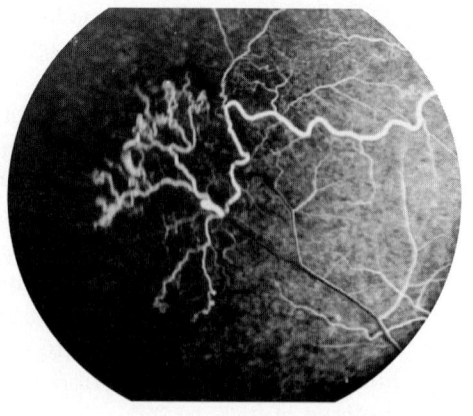

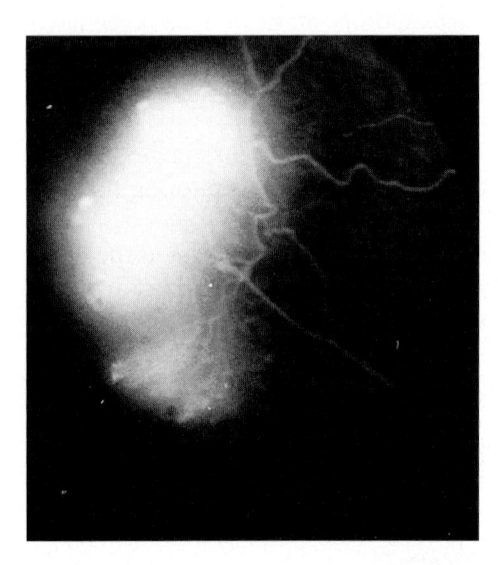

Figure 16-4 Late phase fluorescein angiogram of the peripheral neovascular proliferation ("sea fan") in a patient with proliferative sickle retinopathy.

Figure 16-5 Sea fan in a patient with SC hemoglobinopathy. Note the vitreous hemorrhage inferiorly.

Courtesy H. Logan Brooks, M.D., Tallahassee.

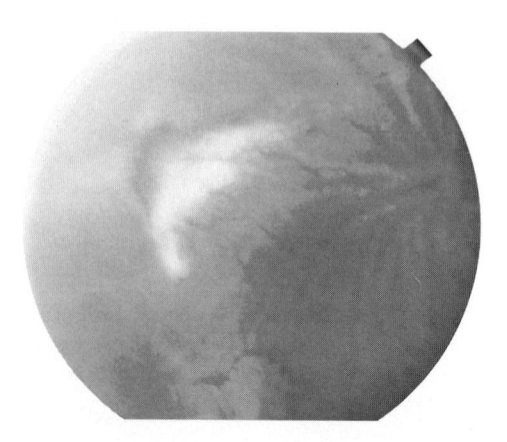

brate *Gorgonia flabellum*.[47] They are usually fed by one or more arterioles and drained by one or more venules. Patches of fibrovascular tissue may coalesce[33] and are seen in the equatorial zone at the junction of ischemic and nonischemic retina, being perhaps more common in the superotemporal quadrant.[2,33] They generally grow anteriorly toward the preequatorial ischemic retina,[33] probably in response to hypoxia and the production of an angiogenic factor by ischemic retina.[2] At times this purposeless proliferation of vessels forms "brushlike" arborizations. Patches of neovascularization occur on the surface of the retina or extend into the vitreous.[33] With leakage these abnormal vessels acquire a covering of white fibrous tissue that can obscure the underlying vessels. They leak fluorescein profusely[33] (Figs. 16-3 and 16-4). Proliferative sickle retinopathy is more common and more severe in sickle cell hemoglobin C disease and sickle thalassemia than in homozygous sickle cell disease[12,13,47] It is rare in heterozygous sickle cell trait (AS).

Vitreous hemorrhage (Stage IV) results from the chronic transudation of plasma, which leads to syneresis of the vitreous and tractional elevation.[7] Hyaloidioangioretinal adhesions transmit tractional forces to the neovascular channels, some of which may grow on the posterior surface of the vitreous. Vitreous hemorrhage occurs (as with "sea fans"), most commonly with SC disease, then S-thalassemia, and rarely SS disease. Hemorrhage is frequently localized to the surface of the retina and to the cortical vitreous adjacent to the responsible patch of neovascularization (Fig. 16-5). The vitreous hemorrhages can be asymptomatic.[33]

Retinal detachment (designated Stage V) is the most severe stage in sickle cell retinopathy. It is divided into 4 substages in accordance with the extent of the detachment.[7]

The detachments can be rhegmatogenous or nonrhegmatogenous. Localized retinoschisis or localized full-thickness retinal detachments also may be found.[7] Retinal ischemia, atrophy, and traction can result in the development of retinal breaks (which may be difficult to identify amid the associated fibrous tissue and hemorrhage) that are horseshoe shaped or round.[7] The breaks often appear adjacent to neovascularization.[33] (Fig. 16-6). It should be remembered that rhegmatogenous retinal detachment may also occur in patients with sickle hemoglobinopathies who do not have proliferative sickle retinopathy.[7] (PSR is uncommon in individuals under 20 years of age, and early detection is important.[29])

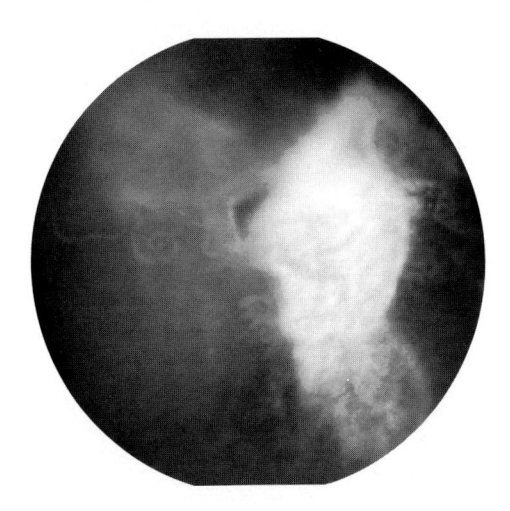

Figure 16-6 Rhegmatogenous retinal detachment in a patient with proliferative sickle retinopathy. Note the tear at the base of the sea fan.

Courtesy H. Logan Brooks, M.D., Tallahassee.

AS and systemic disease can, unfortunately, produce retinal vascular proliferation,[33] and this has been described recently[3] in patients with HbAC.

The differential diagnosis of proliferative sickle cell retinopathy is extensive. It includes, but is not limited to, the following: many of the proliferative retinopathies, some of the anomalous vascular formations, cases of peripheral arteriovenous communication, entities displaying chalk-white vessels and/or isolated vessel segments, conditions with fluffy exudates in the vitreous, entities with peripheral vitreous haze, disorders with pigmented chorioretinal scars, unexplained vitreous hemorrhage and/or retinal detachment, and rubeosis iridis. If the physician maintains a high index of suspicion, careful ophthalmic evaluation and appropriate laboratory studies may result in recognition of sickling hemoglobinopathies before systemic manifestations occur.

GLAUCOMA SECONDARY TO HYPHEMA

Elevation of the intraocular pressure by sickled erythrocytes can follow ocular trauma in any form of sickle cell hemoglobinopathy, including sickle cell trait. Black patients with hyphema should undergo an immediate screening for the presence of sickle hemoglobinopathy followed by a definitive hemoglobin electrophoresis.[21] Glaucoma is frequently associated with a sickle cell hyphema and generally responds poorly to medical management.[24] Complications (local and systemic) can occur as a result of therapy. Systemic dehydrating agents may increase hemoconcentration and viscosity in the vulnerable microvasculature. Carbonic anhydrase inhibitors create the risk of both hemoconcentration and systemic acidosis and can worsen sickling.[21] Early anterior chamber paracentesis may be the most attractive approach for this type of hyphema-induced secondary glaucoma,[21] which can cause central retinal artery occlusion.[45]

As is true of the other proliferative vitreoretinopathies, glaucoma may also follow anterior segment neovascularization.[21]

TREATMENT

To treat proliferative sickle cell retinopathy, one must address neovascularization, vitreous hemorrhage, and retinal detachment. Variations in presentation and personal bias make it inappropriate to imply complete congruity among retinal specialists as to the management of this multifaceted disorder.

Neovascularization

In the past "sea fans" were treated successfully with diathermy, which achieves therapeutic cure by heat-obliterating feeder vessels to the neovascular patches; however, this modality is associated with a high complication rate (e.g., scleral necrosis and anterior segment necrosis).[2,33,46]

Cryotherapy is another technique of treatment. Both a single freeze-thaw method and a triple freeze-thaw method have been used. The triple freeze-thaw method has been abandoned, however, because of the high percentage of resultant retinal detachments.[33,46]

Photocoagulation is the most widely accepted treatment modality. The xenon arc laser has largely been replaced by the argon laser. Argon laser photocoagulation can be focal or scatter.

Direct focal treatment with xenon arc photocoagulation has been reported.[19,33,46] Neovascular lesions were treated directly if flat; if elevated, feeder vessels were treated. Complications included immediate vitreous hemorrhage, peripheral field loss, choroidal neovascularization, preretinal hemorrhage, vitreoretinal traction, retinal detachment and effects of retrobulbar anesthesia.

Direct focal argon laser photocoagulation has been efficacious for infarcting neovascular lesions. Elevated neovascularizations are infarcted by treating the feeder vessels and not the neovascularization itself; if the neovascularization is treated directly, hemorrhage, retinal detachment from vitreous traction, and/or macular pucker can occur.[19,33,46]

The basic underlying systemic disorder persists, and thus after photocoagulation new sea fans may make their appearance. Jacobson et al.[26] have noted that proliferative sickle cell retinopathy can progress unilaterally while the fellow eye continues to manifest only background sickle cell retinopathy. These authors consider that a difference in ocular perfusion may exist between the two eyes, and they stress the evolution of new sea fans in eyes with proliferative sickle cell retinopathy, advocating regular follow-up so new proliferative neovascularizations can be detected. They believe that the usefulness of feeder vessel photocoagulation has been established, but they recognize that scatter photocoagulation may be both safer and more efficacious.

In a randomized prospective clinical trial of argon laser photocoagulation for proliferative sickle cell retinopathy, Farber et al.[19] noted a reduction of prolonged visual acuity loss, vitreous hemorrhage, and complications associated with photocoagulation. They recognized that small intense localized burns in the feeder vessel technique could render the retina susceptible to damage, so they limited their scatter technique to the areas of neovascularization and did not treat the entire 360 degrees. They noted that their local scatter photocoagulation did not prevent new sea fans from developing and, in this regard, felt it likely that 360-degree scatter treatment would be more effective. Because of the low morbidity rate, they recommended scatter treatment.[19]

Peripheral circumferential retinal scatter photocoagulation using argon laser has been employed by Magargal of the Wills Eye Hospital Retinal Vascular Unit.[19,33,46] Treatment is applied to zones of capillary nonperfusion demonstrated angiographically.

Circumferential retinal scatter photocoagulation appears to have fewer complications than experienced with other treatment techniques; it is used to reduce the need for retreatment of sea fans and (hopefully) to eliminate de novo neovascularization.[19,33,46] Support for it is also derived from its effectiveness in the management of other proliferative retinopathies such as diabetes and ischemic central retinal vein obstruction. The principle is based on treating the peripheral nonperfused retina in an effort to eradicate areas of retinal ischemia (which are thought responsible for the vasoproliferative substance causing the neovascularizations). Despite the fact that autoinfarction of retinal neovascularization can occur, proliferative sickle cell retinopathy generally is viewed as a dynamic disorder whose course should be interrupted.[19,33,47]

Vitreous Hemorrhage

Proliferative sickle cell retinopathy may lead to vitreous hemorrhage, and this is often associated with rhegmatogenous and/or traction retinal detachment. Vitrectomy and scleral buckling procedures in patients with sickle cell disease are extremely challenging both systemically and ocularly.[33,46]

Systemically, sickling is an ever-present danger with associated thromboembolic complications such as pulmonary or cerebral embolism and thrombosis.[33,46]

Vitreous hemorrhage is initially managed with 45-degree bedrest in an attempt to obtain gravitational settling of the blood and permit photocoagulation techniques. Longstanding vitreous hemorrhages can be managed by pars-plana vitrectomy. In these cases the peripheral vitreous is removed to uncover perfusing sea fans. Endophotocoagulation, intraoperative or postoperative indirect laser photocoagulation, and postoperative fundus contact lens laser photocoagulation can be employed. Unfortunately, an opaque vitreous skirt sometimes obscures potentially devastating "sea fans."[33,46]

Retinal Detachment

Retinal detachments can be rhegmatogenous, tractional, or exudative. All are capable of causing permanent visual loss; thus, to avoid the necessity of vitrectomy and scleral buckling procedures, emphasis is placed on the early treatment of sickle cell retinopathy.

Because of the high potential for serious complications, surgery is delayed in patients with sickle cell disease who have a tractional retinal detachment unless disconcerting progression is demonstrated or the macula is threatened.[9]

Many of the steps employed in a scleral buckling procedure can promote the sickling process. Scleral buckling in individuals with the sickling hemoglobinopathies increases the risk of anterior segment ischemia.[33,42,46] This syndrome is characterized by striate keratopathy, corneal edema, conjunctival edema, irregular dilation of the pupil with shrinkage toward the area of greatest necrosis, cataract formation, and hypotony.[33,47]

Various techniques have been utilized to try to reduce intravascular sickling in the anterior ciliary and long posterior ciliary arteries. These include the following: use of a local anesthetic without sympathomimetics, dilation only with parasympatholytics, maintenance of lower intraocular pressure (for therapeutic complications see "Glaucoma Secondary to Hyphema," p. 218), avoidance of rectus muscle detachment (or traction), avoidance of a long posterior ciliary vessel manipulation, drainage of subretinal fluid to lower the intraocular pressure, avoidance when possible of the encircling band, avoidance of dehydration, and use of supplemental oxygen and partial exchange blood transfusions. The complications associated with such transfusions, however, which include transfusion reaction, septicemia, and transmission of hepatitis B, cyclomegalovirus, or acquired immune deficiency syndrome, must be integrated in the decision-making process. Consultation with a hematologist is advised, and the patients should be apprised of the risk/benefit ratio of such action.[9,33,46]

Repair of rhegmatogenous retinal detachments in patients with proliferative sickle cell retinopathy carries a guarded prognosis. The breaks are often at the base of the neovascular fronds and difficult to localize and treat. Additionally, iatrogenic breaks may occur. Extensive or high scleral buckles usually are required to relieve the vitreous traction; and since the disease process is in the peripheral retinal, vitrectomy surgery is often difficult and associated with complications.[25,31] Elevated IOP can lead to intraoperative arteriolar occlusion. Expandable gas may have unpredictable effects on the IOP and induce sickling; thus, unless absolutely necessary, ordinary air is preferred to such gasses.[8]

CONCLUSIONS

Even with appropriate clinical decision making, proliferative sickle cell retinopathy can lead to significant visual morbidity. It is ideally best interrupted early in its course.[22] Accurate clinical decision making is critical. There is no perfect approach to the problem, but it would seem that peripheral retinal scatter photocoagulation is gaining in acceptance and may prove to be as close to ideal as currently available. The advent of the indirect laser may further facilitate this treatment approach.

A commercially available test for hemoglobin S should be performed whenever sickling retinopathy is suspected, and a single negative screening test should not be accepted as diagnostic in the presence of suggestive clinical signs. Under these circumstances hemoglobin electrophoresis should be ordered.

REFERENCES

1. Acheson RW, et al: Iris atrophy in sickle cell disease. *Br J Ophthalmol* 70(7):516-521, 1986.
2. Augsburger JJ, Goldberg RE, Magargal LE: Retinal and choroidal vascular abnormalities and fluorescein angiography. In Harley RD (ed): *Pediatric ophthalmology,* ed 2, Philadelphia 1983, WB Saunders.
3. Bresnick GH, et al: Retinal ischemia in diabetic retinopathy, *Arch Ophthalmol* 93:1300-1310, 1975.
4. Carney MD, Jampol LM: Epiretinal membranes in sickle cell retinopathy, *Arch Ophthalmol* 105(2):214-217, 1987.
5. Cohen SB, et al: Diagnosis and management of ocular complications of sickle hemoglobinopathies. I, *Ophthalmic Surg* 17(1):57-59, 1986.
6. Cohen SB, et al: Diagnosis and management of ocular complications of sickle hemoglobinopathies. II, *Ophthalmic Surg* 17(2):110-116, 1986.
7. Cohen SB, et al: Diagnosis and management of ocular complications of sickle hemoglobinopathies. III, *Ophthalmic Surg* 17(3):184-188, 1986.
8. Cohen SB, et al: Diagnosis and management of ocular complications of sickle hemoglobinopathies. IV, *Ophthalmic Surg* 17(5):312-315, 1986.
9. Cohen SB, et al: Diagnosis and management of ocular complications of sickle hemoglobinopathies. V, *Ophthalmic Surg* 17(6):369-374, 1986.
10. Condon PI, Serjeant GR: Ocular findings in elderly cases of homozygous sickle cell disease in Jamaica, *Br J Ophthalmol* 60:361-364, 1976.
11. Condon PI, Serjeant GR: Ocular findings in hemoglobin SC disease in Jamaica, *Am J Ophthalmol* 74:921-931, 1972.
12. Condon PI, Serjeant GR: Ocular findings in homozygous sickle cell anemia in Jamaica, *Am J Ophthalmol* 73:533-543, 1972.
13. Condon PI, Serjeant GR: Ocular findings in sickle cell thalassemia in Jamaica, *Am J Ophthalmol* 74:1105-1109, 1972.
14. Condon PI, et al: Recurrent visual loss in homozygous sickle cell disease, *Br J Ophthalmol* 69(9):700-706, September 1985.
15. Cook WC: A case of sickle cell anemia with associated subarachnoid hemorrhage, *J Med* 1:541, 1930.
16. Cruess AF, et al: Peripheral circumferential retinal scatter photocoagulation for treatment of sickle cell retinopathy, *Ophthalmology* March 1983.

17. Deliyannis GA, Tavlarakis N: Sickling phenomenon in Northern Greece, *Br Med J* 2:299-301, 1955.
18. Dowhan TP, Bodnar ME, Daniels MB: Optociliary shunts and sickle retinopathy in a woman with sickle cell trait, *Ann Ophthalmol* 22(2):66-69, 1990.
19. Farber MD, et al: A randomized clinical trial of scatter photocoagulation of proliferative sickle cell retinopathy, *Arch Ophthalmol* 109(3):363-367, 1991.
20. Gagliano DA, Goldberg MF: The evolution of salmon-patch hemorrhages in sickle cell retinopathy, *Arch Ophthalmol* 107(12):1814-1815, 1989.
21. Goldberg MF: The diagnosis and treatment of secondary glaucoma after hyphema in sickle cell retinopathy, *Am J Ophthalmol* 87:43-49, 1979.
22. Goldberg MF: Natural history of untreated proliferative sickle cell retinopathy, *Arch Ophthalmol* 85:428-437, 1971.
23. Goldberg RE, Tomer T: Fundus abnormalities associated with sickle cell hemoglobin, *J Albert Einstein Med Center,* vol 20, Autumn 1972.
24. Greenwald MJ, Crowley TM: Sickle cell hyphema with secondary glaucoma in a non-black patient, *Ophthalmic Surg* 16(3):170-171, 1985.
25. Herrick JB: Peculiar elongated and sickle-shaped red corpuscles in a case of severe anemia, *Arch Intern Med* 6:517-521, 1910.
26. Jacobson MS, et al: A randomized clinical trial of feeder vessel photocoagulation of sickle cell retinopathy, *Ophthalmology* 98:581-585, 1991.
27. Jampol LM, et al: Calcification of Bruch's membrane in angioid streaks with homozygous sickle cell disease, *Arch Ophthalmol* 105(1):93-98, 1987.
28. Jampol LM, et al: An update on vitrectomy surgery and retinal detachment repair in sickle cell disease, *Arch Ophthalmol* 100:591-593, 1982.
29. Kimmel AS, et al: Proliferative sickle cell retinopathy under age 20: a review. *Ophthalmic Surg* 18(2):126-128, 1987.
30. Kimmel AS, Magargal LE, Tasman WS: Proliferative sickle retinopathy and neovascularization of the disc: regression following treatment with peripheral retinal scatter laser photocoagulation. *Ophthalmic Surg* 17(1):20-22, 1986.
31. Morgan CM, D'Amico DJ: Vitrectomy surgery in proliferative sickle cell retinopathy, *Am J Ophthalmol* 104(2):133-138, 1987.
32. Nagpal KC, et al: Angioid streaks and sickle hemoglobinopathies, *Br J Ophthalmol* 60:31-34, 1976.
33. Nagpal KC, Goldberg MF, Rabb MF: Ocular manifestations of sickle hemoglobinopathies, *Surv Ophthalmol* 21(5):391-411, 1977.
34. Neel JV: The inheritance of sickle cell anemia, *Science* 110:64-66, 1949.
35. Pauling L, et al: Sickle cell anemia, a molecular disease, *Science* 110:543-548, 1949.
36. Peachy NS, et al. Electroretinographic findings in sickle cell retinopathy, *Arch Ophthalmol* 105(7):934-938, 1987.
37. Peachy NS, et al: Correlation of electroretinographic findings and peripheral retinal nonperfusion in patients with sickle cell retinopathy, *Arch Ophthalmol* 108(8):1106-1109, 1990.
38. Rodgers GP: Recent approaches to the treatment of sickle cell anemia, *JAMA* 265(16):2097-2102, 1991.
39. Roth SE, et al: Central retinal-artery occlusion in proliferative sickle cell retinopathy after retrobulbar injection, *Ann Ophthalmol* 20(6):221-224, 1988.
40. Roy MS, et al: Retroequatorial red retinal lesions in sickle cell anemia, *Ophthalmologica* 195(1):26-30, 1987.
41. Roy MS, et al: Conjunctival sign in sickle cell anemia: an in-vivo correlate of the extent of red cell heterogeneity, *Br J Ophthalmol* 69(8):629-632, 1985.
42. Ryan SJ Jr, Goldberg MF: Anterior segment ischemia following scleral buckling in sickle cell hemoglobinopathies, *Am J Ophthalmol* 72:35-50, 1971.
43. Serjeant BE, et al: Blood rheology and proliferative retinopathy in homozygous sickle cell disease, *Br J Ophthalmol* 70(7):522-525, 1986.

44. Slavin ML, Barondes MJ: Ischemic optic neuropathy in sickle cell disease, *Am J Ophthalmol* 105(2):212-213, 1988.
45. Sorr EM, Goldberg RE: Traumatic central retinal artery occlusion with sickle cell trait, *Am J Ophthalmol* 80(4):648-652, 1975.
46. Stephens RF: Proliferative sickle cell retinopathy: the disease and a review of its management, *Ophthalmic Surg* 18(3):222-231, 1987.
47. Taliaferro WH, Huck JG: The inheritance of sickle cell anemia in man, *Genetics* 8:594-598, 1923.
48. Welch RB, Goldberg MF: Sickle cell hemoglobin and its relation to fundus abnormality, *Arch Ophthalmol* 75:353-362, 1966.
49. Westrich DJ, Feman SS: Macular arteriolar occlusions in sickle cell beta-thalassemia, *Am J Ophthalmol* 101(6):739-740, 1986.

17

Retinopathy of Prematurity

J. Arch McNamara

Retinopathy of prematurity (ROP) is likely to rise in its incidence as the ability to save increasingly more premature infants continues. Now a fetus at or beyond 25 weeks of gestation or with an expected weight of 700 g (1.54 pounds) or more has a greater than 50% chance of survival.[1] It is these very small infants who are most susceptible to retinopathy of prematurity. Campbell et al.[2] found that the incidence of acute retinopathy of prematurity among surviving prematures weighing less than 1000 g (2.2 pounds) at birth was three times that of survivors with birth weights between 1001 and 1500 g (3.3 pounds). In pooling the data of five studies,[2-6] it was found that 32% of infants with birth weight of less than 1000 g and 7% of infants with birth weight between 1001 and 1500 g develop acute retinopathy of prematurity. Fortunately, most cases of acute retinopathy of prematurity undergo regression. In the minority of cases that progress, various treatment modalities can lead to regression or stabilization of the disease.

The incidence of ROP in the population of infants at risk (those less than 1500 g and/or 30 weeks gestational age) ranges from 16% to 56%.[7-10] If retinopathy of prematurity is to develop, it usually occurs between 35 to 45 weeks of conceptive age.[11] Most infants who develop retinopathy of prematurity undergo regression of their disease. In those who undergo regression, retinopathy of prematurity lasts approximately 15 weeks.[11] Infants who go on to regression from mild retinopathy of prematurity (less than stage 2+) usually undergo complete resolution.[12] There is an increased incidence of strabismus in those infants compared to a normal full-term population, but this may be due to CNS effects.

The first and most reliable sign of regression is the growth of vessels beyond the ridge (Fig. 17-1). The vessels penetrate into the avascular retina as an arteriole with an accompanying venule. As the vessels grow beyond the ridge, the dilation and tortuosity of vessels just posterior to the shunt and in the posterior pole diminish. The finding of a peripheral retinal detachment, especially if seen with dilated tortuous vessels, is an important forerunner of serious cicatricial changes.

The incidence of progression to the advanced stages of retinopathy of prematurity represents a small minority. Of 1849 consecutive admissions to a university neonatal intensive care unit, Kalina and Karr[3] found 140 infants to have

Retinopathy of prematurity

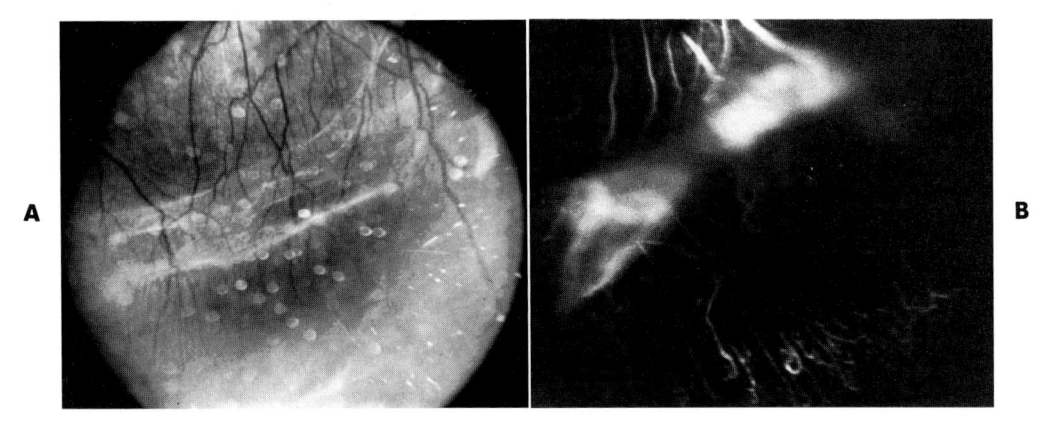

Figure 17-1 A, Regressed ROP. A ridge is no longer present but has been replaced by a vitreoretinal membrane. Vessels are present beyond the former ridge. **B,** Fluorescein angiogram showing vessels growing beyond the ridge into the peripheral avascular retina.

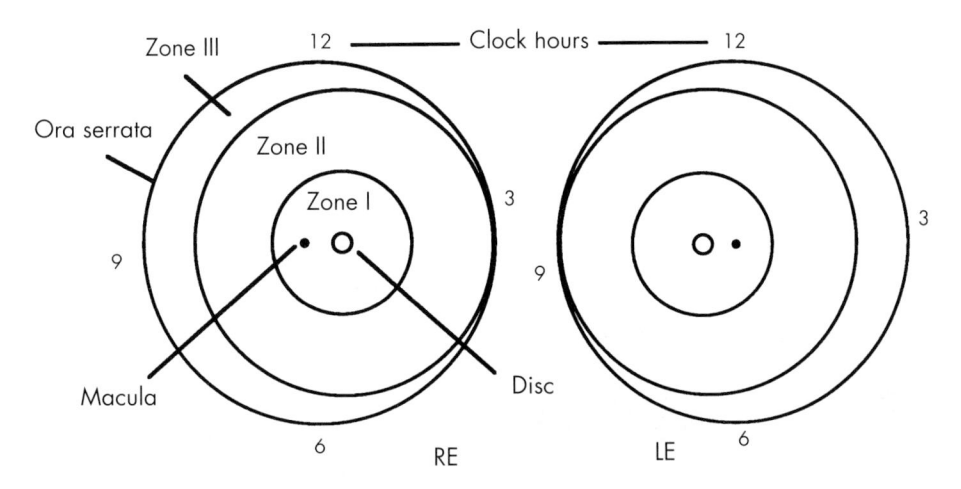

Figure 17-2 Retina of the right eye *(RE)* and left eye *(LE)* showing zone borders and clock hours employed to describe the location and extent of retinopathy of prematurity.

active retinopathy of prematurity. Twenty percent of the 140 infants developed some anatomic features of "cicatricial" retinopathy of prematurity. Very low birth weight is an important prognostic sign regarding progression to advanced retinopathy of prematurity. In Tasman's study on the natural history of retinopathy of prematurity,[9] all babies who became blind were under 1000 g (2.2 pounds).

A classification system for acute retinopathy of prematurity, devised by 23 ophthalmologists from 11 countries, was published and widely accepted in 1984.[14] It clearly defined the location of the disease in the retina as well as the extent of the developing vasculature that was involved.

For the purpose of defining location the retina is divided into three zones, with the optic nerve as the center since retinal vascular growth proceeds from the disc toward the ora serrata (Fig. 17-2). Zone I consists of a circle whose radius extends from the disc to twice the distance from the disc to the center

Figure 17-3 Stage 1, Demarcation line. The posterior vascularized retina is separated from the anterior avascular retina by a thin line.

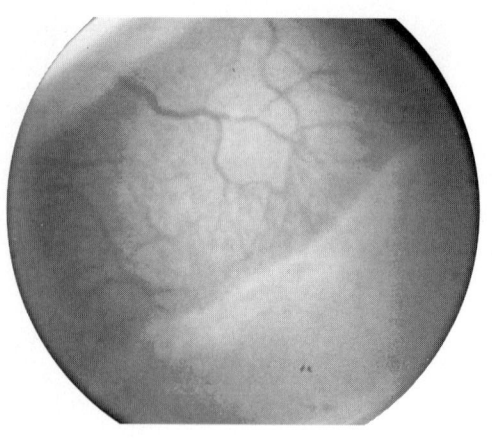

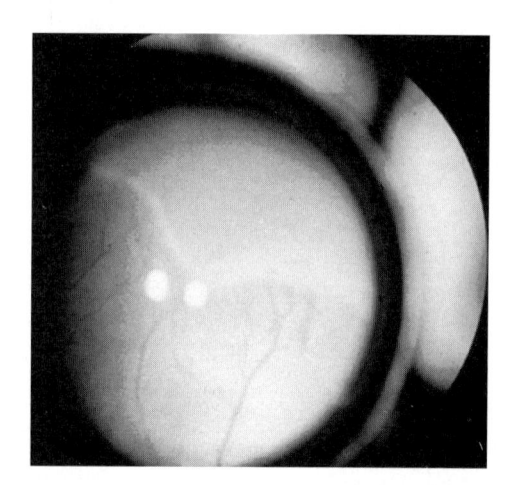

Figure 17-4 Stage 2, Ridge, The line of Stage 1 has thickened and grown out of the plane of the retina.

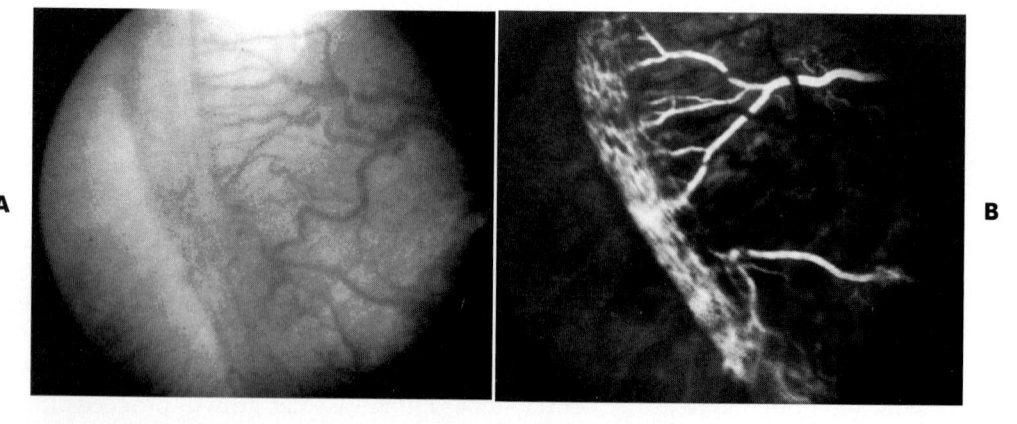

Figure 17-5 A, Stage 3, Ridge with extraretinal fibrovascular proliferation. **B,** Fluorescein angiogram showing vascularization within and above the ridge.

of the macula (twice the disc-fovea distance in all directions from the optic nervehead). Zone II extends from the edge of Zone I peripherally to a point tangential to the nasal ora serrata and around to an area near the temporal anatomic equator. Zone III is the residual temporal crescent of retina anterior to Zone II. This is vascularized last in the premature eye and is the zone most frequently involved with ROP. The extent of disease is specified as hours of the clock (Fig. 17-2).

The second parameter specified in the 1984 classification was staging of the disease (i.e., the degree of abnormal vascular response observed). Four stages were recognized, and the eye as a whole received the stage of the most severe manifestation present.

Stage 1 (demarcation line) is defined as a thin but definite structure that separates avascular retina anteriorly from vascularized retina posteriorly (Fig. 17-3). Abnormal branching or arcading of vessels is seen leading up to the line. It is flat and white and is in the plane of the retina. Stage 2 (ridge) is present when the line of Stage 1 has grown, has height and width, and occupies a volume extending up out of the plane of the retina (Fig. 17-4). The ridge may be pink or white. Vessels may leave the plane of the retina to enter it. Small tufts of new vessels may be seen on the surface of the retina posterior to the ridge. These vessels do not constitute fibrovascular growth, which is a necessary condition for Stage 3 ROP. Stage 3 (ridge with extraretinal fibrovascular proliferation) exists when extraretinal fibrovascular proliferation is added to the ridge of Stage 2 ROP (Fig. 17-5). Stage 3 is arbitrarily further subdivided into mild, moderate, and severe. Stage 4 (retinal detachment) is the addition of retinal detachment to Stage 3 findings. The retinal detachment is caused by tractional forces.

Progressive vascular incompetence, occurring along with the changes at the edge of the abnormally developing retinal vasculature, is noted by increasing dilation and tortuosity of the peripheral retinal vessels, iris vascular engorgement, pupillary rigidity, and vitreous haze. When the vascular changes are so marked that the posterior veins are enlarged and the arterioles tortuous, a plus sign is added to the ROP stage number ("plus" disease) (Fig. 17-6).

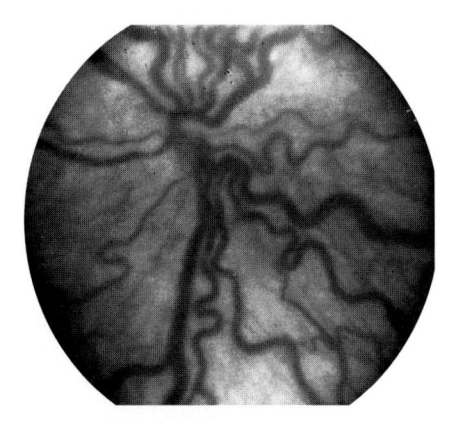

Figure 17-6 "Plus" disease. Dilation of retinal veins and tortuosity of retinal arterioles in the posterior pole, same patient as in Figure 17-5.

Subsequent to the initial International Classification of Retinopathy of Prematurity report, completion of the classification of ROP led to the publication of the classification of retinal detachment.[15] Stage 4 was expanded to Stage 4A and Stage 4B. Stage 4A (Fig. 17-7) represents extrafoveal retinal detachment that is a concave traction type of retinal detachment in the periphery without involvement of the macula. These detachments are generally located in anterior Zone II or Zone III. Stage 4B (Fig. 17-8) classifies a partial retinal detachment including the fovea that usually extends in the form of a fold from the disc through Zone I to involve Zone II and Zone III. Stage 5 (Fig. 17-9) retinal detachments are total and always funnel shaped. Stage 5 is subdivided based on the shape of the funnel. The funnel is divided into anterior and posterior parts, allowing for four subdivisions depending on whether the funnel is open or narrow in both parts of the funnel.

Although not part of the classification, the committee recognized that regression is the most common outcome of ROP. The various patterns of regression were thought to be too myriad to classify (Fig. 17-10), but they were listed (Table 17-1).

Figure 17-7 Stage 4A, Extrafoveal retinal detachment.

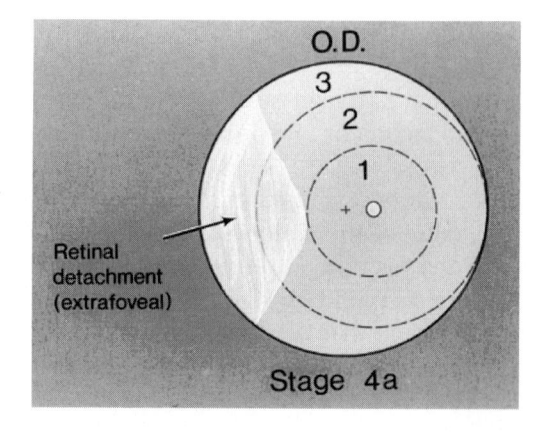

Figure 17-8 Stage 4B, Subtotal retinal detachment involving the fovea.

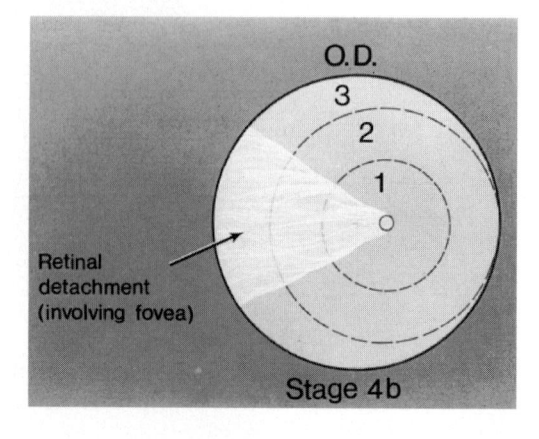

Retinopathy of prematurity

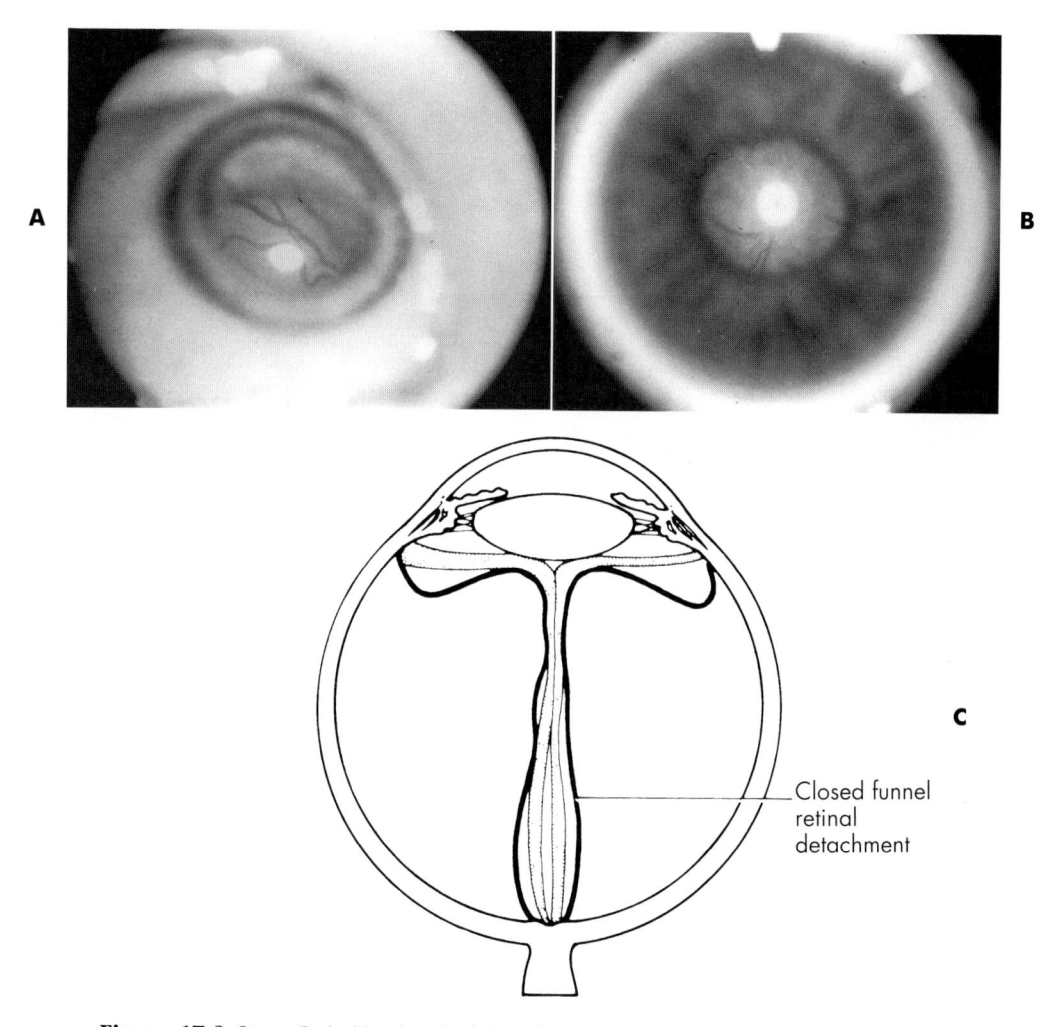

Figure 17-9 Stage 5. **A,** Total retinal detachment with an open funnel. **B,** Total retinal detachment with a closed funnel. A membrane is present behind the lens. **C,** Total retinal detachment closed both anteriorly and posteriorly. Note the retrolental membrane.

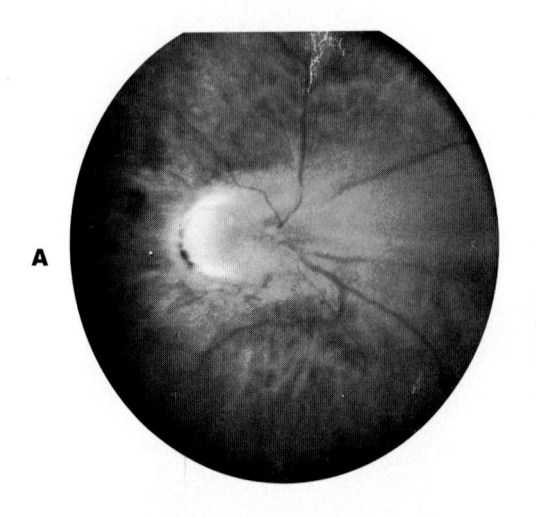

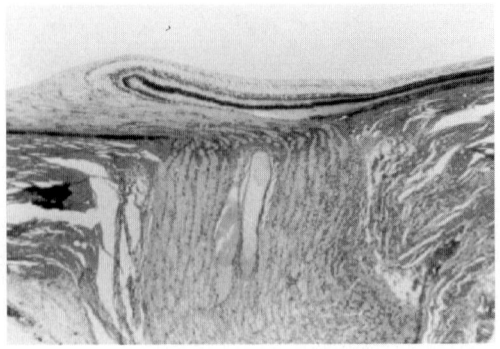

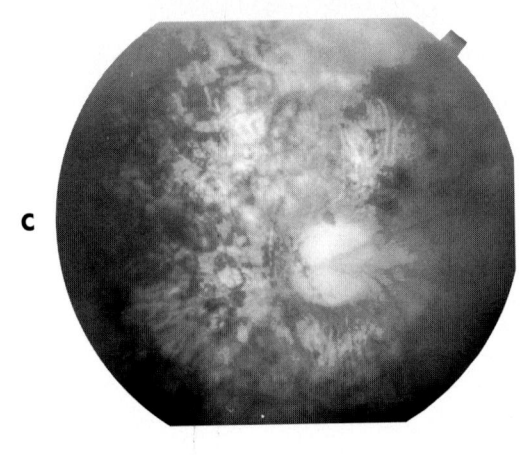

Figure 17-10 A, Temporally dragged retina with straightening of the vessels of the temporal vascular arcades. **B,** Histopathologic specimen of temporal dragging of the retina. The disc is not displaced. **C,** Severe temporal shifting of the retina, leaving behind a thinned nasal portion with extensive pigmentary disruption.

Table 17-1 Patterns of Regressed Retinopathy of Prematurity

	Peripheral	*Posterior*
Vascular	Failure to vascularize peripheral retina	Vascular tortuosity
	Abnormal nondichotomous branching of retinal vessels	Straightening of blood vessels in temporal arcade
	Vascular arcades with circumferential interconnection	Decrease in angle of insertion of major temporal arcade
	Telangiectatic vessels	
Retinal	Pigmentary changes	Pigmentary changes
	Vitreoretinal interface changes	Distortion and ectopia of macula
	Thin retina	Stretching and folding of macula in macular region leading to periphery
	Peripheral folds	
	Vitreous membranes with or without attachment to retina	Vitreoretinal interface changes
	Latticelike degeneration	Vitreous membranes
	Retinal breaks	Dragging of retina over disc
	Traction or rhegmatogenous retinal detachment	Traction or rhegmatogenous retinal detachment

DIFFERENTIAL DIAGNOSIS

The differential diagnosis of retinopathy of prematurity differs depending on the stage of the disease. In its earlier stages conditions that lead to peripheral retinal vascular changes and retinal dragging should be considered. In its more advanced stages the differential diagnosis of a white pupillary reflex must be considered.

The clinical setting often gives the diagnosis. Infants with retinopathy of prematurity typically will be premature and of low birth weight with a history of variable oxygen exposure. There will be no hereditary pattern.

Familial exudative vitreoretinopathy is an autosomal dominant peripheral fundus disorder that is asymptomatic in 80% of cases. Peripheral nonvascularization with straightening and anastomosis of the vessels occurs in a fibrillar pattern at the junction between perfused and nonperfused retina (Fig. 17-11). Dragging of the retina may occur (Fig. 17-12). Regression, as seen in retinopathy of prematurity, typically does not develop in familial exudative vitreoretinopathy. The peripheral retina remains avascular but progression to more severe changes such as tractional retinal detachment and neovascular glaucoma may occur.[16] Patients with familial exudative vitreoretinopathy are normally full term at birth with no history of respiratory difficulties and supplemental oxygen exposure. If familial exudative vitreoretinopathy is suspected in an older child or adult, examination of asymptomatic family members often reveals peripheral fundus lesions.

Incontinentia pigmenti (Bloch-Sulzberger syndrome) is an X-linked dominant condition that may simulate retinopathy of prematurity in female infants. The disease is lethal in males. In the first month infants may have dilated tortuous retinal vessels with peripheral retinal nonperfusion. Hemorrhage may be present at the junction of vascularized and avascularized retina. Other ocular anomalies include strabismus, cataract, myopia, nystagmus, blue sclera, and corneal opacities. Vesicular skin eruptions (Fig. 17-13) that later turn into depigmented areas are seen. CNS disorders include seizures, spastic paralysis, and mental retardation.

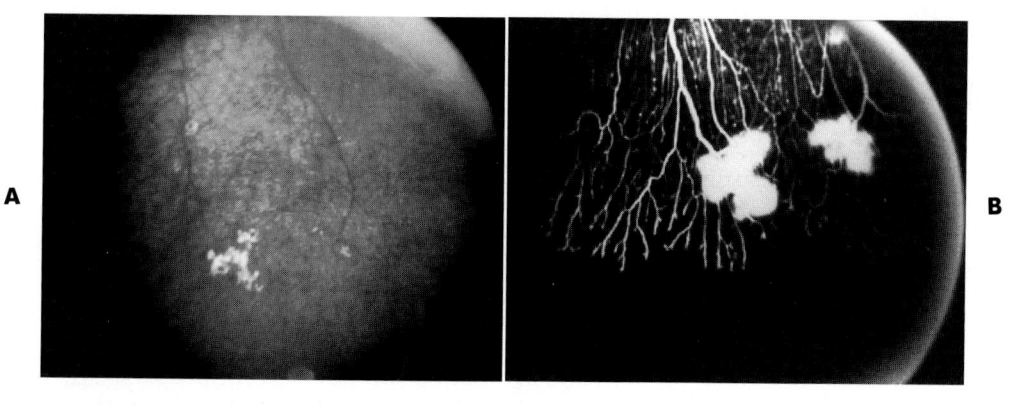

Figure 17-11 A, Clinical photograph and **B,** fluorescein angiogram showing peripheral retinal nonvascularization, straightening of the vessels, exudation, and neovascularization in a patient with familial exudative vitreoretinopathy.

Figure 17-12 Temporal retinal dragging in a patient with familial exudative vitreoretinopathy.

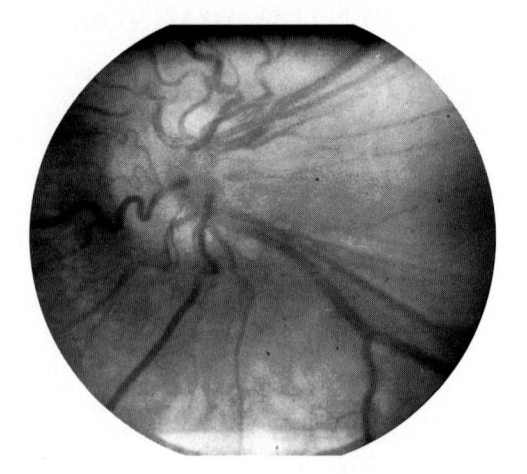

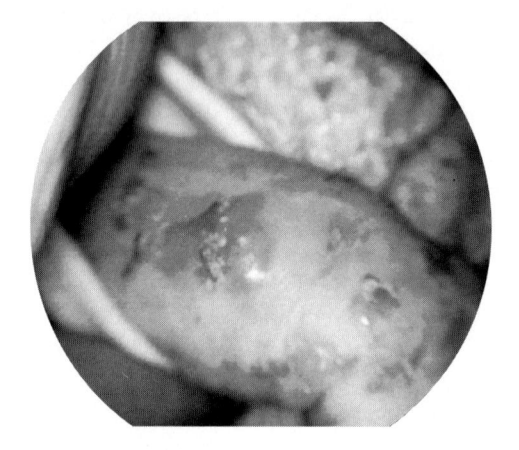

Figure 17-13 Vesicular skin eruptions in a patient with incontinentia pigmenti (Bloch-Sulzberger syndrome).

Patients with X-linked retinoschisis may develop a dragged retina in the first year of life. The dragging may be associated with vitreous hemorrhage. Examination of the fellow eye and electroretinography (showing a decreased b wave) are helpful in making the diagnosis. Family history is frequently positive.

The differential diagnosis of Stage V retinopathy of prematurity is that of a white pupillary reflex (leukokoria). This includes congenital cataract, persistent hyperplastic primary vitreous, retinoblastoma, ocular toxocariasis, intermediate uveitis, Coats' disease, advanced X-linked retinoschisis, and vitreous hemorrhage.

DIAGNOSTIC APPROACH

Careful screening of infants at risk for retinopathy of prematurity is essential. Examinations usually take place in the intensive care nursery (ICN) with monitoring of the infant by the ICN staff. To avoid the risk of vomiting and aspiration, examination should take place no sooner than 1 hour after feeding. We use homatropine hydrobromide 2% and phenylephrine hydrochloride 2.5%, 3, 2, and 1 hours before examination. This allows for an adequate interval of dilation and will frequently overcome iris vascular engorgement in cases of severe Stage 3+ retinopathy of prematurity. Topical anesthesia with proparacaine hydrochloride 0.5% or tetracaine hydrochloride 0.5% is administered, and a lid speculum is inserted. Anterior segment examination followed by indirect ophthalmoscopy with a 20- or 28-diopter lens is then performed.

The degree of dilation should be noted on anterior segment examination. Poor dilation may reflect iris vascular engorgement implying very active ROP. This is often mistaken for iris neovascularization. On indirect ophthalmoscopy the zone should be graded and the stage noted for each clock hour.

Infants who should be examined are those weighing less than 1251 g (2.75 pounds) at birth and those requiring oxygen in excess of room air at some time during the first 7 days of life. The first examination should take place at 4 to 6 weeks of chronologic age. Infants at particularly high risk are those who are less than 1000 g at birth and those born at less than 28 weeks of gestation. Depending on the stage, follow-up examinations should then be carried out every 1 to 2 weeks until one of the following occurs:

1. Complete retinal neovascularization
2. Two successive 2-week examinations show Stage 2 ROP in Zone III (infants should then be followed every 4 to 6 weeks until fully vascularized; however, a stage 3 retina may require reexamination in less than a week)
3. Prethreshold ROP (follow-up should then be done every week until threshold ROP develops or regression occurs)
4. Regressing ROP (when two successive 2-week examinations have shown regression, examinations should be done every 4 to 6 weeks)

If threshold stage 3+ ROP is detected, treatment should be delivered within 72 hours.

If vitreous hemorrhage or severe stage 5 ROP with an anterior closed funnel configuration is present, ultrasonography should be performed. Ultrasonography can help determine whether a retinal detachment exists behind vitreous hemorrhage. In advanced Stage 5 ROP the configuration of the entire funnel-shaped retinal detachment can be evaluated. The anterior and posterior parts of the funnel can be graded as open or closed. This is helpful for providing prognosis and in planning surgery.

MANAGEMENT

Cryotherapy

Cryotherapy is currently accepted as the standard treatment for advanced "active" retinopathy of prematurity. Several pilot studies paved the way for the multicenter trial of cryotherapy for retinopathy of prematurity (CryoROP).[17-19] This study has proven the effectiveness of cryotherapy for reducing the likelihood of an "unfavorable outcome" when children with "threshold" disease are treated. An unfavorable outcome was defined for the purposes of the CryoROP study as the presence of (1) a retinal fold involving the macula, (2) a retinal detachment involving Zone I of the posterior pole, or (3) retrolental tissue or "mass." Threshold disease was defined as five contiguous or eight accumulated clock hours of Stage 3 ROP with "plus" disease (according to the ICROP)[14] (Fig. 17-14). At threshold the risk of blindness without treatment approaches 50% and is the level of disease at which treatment should be applied. When threshold disease is present, treatment should be performed within 72 hours of detection.

There are contraindications to treatment. If the fundus view is obscured by anterior segment changes or vitreous hemorrhage, cryotherapy should not be applied. Ultrasonography should be performed when there is no fundus view.

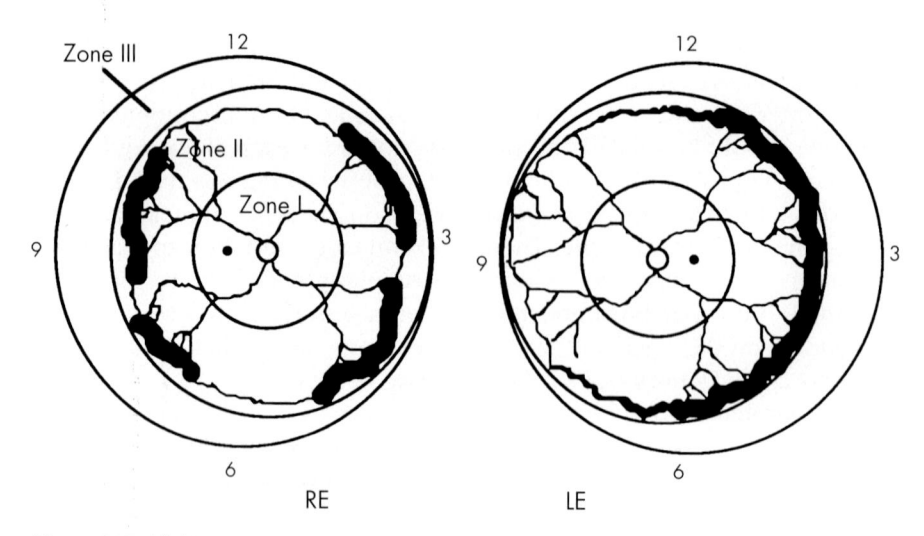

Figure 17-14 Two representative eyes that have reached, threshold disease. Right eye *(RE)*, At least eight cumulative clock hours of Stage 3. Left eye *(LE)*, At least five contiguous clock hours of Stage 3. The thin line of retinopathy of prematurity represents Stage 1 or 2, the broader sketched line Stage 3.

If obscuring vitreous hemorrhage is present during the active stage of ROP, vitrectomy should be considered to clear the view for treatment. If anterior segment changes, such as corneal opacity or cataract, are present in both eyes or in a fellow eye when the other eye is blind, and if retinal detachment is seen on ultrasound, combined anterior segment and vitreous surgery should be considered.

The infant's systemic status may sometimes preclude treatment. Cryotherapy can be stressful. There was a 9% incidence of bradycardia during treatment in the CryoROP study.[18] Brown et al.[20] reported three incidences of respiratory arrest and one of cardiopulmonary arrest in 80 consecutive infants treated with cryotherapy for ROP. If the neonatologist believes that treatment may be too stressful for the infant, then it should be deferred.

Cryotherapy can be applied using a topical anesthetic, local infiltration, or general anesthesia. If a topical or local infiltration is used, intravenous analgesic and sedative medication can be given. With topical anesthesia the ballooning of the conjunctiva associated with subconjunctival infiltration does not occur. The swelling of the conjunctiva from infection of a local anesthetic added to the edema that occurs during cryotherapy sometimes obscures the cornea, necessitating termination of the procedure. For topical anesthesia proparacaine hydrochloride 0.5% or tetracaine hydrochloride 0.5% can be applied to the cornea every 20 minutes during treatment. Local infiltration anesthesia can be given by injecting 0.5 ml of lidocaine hydrochloride 1% into the subconjunctival space. To avoid possible cardiopulmonary complications, no more than 0.5 ml should be injected.[20] General anesthesia can be used and was in 28% of cases in the CryoROP study.[18] For the administration of general anesthesia the infant usually must be removed from the nursery and transported to the operating room. Separation from the staff familiar with the infant and all the risks present in general anesthesia are factors that need to be considered.

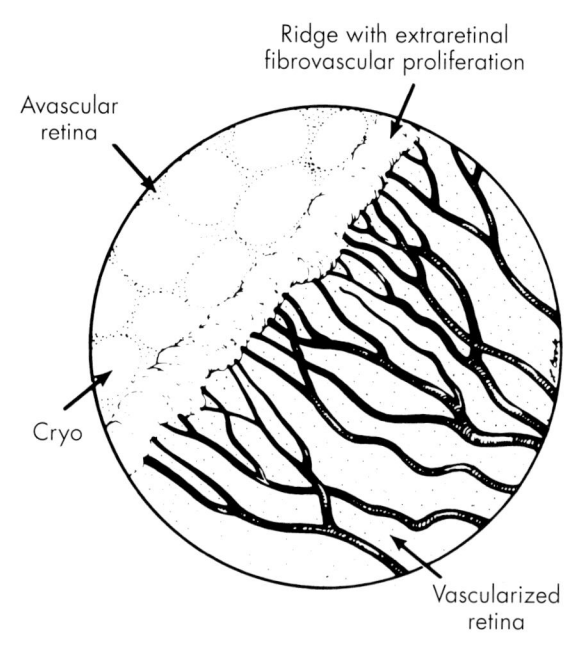

Figure 17-15 Cryotherapy anterior to the ridge in a zone of avascular retina.

Before cryotherapy the pupils are dilated. Homatropine hydrobromide 2% and phenylephrine hydrochloride 2.5% drops instilled 3, 2, and 1 hours preoperatively provide adequate dilation.

After a lid speculum is inserted, cryotherapy may proceed under indirect ophthalmoscopic viewing. A standard retinal or neonatal cryoprobe is used. It is best to start treatment nasally since pressure from the cryoprobe will soften the globe and thus facilitate treatment temporally, where the avascular zone is usually more posterior. Contiguous spots of cryotherapy should be applied throughout the avascular retina anterior to the ridge and extraretinal fibrovascular proliferation. It usually takes just a few seconds for the avascular retina to whiten from the cryotherapy. This whitening is the endpoint for treatment (Fig. 17-15). Typically 30 to 50 applications of cryotherapy are necessary (depending on the extent of avascular retina) to complete treatment. Care should be taken to avoid prolonged scleral depression, which increases the IOP and risk for central retinal artery occlusion.

Most often treatment can be accomplished without making conjunctival incisions. When threshold disease is present in Zone I or posterior Zone II, it may not be possible to treat the entire avascular zone without a conjunctival incision. A small incision 4 mm posterior to the limbus within the center of the quadrant is adequate to allow the cryoprobe tip to fit. One to four incisions may be made depending on the extent of disease. These incisions need not be sutured if they are less than 3 to 4 mm in length.

Occasionally during treatment corneal clouding will obscure the view. Removing the lid speculum and waiting several minutes often result in clearing. If waiting fails, the epithelium may be removed with a cotton-tipped swab soaked in cocaine hydrochloride 4% solution. This provides excellent topical anesthesia as well.

Vitreous hemorrhage may also occur during treatment, necessitating termination of the procedure. This is usually due to bleeding from a florid area of extraretinal fibrovascular proliferation caused by pressure on the globe from the cryoprobe. Completion of treatment should be done when the vitreous hemorrhage clears.

The desired outcome after cryotherapy is regression of both "plus" disease and extraretinal fibrovascular proliferation (Fig. 17-16). In the 1-year outcome assessment paper of the CryoROP study[19] 47% of control eyes (no treatment)

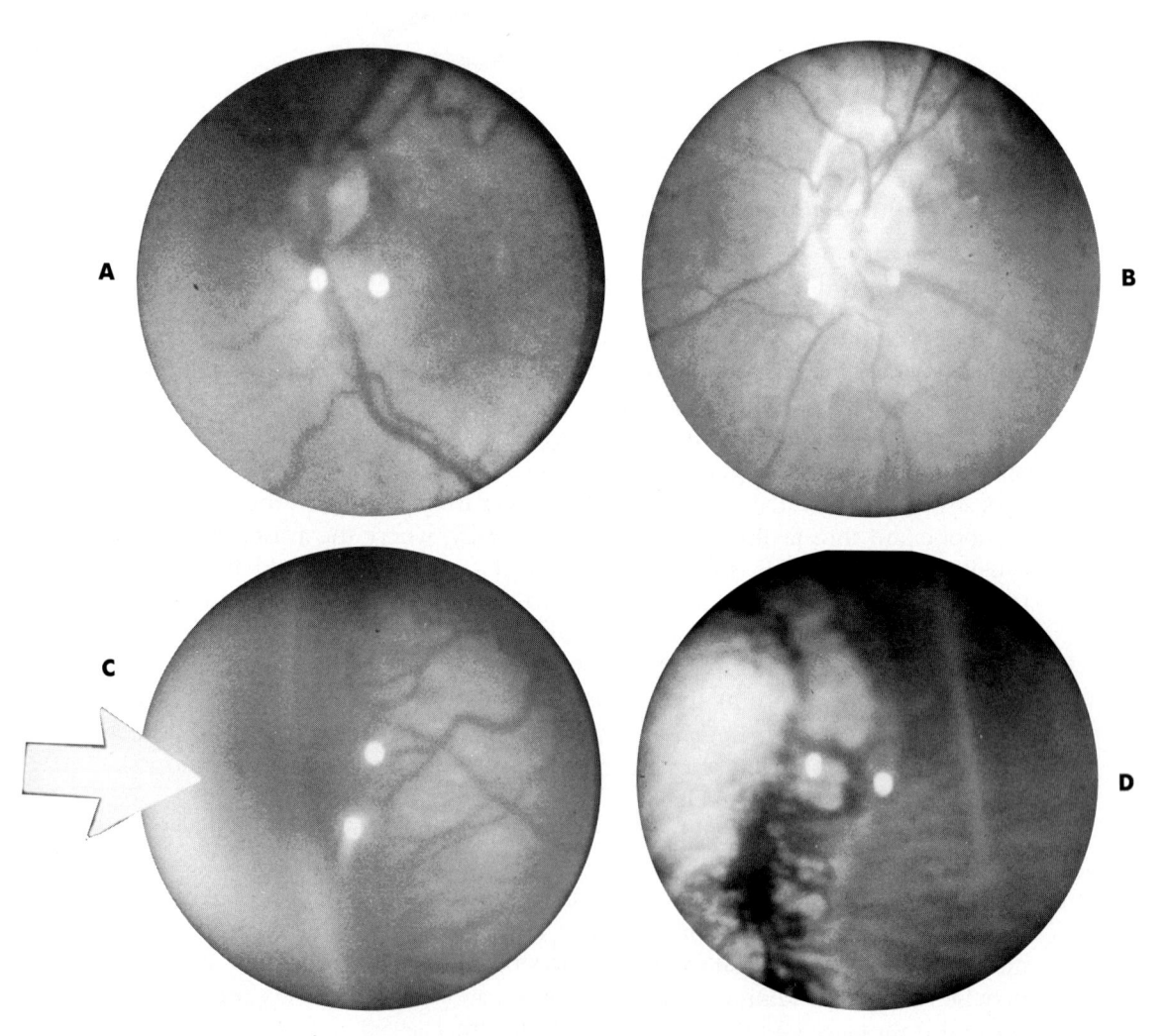

Figure 17-16 A, Preoperative and **B,** postoperative appearance of the posterior pole in an infant treated for threshold retinopathy of prematurity with cryotherapy. Note the regression of "plus" disease after treatment. The *arrow* in **C** indicates an avascular zone in this preoperative eye. **D** is the postoperative appearance of the retinal periphery in the same eye (of an infant). Note the regression of extraretinal fibrovascular proliferation and the cryotherapy scarring.

and 26% of treated eyes had an unfavorable structural outcome. Using grating acuity testing, a reduction in unfavorable functional outcome of 38% was seen.

A reduction in both "plus" disease and extraretinal fibrovascular proliferation should be seen by 1 week after treatment.

Both systemic and ocular complications may occur during cryotherapy for retinopathy of prematurity. Systemic complications may be life threatening. In the CryoROP study[18] 9% of infants suffered bradycardia, arrhythmia, or significant apnea during administration of anesthesia and cryotherapy. An additional 1% experienced acquired or increased cyanosis. One infant had a seizure during treatment. These severe systemic complications underscore the need to have infants carefully monitored by a neonatologist or anesthesiologist during treatment.

All patients treated with cryotherapy have periorbital edema, conjunctival injection, and chemosis. The periorbital edema usually subsides in a few days whereas the conjunctival injection and chemosis take 1 to 2 weeks to regress. The most frequent and disconcerting ocular complication in the CryoROP study was intraocular hemorrhage. Retinal, preretinal, and vitreous hemorrhage occurred in 22% of treated eyes.[18] Sometimes intraocular hemorrhage may prevent completion of treatment. In such cases treatment is aborted and the eye is carefully followed for clearing of the hemorrhage so treatment can be completed. Conjunctival or subconjunctival hematoma occurred in 12% of treated eyes, and unintended conjunctival laceration in 5% of eyes. These complications are self-limited and do not lead to long-term problems.

Central retinal artery occlusion may occur from excessive pressure on the globe during cryotherapy. In the CryoROP study[18] there was one instance of transient closure of the central retinal artery.

Late-onset retinal detachment following cryotherapy has been reported.[21] Breaks are found at the border of cryotherapy-treated and untreated retina. It is postulated that the retinal breaks occur because of inability of the treated retina to stretch as the eye grows. These detachments are treated by standard scleral buckling techniques.

Since treatment is delivered with a probe that needs to be pressed onto the globe, there is potential for severe injury such as perforation of the globe, laceration or avulsion of an eye muscle, and injury to the orbital wall. Care should be taken to limit pressure on the globe and adnexal structures.

Laser Photocoagulation

Photocoagulation was actually the first modality of treatment of the anterior avascular zone for acute retinopathy of prematurity. In 1967 Nagata et al.[22] used xenon arc photocoagulation to induce regression of acute ROP. This method was difficult to deliver, however, and was supplanted by cryotherapy, which was first reported to induce regression by Yamashita[23] in 1973.

In the late 1980s indirect ophthalmoscopic delivery systems for laser photocoagulation became available. Shortly thereafter, McNamara et al.[24] and Iverson et al.[25] compared laser photocoagulation to cryotherapy in prospective randomized trials. Landers et al.[26] also reported on the use of argon laser for threshold ROP. These investigators used the same threshold criteria as the CryoROP study for determining which infants would be treated.

Clear media are even more essential for treating threshold retinopathy of prematurity with laser photocoagulation than they are for cryotherapy. Anterior segment changes, such as cataract and corneal clouding, and vitreous hemorrhage may preclude laser treatment and yet the media may be clear enough for cryotherapy to be performed.

Systemic contraindications seem to be fewer with laser photocoagulation than with cryotherapy. Laser treatment is less stressful systemically; I have been refused permission by the neonatologist to perform cryotherapy because of cardiopulmonary complications and have been asked to perform laser photocoagulation instead.

Laser photocoagulation delivered by the indirect ophthalmoscope can be performed under topical or general anesthesia. There is no need for local infiltration anesthesia since only gentle manipulation of the globe with a scleral depressor is necessary. McNamara et al.[24] used topical anesthesia whereas Iverson et al.[25] and Landers et al.[26] used general. Transient bradycardia occurred in three patients (19%) treated with laser and three (25%) treated with cryotherapy in the McNamara study. Bradycardia resolved when the scleral depressor or cryoprobe was removed for several seconds. No other systemic complications occurred. McNamara et al.[24] believe that the potential complications of general anesthesia outweigh the small risk of potential complications with topical anesthesia for laser photocoagulation.

Before laser photocoagulation the pupils are dilated. Homatropine hydrobromide 2% and phenylephrine hydrochloride 2.5% drops instilled 3, 2, and 1 hours preoperatively provide adequate dilation. If topical anesthesia is to be used, treatment can be performed in the operating room or, if a portable diode laser is used, in the nursery. Proparacaine hydrochloride 0.5% is applied to the globe. A lid speculum is placed. Gentle manipulation with a scleral depressor to position the globe for viewing of the peripheral retina is performed. While viewing the peripheral retina through the indirect ophthalmoscope, one can see the laser aiming beam. When the aiming beam is in focus on the peripheral avascular retina, laser discharge is accomplished by pressing a foot pedal. To avoid laser burns to unwanted areas (e.g., posterior vascularized retina, cornea, iris, and lens), care should be taken to assure that the aiming beam is focused before discharge. Spots should be placed one to one half burn width apart with a dull white laser photocoagulation mark as the end point. With the argon laser the initial power setting should be 200 mW at 0.1-second duration. The power can then be gradually increased to achieve the appropriate laser mark in the fundus. With the diode laser the initial power setting should be slightly lower (150 mW) with a longer duration (0.2 second) to avoid choroidal hemorrhage and Bruch's membrane rupture. The entire anterior avascular retina should be treated. If infant movement under topical anesthesia precludes adequate focusing of the laser, the neonatologist or anesthesiologist may administer intravenous sedation such as fentanyl citrate. Infants should be monitored by a neonatologist and/or anesthesiologist during treatment.

All patients in McNamara's, Iverson's, and Landers' series[24-26] were treated with argon laser. At the time of those studies there were no portable laser units available. More recently portable diode (Fig. 17-17) and argon lasers have been manufactured. The portable laser has the advantage that it can be brought directly into the nursery. This avoids costly and sometimes hazardous transfer of

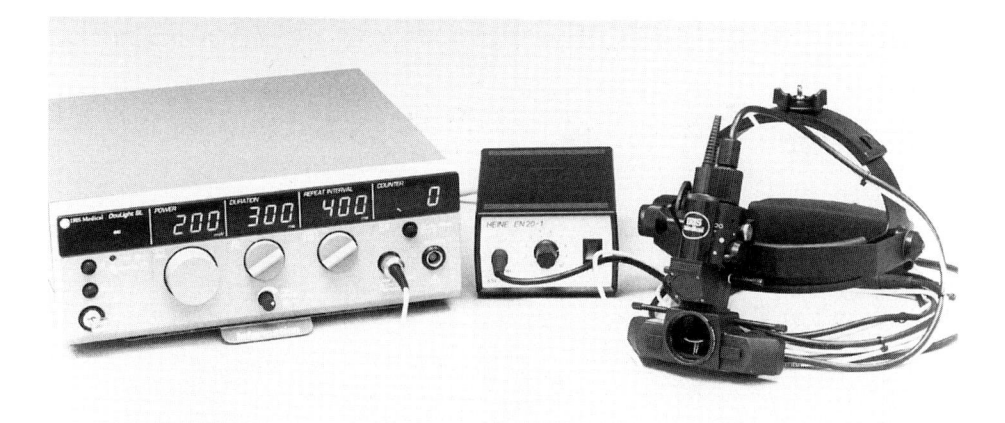

Figure 17-17 IRIS Medical Inc Oculight SLx portable diode laser with an indirect ophthalmoscope delivery unit.

the infant to a facility where a free-standing laser is available. For safety reasons treatment should be performed in an isolated area of the nursery. McNamara et al.[27] have reported on the use of a portable diode laser as compared to cryotherapy for treating threshold ROP. As with argon laser, the portable diode laser seems to be equally effective as cryotherapy, easier to administer, and responsible for fewer side effects than cryotherapy.

Laser photocoagulation for threshold retinopathy of prematurity seems to be as effective as cryotherapy (Tables 17-2 and 17-3 and Fig. 17-18). To date there is still no statistically significant study to prove efficacy, but pilot studies[24-27] have shown favorable trends.

As with cryotherapy, both systemic and ocular side effects may occur with laser photocoagulation for retinopathy of prematurity. It was mentioned above that bradycardia during treatment, presumably from scleral depression, can occur. Releasing the depressor usually leads to resolution of the bradycardia.

Mild conjunctival injection from scleral depression may be present for a day or so after laser photocoagulation. This is much less than the anterior segment changes that typically occur after cryotherapy. Additionally, conjunctival incisions are never needed for laser photocoagulation since posterior treatment is easily delivered. Conjunctival incisions are frequently necessary for treating Zone I disease with cryotherapy.

Anterior segment burns to the cornea, iris, or lens may occur with laser. Landers et al.[26] noted small burns to the pupil margin in 5 of 15 laser-treated eyes. This complication may be diminished by limiting infant movement with sedation if necessary, although all of the Landers babies were treated under general anesthesia. Assuring a clearly focused aiming beam on the retina is essential. Diode laser has the theoretical advantage of lessening the likelihood of lens burns in premature infants with persistent tunica vasculosa lentis. The diode laser, emitting at 810 nm, is not absorbed by the hemoglobin in those vessels whereas argon green, emitting at 514 nanometers, is absorbed by hemoglobin.

Intraocular hemorrhage may occur with laser photocoagulation. There were three instances of mild vitreous hemorrhage in each of the laser-treated and cryotherapy-treated groups in McNamara's study.[24] These resolved within 1

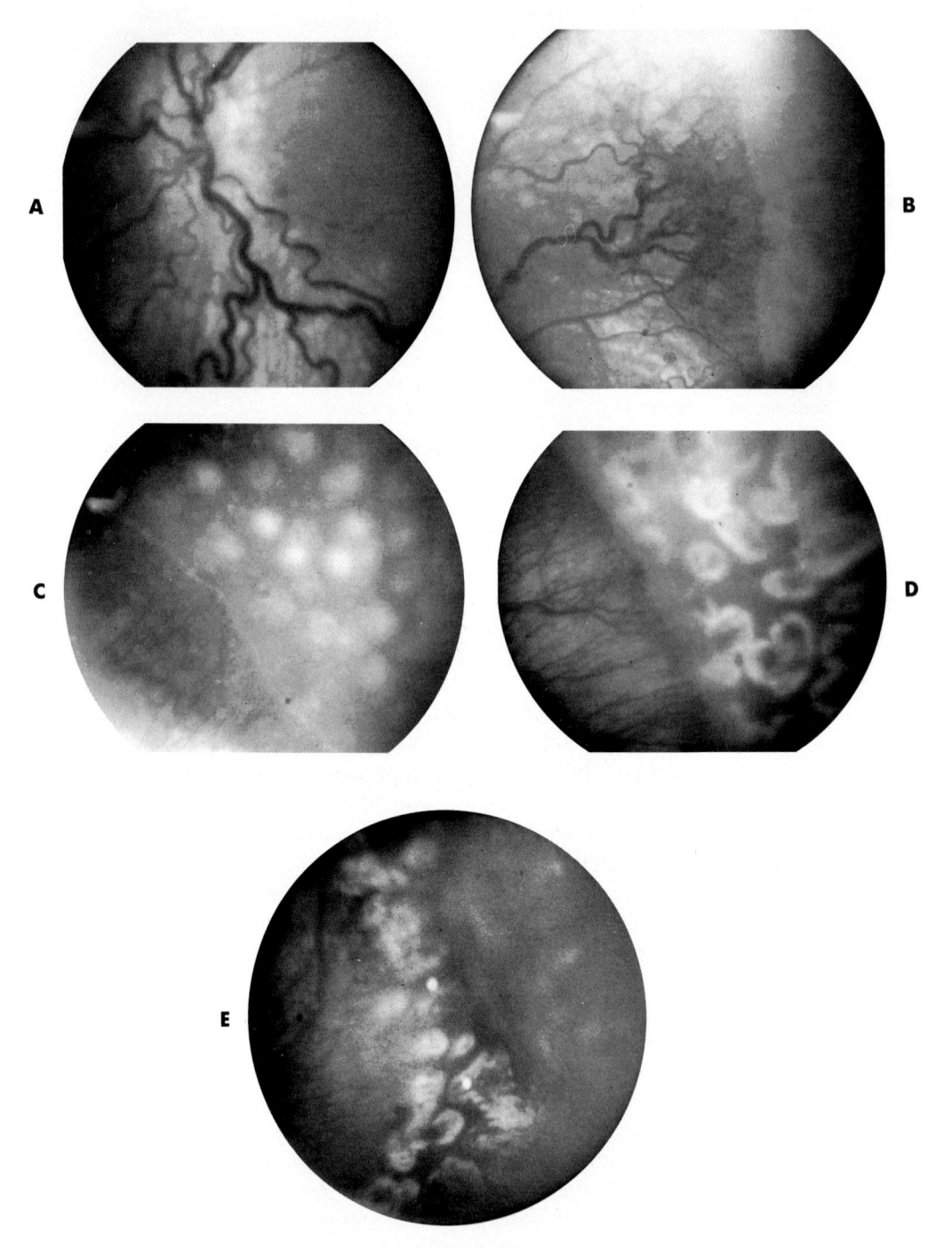

Figure 17-18 A, Severe "plus" disease in the posterior pole of an infant with Zone I threshold retinopathy of prematurity. **B,** Peripheral neovascularization in Zone I. **C,** Peripheral retina immediately after argon laser photocoagulation. **D,** Peripheral retina 1 week after argon laser photocoagulation. **E,** Peripheral retina 1 month after argon laser photocoagulation. Note the complete regression of neovascularization.

Table 17-2 Pooled Data from Three Studies Using Indirect Ophthalmoscopic Delivery of Argon Laser Photocoagulation for Treating Threshold Retinopathy of Prematurity

	Argon laser photocoagulation *Favorable (%)*	*Argon laser photocoagulation* *Unfavorable (%)*	*Cryotherapy* *Favorable (%)*	*Cryotherapy* *Unfavorable (%)*
McNamara et al.[24]	15 (94)	1 (7)	9 (75)	3 (25)
Iverson et al.[25]	6 (100)	0 (0)	5 (83)	1 (17)
Landers et al.[26]	11 (73)	4 (27)	—	—
Total	32 (86)	5 (14)	14 (78)	4 (22)

Table 17-3 Results of Treatment for 28 Infants Treated with Diode Laser Photocoagulation (24 fellow eyes treated with cryotherapy)

Outcome	*Diode laser photocoagulation (%)*	*Cryotherapy (%)*
Favorable	25	20
Unfavorable	3	4
Total	28	24

From McNamara JA, et al: *Arch Ophthalmol* 110:1714-1716, 1992.

week. Choroidal hemorrhages with associated ruptures in Bruch's membrane are a known complication of laser treatment. Appropriate burn intensity will decrease their likelihood.

Late-onset retinal detachment has been reported after cryotherapy[21] and is a potential complication after laser. The risk is probably less since laser is placed in a scatter pattern with intervening areas of untreated retina. This may allow the retina to grow and stretch better, thus decreasing the likelihood of breaks at the border of treated and untreated retina.

Scleral Buckle

Cryotherapy and laser photocoagulation do not cure all cases of threshold retinopathy of prematurity. Progression to Stage 4 or 5 may occur, and some infants may present with these more advanced stages.

The more advanced stages represent retinal detachment from peripheral only to total.[15] Retinal detachments in retinopathy of prematurity are most often serous and tractional (Fig. 17-19). Rhegmatogenous retinal detachments are rare but may present years later as a delayed complication of the disease or at the border between cryotherapy treated and untreated retina.[21] Exuberant extraretinal fibrovascular proliferation may lead to serous fluid accumulation. With progressive fibrous proliferation, tractional detachment of the retina can occur. This proliferation is often circumferential and the retina may detach as if a purse string were being tightened.

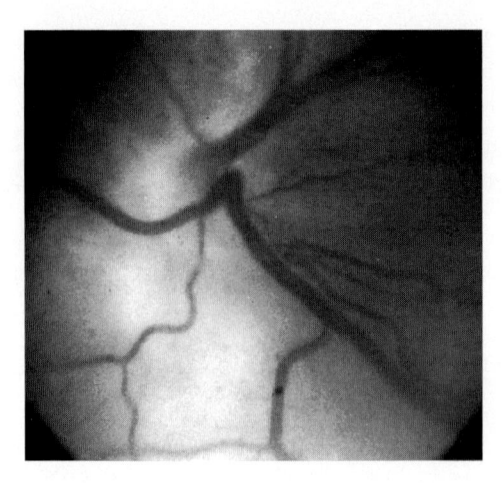

Figure 17-19 Stage 5 retinopathy of prematurity, total retinal detachment. The detachment is shallow with an open funnel configuration. Note the loss of choroidal vascular pattern because of the subretinal fluid.

The indications for scleral buckling surgery are Stage 4B or open funnel Stage 5 retinal detachment. When the fovea detaches, progressive damage to photoreceptors may occur, thus precluding visual development.

Stage 4A retinopathy of prematurity may regress spontaneously or as a result of cryotherapy or laser photocoagulation. These detachments should be followed closely but need not be repaired. When involvement of the fovea is imminent (Stage 4B), scleral buckling should be considered.

A closed or partially closed funnel Stage 5 retinal detachment is not amenable to scleral buckling since apposition of the choroid and retinal pigment epithelium to the retina cannot occur because fibrous tissue elevates the retina. These more severe forms of retinal detachment may be treated with vitreous surgery.

Vitreous hemorrhage is a relative contraindication to scleral buckling surgery. If the hemorrhage is mild and an adequate view is still present allowing staging and appreciation of the amount of fibrous proliferation, then scleral buckling may be performed. If the hemorrhage is too dense or there is any concern that a funnel-shaped retinal detachment is present, vitrectomy should be considered.

As always, the infant's systemic condition should be considered. Scleral buckling is performed under general anesthesia, and any contraindications to this form of obtundation will necessitate delaying the surgery.

Scleral buckling for retinopathy of prematurity is performed under general anesthesia in the operating room. An anesthesiologist skilled in handling pediatric cases, and possibly a neonatologist familiar with the patient, should be in attendance.

Before surgery, the pupils are dilated. Homatropine hydrobromide 2% and phenylephrine hydrochloride 2.5% drops instilled 3, 2, and 1 hours preoperatively provide adequate dilation. After a pediatric lid speculum is inserted, a 360-degree conjunctival peritomy is performed. The rectus muscles are bridled with 4-0 silk sutures. The sclera should be inspected for thin areas. The standard instruments for adult scleral buckling procedures are too large, so a Halstead malleable retractor can be used to expose the sclera in each quadrant.

If cryotherapy was not performed to the avascular peripheral retina before the procedure or if it was performed but the results were inadequate, it should be repeated as described above.

Scleral buckling can be accomplished with either an implant or an exoplant. If an implant is performed, the surgeon should be highly skilled in preparing a scleral bed since the sclera in these infants is extremely thin and perforation during preparation of the scleral flaps may occur.

The globe should be encircled with a band. A 2 mm width no. 40 band or a 2.5 mm no. 240 band can be used. The latter provides a broader area of indentation but may be too large for smaller eyes. If a localized area of greater height is desired (e.g., over a broader area of extraretinal fibrovascular proliferation with greater elevation), then a segment of no. 219 strip (4.5 mm width) can be placed (Fig. 17-20). The silicone element(s) are secured with a single 5-0 nylon mattress suture in each quadrant. The ends of the band are secured to each other with a Watzke sleeve or 5-0 nylon suture.

Various investigators[28-31] differ regarding drainage of subretinal fluid. At the Wills Eye Hospital we usually attempt to drain subretinal fluid. If the retina is very shallowly detached and the buckle almost approximates the choroid and retinal pigment epithelium to the retina when it is drawn up, we will not attempt drainage.

When the buckle is cinched, the intraocular pressure should be assessed. If it is too high, anterior chamber paracentesis can be performed. Alternatively, or in addition to paracentesis, acetazolamide (5 mg/kg) can be given intravenously to lower the pressure. The central retinal artery should be checked by indirect ophthalmoscopy for lack of pulsation to assure that the pressure is not left too high.

At the end of the procedure the bridle sutures are removed, the conjunctiva is closed with absorbable sutures, and antibiotic and steroid medications are applied.

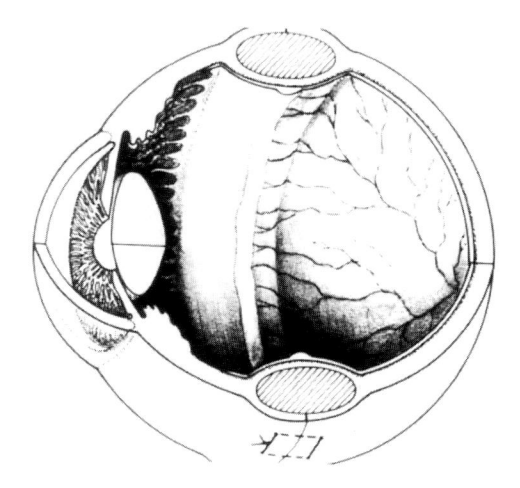

Figure 17-20 Scleral buckle for retinopathy of prematurity. Note that the buckle is placed over the extraretinal fibrovascular proliferation, where traction is the greatest.

Table 17-4 Data From Four Studies Using Scleral Buckling Surgery to Treat Stages 4B and 5 Retinopathy of Prematurity

Investigator	Average age at surgery (months)	No. reattached per total operated (%)	Vision in eyes with reattached retinas
McPherson et al.[28]	3	24/32 (75)	—
Topilow et al.[29]	4	5/7 (71)	—
Greven and Tasman[30]	8	13/22 (54)	≥20/400: 4 of 10 with ≥ 18 months of follow-up
Noorily et al.[31]	4	10/15 (67)	Fix and follow: 2 LP:8

LP, Light perception.

Since these eyes are often very small when operated on, the buckle is frequently transected or removed in the operating room under general anesthesia 6 to 12 months after the original operation. This will facilitate growth and prevent erosion of the scleral buckle into the eye.

Anatomic success after scleral buckling for retinal detachment in ROP is defined as macular reattachment (full attachment of retina between the temporal vascular arcades).

The success rate varies; in the larger studies in the literature[28-31] it is between 54% and 75% (Table 17-4). Greater reattachment rates have been achieved in all studies when additional vitreous or scleral buckling surgery was performed.

Although the anatomic success rates in these studies are encouraging, the visual results are disappointing. One must bear in mind, however, that without reattachment no vision is possible. The reasons for poor visual results in these infants remain speculative. Some infants (as one in Greven and Tasman's[30] series) may have had cerebral dysfunction (e.g., intraventricular hemorrhage) as a result of the complications of prematurity. The maculas in these infants were immature to begin with and detachment may have had a more devastating effect on photoreceptors and their development than in an adult. Amblyopia likely played a role as well.

The complications of scleral buckling surgery for ROP in infants are similar to those that can occur in adults, with some special considerations for the infant eye. The premature infant's eye is significantly smaller than the adult eye. Full adult size of the globe is not attained until 3 years of age. A 34-week-gestation infant's eye is 15 mm in diameter (Fig. 17-21). The sclera is thin, and this must be constantly borne in mind when depressing, cutting a bed, and passing sutures.

Cryotherapy done during a scleral buckling procedure carries the same risks of complications as mentioned above. Corneal clouding and central retinal artery occlusion may occur with prolonged depression during cryotherapy; this should be avoided.

Perforation of the thin infant globe can occur while preparing a scleral bed and during passage of sutures for securing the buckling element. Dissection of scleral beds is technically difficult and should be attempted only by highly experienced surgeons. Similarly, great care should be taken when passing sutures

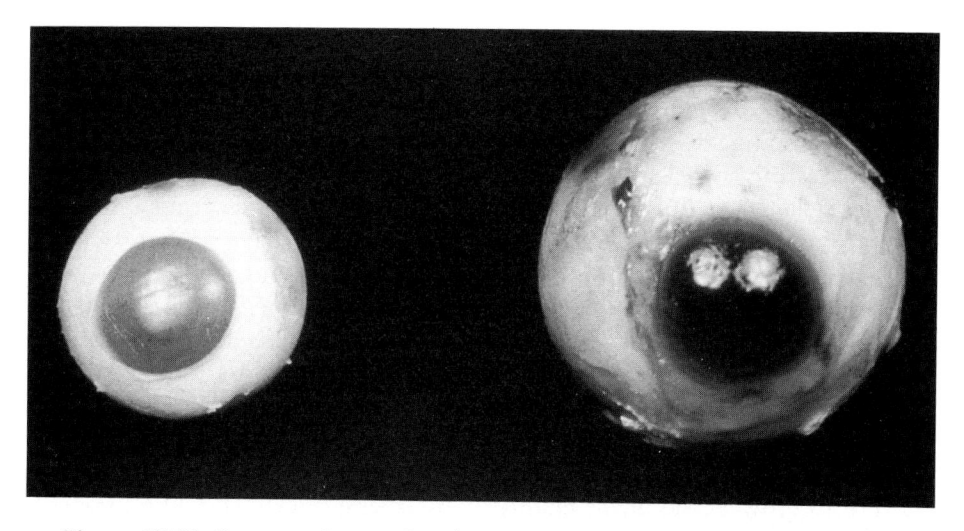

Figure 17-21 Gross specimens of a 34-week-gestation infant eye and an adult eye. Courtesy James Bolling, M.D., Jacksonville Fla.

through the sclera. If perforation occurs during passage of a suture, the suture should be removed and replaced so the buckling element will cover the perforation. Indirect ophthalmoscopy should be done immediately to determine whether there has been retinal damage. It is possible that the retina may have been detached in the area of perforation and fortuitous drainage may occur. If retinal perforation has occurred, cryotherapy should be applied.

A decision to drain subretinal fluid must be made carefully since the risks are significant. If there is only very shallow fluid and if the buckle provides adequate height, drainage may not be necessary. The risks of drainage are perforation, incarceration, hemorrhage, and infection. Perforation can be minimized by choosing a drainage site over bullous retina. If perforation occurs, it should be managed by buckling and cryotherapy as mentioned above. Drainage under the buckle obviates the need to add an additional buckling element over a perforation at a drainage site. Incarceration is less likely with tractional retinal detachment than with the rhegmatogenous variety. This is due to the retina's being pulled inward by tractional forces. Nonetheless, if it does occur, it should be treated with cryotherapy and buckled. Hemorrhage may occur from the choroid during drainage. This can be minimized by diathermizing the choroid prior to drainage. When the globe is entered, the possibility of intraocular infection increases. Endophthalmitis after scleral buckling is extremely rare. It should be managed with standard techniques including injection of intravitreal antibiotics.

Careful attention to the intraocular pressure at the end of the procedure is important. If the pressure is left too high, central retinal artery occlusion may occur. As mentioned above, the pressure should be normalized and the central retinal artery should be checked for the desired absence of pulsations.

In the small infant eye a buckle may induce angle closure glaucoma during the postoperative period. The cornea should be assessed for clarity and the intraocular pressure can be checked with a Tono-Pen. If angle closure glaucoma develops, the scleral buckle must be loosened.

A tight buckle may also induce anterior segment necrosis. This is manifested by corneal edema without high intraocular pressure, chemosis and a cellular reaction in the anterior chamber. The buckle should be loosened or removed.

Scleral buckle infection, manifested by conjunctivitis overlying the buckle and a clear cornea in mild cases or intraocular inflammation in more severe cases, is managed by removal of the buckle and administering antibiotics.

Extrusion of the scleral buckle because sutures have given way is managed by resecuring the buckle or by removal if it is no longer necessary.

Although not a complication per se, nonattachment of the retina is an undesired result. This may be due to the disease process itself (persistent or progressive tractional detachment) but also may be due to a loose buckle. If the height of the buckle seems inadequate, revision of the scleral buckling procedure should be done.

As mentioned above, the scleral buckle may cause erosion or failure of the eye to grow as the infant matures. The scleral buckle should be transected or removed at 6 to 12 months.

Vitrectomy

With progressive severity of ROP, the surgical techniques for attempted repair become more complicated and the visual results worse. Vitreous surgery techniques are used to treat severe Stage 4B and Stage 5 retinal detachments. Since the surgery is complicated and the visual results are poor, patients should be selected carefully. Infants with good regression of ROP and a good potential for vision in one eye, but with severe Stage 4B or 5 in the fellow eye, should probably not undergo surgery. The indications for vitrectomy are bilateral advanced disease with at least severe Stage 3 ROP in the fellow eye. Stage 4B eyes with severe tractional detachment and Stage 5 eyes with closed or partially closed funnel-shaped retinal detachment may be helped with open-sky or closed vitrectomy.

Eyes with obvious buphthalmos and glaucoma will have a poor visual result and should not be operated on. Eyes with opaque corneas have a poor prognosis; there may have been prior glaucoma that caused the corneal opacification. High intraocular pressure at the time of immediate preoperative evaluation is a relative contraindication to surgery. Permanent optic nerve and retinal damage may have occurred and will result in a poor visual prognosis even if the retina is reattached. NLP vision (no response to a bright light) is a relative contraindication to surgery. Bound-down iris prevents the pupil from reacting to light, and a totally detached retina with epiretinal membrane formation may prevent the child from wincing to a bright light. Some infants may, however, regain useful vision even if there is apparent NLP vision preoperatively.[32]

As with other forms of surgery, the infant's systemic condition should be considered. Vitreous surgery is performed under general anesthesia, and any contraindications to this form of anesthesia will necessitate delaying the surgery.

Vitreous surgery for far advanced ROP has evolved and is continuing to do so. A few dedicated surgeons, notably Machemer, Schepens, Charles, Trese, Hirose, Tasman, and deJuan,[32-39] have contributed greatly to our understanding of the surgical pathoanatomy and the development of surgical techniques for far advanced ROP.

The timing of surgery is still in question. It seems, however, that it would be best for the active stage to be quiescent before vitreous surgery is undertaken. If there is persistent "plus" disease with engorgement of the iris vasculature and tortuosity and dilation of the retinal vessels, then the likelihood is very high that intraoperative hemorrhage may occur that cannot be controlled. With the high level of awareness of this disease and widespread knowledge of the CryoROP study results, most patients have already had ablative therapy prior to presenting with advanced retinal detachment. The detachment occurs because of failure of the ablation to arrest the progression of tractional retinal detachment. Nonetheless, ablative therapy usually induces regression of severe "plus" disease, making subsequent vitreous surgery safer. Patients still present with severe Stage 4B and Stage 5 retinal detachments without having undergone ablative therapy, however. If there is persistent and severe "plus" disease, Trese[40] recommends a two-step approach. Patients are initially treated by cryotherapy to the peripheral avascular retina, which usually does not detach since the configuration of these severe retinal detachments is such that a peripheral trough forms, with the more anterior avascular retina remaining attached. In approximately 3 weeks, "plus" disease has generally regressed to the point that vitreous surgery can proceed.

There are two approaches to vitreous surgery in infants with advanced ROP: open-sky vitrectomy and closed vitrectomy. Each has advantages and disadvantages. The main advantage to open-sky vitrectomy (vitreous surgery through a trephined opening in the cornea) is easy access and visualization of the anterior retina and epiretinal membranes. The disadvantages are lack of control of intraocular pressure and difficulty in posterior manipulation. Closed vitrectomy has the advantages of intraocular pressure maintenance, minimal tissue distortion, and good visualization in the posterior pole. The disadvantages are poor visualization in the retinal periphery and restricted manipulation of instruments. The main goal of vitreous surgery for severe Stages 4B and 5 ROP is mechanical release of vitreoretinal traction. This can be accomplished with either form of surgery.

Before a vitrectomy the patient should be examined under anesthesia—including biomicroscopy, corneal diameter measurement, tonometry, indirect ophthalmoscopy, fundus photography, A- and B-scan ultrasonography, and visualization with the operating microscope. Findings as mentioned above (e.g., severely elevated IOP and corneal opacity) may be present that would preclude surgery.

The technique of open-sky vitrectomy was pioneered by Schepens[34-35] and has been modified by Hirose[32] and Tasman.[38] This operation is most appropriate for Stage 5 retinal detachment with a narrow open funnel. A Flieringa ring is sewn to the sclera to provide support. A corneal trephine 2 to 3 mm less than the diameter of the cornea is used to remove a corneal button. Most often a 7 mm trephine is used. The corneal button is stored in McCarey-Kaufman media for later repositioning. Iris sphincterotomies are cut at 6 and 12 o'clock. The lens is then extracted with a cryoprobe. When the lens is removed, epiretinal fibrous proliferation can be clearly seen on the surface of the detached retina. Starting peripherally, near the ora serrata, Vannas scissors cut into the epiretinal tissue to establish a cleavage plane (Fig. 17-22). By sharp dissection, the tissue is freed up toward the center. It is then removed from the surface of the

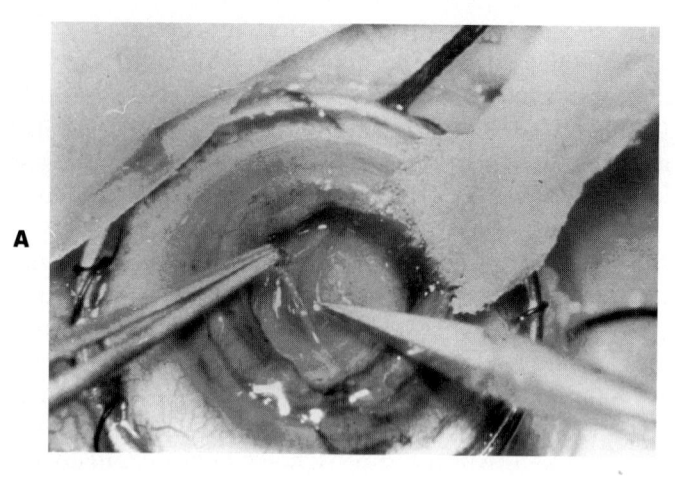

Figure 17-22 A, Dissection of retrolental epiretinal tissue using a two-handed technique. **B,** Corresponding diagram.

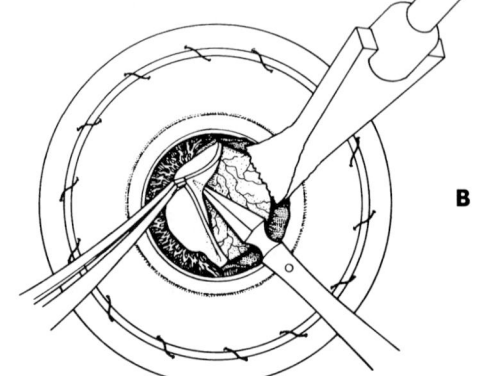

retina. Great care must be taken, especially in the periphery (where the retina is thinnest), to avoid making an inadvertent retinotomy. After the tissue is removed from the surface of the retina anteriorly, sodium hyaluronate can be gently injected into the funnel to open it up and facilitate posterior dissection. Special curved long-bladed scissors and forceps are used in the funnel to remove posterior proliferation. External drainage of subretinal fluid can be done, but this is not essential since the goal is to release traction. Subretinal fluid will resorb spontaneously over several weeks if adequate traction is released. When dissection is complete, the iridotomies are closed with 10-0 proline sutures. The corneal button is replaced and secured with interrupted sutures. (We usually remove the sutures 3 months after surgery.)

Machemer (Treister and Machemer[33]) first described closed vitrectomy for the retinal detachment associated with ROP. Charles,[36] Trese,[37,40] and deJuan[39,41] refined the indications and technique. As newer instrumentation is developed and our understanding of this disease increases, further evolution of vitrectomy techniques will occur.

The entry site for closed vitrectomy remains controversial. Entering at the limbus anterior to the iris helps avoid the possibility of making a retinal break in anteriorly detached and dragged retina. With the instruments so far anterior, however, the cornea may develop folds, limiting visualization. Entering through the pars plicata 1 to 2 mm posterior to the iris improves visualization but adds the risk of creating anterior retinal breaks. I prefer the posterior approach and direct the sclerotomy blade into the lens parallel with the iris. Two or three ports may be utilized. In the three-port system a blunt-tipped 2 mm infusion cannula is sewn into the anterior chamber at the limbus inferotemporally. The remaining two ports are created in the superior quadrants and are utilized for a fiberoptic light pipe and various vitrectomy instruments (suction/cutter, membrane peeler/cutter, scissors, diathermy). In a two-port system a 20-gauge end-irrigating light pipe is used through one of the superior sclerostomy sites to provide both irrigation and illumination. When one is in the anterior chamber with the vitreous cutter, the soft infant lens is removed by suction and cutting. The retrolental tissue is then grasped in the center with tissue forceps, lifted, and incised with a microvitreoretinal blade or scissors. After a plane has been created, further dissection with forceps and a membrane peeler/cutter can be accomplished. Flaps of cut membrane are removed with the vitreous cutter. Great care should be taken not to create a retinal break in the thin periphery. All the fibrous tissue need not be removed since the goal of surgery is Zone I reattachment. A retinal break in the periphery will likely result in nonattachment.[39] With the hole in the retrolental tissue enlarged as much as possible the dissection is carried further posteriorly. A narrow configuration posteriorly is more difficult to dissect because of the greater accumulation of fibrous proliferation. Dissection must be performed since peeling can cause retinal breaks. As the dissection is carried posteriorly, a peripheral trough configuration may become apparent. If the trough is not too tight, opening it with a "pic," forceps, or membrane peeler/cutter may be possible. Scleral depression by the assistant frequently aids this dissection. If the trough is too tight, dissection should be avoided to prevent creating a retinal break. When as much membrane as possible has been removed, the operation is finished. Drainage of subretinal fluid is not necessary. At the end of the operation, air is injected into the vitreous cavity to help maintain retinal separation as the subretinal fluid is resorbing. The entry sites are closed with 9-0 absorbable Vicryl sutures.

In selected cases with posterior proliferation and an attached peripheral retina the lens may be spared.[42] A two-port system as mentioned above is utilized. Incisions should be directed parallel with the visual axis, and great care must be taken to avoid moving the instruments across the midline since the lens may be struck. Saving the lens in this age group highly susceptible to amblyopia is desirable.

Surgical results have gradually improved, but most investigators are reporting an anatomic success rate (reattachment of at least the posterior retina) with either technique (open-sky or closed vitrectomy) of only about 40%. The complicated pathoanatomy and the high likelihood of inducing a retinal break during surgery combine to produce this encouraging, but low, rate of success.

The visual results are even more disappointing. One half or fewer of the patients whose retinas were reattached in the studies quoted above had "fix and follow" vision or better. In a more standardized assessment of visual acuity in infants who were enrolled in the CryoROP study and who developed retinal detachment, it was found that only 2 eyes of one infant out of 71 eyes that were vitrectomized had pattern vision at the lowest measurable threshold.[43] None of the 58 control eyes with retinal detachment that did not undergo vitrectomy had pattern vision. These results underscore the authors' suggestions that efforts are well spent in attempting to prevent retinal detachment in ROP.

Aside from massive hemorrhage and infection, the most disastrous complication in eyes undergoing vitrectomy for far advanced ROP is retinal break formation. Retinal breaks most often occur anteriorly in the region of the pars plana during dissection of the tenacious epiretinal membrane. When a retinal break is created, the case is almost certainly lost since flattening of the retina to allow for adequate cryotherapy to the break and scleral buckling is almost impossible. In none of the cases of Zilis et al.[39] in which a retinal break was noted during surgery did reattachment occur. Sometimes a retinal break is not seen, but *schlieren* (small masses or streaks occurring when two clear fluids of different optical densities mix) are present. A retinal break has to be assumed in those cases.

Bleeding during both open-sky and closed vitrectomy is a frequent problem. Most often eyes are operated on when the active phase of ROP has subsided. If some degree of "plus" disease is still present at surgery, however, hemorrhage is much more likely. Intraocular diathermy is usually sufficient to stop bleeding. Blacharski and Charles[44] have used intravitreal thrombin to control bleeding during vitrectomy for stage 5 ROP.

CONCLUSION

The increased survival rate of low–birth weight infants has led to an increased incidence of retinopathy of prematurity. Great strides have been made with the advent of the International Classification of the disease. The information obtained to date from the CryoROP study has shown that treatment is beneficial. Laser photocoagulation has been at least as successful as cryotherapy in several studies and is easier and possibly safer to administer. For more advanced disease, favorable reattachment results are being obtained. The management of retinal detachment in ROP remains controversial, however, since the visual results are so poor. Efforts should certainly be directed at preventing the later stages of this formidable disease.

References

1. Hack M, Fanaroff AA: Outcomes of extremely-low-birth-weight infants between 1982 and 1988, *N Engl J Med* 321:1642-1647, 1989.
2. Campbell PB, Bull MJ, Ellis FD, et al: Incidence of retinopathy of prematurity in a tertiary newborn intensive care unit, *Arch Ophthalmol* 101:1686-1688, 1983.
3. Kalina RE, Karr DJ: Retrolental fibroplasia. Experience over two decades in one institution, *Ophthalmology* 89:91-95, 1982.
4. Petersen RA: Six years experience with retrolental fibroplasia in the Joint Program for Neonatology at Harvard Medical School. Read before the Retinopathy of Prematurity Conference, Washington DC, December 1981.
5. Pomerance JJ: Incidence of retrolental fibroplasia. Read before the Retinopathy of Prematurity Conference, Washington DC, December 1981.
6. Sniderman SH, Riedel PA, Bert MA, et al: Factors influencing the incidence of retrolental fibroplasia. Read before the Retinopathy of Prematurity Conference, Washington DC, December 1981.
7. Kingham JD: Acute retrolental fibroplasia, *Arch Ophthalmol* 95:39-47, 1977.
8. Schulenburg WE, Prendiville A, Ohri R: Natural history of retinopathy of prematurity, *Br J Ophthalmol* 71:837-843, 1987.
9. Tasman WS: The natural history of retinopathy of prematurity, *Ophthalmology* 91:1499-1503, 1984.

10. Zak TA: Retinopathy of prematurity; an update on retrolental fibroplasia, *NY State J Med* 82:1795-1796, 1982.
11. Flynn JT, Bancalari E, Bachynski BN, et al: Retinopathy of prematurity. Diagnosis, severity, and natural history, *Ophthalmology* 94:620-629, 1987.
12. Schaffer DB, Quinn GE, Johnson L: Sequelae of arrested mild retinopathy of prematurity, *Arch Ophthalmol* 102:373, 1984.
13. Reference deleted in proofs.
14. Committee for the Classification of Retinopathy of Prematurity: An international classification of retinopathy of prematurity, *Arch Ophthalmol* 102:1130-1134, 1984.
15. The International Committee for the Classification of the Late Stages of Retinopathy of Prematurity. An international classification of retinopathy of prematurity. II. The classification of retinal detachment, *Arch Ophthalmol* 105:906-912, 1987.
16. Tasman WS: Late complications of retrolental fibroplasia, *Trans Am Acad Ophthalmol Otolaryngol* 86:1724-1740, 1979.
17. Cryotherapy for Retinopathy of Prematurity Cooperative Group: Multicenter trial of cryotherapy for retinopathy of prematurity: preliminary results, *Arch Ophthalmol* 106:471-479, 1988.
18. Cryotherapy for Retinopathy of Prematurity Cooperative Group: Multicenter trial of cryotherapy for retinopathy of prematurity: three-month outcome, *Arch Ophthalmol* 108:195-204, 1990.
19. Cryotherapy for Retinopathy of Prematurity Cooperative Group: Multicenter trial of cryotherapy for retinopathy of prematurity: one-year outcome: structure and function, *Arch Ophthalmol* 108:1408-1416, 1990.
20. Brown GC, Tasman W, Naidoff M, et al: Systemic complications associated with retinal cryoablation for retinopathy of prematurity, *Ophthalmology* 97:855-858, 1990.
21. Greven CM, Tasman W: Rhegmatogenous retinal detachment following cryotherapy for retinopathy of prematurity, *Arch Ophthalmol* 107:1017-1018, 1989.
22. Nagata M, Kobayashi Y, Fukuda H, et al: Photocoagulation for the treatment of retinopathy of prematurity, *Jpn J Clin Ophthalmol* 22:419, 1968.
23. Yamashita Y: Studies on retinopathy of prematurity. III. Cryocautery for retinopathy of prematurity, *Jpn J Clin Ophthalmol* 26:385-393, 1972.
24. McNamara JA, Tasman W, Brown GC, et al: Laser photocoagulation for stage 3+ retinopathy of prematurity, *Ophthalmology* 98:576-580, 1991.
25. Iverson DA, Trese MT, Orgel IK, et al: Laser photocoagulation for threshold retinopathy of prematurity, *Arch Ophthalmol* 109:1342-1343, 1991.
26. Landers MB III, Toth CA, Semple C, et al: Treatment of retinopathy of prematurity with argon laser photocoagulation, *Arch Ophthalmol* 110:44-47, 1992.
27. McNamara JA, Tasman W, Vander JF, et al: Diode laser photocoagulation for retinopathy of prematurity: preliminary results, *Arch Ophthalmol* 110:1714-1716, 1992.
28. McPherson AR, Hittner HM, Lemos R: Retinal detachment in young premature infants with acute retrolental fibroplasia: thirty-two new cases, *Ophthalmology* 89:160-169, 1982.
29. Topilow HW, Ackerman AL, Wang FM: The treatment of advanced retinopathy of prematurity by cryotherapy and scleral buckling surgery, *Ophthalmology* 92:379-387, 1985.
30. Greven C, Tasman W: Scleral buckling in stages 4B and 5 retinopathy of prematurity, *Ophthalmology* 97:817-820, 1990.
31. Noorily SW, Small K, deJuan E, Machemer R: Scleral buckling surgery for stage 4B retinopathy of prematurity, *Ophthalmology* 99:263-268, 1992.
32. Hirose T, Schepens CL, Katsumi O, et al: Open sky vitrectomy in stage 5 ROP: anatomical and visual results. Presented at the annual meeting of the American Academy of Ophthalmology. New Orleans, 1989.
33. Treister G, Machemer R: Results of vitrectomy for rare proliferative and hemorrhagic diseases, *Am J Ophthalmol* 84:394-412, 1977.
34. Schepens CL: Clinical and research aspects of subtotal open-sky vitrectomy. *Am J Ophthalmol* 91:143-171, 1981.

35. Hirose T, Schepens CL, Lopansri C: Subtotal open-sky vitrectomy for severe retinal detachment as a late complication of ocular trauma. *Ophthalmology* 88:1, 1981.
36. Charles S: *Vitreous microsurgery,* Baltimore, 1987, Williams & Wilkins, p 158.
37. Trese MT: Visual results and prognostic factors for vision following surgery for stage V retinopathy of prematurity, *Ophthalmology* 93:574-579, 1986.
38. Tasman WS, Borrone RN, Bolling J: Open sky vitrectomy for total retinal detachment in retinopathy of prematurity, *Ophthalmology* 94:449-452, 1987.
39. Zilis JD, deJuan E, Machemer R: Advanced retinopathy of prematurity. The anatomic and visual results of vitreous surgery, *Ophthalmology* 97:821-826, 1990.
40. Trese MT: Surgical therapy for stage V retinopathy of prematurity: a two-step approach, *Graefes Arch Clin Exp Ophthalmol* 225:266-268, 1987.
41. deJuan E Jr, Machemer R: Retinopathy of prematurity. Surgical technique, *Retina* 7:63-69, 1987.
42. Maguire AM, Trese MT: Lens-sparing vitreoretinal surgery in infants, *Arch Ophthalmol* 110:284-286, 1992.
43. Quinn GE, Dobson V, Barr CC, et al: Visual results in infants after vitrectomy for severe retinopathy of prematurity. *Ophthalmology* 98:5-13, 1991.
44. Blacharski PA, Charles ST: Thrombin infusion to control bleeding during vitrectomy for stage V retinopathy of prematurity, *Arch Ophthalmol* 105:203-205, 1987.

18

Retinal Arterial Macroaneurysms

James F. Vander

Retinal arterial macroaneurysms rarely occur in patients under the age of 60 years and are seen in women more than men (about 75% of cases).[1] Visual loss is the most common presenting symptom, although many patients are asymptomatic.[2] Loss of vision may occur gradually when due to edema and exudate, or suddenly if vitreous hemorrhage is present. The majority of macroaneurysms eventually thrombose, fibrose, and involute spontaneously.[3] The prognosis for vision depends on the location of the hemorrhage and exudate as well as the severity and duration of macular involvement. Intraretinal hemorrhage is likely to resolve, with recovery of vision, whereas subretinal hemorrhage may lead to photoreceptor dysfunction and scarring. Preretinal hemorrhage can cause epiretinal membrane formation. Chronic macular edema usually results in a permanent visual deficit as well. Of patients presenting with macular involvement, as many as 50% are left with vision of 20/200 or worse.[4]

CLINICAL FINDINGS

Arterial macroaneurysms appear typically as round or fusiform dilations of the arterial walls (Fig. 18-1) with enlargement up to several times the size of normal.[1] Multiple macroaneurysms are present in as many as 20% of cases, with involvement of one or more vessels (Fig. 18-2). They are most common along the temporal arcades, with an even distribution between the superior and inferior arteries. Hemorrhage is present in about 50% of cases. This may be subretinal, intraretinal, preretinal, intravitreal, or any combination of these positions. Simultaneous subretinal and preretinal hemorrhage is present in up to 40% of cases and is highly suggestive of arterial macroaneurysm (Fig. 18-3). Recurrent hemorrhage from the same macroaneurysm is rare. After hemorrhaging, focal narrowing or a kink in the vessel wall may be the only sign of the source of the hemorrhage. Bilateral macroaneurysms are infrequently present.

Intraretinal exudate is a common finding, either in a circinate pattern or diffusely in the macula, regardless of the location of the macroaneurysm (Fig. 18-4). Other findings include pulsation of the macroaneurysm, which may suggest impending hemorrhage, and, rarely, branch retinal artery occlusions (Fig. 18-5).

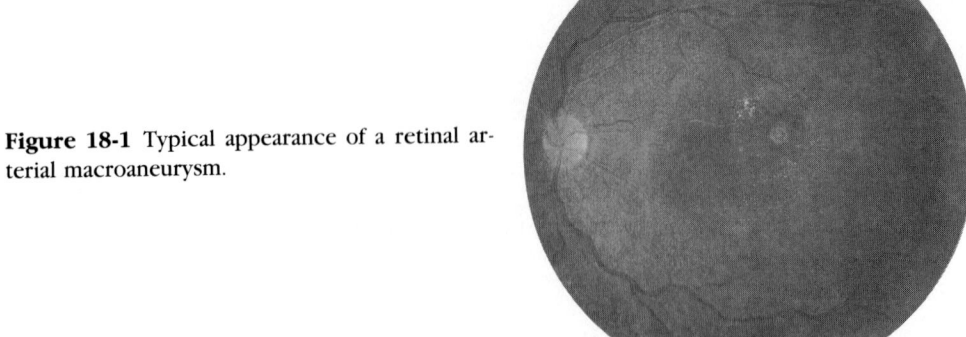

Figure 18-1 Typical appearance of a retinal arterial macroaneurysm.

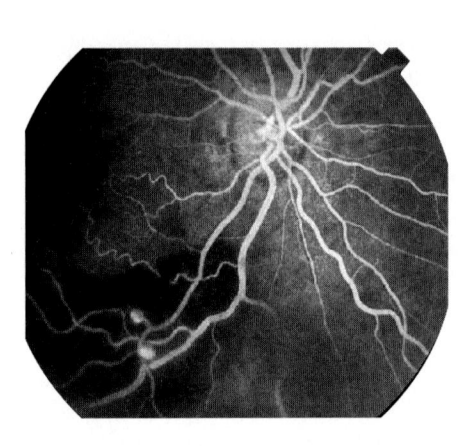

Figure 18-2 Fluorescein angiogram of a patient with multiple macroaneurysms along the same branch retinal arteriole. The hypofluorescent area is the result of a large subretinal hemorrhage.

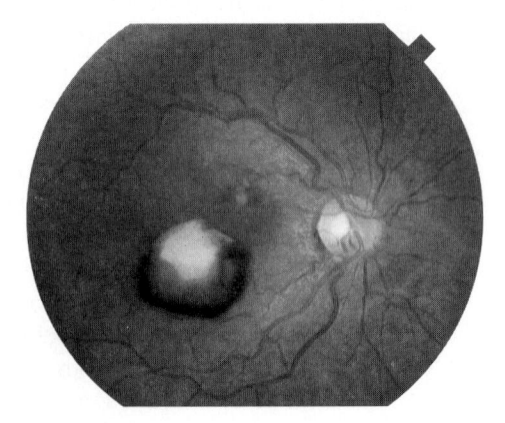

Figure 18-3 Simultaneous preretinal and subretinal hemorrhage from a retinal arterial macroaneurysm.

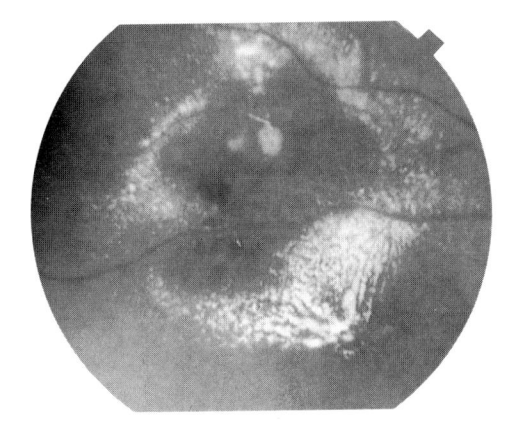

Figure 18-4 Lipid exudate surrounding a retinal arterial macroaneurysm. Note the white appearance of the macroaneurysm.

Figure 18-5 Branch retinal artery occlusion that occurred spontaneously distal to a retinal arterial macroaneurysm.

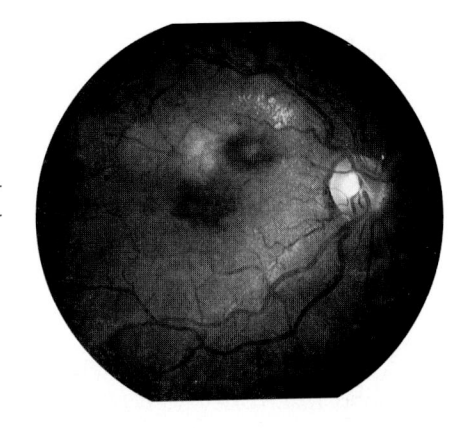

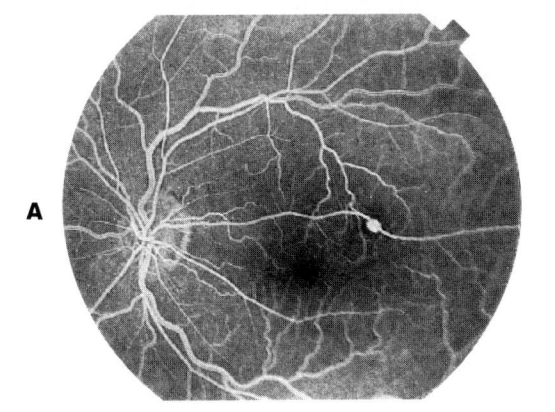

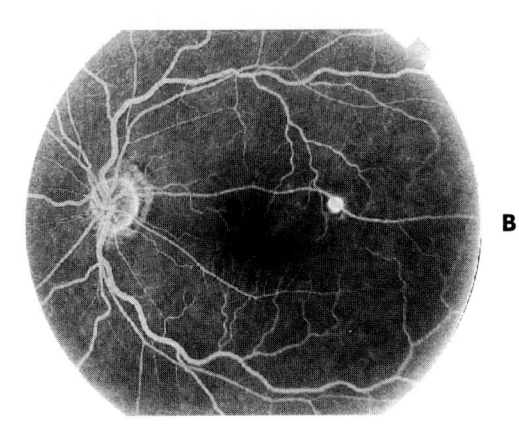

Figure 18-6 A, Hyperfluorescence of a retinal arterial macroaneurysm during the early phase of a fluorescein angiogram. **B,** Slight staining around the macroaneurysm in the recirculation phase.

Figure 18-7 A, Retinal microvascular changes around an arterial macroaneurysm producing macular edema and exudate. **B,** Multiple microaneurysms during the early transit phase of a fluorescein angiogram. **C,** Late hyperfluorescence in areas of macular edema.

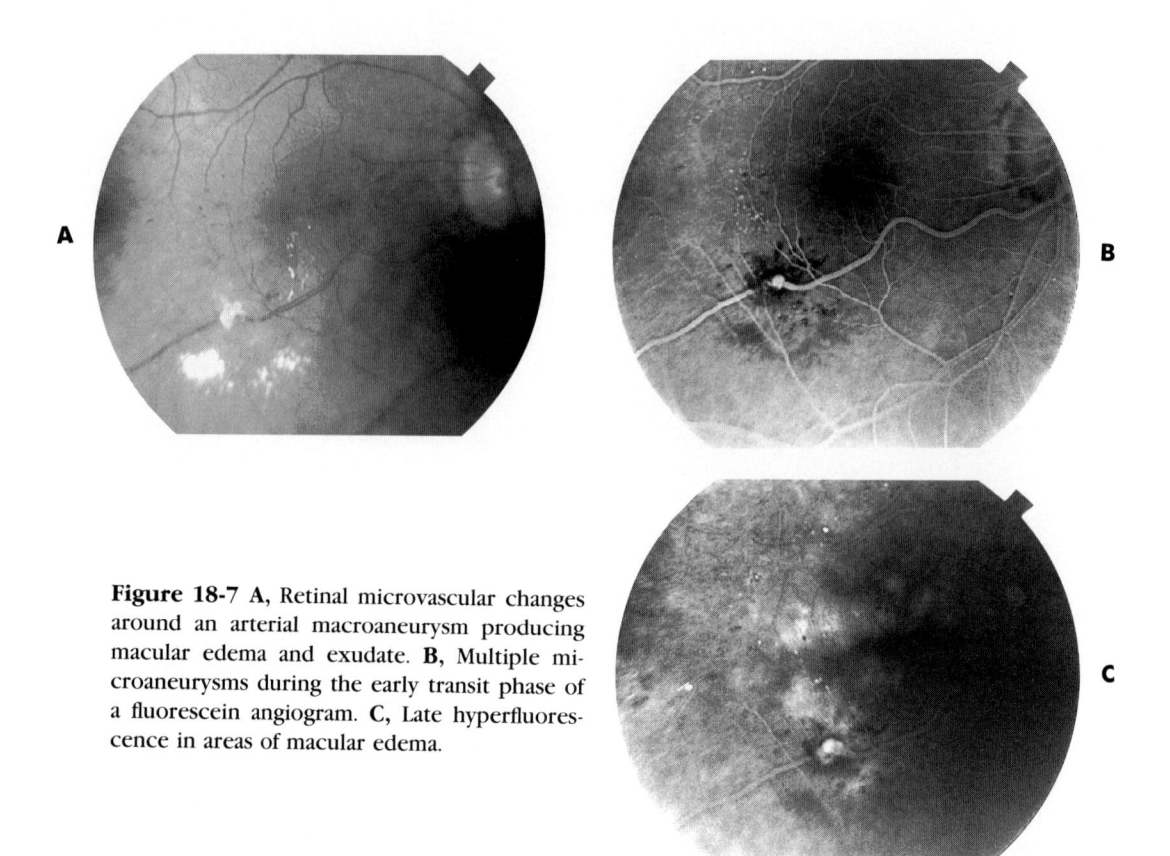

Immediate uniform filling is the typical fluorescein angiographic appearance of a macroaneurysm (Fig. 18-6) although irregular filling may occur and presumably is due to partial or complete obliteration of the lumen by thrombosis or endothelial cell proliferation.[6] Leakage of dye is common either from the aneurysm or the proximal artery wall. Blockage of fluorescence from hemorrhage is frequently present. In addition, capillary microaneurysms, nonperfusion, and intraretinal microvascular abnormalities may occur around the macroaneurysm (Fig. 18-7). Retinal arterial macroaneurysms are similar histologically to the intracerebral miliary aneurysms occurring in elderly hypertensive patients.[7,8] Loss of the muscular coat with thinning and fibrosis of the vessel wall results in decreased elasticity and increased susceptibility to dilation from intraluminal pressure. It is not known whether the abnormal capillary permeability frequently seen surrounding a retinal arterial macroaneurysm is a precursor to the macroaneurysm or a secondary response.

DIFFERENTIAL DIAGNOSIS

The differential diagnosis of retinal arterial macroaneurysm includes retinal telangiectasis, venous macroaneurysms after retinal vein occlusion, diabetic retinopathy, acquired and congenital retinal capillary hemangioma, retinal cavernous hemangioma, age-related macular degeneration, and choroidal melanoma.[9,10]

Congenital retinal telangiectasis may present with macular edema and exudation similar to that seen in retinal arterial macroaneurysm. The former condition, however, tends to occur in younger men and usually shows multiple dilated aneurysmal vessels.[11]

Aneurysmal dilation of the retinal venules can occur after branch retinal vein obstruction and has a similar appearance to retinal arterial macroaneurysm. Careful examination, however, should reveal the venous nature of the aneurysm. Fluorescein angiography will confirm this finding and will likely demonstrate other features of a prior venous obstruction. Since the intraluminal pressure is much lower than on the arterial side, a large vitreous or subretinal hemorrhage would not be likely to result from a venous macroaneurysm.[12]

The presence of a clinically apparent retinal arterial macroaneurysm generally makes distinguishing between the associated microvascular abnormalities of macroaneurysm and those of diabetes fairly straightforward. In older patients with a history of diabetes and hypertension, however, both entities must be considered when a vitreous hemorrhage obscures visualization of the fundus detail. The presence of diabetic retinopathy in the fellow eye may be a helpful clue.

Congenital retinal hemangioma is found in younger patients, usually with other manifestations of the von Hippel–Lindau syndrome. The characteristically dilated feeder and draining vessels give this lesion an appearance quite distinct from that of a retinal arterial macroaneurysm. An acquired retinal hemangioma, however, generally does not have these dilated vessels and could be confused with a macroaneurysm.[13] Unlike a macroaneurysm, the distal vessel draining an acquired hemangioma is venous and can be seen clinically or angiographically to return flow to the optic disc. The acquired hemangioma tends to occur in the peripheral retina and to be larger and more elevated from the retinal surface than a macroaneurysm.

The retinal cavernous hemangioma is rare and typically has numerous saccular vascular cavities that appear like a "bunch of grapes." Fluorescein angiography demonstrates fairly slow filling, often with a horizontal layering of dye caused by serum erythrocyte separation in these low-flow channels.[13]

Subretinal hemorrhage in elderly patients is frequently the result of age-related macular degeneration. The presence of drusen, pigmentary alteration, or other features of macular degeneration in the fellow eye is helpful in distinguishing this entity from retinal arterial macroaneurysm. It becomes especially helpful if the hemorrhage is large and has resulted in breakthrough bleeding into the vitreous cavity that obscures visualization of the retina.

In patients with a large subretinal and vitreous hemorrhage, ultrasound may demonstrate a subretinal echodense mass that could be confused with a choroidal neoplasm, especially a melanoma.[10] Ultrasound of a subretinal hemorrhage, however, tends to show higher internal reflectivity than a melanoma and would not produce characteristic choroidal excavation.

TREATMENT

Since the majority of macroaneurysms resolve spontaneously, with variable visual results, the indications for photocoagulation remain unclear.[1] Patients with good vision and no macular involvement should probably be followed. In addi-

Figure 18-8 Vision is 20/200.

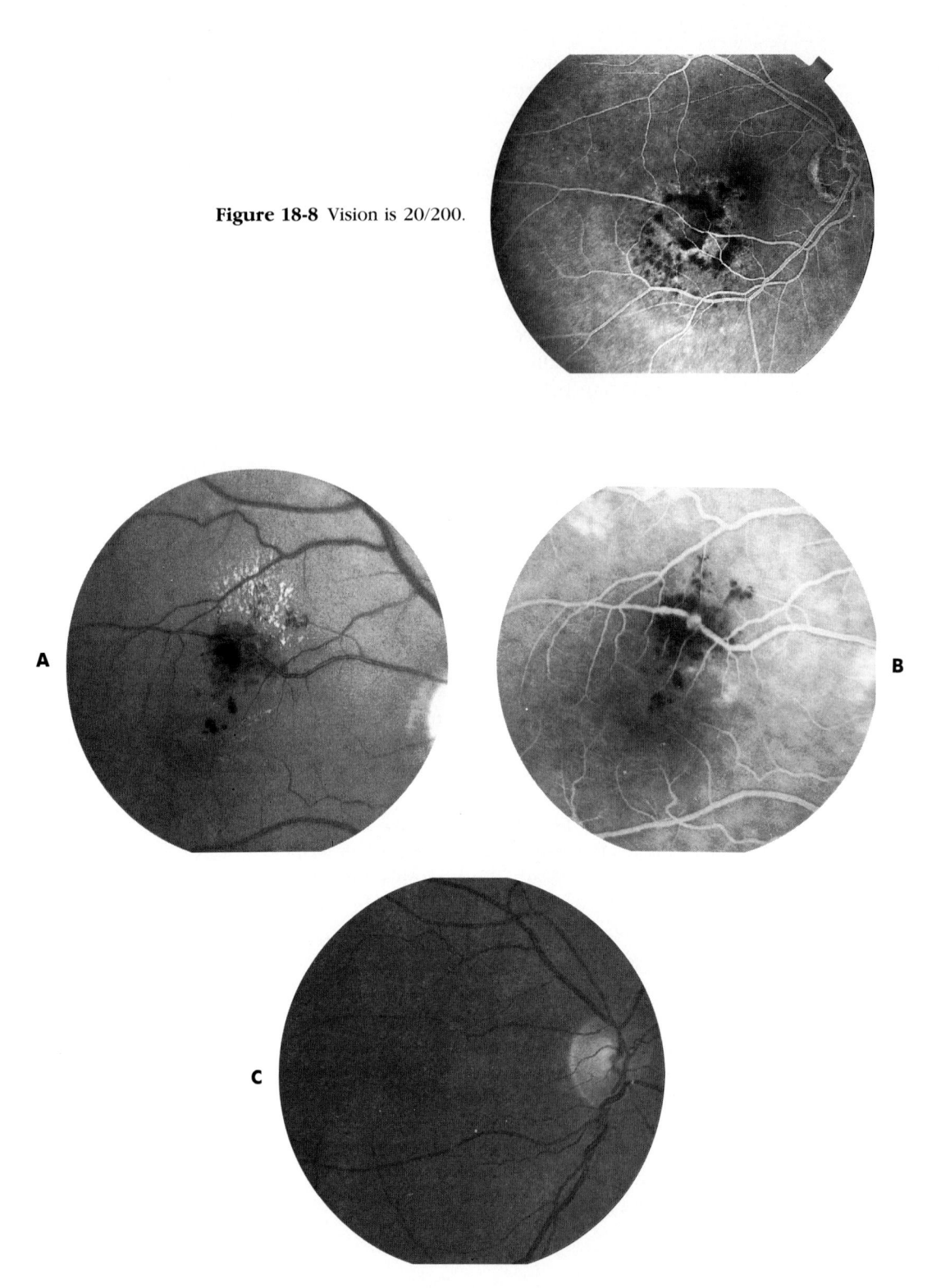

Figure 18-9 A, Macular edema with exudates from a retinal arterial macroaneurysm reducing vision to 20/40. **B,** Pretreatment fluorescein angiogram showing the retinal arterial macroaneurysm along with a few associated microaneurysms. **C,** Five months later the edema has resolved and the exudates are nearly completely resorbed. Vision returned to 20/20.

tion, patients with decreased vision on the basis of intraretinal or preretinal hemorrhage should be followed to allow for spontaneous improvement. Visual recovery after subretinal hemorrhage is variable, with some patients improving dramatically despite large hemorrhages. In some cases, though, extensive retinal and RPE damage may develop and limit the final visual acuity (Fig. 18-8). Using vitrectomy techniques in conjunction with fibrinolytic agents (e.g., tissue plaminogen activator), it is technically possible to remove such hemorrhages.[14] The benefits of such surgery for patients with retinal arterial macroaneurysm remain unproven, however.

Patients with edema, exudate, or retinal detachment should probably be treated, especially if deterioration of vision is documented (Fig. 18-9). Other possible indications are obvious growth, onset of pulsations (which may be a sign of impending rupture), or, rarely, recurrent hemorrhage from the same macroaneurysm.

Treatment modalities include direct and indirect photocoagulation of the lesion. Direct treatment involves use of argon green or dye yellow wavelengths at low energies to create light burns on the lesion. Artery occlusion may occur directly after these applications. Indirect treatment potentially avoids this complication and the theoretic risk of rupture and hemorrhage. It consists of surrounding the macroaneurysm with a laser grid and would be expected to be most helpful in cases of edema or exudation secondary to the microvascular changes associated with retinal arterial macroaneurysm. Retinal traction and an increase in retinal exudation are potential complications of this form of treatment.

Up to 75% of patients with retinal arterial macroaneurysm have systemic arterial hypertension. The blood pressure should be checked for patients with newly diagnosed macroaneurysm and appropriate treatment instituted if hypertension is present.

References

1. Rabb MF, Gagliamo DA, Teske MP: Retinal arterial macroaneurysms, *Surv Ophthalmol* 33:73, 1988.
2. Lavin MJ, Marsh RJ, Peart S, Rehman A: Retinal arterial macroaneurysms: A retrospective study of 40 patients, *Br J Ophthalmol* 71:817, 1987.
3. Robertson D: Macroaneurysms of the retinal arteries, *Trans Am Acad Ophthalmol Otolaryngol* 77:OP55, 1973.
4. Schatz H, Gitter K, Yannuzi L, Irvine A: Retinal arterial macroaneurysms: a large collaborative study. Presented at the annual meeting of the American Academy of Ophthalmology, Chicago, November 1980.
5. Lewis RA, Norton EWD, Gass JDM: Acquired arterial macroaneurysms of the retina, *Br J Ophthalmol* 60:21, 1976.
6. Gass JDM: A fluorescein angiographic study of macular dysfunction secondary to retinal vascular disease. V. Retinal telangiectasis, *Arch Ophthalmol* 80:592, 1968.
7. Cleary PE: Retino-vascular malformations, *Trans Ophthalmol Soc UK* 96:213, 1976.
8. Russell RWR: Observations on intracerebral aneurysms, *Brain* 86:425, 1963.
9. Spalter HF: Retinal macroaneurysms: a new masquerade syndrome, *Trans Am Ophthalmol Soc* 80:113, 1982.
10. Perry HD, Zimmerman LE, Benson WE: Hemorrhage from isolated aneurysm of a retinal artery: report of two cases simulating malignant melanoma, *Arch Ophthalmol* 95:281, 1977.
11. Gass JDM: *Stereoscopic atlas of macular diseases: diagnosis and treatment*, ed 3, St Louis, 1987, Mosby, p 384.

12. Sanborn GE, Magargal LE: Venous macroaneurysm associated with branch retinal vein obstruction, *Ann Ophthalmol* 16:464, 1984.
13. Shields JA, Shields CL: *Intraocular tumors: a text and atlas,* Philadelphia, 1992, WB Saunders, p 393.
14. Vander JF: Tissue plasminogen activator irrigation to facilitate removal of subretinal hemorrhage during vitrectomy, *Ophthalmic Surg* 23:361, 1992.

19

Radiation Retinopathy

James J. Augsburger

Radiation retinopathy is an uncommon retinal vascular disorder whose hallmarks are (1) a prior history of ionizing ocular irradiation, (2) a latent interval between the irradiation and development of the disorder, and (3) characteristic retinal vascular abnormalities in the field of irradiation.[1-6] In this chapter I will describe the clinical spectrum of radiation retinopathy, discuss the mechanism by which ionizing radiation causes the disorder, identify factors influencing the development and severity of the condition, mention the pertinent differential diagnosis, comment on the natural history of untreated cases, review current management, and emphasize preventive measures that can be taken to avoid the disorder or minimize its severity.

CLINICAL FEATURES

Symptoms

The presenting symptoms in patients with radiation retinopathy range from none at all to abrupt and severe loss of vision.[1-6] The typical patient presents with blurred or dimmed central vision and/or an apparent scotoma in the visual field. In advanced cases the affected eye can become blind and painful as a consequence of radiation-induced ocular ischemia or neovascular glaucoma, or both.[4,7]

Ophthalmoscopy

The earliest ophthalmoscopically visible features of radiation retinopathy are retinal microaneurysms, intraretinal microvascular abnormalities, retinal edema, intraretinal exudates, and blot, dot, and linear intraretinal hemorrhages.[1-6] In more advanced cases one can observe large vessel obstructions (both arterioles and venules of the retina), neovascularization of the retina and/or disc, and preretinal and intravitreal hemorrhages. Diffuse depigmentation of the retinal pigment epithelium is another common clinically observed feature.[3,8]

Radiation retinopathy can be categorized as background, preproliferative, or proliferative.

Background Radiation Retinopathy (Figs. 19-1 and 19-2). Radiation retinopathy is classifiable as *background* when it consists of one or more clinically identifiable retinal capillary microaneurysms associated with biomicroscopically evident retinal edema (focal or diffuse) and/or intraretinal exudates (with or without dot, blot, or linear intraretinal hemorrhages, one to a few retinal cotton-wool spots, and minor scattered nonaneurysmal microvascular abnormalities). Eyes treated by conventional fractionated external beam radiation appear more likely to develop retinopathy characterized by multiple cotton-wool spots and linear retinal hemorrhages (Fig. 19-1) whereas eyes treated by episcleral plaque radiation appear more likely to develop retinopathy typified by prominent intraretinal and subretinal exudates[4] (Fig. 19-2).

Preproliferative Radiation Retinopathy (Fig. 19-3). Radiation retinopathy is classifiable as *preproliferative* when it consists of any or all of the features of background disease plus retinal venous beading, numerous retinal cotton-wool spots, and prominent nonaneurysmal intraretinal microvascular abnormalities.

Proliferative Radiation Retinopathy (Fig. 19-4). Radiation retinopathy is classifiable as *proliferative* when it includes one or more extraretinal fibrovascular proliferations (neovascularization) arising from the optic disc (neovascularization of the disc, NVD) and/or extrapapillary retina (neovascularization of the retina, NVR).

Radiation retinopathy is commonly associated with radiation-induced optic papillopathy.[9] Acute radiation papillopathy is characterized by hyperemic optic disc swelling, circumpapillary exudative subretinal fluid, circumpapillary intraretinal exudates, and epipapillary and peripapillary retinal hemorrhages (Fig. 19-5) associated with an acute ipsilateral decrease in visual acuity. In some pa-

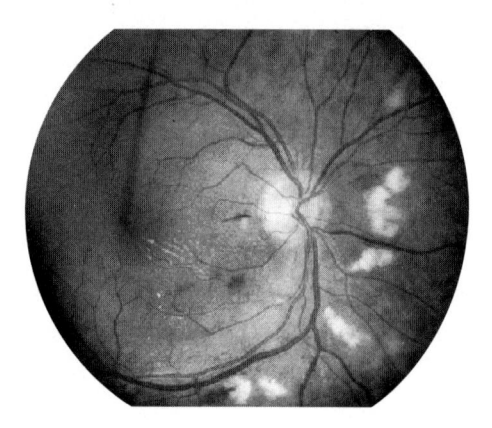

Figure 19-1 Background radiation retinopathy following external beam radiotherapy for nasopharyngeal carcinoma. The principal manifestations of this retinopathy are cotton-wool spots and linear retinal hemorrhages around the disc.

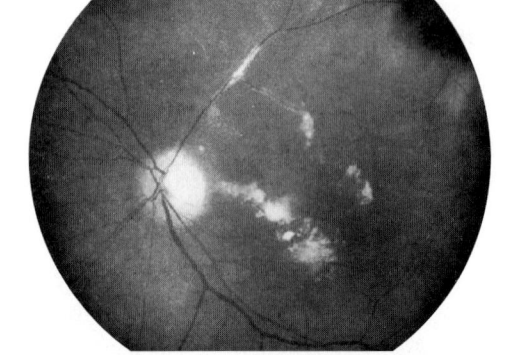

Figure 19-2 Exudative macular background radiation retinopathy following radioactive episcleral plaque therapy for a superotemporal midzone choroidal malignant melanoma.

Radiation retinopathy

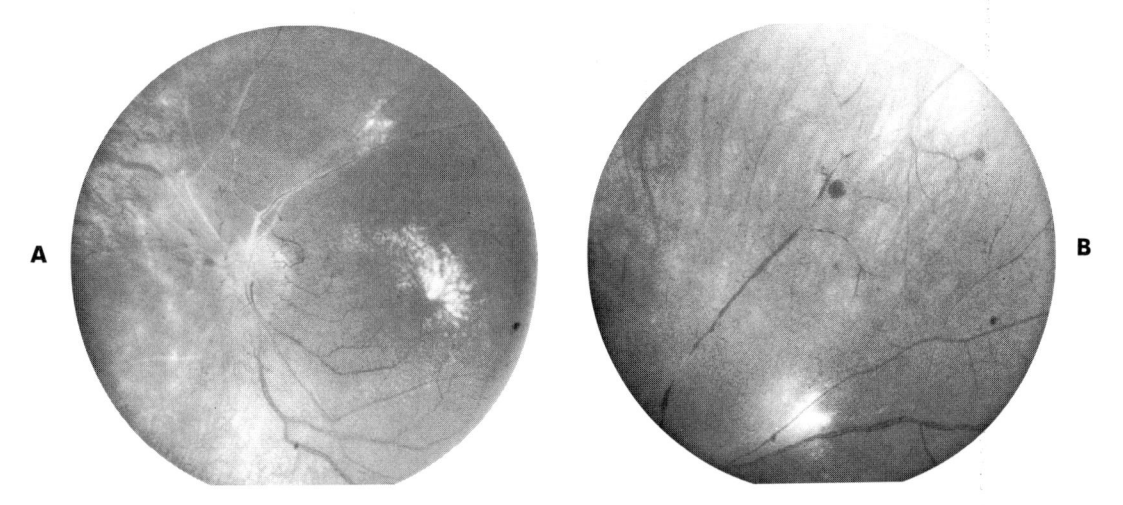

Figure 19-3 Preproliferative radiation retinopathy following cobalt-60 plaque therapy for a superonasal midzone choroidal malignant melanoma. **A,** Posterior pole view showing disc pallor, marked attenuation and sclerosis of the retinal arterioles and venules, and prominent macular exudates. **B,** Superotemporal midzone view showing segmentation of the larger retinal blood vessels and prominent blot retinal hemorrhages.

Figure 19-4 Proliferative radiation retinopathy following external beam radiotherapy for a nasopharyngeal carcinoma (same case as Figure 19-1 but 6 months later). Note the neovascularization in the disc and the preretinal hemorrhage along the course of the inferotemporal branch retinal vessels.

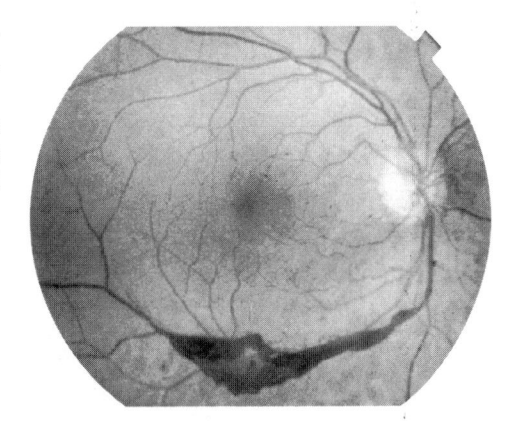

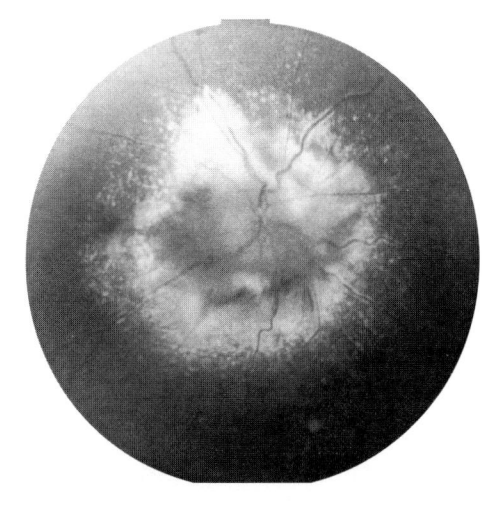

Figure 19-5 Severe radiation optic papillopathy 13 months after radioactive episcleral plaque therapy for a primary choroidal malignant melnoma. The disc is congested and elevated, surrounded by retinal hemorrhages and a thick ring of intraretinal and subretinal exudates.

tients undergoing ocular radiotherapy, especially ones treated by an episcleral radioactive plaque or charged-particle beam irradiation for a choroidal melanoma just nasal to the optic disc, radiation papillopathy occurs as a separate disorder without any of the extrapapillary features of classic radiation retinopathy.[9]

Radiation retinopathy is also commonly associated with clouding or opacification of the lens (radiation cataract).[3] The classic radiation cataract begins as a posterior subcapsular plaque that can become diffuse and dense. In addition, eyes with advanced radiation retinopathy commonly develop neovascularization of the iris.[3,7] The iris neovascularization, in turn, commonly leads to intractable neovascular glaucoma.

Fluorescein Angiography

Fundus fluorescein angiography is commonly used in evaluating and recording the retinal vascular abnormalities that characterize radiation retinopathy.[2,4,5] It enables one to distinguish between small blot and dot intraretinal hemorrhages and capillary microaneurysms. It also enhances the detection of nonaneurysmal intraretinal microvascular abnormalities and small foci of extraretinal fibrovascular proliferation, shows foci of retinal capillary nonperfusion, reveals leakage of fluorescein from radiation-damaged retinal capillaries, venules, and arterioles, and confirms intraretinal fluorescein accumulation focally or diffusely in areas of retinal edema. The earliest fluorescein angiographically identifiable changes of radiation retinopathy appear to be focal capillary closure, capillary microaneurysms, and irregular dilation and telangiectasis of the neighboring microvasculature (intraretinal microvascular abnormalities, IRMAs)[2,4-6,10] (Fig. 19-6). The microaneurysms tend to develop from the retinal capillaries that border zones of retinal capillary nonperfusion and to leak fluorescein by the late phase frames of the angiogram. The dilated telangiectatic retinal blood vessels may represent capillary collaterals that divert blood around obstructed capillary beds. Depending on the extent of breakdown of the inner blood-retina barrier, one can also see variable amounts of progressive fluorescein accumulation in areas of focal or diffuse retinal edema by the late-phase frames.

In eyes with preproliferative radiation retinopathy, fluorescein angiography typically reveals broad zones of confluent retinal capillary nonperfusion, generalized retinal arteriolar attenuation, and prominent intraretinal microvascular abnormalities bordering the zones of retinal capillary nonperfusion[2,4-6,10] (Fig. 19-7). It also accentuates foci of extraretinal fibrovascular proliferation and shows progressive fluorescein leakage from the abnormal new vessels into the adjacent vitreous by the late-phase frames.[2,4-6,10]

HISTORY OF IONIZING OCULAR IRRADIATION

The sine qua non of radiation retinopathy is a history of prior ocular ionizing radiotherapy.[1-6] That therapy may have been intended for the eye (e.g., in patients with metastatic carcinoma to the choroid or a primary posterior uveal melanoma),[11-23] or it may have been inadvertent (associated with conventional external beam radiation therapy to an intracranial tumor)[24-31] or unavoidable (whole orbital irradiation for lymphoma of the orbit).[32,33]

The interval between ocular irradiation and the onset of symptoms and signs

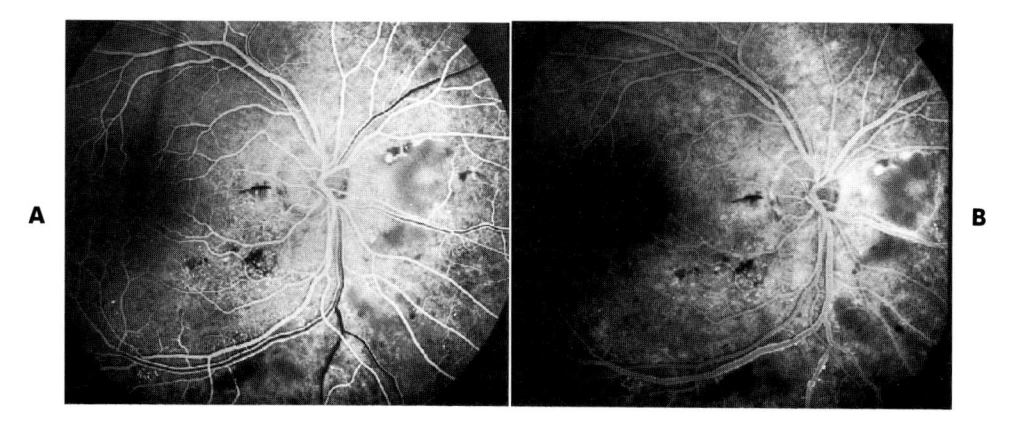

Figure 19-6 Fluorescein angiogram of background radiation retinopathy (same case as in Figure 19-1). **A,** Laminar venous phase frame showing multiple small foci of retinal capillary nonperfusion corresponding to cotton-wool spots, hypofluorescent linear and dotlike figures corresponding to intraretinal hemorrhages, and numerous retinal capillary microaneurysms. **B,** Late venous phase frame showing prominent beading in the major inferior branch retinal vein and early leakage from many of the microaneurysms.

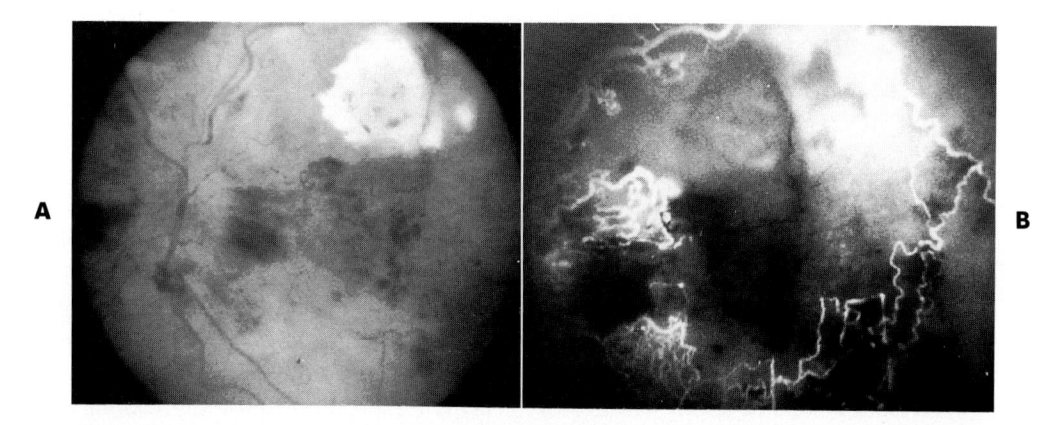

Figure 19-7 Ischemic radiation retinopathy following radioactive episcleral plaque therapy for a retinoblastoma. **A,** Regressed white retinal tumor in the superior macula, prominent linear and blotlike intraretinal hemorrhages, and marked irregularities in caliber of the remaining large retinal blood vessels. **B,** Venous phase frame of the fluorescein angiogram showing extensive confluent retinal capillary nonperfusion and severe irregularities of the remaining retinal blood vessels.

of radiation retinopathy can be as short as 1 to 3 months or as long as 10 to 20 years.[4,6] In general, however, it is uncommon for radiation retinopathy to develop within the first 6 months after ocular irradiation or more than 5 years after that treatment. The average latent interval between ocular irradiation and detection of radiation retinopathy in the largest reported series of cases to date from a single institution[4] was about 15 months following cobalt-60 plaque therapy and approximately 19 months following conventional fractionated external beam radiotherapy.

DIFFERENTIAL DIAGNOSIS[1,2-4,6]

Diabetic retinopathy is the condition that most closely resembles radiation retinopathy. Unlike its radiation-induced counterpart, however, it is almost exclusively a bilateral disorder. It also is usually symmetric in extent and severity between the two eyes. Affected patients often have a long-standing history of recognized diabetes mellitus but not of prior ocular irradiation (which is the hallmark of radiation retinopathy).

Other retinal vascular disorders that must be included in the differential diagnosis of radiation retinopathy include branch and central retinal vein obstructions, hypertensive retinopathy, the retinopathies of various systemic vasculitides, and the retinopathy of AIDS (acquired immune deficiency syndrome).[34]

MECHANISM OF DEVELOPMENT

The precise mechanism by which ionizing radiation causes radiation retinopathy is unknown. It appears, however,[4-6,12,35] to be principally through damage of the retinal vascular endothelial cells. If such damage is not too severe, the cells remain viable but lose the integrity of their intercellular tight junctions (zonulae occludentes). When this happens, the affected retinal blood vessels become abnormally permeable to larger molecules and retinal edema begins to develop. If the radiation-induced damage is marked, the affected cells die and their corresponding vascular channels become occluded.

FACTORS INFLUENCING OCCURRENCE AND SEVERITY

Factors currently recognized to influence the occurrence of radiation retinopathy include (1) the total retinal radiation dose,[36-38] (2) the fractional radiation dose (in conventional external beam radiotherapy),[36] (3) associated diabetes mellitus,[39] and (4) adjunctive chemotherapy.[40]

The higher the total dose of radiation to the retina, the higher is the probability of developing radiation retinopathy. In external beam radiotherapy, radiation retinopathy occurs rarely when the retinal radiation dose is 30 Gy* or less, develops in about half the eyes receiving a total dose of approximately 50 Gy, and afflicts the great majority of eyes receiving 80 Gy or more.[35,36] Similarly, in episcleral radioactive plaque therapy, radiation retinopathy and papillopathy usually do not develop if the radiation dose to the macula and optic disc is less than 50 Gy.[4,14]

For a particular retinal radiation dose delivered by fractionated external beam radiotherapy, the higher the fractional dose the greater the likelihood of developing radiation retinopathy.[36] Radiation dose fractions in the range of 200 cGy are rarely associated with radiation retinopathy, but fractions in excess of 250 cGy are likely to cause retinal vascular problems.

For a particular retinal radiation dose, patients with diabetes mellitus appear to have a substantially increased risk of developing radiation retinopathy compared to patients without this systemic disorder.[39] Presumably, the increased risk is due to underlying retinal vascular abnormalities in the diabetic retina (which may or may not be visible ophthalmoscopically) that are accentuated

---

*1 Gy (gray) is equal to 100 rads.

by the damaging effects of ocular irradiation. Diabetics with preexisting clinical diabetic retinopathy are at particularly high risk of developing a severely ischemic or proliferative diabetic-radiation retinopathy following therapeutic ocular irradiation.[4]

For a particular retinal radiation dose, patients who receive adjunctive chemotherapy appear to be at substantially increased risk of developing radiation retinopathy.[40] The precise mechanism by which chemotherapy exerts its synergistic effect is currently unknown. Moreover, it is not known whether this effect is a generic result of chemotherapy or a specific result of certain chemotherapeutic agents or combinations of drugs.

Bone marrow transplantation[41] and simultaneous external beam radiotherapy with hyperbaric oxygen therapy[42] may also influence the probability of radiation retinopathy. The greater the number of adverse prognostic factors in a given patient, the greater is the likelihood that radiation retinopathy will develop.

The same factors that influence the development of radiation retinopathy appear also to influence its severity.[4,6] Two additional factors may have an effect[4,35]: (1) the area of retina encompassed in the field of treatment and (2) the technique of ocular irradiation (i.e., conventional fractionated external beam radiotherapy versus episcleral radioactive plaque). If only a small portion of the retina receives a substantial radiation dose and the macula and optic disc absorb but a fraction of this, the retinopathy is likely to be extramacular, relatively mild, and visually unimportant. Such a circumstance occurs in many patients undergoing external beam radiotherapy for a paranasal sinus malignancy or intracranial neoplasm and in most patients with a small peripheral intraocular neoplasm managed by an episcleral plaque. By contrast, if the whole retina or a substantial portion (including the disc and macula) is irradiated, the retinopathy is likely to be much more pronounced and more damaging visually.

When an episcleral plaque is used to treat an intraocular tumor, my radiation oncology colleagues and I try to select or fabricate a plaque that is 5 to 6 mm larger than the largest linear diameter of the tumor. Such a plaque provides a safety margin of apparently normal tissue around the tumor 2.5 to 3 mm wide. The entire area underlying the plaque receives a radiation dose that is at least equal to the target dose to the tumor apex. For choroidal melanoma that is usually 80 to 100 Gy. For retinoblastoma it is 40 to 45 Gy. In my opinion radiation retinal vascular effects that occur in the tumor and within the safety margin around the tumor following episcleral plaque therapy should be categorized as *radiation tumor vasculopathy* (i.e., expected effects of the irradiation) and not radiation retinopathy.[6] (See also "Complication or Expected Side Effect?" at the end of this chapter.) Because the target radiation dose is substantially higher for choroidal melanomas than for retinoblastomas, the frequency of radiation tumor vasculopathy is substantially greater following melanoma treatment.

INCIDENCE

Radiation retinopathy appears to be a relatively uncommon condition. Its precise frequency, however, is not currently known. To estimate the true frequency, one must follow patients treated for different forms of the disorder prospectively and compute an incidence curve by actuarial methods. This has not been done for patients treated by conventional fractionated external beam radiotherapy. Consequently, there are no published actuarial estimates of the cumulative probabilities of developing radiation retinopathy over time following conventional external beam radiotherapy. Currently available estimates of its frequency following external beam radiotherapy[13,15-20,23] are all simple proportions of evaluated cases having retinopathy at the time of survey. These proportions do not take into account losses to follow-up because of death or other circumstances, differences in length of follow-up among evaluable patients in the surveyed groups, or differences in potentially important prognostic factors for radiation retinopathy (e.g., total retinal radiation dose and fractional dose) among members of the groups.

There are also no published actuarial estimates of the probability of developing radiation retinopathy after episcleral plaque therapy of intraocular tumors. My clinical experience with plaque treatment of choroidal melanomas is sufficient, however, to allow me to compute such a curve. I reviewed my personal experience with ^{60}Co plaque radiotherapy (460 cases, May 1976 to December 1985) and ^{125}I plaque radiotherapy (100 cases, May 1982 to December 1990). The tumors in both groups were treated by target doses of 80 to 100 Gy to the tumor apex and 300 to 450 Gy to the tumor base. The thicker the tumor and the closer to the disc and macula, the higher was the radiation dose delivered to the disc and macular retina. The survey date for my analysis was January 1992.

Among the 459 evaluable cases in the ^{60}Co group, 201 (43.8%) developed radiation retinopathy during available follow-up. Thirty of these 201 patients also developed radiation papillopathy. In addition, seven patients (1.5%) developed radiation papillopathy without evidence of extrapapillary retinopathy. By life-table analysis (Fig. 19-8), the cumulative 3-year and 5-year postirradiation probabilities of developing radiation retinopathy (with or without papillopathy) were 39.3% (SE = 2.6%) and 53.1% (SE = 2.8%) respectively. The median time from irradiation to diagnosis of radiation retinopathy was 52.8 months. The cumulative 3-year and 5-year probabilities of developing radiation papillopathy in the ^{60}Co plaque group were 7.9% (SE = 1.5%) and 9.9% (SE = 1.7%).

Of the 87 evaluable cases treated by ^{125}I plaque (the total being substantially less than 100 cases because patients with less than 1 year of follow-up were considered nonevaluable in this analysis), 25 (28.7%) developed radiation retinopathy during available follow-up. Four of these 25 patients also developed radiation papillopathy. In addition, three patients (3.4%) had radiation papillopathy without evidence of extrapapillary retinopathy during available follow-up. By life-table analysis (Fig. 19-8), the cumulative 3-year and 5-year probabilities of developing radiation retinopathy (with or without papillopathy) were 32.2% (SE = 6.3%) and 61.4% (SE = 9.9%). The difference between the cumulative actuarial curves for radiation retinopathy following ^{60}Co plaque versus ^{125}I plaque is neither substantial nor statistically significant (P > 0.1, Mantel-Haenszel test).

Incidence curves for radiation retinopathy following charged-particle (proton or helium ion) beam irradiation for choroidal and ciliary body melanomas are not currently available.

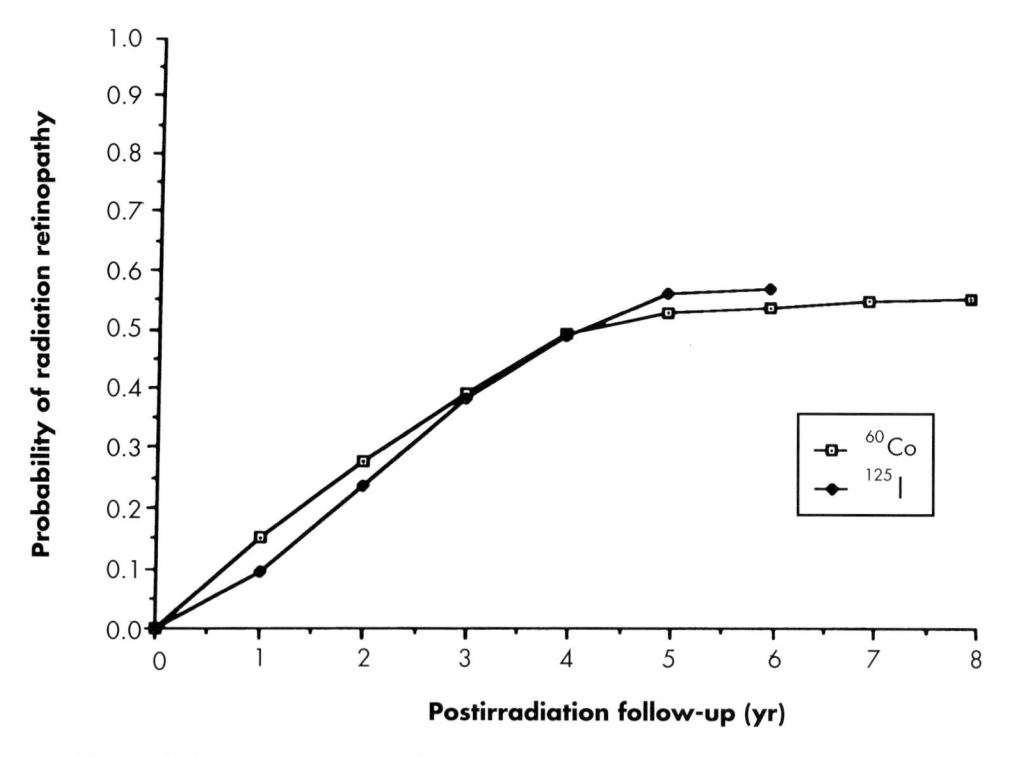

Figure 19-8 Cumulative actuarial probabilities of developing radiation retinopathy following cobalt-60 or iodine-125 plaque therapy for a choroidal or ciliary body malignant melanoma.

NATURAL HISTORY

The natural history of radiation retinopathy is quite varied.[5] After detection and diagnosis some patients show stabilization of the retinal abnormalities and a gradual return of retinal function.[43] At the other end of the spectrum, some show progressive retinal vasoobliteration, progressive accumulation of intraretinal hemorrhages, exudates, and cotton-wool spots, and eventual development of extraretinal fibrovascular proliferation leading to recurrent intravitreal hemorrhages, tractional retinal detachment, and severe visual loss.[4,10] In any individual case it is extremely difficult if not impossible to predict the natural history of the retinopathy. If the disorder is going to worsen progressively, it usually does so within 3 to 6 months after its initial detection.[4] Consequently, it is prudent for the ophthalmologist to monitor closely over the first year any patient with early signs to see whether the retinopathy is self-limited or progressive and in need of therapeutic intervention.

If acute radiation papillopathy develops in combination with radiation retinopathy or as a separate condition, its acute features usually begin to wane over a 3- to 12-month interval.[9] In the typical case, vision decreases to the range of counting fingers or no light perception and the disc gradually becomes pale and atrophic. In occasional patients with mild papillopathy, vision in the affected eye will improve to some extent as the disc edema resolves.[9] Even in such favorable circumstances, however, it usually does not recover to the pretreatment level.

MANAGEMENT

The management of radiation retinopathy ranges from observation alone to enucleation of the affected eye if it becomes blind and painful.[4,7] The most commonly employed option today, however, is photocoagulation.[44] The same general guidelines and techniques used to treat diabetic retinopathy with laser (i.e., Diabetic Retinopathy Study[45] [DRS] and Early Treatment Diabetic Retinopathy Study[46] [ETDRS] guidelines) are used to treat patients with radiation retinopathy. As with diabetic retinopathy, treatment recommendations differ according to the type and extent of the retinopathy.

No clinical trials of alternative treatments or of treatment versus no treatment have been performed for radiation retinopathy. Because of the rarity of the condition and its wide spectrum of presentations, both of which limit the feasibility of a clinical trial, no therapeutic studies are likely to be organized in the foreseeable future.

TREATMENT

Background Radiation Retinopathy

For background radiation retinopathy with focal macular edema or hard exudates involving or threatening the central macula, focal photocoagulation is generally applied to the leaking sites identified at fluorescein angiography[44] (Fig. 19-9). The argon green laser is still the most commonly employed tool for such treatments at the time of this writing, but dye lasers that can be set at yellow wavelengths are gradually becoming more popular for treating intraretinal vascular abnormalities. Typical laser settings are 50 to 100 μm burn diameter and 0.05 to 0.1 second exposure duration. Identified retinal capillary microaneurysms should whiten or darken in response to treatment. If the macular edema or hard exudates persist, retreatment may be necessary within 1 to 3 months.

For background retinopathy with diffuse macular edema, grid laser photocoagulation to the edematous retina plus focal treatment to identified microaneurysms and other intraretinal microvascular abnormalities is usually employed[44] (Fig. 19-10). The same laser settings indicated above are generally used in this type of treatment, and individual laser burns are spaced about one burn diameter apart throughout the entire zone of edematous retina. Each burn is intended to be gray-white in intensity rather than opaque white. If the macular edema extends beneath the fovea, the grid treatment should approach within about 0.5 mm of the foveola but not involve the foveal zone proper. As with focal treatment, grid laser can be repeated within 1 to 3 months if the diffuse macular edema persists.

For background retinopathy with no macular edema or hard exudates and evidence of confluent retinal capillary nonperfusion in the macular retina, no treatment is currently available. Such patients must be monitored, however, for the subsequent development of proliferative retinopathy.

Proliferative Radiation Retinopathy

In the case of proliferative retinopathy, one treats all the zones of retinal ischemia with scatter retinal photocoagulation[7,44] (Fig. 19-11), usually employing burn spot sizes of 500 to 1000 μm and spacing the burns one to two burn diameters apart. If the radiation retinopathy is generalized in all quadrants of

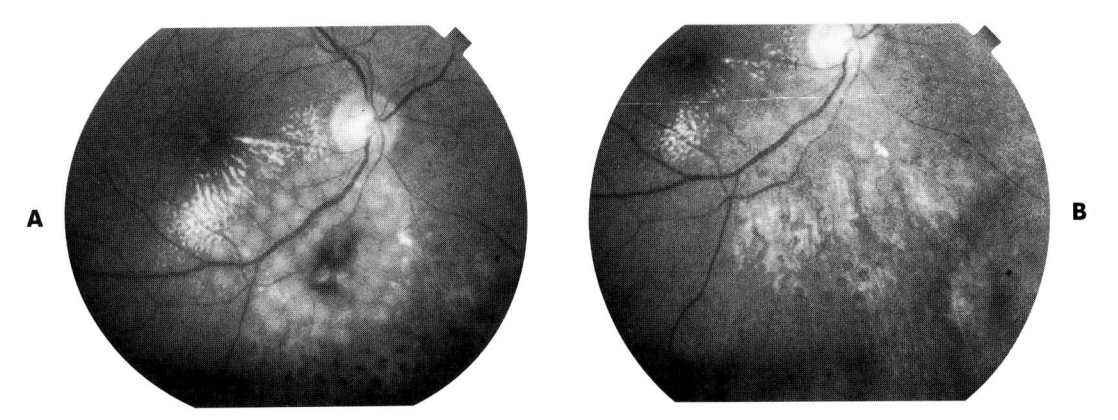

Figure 19-9 Focal and grid photocoagulation for exudative background radiation retiniopathy following iodine-125 plaque therapy for a choroidal melanoma. **A,** Immediately following argon laser treatment, showing the grid of white retinal burns scattered over the entire area of exudation. **B,** Same area of the fundus 3 months after laser treatment. Blood and most of the exudates have resorbed.

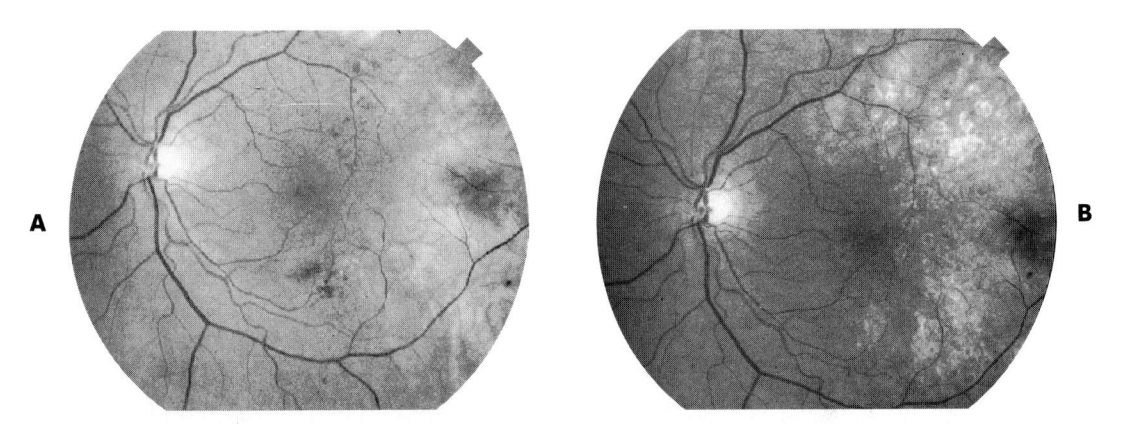

Figure 19-10 Focal and grid laser photocoagulation for radiation retinopathy with diffuse macular edema following iodine-125 plaque therapy for a temporal midzone choroidal melanoma. **A,** Pretreatment appearance of the macula. Note the retinal hemorrhages above and below the fovea and the diffuse macular edema. **B,** Six months after focal and grid laser treatment, showing resorption of the hemorrhages and resolution of the edema.

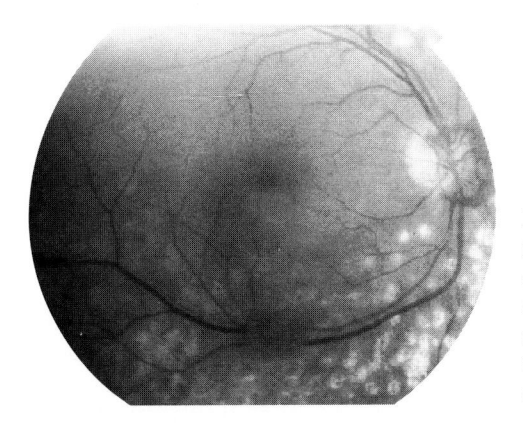

Figure 19-11 Scatter retinal photocoagulation for proliferative radiation retinopathy (same case as in Figure 19-4), showing resorption of preretinal hemorrhages and stabilization of prepapillary and preretinal neovascularization following scatter laser treatment to the nasal and inferior quadrants of the fundus.

the fundus, complete panretinal photocoagulation should be performed.[44] In addition, one can treat discrete foci of extraretinal fibrovascular proliferation directly in attempt to hasten the involution of these abnormal vessels. If this is successful, it should be possible to see involution or stabilization of all neovascularization of the retina and optic disc. The scatter retinal photocoagulation can be supplemented if the retinopathy persists or worsens.

If proliferative radiation retinopathy is complicated by recurrent or massive intravitreal hemorrhage or development of a tractional or rhegmatogenous retinal detachment, a complete posterior vitrectomy must be performed.[44] Focal and scatter laser therapy (endophotocoagulation or indirect ophthalmoscope laser therapy) can be performed at the time of this surgery to reduce the chance of recurrent bleeding or retinal detachment.

Radiation Papillopathy

There is no treatment recognized effective in stabilizing or reversing the visual effects of radiation papillopathy. At present, all one can do is hope that the visual loss attributable to this condition will not become too severe.

PREVENTIVE MEASURES

Ophthalmologists should work with radiation oncologists in the design of irradiation treatment plans that intentionally or potentially affect one or both eyes. By working together in this way, the ophthalmologist can help ensure that the ocular radiation dose is as limited as reasonably possible[35] and thus minimize the likelihood of the patient's developing radiation retinopathy.

Ophthalmologists should also encourage their radiation oncology colleagues to advise patients undergoing ocular irradiation or irradiation of the orbit, paranasal sinuses, or pituitary region of the potential risk of developing radiation retinopathy in the future. Furthermore, the ophthalmologist should be aware of the synergistic impacts of diabetes mellitus and adjunctive chemotherapy on the occurrence of radiation retinopathy in such patients and advise their radiation therapy colleagues appropriately.

COMPLICATION OR EXPECTED SIDE EFFECT?

When radiation-induced retinal vascular abnormalities occur following radiation therapy that intentionally includes the macula and/or optic disc in the treatment field (e.g., external beam radiotherapy for a malignant orbital tumor directly behind the globe, or episcleral plaque therapy or charged-particle beam irradiation for a posterior choroidal malignant melanoma), they should be regarded as expected consequences of the irradiation (side effect) and not as treatment complications.[6] By contrast, when radiation-induced retinal vascular abnormalities occur following irradiation that was planned to avoid substantial ocular radiation exposure (e.g., irradiation of a tumor of the pituitary fossa or paranasal sinuses), they should rightly be considered true complications of the treatment.

SUMMARY

Radiation retinopathy is a distinct clinical entity with characteristic ophthalmoscopic and fluorescein angiographic features. It can be categorized as background, preproliferative, or proliferative. Patients who receive an excess of 30 Gy to the eye by conventional photon teletherapy should probably be examined at least once yearly for 5 years or more following the irradiation to screen for radiation retinopathy. Patients who receive 50 Gy or more to the eye by external beam radiotherapy should be followed even more closely. Patients undergoing ocular irradiation by episcleral plaque or charged-particle beam for an intraocular tumor must be advised of the relatively high risk of developing subsequent radiation retinopathy. They should be followed on a close regular basis for tumor monitoring as well as screening to detect radiation retinopathy and the other complications and side effects of radiotherapy. Focal, grid, or scatter laser therapy can be used to treat selected patients with this disorder.

References

1. Chee PHY: Radiation retinopathy, *Am J Ophthalmol* 66:860-865, 1968.
2. Hayreh SS: Post-radiation retinopathy: a fluorescence fundus angiographic study, *Br J Ophthalmol* 54:705-714, 1970.
3. MacFaul PA, Bedford MA: Ocular complications after therapeutic irradiation, Br J Ophthalmol 54:237-247, 1970.
4. Brown GC, Shields JA, Sanborn G, et al: Radiation retinopathy, *Ophthalmology* 89:1494-1501, 1982.
5. Archer DB, Amoaku WMK, Gardiner TA: Radiation retinopathy: clinical, histopathological, ultrastructural, and experimental correlations, *Eye* 5:239-251, 1991.
6. Schachat AP: Radiation retinopathy. In Ryan SJ (ed): *Retina*, St Louis, 1989, Mosby, pp 541-545.
7. Augsburger JJ, Roth SE, Magargal LE, Shields JA: Panretinal photocoagulation for radiation-induced ocular ischemia, *Ophthalmic Surg* 18:589-593, 1987.
8. Ehlers N, Kaae S: Effects of ionizing radiation on retinoblastoma and on the normal ocular fundus in infants: radiation effects in the normal ocular fundus, *Acta Ophthalmol* 65(suppl 181):47-62, 1987.
9. Brown GC, Shields JA, Sanborn G, et al: Radiation optic neuropathy, *Ophthalmology* 89:1489-1493, 1982.
10. Amoaku WMK, Archer DB: Fluorescein angiographic features, natural course and treatment of radiation retinopathy, *Eye* 4:657-667, 1990.
11. Bedford MA, Bedotto C, MacFaul PA: Radiation retinopathy after the application of a cobalt plaque: report of three cases, *Br J Ophthalmol* 54:505-509, 1970.
12. Egbert PR, Farjado LF, Donaldson SS, Moazed K: Posterior ocular abnormalities after irradiation for retinoblastoma: a histopathological study, *Br J Ophthalmol* 64:660-665, 1980.
13. Shields JA, Augsburger JJ, Brady LW, Day JL: Cobalt plaque therapy of posterior uveal melanomas, *Ophthalmology* 89:1201-1207, 1982.
14. Cruess AF, Augsburger JJ, Shields JA, et al: Visual results following cobalt plaque radiotherapy for posterior uveal melanomas, *Ophthalmology* 91:131-136, 1984.
15. Packer S, Rotman M, Salanitro P: Iodine-125 irradiation of choroidal melanoma: clinical experience, *Ophthalmology* 91:1700-1708, 1984.
16. Moura RA, McPherson AR, Easley J: Malignant melanoma of the choroid: treatment with episcleral ^{198}Au plaque and xenon-arc photocoagulation, *Ann Ophthalmol* 17:114-125, 1985.

17. Förster MH, Bornfeld N, Shulz U, et al: Complications of local β-irradiation of uveal melanomas, *Graefes Arch Ophthalmol* 224:536-541, 1986.
18. Lommatzsch PK: Results after β-irradiation (^{106}Ru/^{106}Rh) of choroidal melanomas: 20 years' experience, *Br J Ophthalmol* 70:844-851, 1986.
19. Davidorf FH, Pajka JT, Makley TA, Kartha MK: Radiotherapy for choroidal melanoma: an 18-year experience with radon, *Arch Ophthalmol* 105:352-355, 1987.
20. Gragoudas ES, Seddon JM, Egan K, et al: Long-term results of proton beam irradiated uveal melanomas, *Ophthalmology* 94:349-353, 1987.
21. Char DH, Castro JR, Quivey JM, et al: Uveal mealnoma radiation: ^{125}I brachytherapy versus helium ion irradiation, *Ophthalmology* 96:1708-1715, 1989.
22. Balmer A, Gailloud C, De Potter P, et al: Treatment of retinoblastoma and results, *Klin Monatsbl Augenheilkd* 196:374-376, 1990.
23. Char DH, Castro JR, Kroll SM, et al: Five-year follow-up of helium ion therapy for uveal melanoma, *Arch Ophthalmol* 108:209-214, 1990.
24. de Schryver A, Wachtmeister L, Baryd I: Ophthalmologic observations on long-term survivors after radiotherapy for nasopharyngeal tumors, *Acta Radiol Ther Phys Biol* 10:193-209, 1971.
25. Shukovsky LJ, Fletcher GH: Retinal and optic nerve complications in a high dose irradiation technique of ethmoid sinus and nasal cavity, *Radiology* 104:629, 1972.
26. Bagan SM, Hollenhorst RW: Radiation retinopathy after irradiation of intracranial lesions, *Am J Ophthalmol* 88:694-697, 1979.
27. Nakissa N, Rubin P, Strohl R, Keys H: Ocular and orbital complications following radiation therapy of paranasal sinus malignancies and review of literature, *Cancer* 51:980-986, 1983.
28. Midena E, Segato T, Piermarocchi S, et al: Retinopathy following radiation therapy of paranasal sinus and nasopharyngeal carcinoma, *Retina* 7:141-147, 1987.
29. Elsas T, Thorud E, Jetne V, Conradi IS: Retinopathy after low dose irradiation for an intracranial tumor of the frontal lobe, *Acta Ophthalmol* 66:65-68, 1988.
30. Parsons JT, Mendenhall WM, Mancuso AA, et al: Malignant tumors of the nasal cavity and ethmoid and sphenoid sinuses, *Int J Radiat Oncol Biol Phys* 14:11-22, 1988.
31. Amoaku WMK, Archer DB: Cephalic radiation and retinal vasculopathy, *Eye* 4:195-203, 1990.
32. Kinyoun JL, Kalina RE, Brower SA, et al: Radiation retinopathy after orbital irradiation for Graves' ophthalmopathy, *Arch Ophthalmol* 102:1473-1476, 1984.
33. Bessel EM, Henk JM, Whitelocke RA, Wright JE: Ocular morbidity after radiotherapy of orbital and conjunctival lymphoma, *Eye* 1:90-96, 1987.
34. Brown GC, Brown MM, Hiller T, et al: Cotton-wool spots, *Retina* 5:206-214, 1985.
35. Brady LW, Shields JA, Augsburger JJ, et al: Complications from radiation therapy to the eye. In Vaeth JM, Meyer JL (eds): *Radiation tolerance of normal tissues: frontiers of radiation therapy and oncology,* Basel, 1989, S Karger, pp 238-250.
36. Merriam GR, Szechter A, Focht EF: The effects of ionizing radiations on the eye, *Front Radiat Ther Oncol* 6:346-385, 1972.
37. Irvine AR, Alvarado JA, Wara WM, et al: Radiation retinopathy: an experimental model for the ischemic-proliferative retinopathies, *Trans Am Ophthalmol Soc* 79:103-119, 1981.
38. Irvine AR, Wood IS: Radiation retinopathy as an experimental model for ischemic proliferative retinopathy and rubeosis iridis, *Am J Ophthalmol* 103:790-797, 1987.
39. Viebahn M, Barricks ME, Osterloh MD: Synergism between diabetic and radiation retinopathy: case report and review, *Br J Ophthalmol* 75:629-632, 1991.
40. Wara WM, Irvine AR, Neger RE, et al: Radiation retinopathy, *Int J Radiat Oncol Biol Phys* 5:81-83, 1979.
41. Lopez PF, Sternberg P, Dabbs CK, et al: Bone-marrow transplant retinopathy, *Am J Ophthalmol* 112:635-646, 1991.

42. Weaver RG, Chauvenet AR, Smith TJ, Schwartz AC: Ophthalmic evaluation of long-term survivors of childhood acute lymphoblastic leukemia, *Cancer* 58:963-968, 1986.
43. Noble KG, Kupersmith MJ: Retinal vascular remodeling in radiation retinopathy, *Br J Ophthalmol* 68:475-478, 1984.
44. Kinyoun JL, Chittum ME, Wells CG: Photocoagulation treatment of radiation retinopathy, *Am J Ophthalmol* 105:470-478, 1988.
45. Diabetic Retinopathy Study Research Group: Photocoagulation treatment of proliferative diabetic retinopathy: the second report of diabetic retinopathy findings, *Ophthalmology* 85:82-106, 1978.
46. Early Treatment Diabetic Retinopathy Study Research Group: Early photocoagulation for diabetic retinopathy, *Ophthalmology* 98:766-785, 1991.

20

Ocular Ischemic Syndrome

Gary C. Brown

In 1963 Kearns and Hollenhorst [1] published on an entity they called venous stasis retinopathy. Since that time a number of alternative nomenclatures have arisen for this group of ocular symptoms and signs attributable to severe carotid artery obstruction. Included among them are ischemic ocular inflammation,[2] ischemic oculopathy,[3] and the ocular ischemic syndrome.[4] This last term will be used throughout the remainder of the present chapter.

Approximately 5% of people with marked carotid artery stenosis manifest the ocular ischemic syndrome.[1] In general, a 90% or greater stenosis is necessary to induce the symptom complex.[5] It has been estimated[6] that 90% stenosis of the carotid artery reduces the ipsilateral central retinal artery perfusion pressure by about 50%.

Some demographic data can be drawn from a recent large series of patients with the ocular ischemic syndrome.[5] The mean age at the time of presentation is about 65 years, with a range from the 50s to the 80s. Men are affected more than women, by a ratio of about 2:1, but there is no known racial predilection. Approximately 20% of cases are bilateral.

The prevalence of the disease is uncertain. Nevertheless, from the work of Sturrock and Mueller[7] in England, it can be estimated that at least 7.5 cases per million people per year will develop the ocular ischemic syndrome. In actuality, this number is probably low since many cases may go unrecognized.

PRESENTING SYMPTOMS

More than 90% of affected individuals relate a history of recent visual loss in the affected eye(s).[5] In approximately two thirds the loss occurs over a period of weeks or months. Roughly 10% to 15% of patients experience an abrupt visual loss, usually because of the development of acute retinal ischemia with a cherry-red spot.[5] A history of amaurosis fugax is elicited in about 10% of patients. Some people experience prolonged recovery of vision after exposure to bright light, a phenomenon that probably occurs secondary to posterior segment ischemia adversely affecting retinal metabolism.[8]

Pain is encountered in about 40% of cases.[5] It is typically ipsilateral to the affected eye in the orbital region and is characterized as a dull ache. Its causes may be ischemia of the globe, increased intraocular pressure in cases with neovascular glaucoma, ischemia of the ipsilateral dura, or a combination of these mechanisms.

CLINICAL FINDINGS

At the time of presentation, rubeosis iridis (Fig. 20-1) is seen in about two thirds of eyes.[5] Nevertheless, the intraocular pressure (IOP) is increased in only half these eyes, in some cases even if the anterior chamber is closed by fibrovascular tissue. This probably occurs secondary to impaired ciliary perfusion, leading to decreased aqueous production.

Flare is usually seen in the anterior chamber of eyes with rubeosis iridis.[5] In nearly 20% of eyes with the ocular ischemic syndrome a cellular response in the anterior chamber is also present, sometimes in association with mild keratic precipitates. The cellular response rarely exceeds Grade 2 of the Schlaegel classification.[9]

Posterior segment signs[5] include narrowed retinal arteries and dilated (but generally not tortuous) retinal veins (Fig. 20-2). Retinal hemorrhages are seen in about 80% of eyes and are most often of the dot and blot variety, usually most pronounced in the midperiphery. In some cases they are also present in the posterior pole (Figs. 20-3 and 20-4). Microaneurysms are frequently observed in the midperiphery (Fig. 20-5) but, additionally, can be seen in the posterior pole.

Neovascularization of the disc (NVD) (Fig. 20-6) is found in about 35% of eyes whereas neovascularization elsewhere (NVE) (i.e., of the retina) has been noted in 8%.[5] Vitreous hemorrhage can arise from both these forms of neovascularization, and in severe cases fibrovascular proliferation may develop. In about one of eight cases a cherry-red spot appears. This can be due to inner retinal ischemia from an embolus within the central retinal artery, or, alternatively, it can occur when the IOP exceeds the perfusion pressure within the central retinal artery.

Additional posterior segment signs[5] include cotton-wool spots (6%) (Fig. 20-7), spontaneous retinal arterial pulsations (4%), and cholesterol emboli (2%). Anterior ischemic optic atrophy has been associated in 2% of cases.[5] A summary of anterior and posterior segment signs seen with the ocular ischemic syndrome is shown in Table 20-1.

Diseases associated with atherosclerosis are often encountered in patients with the ocular ischemic syndrome.[10] Approximately three fourths of patients have systemic arterial hypertension, and over half are diabetic. Nearly half the patients have ischemic heart disease, and about one fourth have had a stroke by the time they present with ocular symptoms and signs. Nearly one fifth have already required previous bypass surgery for the sequelae of peripheral vascular disease. The annual stroke rate for patients with the ocular ischemic syndrome is about 4%. The 5-year mortality rate is 40%, with two thirds of people succumbing to cardiovascular disease.

Intravenous fluorescein angiography demonstrates several features[5]: Normally the choroid is completely filled within 5 seconds of the first appearance of dye within it. In 60% of eyes there is delayed and patchy choroidal filling

Figure 20-1 Fluorescein angiogram of the iris in an eye with the ocular ischemic syndrome. Leakage of dye is present in the areas of iris neovascularization.

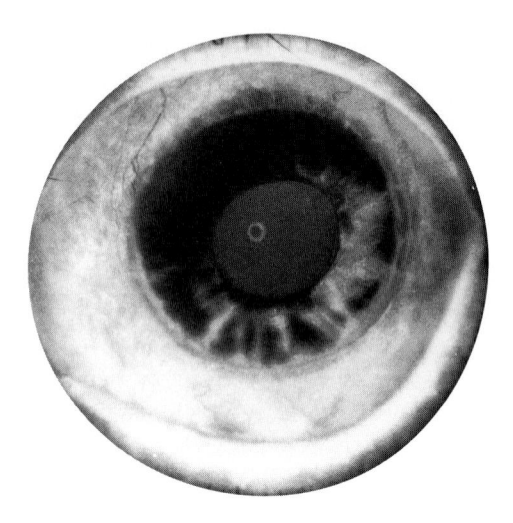

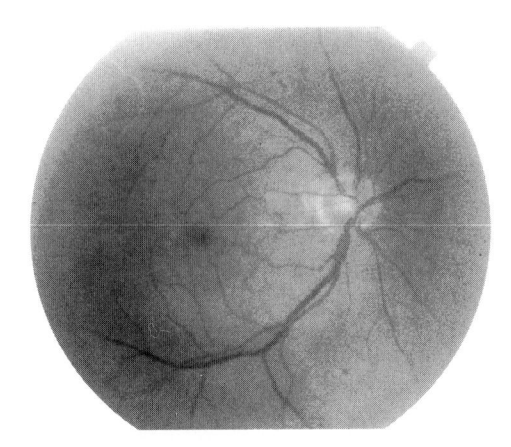

Figure 20-2 Fundus of an eye with the ocular ischemic syndrome. The retinal arteries are narrowed, and the retinal veins slightly dilated but not tortuous. A number of small retinal hemorrhages are scattered throughout the posterior pole.

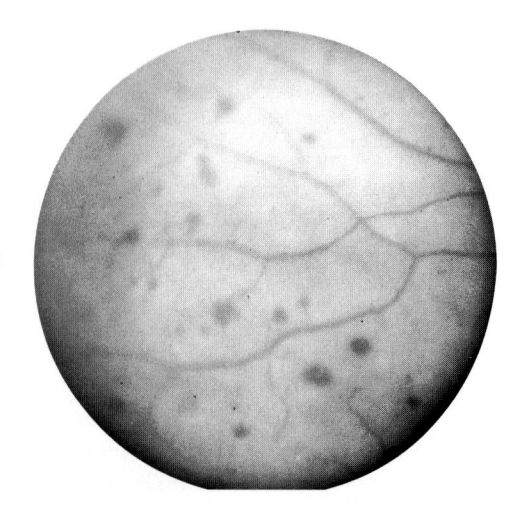

Figure 20-3 Midperipheral dot and blot retinal hemorrhages in an eye with the ocular ischemic syndrome.

Ocular ischemic syndrome

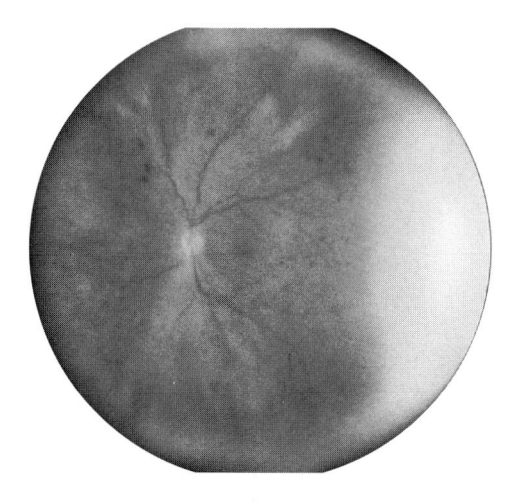

Figure 20-4 Midperipheral retinal hemorrhages in an eye with the ocular ischemic syndrome (equator-plus photograph).

Figure 20-5 Fluorescein angiogram of the midperiphery of an eye with the ocular ischemic syndrome. The numerous foci of hyperfluorescence correspond to microaneurysms. Staining of the retinal vessels can also be seen.

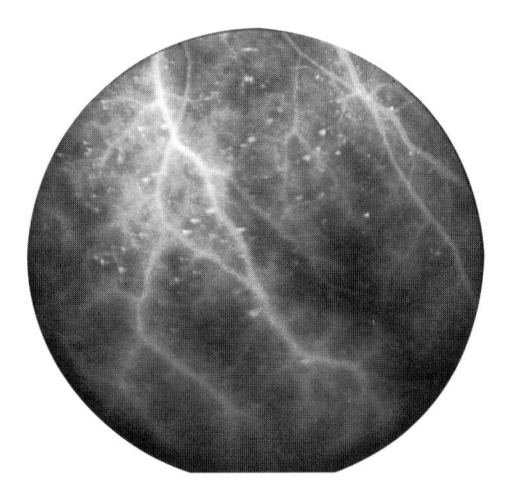

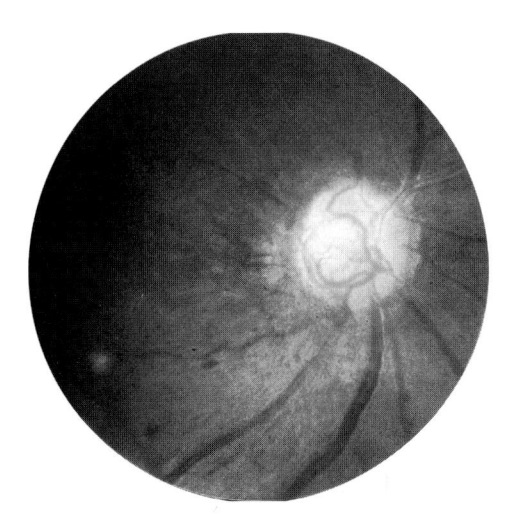

Figure 20-6 Neovascularization of the disc in a nondiabetic patient with the ocular ischemic syndrome. The retinal veins are dilated and slightly beaded.

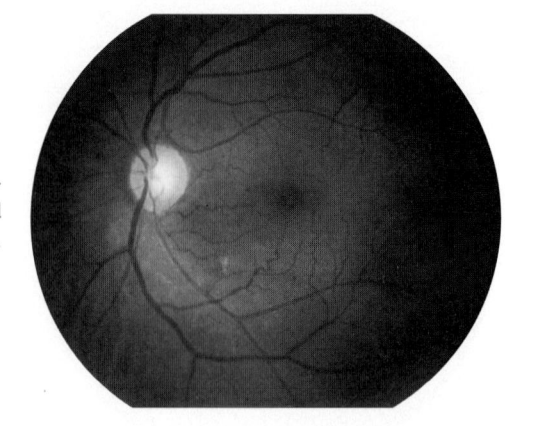

Figure 20-7 A single cotton-wool spot, occasional retinal dot hemorrhages, and mildly dilated retinal veins in an ocular ischemic syndrome eye.

Table 20-1 Signs Associated with the Ocular Ischemic Syndrome

	Percent
Anterior segment	
Rubeosis iridis	67
Neovascular glaucoma (rubeosis and IOP >22 mm Hg)	35
Uveitis (cells and flare)	18
Posterior segment	
Narrowed retinal arteries	Common
Dilated (not tortuous) retinal veins	Common
Retinal hemorrhages	80
Neovascularization	
Of optic disc	35
Of retina	8
Cherry-red spot	12
Cotton-wool spot(s)	6
Vitreous hemorrhage	4
Spontaneous retinal arterial pulsations	4
Retinal arterial emboli	2

From Brown GC, Margaral LE: *Int Ophthalmol* 11:239-251, 1988.

(Fig. 20-8). This is one of the most specific signs for the ocular ischemic syndrome. The retinal arteriovenous transit time (i.e., from the first appearance of dye within the arteries of the temporal vascular arcade until the corresponding veins are completely filled; normal <11 seconds) is prolonged in 95% of eyes. Hyperfluorescent microaneurysms are frequently encountered (Fig. 20-5), and staining of the larger retinal vessels is seen in 85% of eyes (Fig. 20-9). The leakage of dye is generally more prominent in the arteries than in the veins, although both can be involved. A fluorescein angiographic pattern of macular edema is found in about one of six eyes. Discrete retinal capillary nonperfusion is variably present. A summary of the fluorescein angiographic signs seen with the ocular ischemic syndrome is shown in Table 20-2.

Ocular ischemic syndrome 281

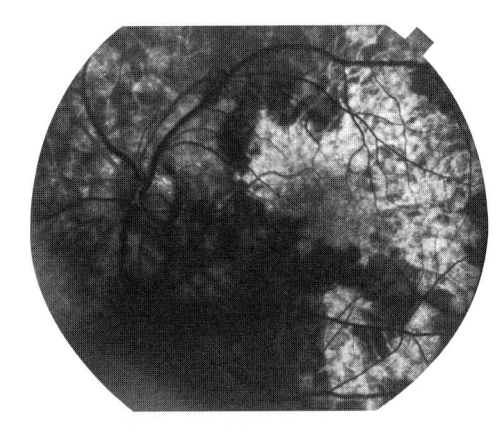

Figure 20-8 Fluorescein angiogram demonstrating patchy delayed choroidal filling in an eye with a severe ipsilateral carotid artery stenosis.

Figure 20-9 Fluorescein angiogram at almost 9 minutes after injection in an eye with the ocular ischemic syndrome and an ipsilateral 100% common carotid artery stenosis. Note the marked staining of the large retinal vessels, particularly the arteries.

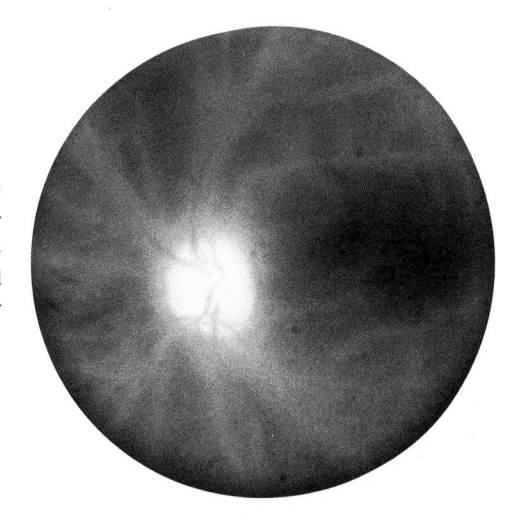

Table 20-2 Fluorescein Angiographic Signs Seen with the Ocular Ischemic Syndrome

	Percent
Delayed and patchy choroidal filling	60
Prolonged retinal arteriovenous transit time (>11 seconds)	95
Retinal vascular staining	85
Macular edema	17
Other	
Microaneurysms	
Retinal capillary nonperfusion	
Hyperfluorescence of disc	

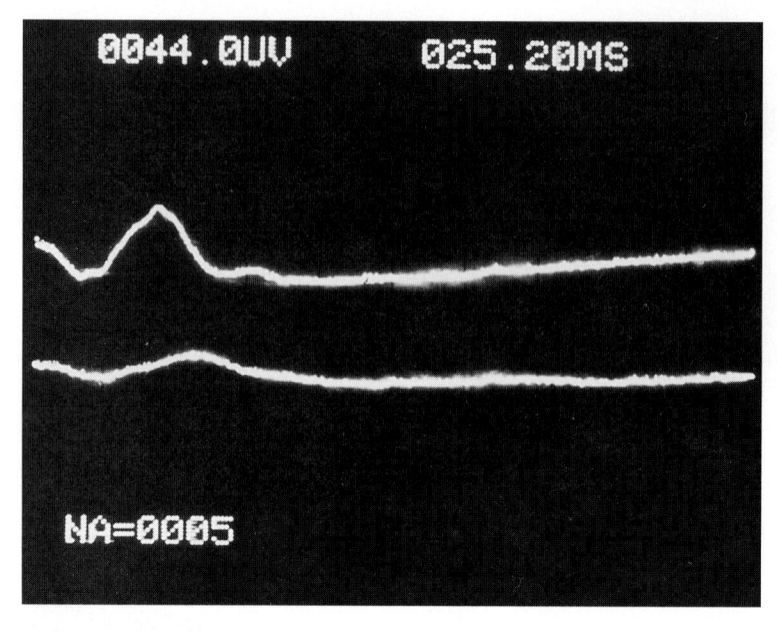

Figure 20-10 Electroretinographic tracings of a normal right eye *(above)* and a left eye *(below)* with the ocular ischemic syndrome. The amplitudes of the a- and b-waves are diminished in the eye with the ocular ischemic syndrome.

Electroretinography (Fig. 20-10) may demonstrate diminution of a- and b-waves.[5,11] The a-wave reflects photoreceptor function and can be compromised with choroidal ischemia. The b-wave most likely corresponds to the function of bipolar and Mueller cells in the inner retina and can be diminished by compromised flow within the retinal vascular system.

DIFFERENTIAL DIAGNOSIS

Most cases of the of the ocular ischemic syndrome occur secondary to carotid artery stenosis. The aortic arch syndrome (obstruction of the major arteries as they branch from the aorta) can produce the same clinical picture as an obstruction more distal within the carotid system.[12] Chronic ophthalmic artery obstruction is also a cause.[5,13,14] Manifestations of the entity have even been seen[15] with embolic obstruction of the central retinal artery on the disc.

The vast majority of cases occur secondary to atherosclerosis. Other causes include dissecting aneurysm, syphilitis aortitis, giant cell arteritis, and Takayasu's disease.

Entities with findings that can closely mimic those seen with the ocular ischemic syndrome include diabetic retinopathy and mild (nonischemic) central retinal vein obstruction. Features that help differentiate between the entities are listed in Table 20-3.

Diabetic retinopathy can be particularly difficult to differentiate since patients with the ocular ischemic syndrome not uncommonly have associated diabetic retinopathy. The presence of severe proliferative retinopathy in one eye and only mild or moderate background changes in the contralateral eye should alert the clinician that a carotid stenosis might be a contributory factor in the

Table 20-3 Features that Differentiate the Ocular Ischemic Syndrome (OIS), Nonischemic Central Retinal Vein Obstruction (CRVO), and Diabetic Retinopathy (DR)

	OIS	*CRVO*	*DR*
Laterality	Unilateral (80%)	Unilateral	Bilateral
Age	50s to 80s	50s to 80s	Variable
Fundus signs			
Veins	Dilated, beaded	Dilated, tortuous	Dilated, beaded
Disc	Normal	Swollen	Normal
Retinal artery perfusion pressure	Decreased	Normal	Normal
Retinal hemorrhages	Mild	Mild to severe	Mild to moderate
Microaneurysms	Midperiphery	Variable	Posterior pole
Hard exudates	None (unless concomitant DR)	Rare	Common
Fluorescein angiography			
Choroidal filling	Delayed	Normal	Normal
Retinal AV transit	Prolonged	Prolonged	Normal
Vessel staining	More arterial	More venous	Usually absent

From Brown GC: In Ryan SJ (ed): *Retina,* St Louis, 1989, Mosby, vol 2, Chapter 88.

eye with severe proliferative disease.[16] It should be remembered that it takes approximately 70% stenosis within a carotid vessel before there is significant compromise of flow. Therefore a mild carotid stenosis would be expected to have little effect on diabetic retinopathy. Although severe carotid stenoses can probably exacerbate proliferative diabetic retinopathy, it is uncertain whether milder degrees have a protective effect on the development of background and/or proliferative changes.

The presence of hard exudates in the fundus suggests diabetic retinopathy and is generally not seen in the ocular ischemic syndrome alone. Microaneurysms can be found with both diseases, but are usually more pronounced in the posterior pole with diabetic retinopathy and in the midperiphery with the ocular ischemic syndrome. Bilaterality is generally the rule with diabetic retinopathy but is encountered in only 20% of cases of the ocular ischemic syndrome.[5] When rubeosis iridis is present in an eye that appears to have only minimal diabetic retinopathy, the ocular ischemic syndrome should be considered. Among all cases of rubeosis iridis, retinal vein obstruction accounts for about a third, diabetic retinopathy for another third, and the ocular ischemic syndrome for another 12%.[17]

Milder, or nonischemic, central retinal vein obstruction can closely mimic the ocular ischemic syndrome. In central retinal vein obstruction the veins tend to be dilated and tortuous because of the outflow obstruction. In the ocular ischemic syndrome, in which there is an inflow obstruction, they are dilated and sometimes beaded but generally not tortuous. The dilation may be a nonspecific response to ischemia. Additionally, the retinal hemorrhages are often more pronounced in eyes with central retinal vein obstruction than eyes with the ocular ischemic syndrome.

Kearns[18] has pointed out a helpful sign to differentiate between central retinal vein obstruction and the ocular ischemic syndrome. Eyes with the OIS have a low retinal arterial perfusion pressure and, consequently, low ophthalmodynamometry readings. In the absence of an ophthalmodynamometer, light digital palpation on the lid of the affected eye will induce retinal arterial pulsations. With CRVO the arterial perfusion pressure is not diminished.

The presence of delayed choroidal filling is found by fluorescein angiography in 60% of eyes with the ocular ischemic syndrome but generally not in eyes with diabetic retinopathy. Staining of the larger retinal vessels is most often absent with diabetic retinopathy but is frequently seen in the ocular ischemic syndrome; staining of the retinal veins can be present in eyes with central retinal vein obstruction.

TREATMENT

The most effective treatment for eyes with the ocular ischemic syndrome is uncertain. The presence of rubeosis iridis implies a particularly grim prognosis, since over 95% of such eyes have a visual acuity of counting fingers or less within a year, with or without treatment.[19] In the largest series of patients reported with the ocular ischemic syndrome,[19] 43% of eyes presented with a visual acuity of 20/20 to 20/50 whereas at the end of 1 year only 24% remained in this group. In the same series 37% of eyes initially had an acuity of counting fingers or worse as compared to 58% of eyes after a year's follow-up.

Ocular therapy, in the form of full scatter laser panretinal photocoagulation, has been shown[19] to cause regression of rubeosis iridis in about 35% of ocular ischemic syndrome eyes. Nevertheless, this may well be just a temporizing procedure unless blood flow can be restored to the eye via an endarterectomy.

When a 100% carotid artery stenosis is present, as occurs in approximately 60% of eyes with the ocular ischemic syndrome,[19] carotid endarterectomy is generally ineffective. This occurs, in part, because a thrombus often propagates proximally from the site of obstruction to the next major vessel. Extracranial-to-intracranial bypass surgery has previously been attempted in such cases. Although it has been shown to benefit visual acuity in about 20% of cases over the short term, at the end of 1 year's follow-up there appears to be no beneficial visual effect in eyes with the ocular ischemic syndrome.[19] Additionally, extracranial-to-intracranial bypass surgery has not been shown to reduce the incidence of ischemic stroke compared to medical treatment.[20]

Carotid endarterectomy is of some benefit in stabilizing and improving vision in selected eyes with the ocular ischemic syndrome.[19,21] The exact percentage of patients who benefit from this therapy is unknown, but it is probably a safe assumption that eyes in which the syndrome is discovered at an earlier stage have a more favorable prognosis. It has been shown[22] that patients with a hemispheric transient ischemic attack, amaurosis fugax, or nondisabling stroke who have a 70% to 99% ipsilateral carotid artery stenosis benefit as a group from carotid endarterectomy. The incidence of subsequent stroke within 2 years of an endarterectomy in these patients is approximately 9%; for a comparable group treated by antiplatelet therapy alone it is approximately 26%. Nearly one third of eyes with the ocular ischemic syndrome have a 70% to 99% ipsilateral carotid stenosis as the cause.[19]

References

1. Kearns TP, Hollenhorst RW: Venous-stasis retinopathy of occlusive disease of the carotid artery, *Proc Mayo Clin* 38:304-312, 1963.
2. Knox DL: Ischemic ocular inflammation, *Am J Ophthalmol* 60:995-1002, 1965.
3. Young LHY, Appen RE: Ischemic oculopathy: a manifestation of carotid artery disease, *Arch Neurol* 38:358-361, 1981.
4. Brown GC, Magargal LE, Simeone FA, et al: Arterial obstruction and ocular neovascularization, *Ophthalmology* 89:139-146, 1982.
5. Brown GC, Magargal LE: The ocular ischemic syndrome: clinical, fluorescein angiographic, and carotid angiographic features, *Int Ophthalmol* 11:239-251, 1988.
6. Kearns TP: Ophthalmology and the carotid artery, *Am J Ophthalmol* 88:714-722, 1979.
7. Sturrock GD, Mueller HR: Chronic ocular ischaemia, *Br J Ophthalmol* 68:716-723, 1984.
8. Jacobs NA, Ridgway AEA: Syndrome of ischaemic ocular inflammation: six cases and a review, *Br J Ophthalmol* 69:681-687, 1985.
9. Schlaegel T: Symptoms and signs of uveitis. In Duane TD (ed): *Clinical ophthalmology*, Hagerstown Md, 1983, Harper & Row, vol 4, pp 1-7.
10. Sivalingam A, Brown GC, Magargal LE, Menduke H: The ocular ischemic syndrome. II. Mortality and systemic morbidity, *Int Ophthalmol* 13:187-191, 1989.
11. Carr RE, Siegel JM: Electrophysiologic aspects of several retinal diseases, *Am J Ophthalmol* 58:95-107, 1964.
12. Bolling J, Goldberg RE, Brown GC: Aortic arch syndrome. In Gold DH, Weingeist TA (eds): *The eye in systemic disease*, Philadelphia, 1990, JB Lippincott, pp 647-649.
13. Madsen PH: Venous-stasis retinopathy insufficiency of the ophthalmic artery, *Acta Ophthalmol* 44:940-947, 1965.
14. Bullock JD, Falter RT, Downing JE, Snyder H: Ischemic ophthalmia secondary to an ophthalmic artery occlusion, *Am J Ophthalmol* 74:486-493, 1972.
15. Magargal LE, Sanborn GE, Zimmerman A: Venous stasis retinopathy associated with embolic obstruction of the central retinal artery, *J Clin Neuroophthalmol* 2:113-118, 1982.
16. Duker J, Colt C, Brown GC, Bosley T: Asymmetric diabetic retinopathy and carotid artery obstructive disease, *Ophthalmology* 97:869-874, 1990.
17. Brown GC, Magargal LE, Schachat A, Shah H: Neovascular glaucoma: etiologic considerations, *Ophthalmology* 91:315-319, 1984.
18. Kearns TP: Differential diagnosis of central retinal vein obstruction, *Ophthalmology* 90:475-490, 1983.
19. Sivalingam A, Brown GC, Magargal LE: The ocular ischemic syndrome. III. Visual prognosis and the effect of treatment, *Int Ophthalmol* 15:15-20, 1991.
20. EC/IC Bypass Study Group: The failure of extracranial-intracranial bypass to reduce the risk of ischemic stroke: results of an international randomized trial, *N Engl J Med* 313:1191-1200, 1985.
21. Johnston ME, Gonder J, Canny CL: Successful treatment of the ocular ischemic syndrome with panretinal photocoagulation and cerebrovascular surgery, *Can J Ophthalmol* 23:114-119, 1988.
22. North American Symptomatic Carotid Endarterectomy Trial Collaborators: Beneficial effect of carotid endarterectomy in symptomatic patients with high-grade carotid stenosis, *N Engl J Med* 325:445-453, 1991.

PART IV

Inflammatory Disease

21

Ocular Toxoplasmosis

David H. Fischer

Toxoplasma, an intracellular obligate protozoal parasite, is one of the more common causes of posterior uveitis and associated visual morbidity.[14,37,48] The clinical findings and suggestive history of toxoplasmosis, with laboratory confirmation, are often characteristic, allowing the clinician to make a diagnosis of ocular infection and afford specific rational treatment.

CLINICAL DIAGNOSIS

The hallmark of toxoplasmosis is retinochoroiditis; the organism creates retinal inflammation with spillover into the vitreous gel and underlying choroid.[12] This is usually in a localized zone within the retinal architecture, but in some cases it can be multifocal. The exact nature of the lesions often depends on the manner in which the disease was acquired. In-utero involvement in a previously healthy noninfected mother who acquires a systemic toxoplasmic infection during pregnancy can lead to the infant's developing the stigmas of ocular and systemic toxoplasmosis.[5,22,25,51] These include retinochoroidal scarring and systemic complications at birth depending on the protozoal load, the time frame in which the infection occurred during pregnancy, and the immune status. Individuals who later develop recurrent toxoplasmic ocular infections have old retinochoroidal scars along the edge of active inflammation in which the inactive tissue cysts break down along the edge of the scarred area. In addition, active trophozoites create contiguous cellular destruction with subsequent tissue loss and resultant inflammation.[38,39] This is almost pathognomonic for toxoplasmic retinochoroiditis. Classically the history includes "spots and floaters," the result of debris entering the vitreous cavity from an infectious nidus with subsequent blurring of vision. Depending on the amount of debris and the site of retinochoroiditis, the clinician generally has only to recognize this presentation and institute appropriate treatment. Laboratory testing may help confirm the diagnosis but is not essential.

Toxoplasmic retinochoroiditis may be unilateral or bilateral, but in recurrent disease it is usually one sided. If looked for diligently, scars can often be noted from past infection in both eyes. A detailed history will disclose that episodes of floaters with blurred vision have occurred in the past, frequently lasting a number of weeks with clearing in 1 to 2 months.

The lesions can range from punctate areas deep in the retina to large geographic zones of retinitis. If they are located in the peripheral retina central, vision is compromised only by the blur caused by vitreous debris from inflammatory cells (Fig. 21-1). If the active lesions are in the macular region, however, central visual loss with potential blindness can result from foveal involvement in the necrotizing granulomatous retinochoroiditis process. If the infectious area is close to the optic nerve, secondary optic neuritis may occur with damage to the nerve fibers in the involved zone and visual field damage with scotomas[11,17,49] (Fig. 21-2). Lesions that involve large vessels along the vascular arcades may, through necrotizing inflammation, develop obstruction of large arteries and veins with all types of vascular complications (Figs. 21-3 and 21-4), including arterial and venous obstruction, vasculitis, and in late cases choroidal neovascularization (Figs. 21-5 and 21-6) with secondary bleeding and exudation. Central involvement creates severe visual loss.

The acquired form of the disease is usually caused by ingestion of oocysts from uncooked meat or by inhalation of the organism, most commonly from the dried aerosolized excreta of cats that have themselves acquired the infection.[19,23,42] Avoidance of rare or uncooked meats and changing cat litter at 24-hour intervals can reduce the spread of the disease. The primary systemic disease is quite common and causes an influenza-like syndrome with lymphadenopathy and malaise, often mistaken for upper respiratory infection. In an estimated 2% to 3% of individuals the blood-borne infection reaches the eye, creating a localized retinochoroiditis.[1,29] The initial ocular infection may go unnoticed, especially if the site is extramacular, with healing over a 6- to 8-week period. In recurrent disease there are often anterior segment findings not seen in primary involvement (Fig. 21-7). Characteristically, granulomatous uveitis occurs with mutton-fat keratic precipitates, mild cellular reaction, occasional hyperemia of the iris vessels, and a ciliary flush. Intraocular pressure will frequently be elevated, a helpful clue indicating that one is dealing with recurrent ocular toxoplasmosis (since other forms of anterior uveitis can cause mild hypotony).[12] It is thought[26] that anterior segment findings may be related to immune reaction to the toxoplasma antigen liberated in the posterior segment during recurrent disease. This anterior involvement is not seen in the primary infection. Care must be taken therefore in evaluating an individual who presents with anterior granulomatous uveitis. The fundus must be carefully examined for zones of retinochoroiditis, indicating posterior segment activity and a diagnosis of recurrent disease. The clinician will generally be rewarded with the underlying cause of the anterior chamber findings and thus will make the correct diagnosis and prescribe correct therapy.

The toxoplasmic infection to the eye may be quite severe; however, because a spectrum of disease exists, some forms are mild and will heal spontaneously without severe scarring in the immune-competent host. Severe involvement can cause development of full-thickness retinal and choroidal tissue loss, leaving a window defect in the sclera if not treated early and aggressively (Fig. 21-8). A chronic form of retinochoroiditis can persist, often causing severe vitritis with large geographic areas of inflammation and necrosis (Fig. 21-9).

The initial onset of "spots and floaters" is due to the cell-mediated response

Ocular toxoplasmosis 291

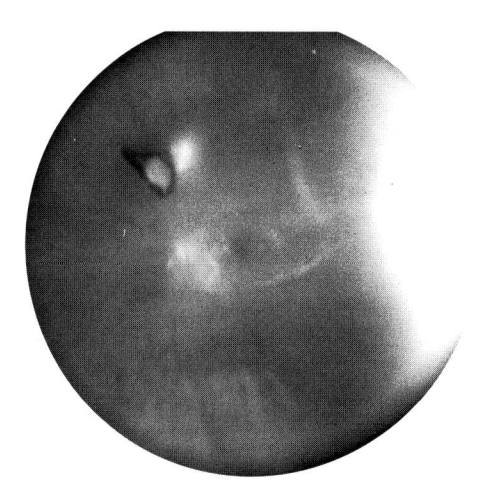

Figure 21-1 Left eye with a lesion approximately four disc diameters in the 11 o'clock area superior and slightly nasal to the optic disc. Note the pigmented chorioretinal scar with a temporal focus of active retinitis (equator-plus photograph). From the patient's standpoint, the lesion itself was asymptomatic; however, the vitreous reaction that can be seen overlying the macular region created floaters and diminished visual function, prompting the patient to seek treatment. Although fundus evaluation showed the characteristic findings of ocular toxoplasmosis, the initial symptoms were "spots and floaters."

Figure 21-2 Healed toxoplasmic retinochoroiditis scar with secondary pigment dispersion. The visual field shows an inferior arcuate defect related to that quadrant.

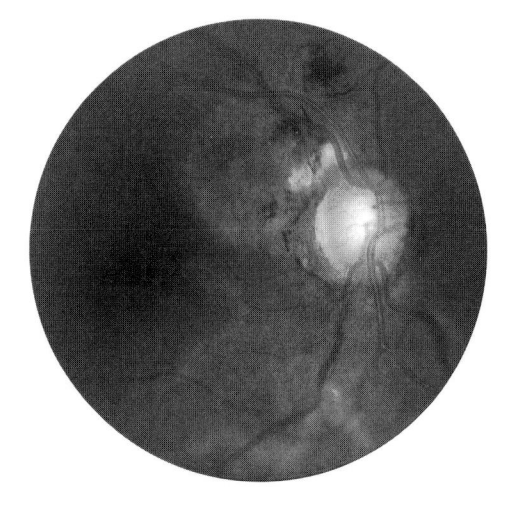

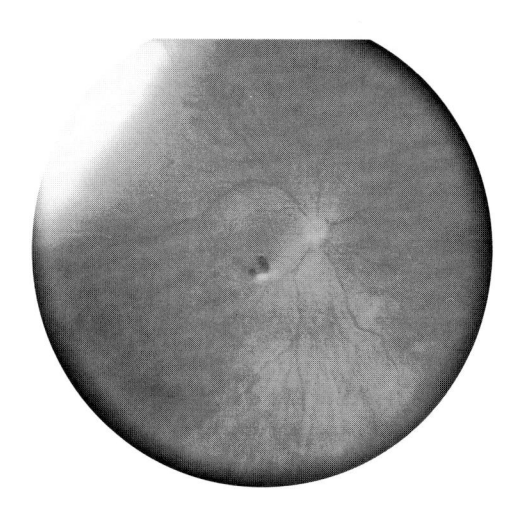

Figure 21-3 Right eye with retinitis and pigment along the inferior arcade (equator-plus wide-angle photograph). An inferotemporal sectoral hemorrhagic venous obstruction is the vascular complication of this inflammatory lesion.

Figure 21-4 Pigmented alteration along the macular edge of the inferior arcade from an old toxoplasmic scar (close-up of the lesion in Figure 21-3). Abutting this arcade is a fluffy retinitis that has created a venous obstruction secondary to acute inflammation.

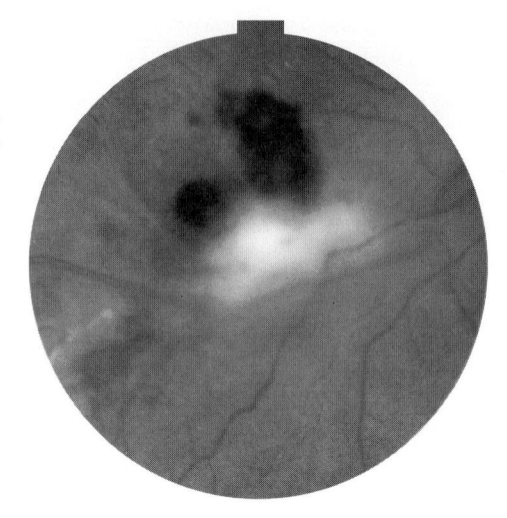

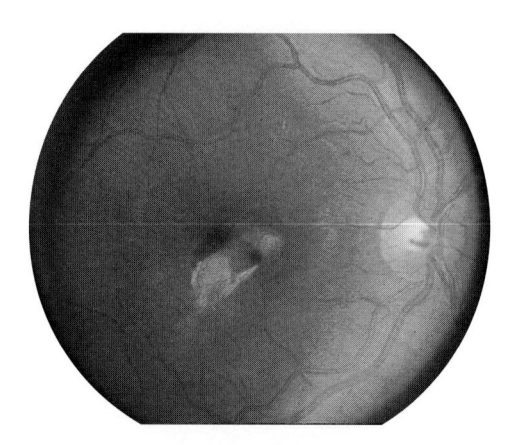

Figure 21-5 Old chorioretinal scar just inferotemporal to fixation. Note the subretinal lesion with secondary serous fluid from a choroidal neovascularization next to the scar and involving fixation.

Figure 21-6 Fluorescein angiogram revealing an active hyperfluorescent cap next to the old chorioretinal scar involving fixation in the patient in Figure 21-5. This choroidal neovascular membrane is an uncommon, but vision-threatening, complication of healed ocular toxoplasmosis.

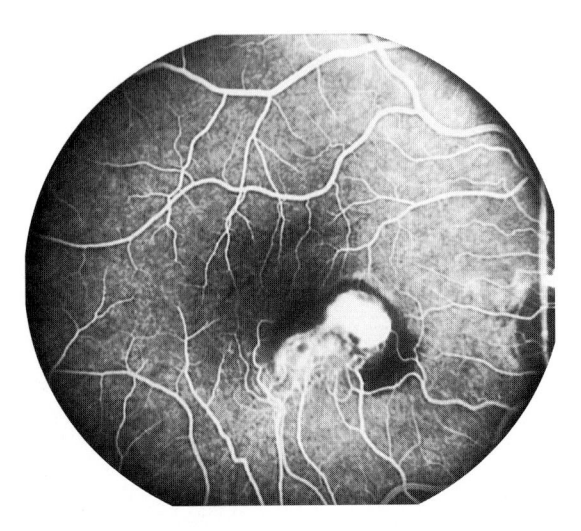

Figure 21-7 Granulomatous keratinic precipitates in the anterior segment with recurrent posterior ocular toxoplasmic retinochoroiditis and secondary glaucoma (high-powered slit-lamp photograph).

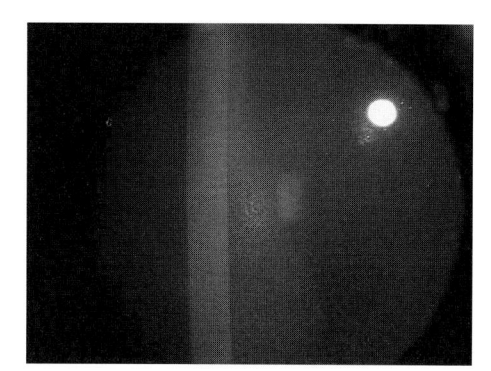

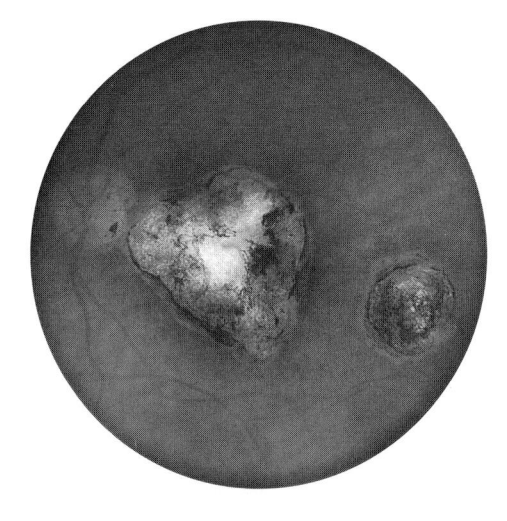

Figure 21-8 A dense macular scar has created irreversible loss of central visual function. White sclera can be seen because the retinal/choroidal inflammation has left a complete but thinned scar ("macular coloboma"). Note the peripheral lesion temporal to the scar, quite common in recurrent ocular toxoplasmic infection.

of the active infection. As the cells are shed into the vitreous cavity, symptoms evolve. Some strains of *Toxoplasma* are more virulent than others and can create a much greater inflammatory response in the eye. This results in greater severity and more damage to the underlying tissues. The vitreous debris may become so extensive that vision is compromised The clinician must search diligently through the vitreous haze looking for the "headlight in the fog" lesion that is the active retinitis. Precipitates will often occur on the back surface of the vitreous face, yielding a characteristic clinical picture (Figs. 21-9 and 21-10). This chronic smoldering manifestation of the disease is labeled endophthalmitic toxoplasmosis. It often accompanies the chronic use of corticosteroids, either orally or periocularly, with no antibiotic coverage. High-dose steroids are immune compromising, allowing the organism to proliferate, retarding healing, and taking 6 to 12 months to clear. For this reason the use of periocular sub-Tenon injections of corticosteroids for toxoplasmosis is contraindicated.[27]

Another characteristic finding that may be helpful in the clinical diagnosis of toxoplasmic retinochoroiditis is a peculiar vasculitis that can be seen in the distribution of vessels around the lesion[2,30,50,53] (Fig. 21-11). It is thought to be caused by immune complex deposition on the vessel walls.[2] Fluorescein angiography reveals good transit of dye through this characteristic vasculitis, which affects both arteries and veins. The clinical findings of vitritis, a focal zone of retinitis, and this secondary vasculitis are generally pathognomonic for ocular toxoplasmosis in the immune-competent host and should be looked for carefully.

Figure 21-9 Large chorioretinal scars with healing from the outer edges inward, especially in the superior lesion. There is still a central necrotic cap of tissue creating chronic posterior vitritis and inflammation. Punctate yellowish precipitates can be seen on the partially detached back surface of the vitreous base, another common finding in the low-grade, chronic, endophthalmitic form of ocular toxoplasmic infection.

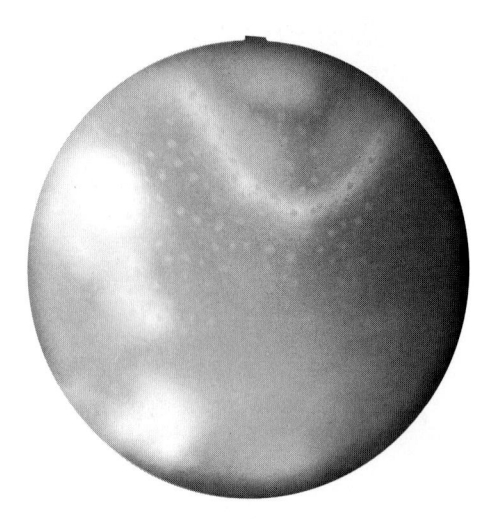

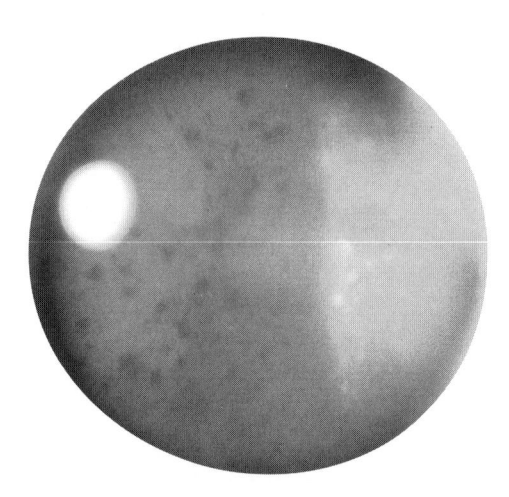

Figure 21-10 Severe exudation of granulomatous cells into the vitreous cavity (slit-lamp photograph). These often obscure the posterior segment in chronic endophthalmitic ocular toxoplasmosis.

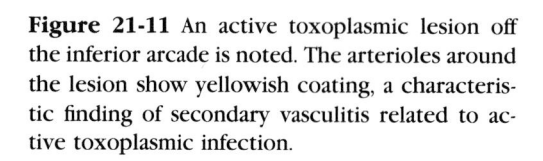

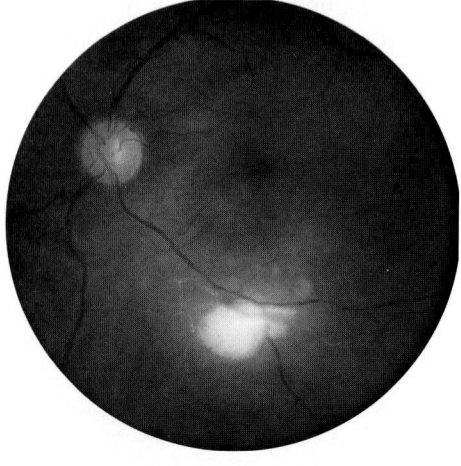

Figure 21-11 An active toxoplasmic lesion off the inferior arcade is noted. The arterioles around the lesion show yellowish coating, a characteristic finding of secondary vasculitis related to active toxoplasmic infection.

LABORATORY DIAGNOSIS

The laboratory diagnosis of ocular toxoplasmosis can be helpful in confirming the clinical diagnosis, but care should be taken with interpretation.[9,18,22] As noted, clinical findings may be characteristic and suggest the appropriate therapy.

If the clinician suspects a primary toxoplasmic infection, serum IgM antibody should be drawn.[7,8] Levels are elevated in the early stages of disease, up to 6 weeks. Serum IgG will then become elevated and remain positive for life.[47] A negative IgM with a positive IgG antibody suggests that toxoplasmosis has been present in the past and confirms the diagnosis of recurrent disease. The IgG level may fall to low titers over the years. Despite newer tests using very specific and sophisticated technology (e.g., the enzyme-linked immunosorbent assay [ELISA]),[22,33,34] one must remember that the local ocular antibody production is often quite small and may not be reflected in the systemic level. Even in undiluted serum, eyes can be teeming with toxoplasmic organisms yet systemic antibody levels are normal. Thus, any positive titer may help the clinician confirm the presence of ocular toxoplasmosis but does not necessarily reflect the severity of the disease. The diagnosis of ocular toxoplasmosis is still a clinical one, with secondary help from the laboratory.

Although not universally available, localized testing using aqueous or vitreous taps can be helpful in delineating local intraocular antibody production with increased antibody levels that may not be reflected in serum levels.[7,8] In the future, with newer techniques such as DNA probes and polymerase chain reaction to amplify minute antigen or antibody levels, the diagnosis may be made in the laboratory using ocular fluids.[3] At present, laboratory confirmation is helpful but not diagnostic.

Another diagnostic parameter is the biopsy of ocular tissues. Although reserved for unusual presentations, or diagnostic and therapeutic dilemmas, it may reveal toxoplasmic organisms within retinal tissues. For the immune-competent individual, however, these aggressive techniques are usually not required; the clinical picture is sufficient.

Ocular toxoplasmosis may also present in the immune-compromised host, but the characteristic patterns are somewhat different.* In AIDS a more diffuse form of toxoplasmic retinochoroiditis has been seen. Multifocal infiltrates and bilaterality may confuse the clinician. A high index of suspicion is indicated with associated systemic findings. Because the individual with AIDS has a poor T-cell response, the infection can become diffuse and bilateral and may mimic endogenous bacterial or fungal endophthalmitis. Biopsy can be of help, through either a partial-thickness eye-wall or a fine-needle aspiration technique (Fig. 21-12).

THERAPY

Therapy for toxoplasmosis may require an increased dosage and duration to control the spread of infection, depending on the specific involvement of retinochoroiditis in the eye and the needs of the patient.[10] A small far-peripheral lesion next to a surrounding scar with vitritis may be asymptomatic or result

---

*References 4, 24, 31, 35, 44, 52.

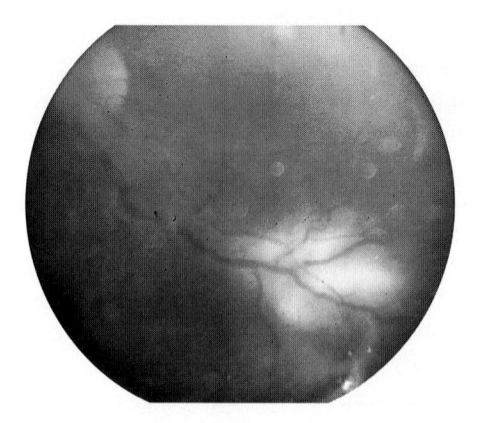

Figure 21-12 Bilateral "endogenous endophthalmitis" in a patient with AIDS. This infection defied diagnosis serologically or through vitreous biopsy. A full-thickness eye-wall biopsy of the lesion disclosed cysts of ocular toxoplasmosis.

only in complaints of "spots and floaters." If the patient is not physiologically compromised and is immune competent, observation may be all that is required by way of therapy. The lesion usually takes 6 to 8 weeks to clear and follows a characteristic pattern of healing. The outer edges start to show firming, and the cells overlying the area of retinitis in greatest number diminish. Healing takes place from the outer edges in toward the center, and after a few weeks one can often see pigmentation along the edges. The center of the lesion is the last part to heal, and finally a retinal scar with pigmentation is noted. Depending on the severity of the infectious process and the immune reaction to the organism, the scar may be so subtle that it cannot be noticed. Conversely, it may be so dense that only bare sclera is seen, with an absolute scotoma and visual field defect in the area. If the scar is quite peripheral, it may be unnoticed; but when it is closer to the optic nerve and important visual structures, the patient is usually quite symptomatic and vision is threatened. Therapy is indicated to stop the infectious process and reduce scarring.

The agents classically used in the treatment of ocular toxoplasmosis are sulfadiazine and pyrimethamine. Both are folic acid antagonists that work on the DNA cycle of the organism in different parts of construction of the protozoal genome. Sulfadiazine is initiated with a loading dose of 4 g, followed by 1 to 2 g orally four times daily, depending on the clinical response, usually over a 4- to 6-week period. It should be discussed with the patient that this medication is not without risks, and the patient should be cautioned to drink at least six to eight glasses of water daily to reduce the risk of kidney stone formation. Patients also should be alerted to call promptly if any side effects such as rash, mucous membrane swelling, or diarrhea are noted. Stevens-Johnson syndrome is a rare complication with the use of sulfa agents. It can be life threatening and requires prompt cessation of the medication with institution of antiinflammatory therapy. Sulfadiazine may be difficult to find in some pharmacies today. Recent unreported evidence has suggested that Bactrim may be effective. This agent (trimethoprim and sulfamethoxazole) is taken only twice daily, aiding medical compliance. Pyrimethamine (Daraprim), the other folic acid antagonist, which is used in conjunction with sulfadiazine, has a loading dose of 75 mg and then is taken 25 mg orally twice daily, usually for the same duration. Although rare, its most feared complication is bone marrow suppression, and treatment with folinic acid is often used concomitantly.[16] Platelet counts should be taken on a weekly basis during the administration of this therapy.

The use of oral corticosteroids to reduce any inflammatory reaction and improve symptoms should be considered.[10,24,27] They can slow the cellular reaction and diminish vitritis; but care should be taken that they are not used to immune-compromise the individual and the eye, causing retardation of the healing process and an indolent necrotic retinitis. Dosage must be tailored to the patient's age, health, and potential ocular morbidity; 20 to 60 mg per day, with a quick taper based on clinical findings, is the standard treatment. The protean complications of prednisone should be discussed with the patient, and dosage reduced promptly if complications occur. Medrol Dospak (methylprednisolone) therapy may be helpful for selected individuals, but treatment requires 3 to 6 weeks with a slow taper. Prednisone may not be required at all in mild cases with antibiotic coverage as the only therapy.

Clindamycin has recently been advocated[20,40,43] as an effective antibiotic for use in cases of toxplasmic retinochoroiditis. Studies have suggested its effectiveness in eradicating the active organism in both animals and humans. As is true of the previously discussed antibiotics, however, it does not cause sterilization of the cysts, which remain in the retina after the active phase of the infection is over. Thus there can be recurrences of ocular toxoplasmosis, and the patient should be warned that symptoms may suddenly reappear. If lesions are in important sight-threatening areas, the use of an Amsler grid or other devices can be helpful in alerting the individual to a recurrence. Prompt treatment will limit scarring and ocular morbidity. This is the rationale for aggressive therapy of ocular toxoplasmosis.

Clindamycin dosage is 150 to 300 mg four times daily, for 4 to 6 weeks with appropriate taper. This medication, however, can cause gastrointestinal problems and rash. An overgrowth of *Clostridium difficile* in the intestinal mucosa may create severe gastroenteritis, which has led to death in some individuals. For this reason, if any diarrhea occurs the medicine should be promptly discontinued. If the medicine must be continued, *C. difficile* can be effectively treated with vancomycin.[45]

Minocycline, a tetracycline derivative, has also been used in rabbits to treat toxoplasmosis and may be a helpful adjunct for individuals who cannot tolerate the classic antibiotics.[33] Clinical studies, however, are lacking. Dosage is 100 mg twice a day over a 3- to 6-week period.

Minocycline and clindamycin act in a different manner from pyrimethamine and sulfadiazine. They block protozoal protein synthesis and act synergistically with the folate antagonists.

Quadruple therapy—sulfadiazine, pyrimethamine, clindamycin, and corticosteroids—has been used in individuals with severe infection. Tailoring the medication is important. Patients with mild disease who are minimally symptomatic, and with minimal chance of severe scarring, may do well taking oral sulfadiazine alone or clindamycin alone. In severe cases, when vision is threatened, more aggressive attempts are necessary to control the infection and inflammatory reaction quickly and prevent scarring. Newer agents that may eradicate both active disease and residual toxoplasmic cysts are on the horizon. In the future such drugs will be available to sterilize the retina, ridding the tissues of cysts that break down into active trophozoites that cause recurrent infection and scarring.[21]

Finally, the use of retinodestructive procedures such as cryotherapy or laser treatment has been advocated in selected cases.[15,22,41] Chronic peripheral lesions can be treated in an outpatient setting with cryotherapy, or more posterior lesions can be managed with cutting cryo techniques. A double freeze-thaw cycle is helpful in destroying the cysts and trophozoites by treating the area of infection and its edges. This may not, however, prevent future recurrences, since ophthalmoscopically all cysts may not be frozen or irradicated. The technique is useful for individuals who cannot take oral prednisone or are allergic to the antibiotics. Vitrectomy surgery may be of use in the treatment of ocular toxoplasmosis if vitritis is chronic and relentless. Done in conjunction with cryotherapy, it can limit the disease, quieting the active process and clearing the media. It is usually reserved for individuals who have had chronic disease for more than 6 months or who require an immediate improvement in vision because of their daily needs. Potential complications of introacular surgery need to be evaluated in relation to medical therapy.

DIFFERENTIAL DIAGNOSIS

The differential diagnosis of ocular toxoplasmosis includes both infectious and immune causes of retinitis with subsequent vitritis and uveitis. The characteristic sequence of events in ocular toxoplasmosis, spots and floaters with retinochoroiditis and asymptomatic periods lasting months to years, is the classic clinical picture. There are, however, individuals who present with clinical parameters suggestive of toxoplasmosis but in whom other diagnoses are tenable. The most common group is viral retinitis. Because both *Toxoplasma gondii* and herpesviruses have a predilection for retinal tissue, clinical findings may be similar, although treatment is very different. The acute retinal necrosis syndrome (ARN) (Fig. 21-13) is one such disease that can occur in immunocompetent

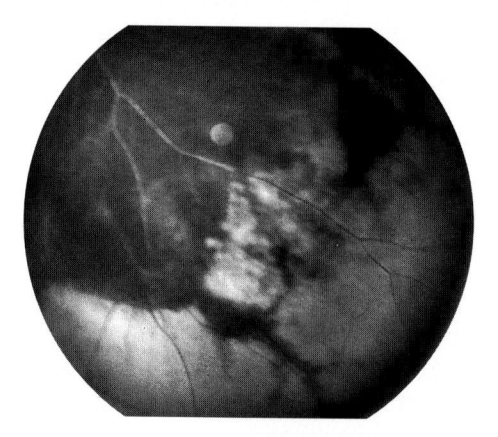

Figure 21-13 The acute retinal necrosis syndrome (ARN) can manifest as large zones of retinitis with secondary vasculitis and bleeding. There may be vitreous involvement in the later phases, and a predilection has been noted for bilaterality in one third of patients. The disease process is usually acute with rapid progression. Severe ocular morbidity results if cases are left untreated.

individuals and may be confused clinically with ocular toxoplasmosis. A sudden onset of both anterior and posterior uveitis with whitish patches, often noted in the peripheral retina with surrounding vasculitis and progressive visual loss over days to weeks, is the hallmark of this disease. The entire retina may become involved with this herpes zoster–type retinal infection, and the eye and useful vision may subsequently be lost. Prompt recognition is paramount. The disease usually follows a much more aggressive course than that of the more indolent toxoplasmic lesions. ARN lesions often spread quite rapidly, and one third are bilateral. No antecedent scars are observed. Antiviral agents such as acyclovir are the suggested form of therapy. ARN is a clinical diagnosis based on laboratory studies that exclude other causes.

Viral retinitis is also found in immunocompromised individuals with acquired immune-deficiency syndrome (AIDS) or those receiving high-dose anti-immune medications such as cyclosporin, prednisone, and immunosuppressive agents for organ transplants and other conditions. These individuals develop a viral retinitis usually secondary to cytomegalovirus[6,13,22,28,46] (Fig. 21-14). The clinical findings, however, are somewhat different from those of ARN or ocular toxoplasmosis. The disease is often indolent, with retinitis spreading quite slowly. There is often only minimum vitreous reaction, and the underlying history is very helpful in placing these individuals in proper perspective. Accurate diagnosis is important since treatment is specific, with antiviral agents for cytomegalovirus (ganciclovir and foscarnet).

Ocular syphilis can mimic the clinical picture of ocular toxoplasmosis. Anterior uveitis, vitritis, and even patchy focal retinitis and pigment epitheliitis may be seen (Figs. 21-15 and 21-16). Usually no active areas are noted next to scars, but vasculitis is not uncommon. A suggestive history of syphilis or venereal disease in the past, confirmed by laboratory testing, helps establish the diagnosis. The VDRL (Venereal Disease Research Laboratories) test is positive in high titers of early systemic disease but may become negative over the years. The FTA-ABS (fluorescent treponemal antibody absorbed) test, however, is positive for life. Late latent and tertiary syphilis may present with ocular or neurologic findings that clinically resemble the disease pattern of ocular toxoplasmosis. With ocular syphilis, laboratory confirmation is helpful in determining the correct diagnosis.

Candida endophthalmitis is included in the differential diagnosis and is usually seen in immune-compromised individuals who have been receiving long-term intravenous therapy or hyperalimentation (Fig. 21-17). Through hematogenous spread from an infected organ, lesions begin as small, light, fluffy spots on the retina but progress to form localized fungal puffballs overlying the retinal surface. The disease is quite insidious; and if the lesions do not involve an area of central vision, patients may complain of only spots and floaters. If the lesions are near the macula or optic nerve, however, visual field and/or central visual defects may be noted. Treatment is with amphotericin or fluconazole—the former either intravenously or intravitreally, the latter orally.

Vasculitis syndromes such as Behçet's disease may at times confuse the clinician and lead to a diagnosis of ocular toxoplasmosis. Close evaluation, however, will show that the vascular defect is primary and the retinal whitening due to infarction rather than inflammation. There is usually minimal vitritis in these conditions, and it is diffuse rather than localized. Vasculitic stigmas (e.g.,

Figure 21-14 If left untreated, cytomegalovirus retinitis in AIDS characteristically follows an indolent progressive course. Often there are zones of punctate pigment alteration, with a "brushfire" leading border. Because of the progressive loss of retinal structure, vitreous cells are rare and symptoms frequently are related to the visual field defects.

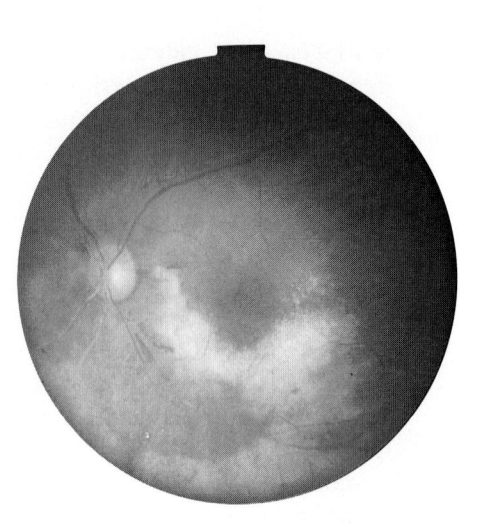

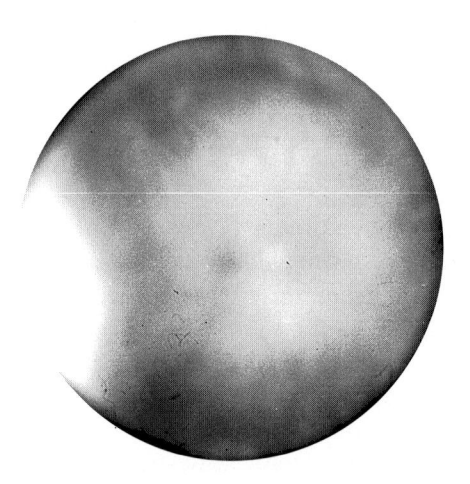

Figure 21-15 Severe vitritis related to an acute loss of vision in a young HIV-positive individual who was found to have ocular syphilis. Initially toxoplasmosis was considered to be the cause of this white lesion in the peripheral retina.

Figure 21-16 Following appropriate treatment, the whitish lesion in Figure 21-15 appears as a focal zone of retinitis and pigment epitheliitis. Healing after antiluetic therapy occurred with pigmentation and mild chorioretinal scarring.

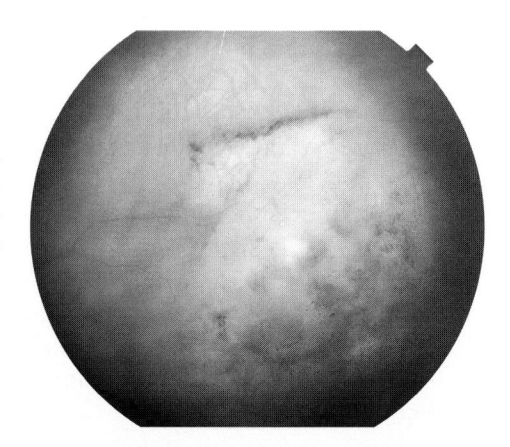

Ocular toxoplasmosis 301

Figure 21-17 Note the whitish lesion just temporal to fixation and a small satellite lesion off the inferior arcade in the left eye of this 55-year-old man who complained of diminished vision following hyperalimentation. Blood cultures revealed *Candida,* and the lesion promptly resolved with fluconazole treatment.

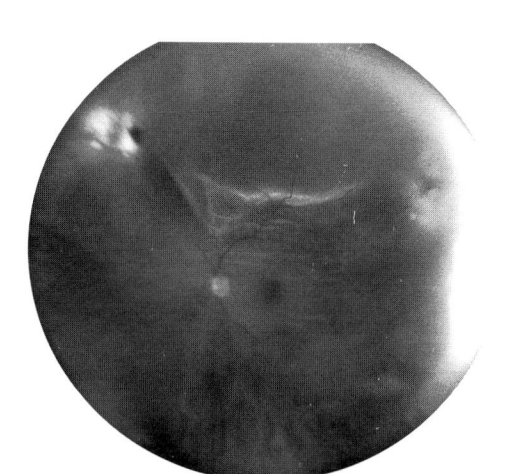

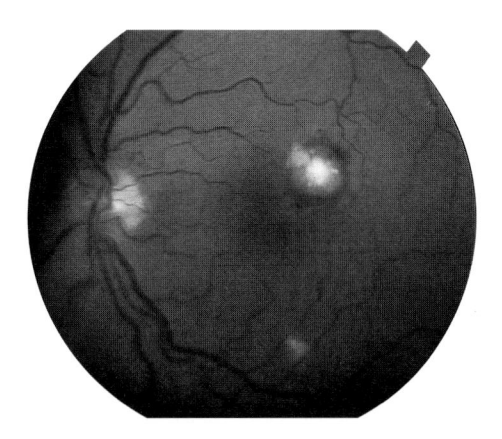

Figure 21-18 Retinal detachment with a retinal break along the edge of the chorioretinal scar superonasally. A past history of ocular toxoplasmosis with lesions in the far-superior nasal quadrant was recorded in this patient who complained of a sudden loss of the inferior field as well as central vision in the left eye. Subretinal fluid had extended down through the macular region with the sudden loss of central vision. Routine scleral buckling resolved the detachment.

phlebitis, dermatologic lesions, oral and genital aphthae, and rheumatologic disease), along with HLA-β5, help make the clinical diagnosis. Treatment is with antiinflammatory and immunosuppressive agents.

Often individuals with ocular toxoplasmosis are quite alert to changes in their symptoms. The start of "spots and floaters" may be a harbinger that toxoplasmosis is occurring. After bouts of the disease, however, the vitreous gel will spontaneously separate, causing similar symptomatology. Patients often present promptly because of the concern for active infection, yet all that has occurred is posterior vitreous gel separation. The clinician should diligently look for any evidence of retinal breaks or tears, since the incidence is slightly higher when posterior vitreous detachment occurs secondary to inactive toxoplasmosis. Retinal detachment can also occur (Fig. 21-18). The breaks may extend from the vitreous base in unaffected areas or follow the edges of old scars. Scleral buckling is effective; and if there is associated severe vitritis, a combination of vitrectomy, internal gas, and endolaser will be effective in healing these detachments.

SUMMARY

Ocular toxoplasmosis in the immune-competent patient has a characteristic clinical picture and usually responds well to medications or the natural course of healing. Treatment must be tailored to the needs of the individual, with concern given to potential side effects of the medications used. Often vision is restored and, depending on the areas affected, the final outcome is quite good. As with all intraocular inflammations, a detailed history, complete ocular physical examination, and appropriate laboratory studies can establish the correct diagnosis and exclude other causes. Treatment goals are prompt control of the infection, decreased intraocular scarring, and prevention of visual loss.

References

1. Akstein RB, Wilson LA, Teutsch SM: Acquired toxoplasmosis, *Ophthalmology* 89:1299-1302, 1982.
2. Braunstein RA, Gass JDM: Branch artery obstruction caused by acute toxoplasmosis, *Arch Ophthalmol* 98:512-513, 1980.
3. Brezin AP, Egwuagu CE, Burnier M Jr, et al: Identification of toxoplasma gondii in paraffin-embedded section polymerase chain reaction, *Am J Ophthalmol* 110(6):599-604, 1990.
4. Cohen SN: Toxoplasmosis in patients receiving immunosuppressive therapy, *JAMA* 211:657-669, 1970.
5. Couvreur J, Desmonts G: Congenital and maternal toxoplasmosis: a review of 300 congenital cases, *Dev Med Child Neurol* 4:519-530, 1962.
6. de Smet MD: Differential diagnosis of retinitis and choroiditis in patients with acquired immunodeficiency syndrome. *Am J Med* 92(suppl 2A):17S-21S, 1992.
7. Desmonts G: Definitive serological diagnosis of ocular toxoplasmosis, *Arch Ophthalmol* 76:839-851, 1966.
8. Desmonts G, Forestier F, Thulliez P, et al: Prenatal diagnosis of congenital toxoplasmosis, *Lancet* 1:500-504, 1985.
9. Eichenwald HF: The laboratory diagnosis of toxoplasmosis, *Ann NY Acad Sci* 64:207-214, 1956.
10. Engstrom RE Jr, Holland GN, Nussenblatt RB, Jabs DA: Current practices in the management of ocular toxoplasmosis, *Am J Ophthalmol* 111(5):601-610, 1991.
11. Folk JC, Lobes LA: Presumed toxoplasmic papillitis, *Ophthalmology* 91:64-67, 1984.
12. Friedmann CT, Knox DL: Variations in recurrent active toxoplasmic retinochoroiditis, *Arch Ophthalmol* 81:481-493, 1969.
13. Gagliuso DJ, Teich SA, Friedman AH, Orellana J: Ocular toxoplasmosis in AIDS patients, *Trans Am Ophthalmol Soc* 88:63-86, 1990.
14. Gass JDM: *Stereoscopic atlas of macular diseases: diagnosis and treatment,* ed 2, St Louis, 1987, Mosby.
15. Ghartey KN, Brockhurst RJ: Photocoagulation of active toxoplasmic retinochroiditis, *Am J Ophthalmol* 89:858-864, 1980.
16. Giles CL: The treatment of Toxoplasma uveitis with pyrimethamine and folinic acid, *Am J Ophthalmol* 58:611-617, 1964.
17. Hayreh SS: Optic disc vasculitis, *Br J Ophthalmol* 56:652-670, 1972.
18. Holliman RE, Stevens RJ, Duffy KT, Johnson JD: Serological investigation of ocular toxoplasmosis, *Br J Ophthalmol* 75(6):353-355, 1991.
19. Krick JA, Remington JS: Toxoplasmosis in the adult: an overview, *N Engl J Med* 298:550-553, 1978.
20. Lakhanpal V, Schocket SS, Nirankari VS: Clindamycin in the treatment of toxoplasmic retinochoroiditis, *Am J Ophthalmol* 95:605-613, 1983.
21. Lopez JS, de Smet MD, Masur H, et al: Orally administered 566C80 for treatment of ocular toxoplasmosis in a patient with the acquired immunodeficiency syndrome (letter), *Am J Ophthalmol* 113(3):331-333, 1992.
22. McCabe RE, Remington JS: Toxoplasma gondii. In Mandell GL, Douglas RG Jr, Bennett JE (eds): *Principles and practice of infectious diseases,* ed 2, New York, 1985, John Wiley & Sons.
23. Miller NL, Frenkel JK, Dubey JP: Oral infections with toxoplasma cysts and oocysts in felines, other mammals, and in birds, *J Parasitol* 58:928-937, 1972.
24. Nicholson DH, Wolchok EB: Ocular toxoplasmosis in an adult receiving long-term corticosteroid therapy, *Arch Ophthalmol* 94:248-254, 1976.
25. Nolan J, Rosen ES: Treatment of active toxoplasmic retinochoroiditis, *Br J Ophthalmol* 52:396-399, 1968.

26. O'Connor GR: The roles of parasite invasion and of hypersensitivity in the pathogenesis of toxoplasmic retinochoroiditis, *Ocular Inflammation Ther* 1:37-46, 1983.
27. O'Connor GR, Frenkel JK: Dangers of steroid treatment in toxoplasmosis: periocular injections and systemic therapy, *Arch Ophthalmol* 94:213, 1976.
28. Parke DW II, Font RL: Diffuse toxoplasmic retinochoroiditis in a patient with AIDS, *Arch Ophthalmol* 104:571-575, 1986.
29. Perkins ES: Ocular toxoplasmosis, *Br J Ophthalmol* 57:1-17, 1973.
30. Rao NA, Font RL: Toxoplasmic retinochoroiditis: electron-microscopic and immunofluorescence studies of formalin-fixed tissue, *Arch Ophthalmol* 95:273-277, 1977.
31. Reynolds ES, Walls KW, Pfeiffer RI: Generalized toxoplasmosis following renal transplantation: report of a case, *Arch Intern Med* 118:401-405, 1966.
32. Rollins DF, Tabbara KF, O'Connor GR, et al: Detection of toxoplasmal antigen and antibody in ocular fluids in experimental ocular toxoplasmosis, *Arch Ophthalmol* 101:455-457, 1983.
33. Rollins DF, Tabbara KF, Ghosheh R, Nozik RA: Minocycline in experimental ocular toxoplasmosis in the rabbit, *Am J Ophthalmol* 93:361-365, 1982.
34. Rothova A, Van Knapen F, Baarsma GS, et al: Serology in ocular toxoplasmosis, *Br J Ophthalmol* 70:615-622, 1986.
35. Ruskin J, Remington JS: Toxoplasmosis in the compromised host, *Ann Intern Med* 84:193-199, 1976.
36. Sabates R, Pruett RC, Brockhurst RJ: Fulminant ocular toxoplasmosis, *Am J Ophthalmol* 92:497-503, 1981.
37. Schlaegel TF Jr: Toxoplasmosis. In Duane TD, Jaeger EA (eds): *Clinical ophthalmology*, Hagerstown Md, 1978, Harper & Row, vol 4.
38. Shimada K, O'Connor GR, Yoneda C: Cyst formation by toxoplasma gondii (RH strain) in vitro, *Arch Ophthalmol* 92:496-500, 1974.
39. Tabbara KF, Nozik RA, O'Connor GR: Clindamycin effects on experimental ocular toxoplasmosis in the rabbit, *Arch Ophthalmol* 92:244-247, 1974.
40. Tabbara KF: Toxoplasmosis. In Duane TD, Jaeger EA (eds): *Clinical ophthalmology*, Hagerstown Md., 1987, Harper & Row, vol 4.
41. Tabbara KF, O'Connor GR: Treatment of ocular toxoplasmosis with clindamycin and sulfadiazine, *Ophthalmology* 87:129-134, 1980.
42. Teutsch SM, Juranek DD, Sulzer A, et al: Epidemic toxoplasmosis associated with infected cats, *N Engl J Med* 300:695-699, 1979.
43. Tate GW Jr, Martin RG: Clindamycin in the treatment of human ocular toxoplasmosis, *Can J Ophthalmol* 12:188-195, 1977.
44. Vietzke WM, Gelderman AH, Grimley PM, Valsamis MP: Toxoplasmosis complicating malignancy: experience at the National Cancer Institute, *Cancer* 21:816-827, 1968.
45. Viteri AL, Howard PH, Dyck WP: The spectrum of lincomycin-clindamycin colitis, *Gastroenterology* 66:1137-1144, 1974.
46. Weiss A, Margo CE, Ledford DK, et al: Toxoplasmic retinochoroiditis as an initial manifestation of the acquired immune deficiency syndrome, *Am J Ophthalmol* 101:248-249, 1986.
47. Weiss MJ, Velazquez N, Hofeldt AJ: Serologic tests in the diagnosis of presumed toxoplasmic retinochoroiditis, *Am J Ophthalmol* 109(4):407-411, 1990.
48. Wilder HC: Toxoplasma chorioretinitis in adults, *Arch Ophthalmol* 48:127-136, 1952.
49. Willerson D Jr, Aaberg TM, Reeser F, Meredith TA: Unusual ocular presentation of acute toxoplasmosis, *Br J Ophthalmol* 61:693-698, 1977.
50. Williamson TH, Meyer PA: Branch retinal artery occlusion in toxoplasma retinochoroiditis, *Br J Ophthalmol* 75(4):253, 1991.
51. Wilson CB, Remington JS, Stagno S, Reynolds DW: Development of adverse sequelae in children born with subclinical congenital toxoplasma infection, *Pediatrics* 66:767-774, 1980.
52. Yeo JH, Jakobiec FA, Iwamoto T, Richard G, Kreissig I: Opportunistic toxoplasmic retinochoroiditis following chemotherapy for systemic lymphoma: a light and electron microscopic study, *Ophthalmology* 90:885-898, 1983.
53. Zimmerman LE: Ocular pathology of toxoplasmosis, *Surv Ophthalmol* 6:832-856, 1961.

22

Ocular Toxocariasis

Carol L. Shields
Jerry A. Shields

BACKGROUND

Epidemiology

Intraocular involvement by *Toxocara canis* is an important cause of childhood blindness.[1] Ocular toxocariasis results from hematogenous invasion of the eye by the second- or third-stage larva of the dog roundworm, *T. canis,* following systemic infestation by this parasite, a condition known as visceral larval migrans (VLM). In most patients with ocular involvement, however, a clearcut history of VLM cannot be elicited.

A historical review of VLM was provided by Sprent in 1958.[2] Following his report, it became apparent that *T. canis* was an important canine parasite, but it was still not recognized that this organism could also affect humans. Clinicians during the 1940s recognized in children several cases of an idiopathic syndrome characterized by fever, hepatosplenomegaly, pneumonitis, and sometimes encephalitis associated with extreme eosinophilia. Exploratory laparotomy in affected patients revealed numerous gray nodules scattered throughout the liver that were shown histologically to be eosinophilic granulomas. In 1952, Beaver et al.[3] reported on three patients with this syndrome in whom liver biopsies revealed nematode larvae within an eosinophilic granuloma. The larvae were later identified as *T. canis* and the syndrome was termed "visceral larval migrans."

T. canis is a parasite of dogs, wolves, and foxes.[4] In puppies 2 to 6 months of age the prevalence is reported to be greater than 80% whereas in dogs older than 1 year the prevalence drops to less than 20%. Schantz et al.[4] have pointed out that between one third and one half of households in the United States have one or more dogs, most of which are infected with *T. canis* as puppies. It is estimated[5] that 20% of dogs in southern England are infected and even well-cared for dogs are capable of acquiring the nematode.

The dogs acquire *T. canis* in several ways: (1) ingestion of infective eggs, (2) ingestion of larvae in tissues of paratenic hosts, (3) transplacental migration, (4) transmammary passage of larvae, and (5) ingestion of late stage larvae or immature adults in the vomitus or feces of infected pups. Within the dog intestine the first- and second-stage larvae exist completely within the protective shell of the egg. Under favorable conditions or through intestinal activity the shell ruptures, liberating the third-stage larvae into the intestine. The motile larvae penetrate the intestinal wall to gain access to lymphatics and the portal circulation. During the course of systemic migration they pass through two or three further molts. Some larvae settle in distant organs such as the liver, lungs, brain, and eyes, producing a syndrome similar to the human disease. Those that reach the lungs of young puppies undergo tracheosophageal migration and are swallowed. When they reach the small intestine, they mature into adult worms. Within the intestine the adult female worm produces eggs, which may be excreted into the soil. The eggs become developed in moist soil and are infective upon being swallowed by puppies, allowing the cycle to be initiated again.

Transmission to humans occurs primarily from the ingestion of embryonated eggs that are present in contaminated soil. The majority of infected patients have a history of geophagia or other forms of pica such as ingestion of clay or grass. The eggs hatch in the human small intestine, and the larvae then migrate into the mucosa to reach the portal circulation. They migrate to the liver, follow vascular channels to the lungs, and then enter the systemic circulation to reach numerous organs, including the liver, lungs, brain, and eyes. The great majority of patients with systemic disease do not have ocular involvement. It has been determined[6] that in the United States VLM is most prevalent in the south central and southeastern regions. From 10% to 30% of soil samples in public playgrounds and parks are contaminated with toxocara eggs.

Clinical Features

Systemic. Children who develop VLM are most often boys between 6 months and 3 years of age at the onset of symptoms. There is usually a history of contact with puppies, and most children are reported by the patients as being geographic.

The symptoms include fever (55%), pallor (40%), coughing or wheezing (20%), lassitude, anorexia, and weight loss.[7] Seizures, usually of the petit mal type, may be an associated symptom, and poliomyelitis and myocarditis have been known to occur. Many children can be infected with *Toxocara canis* but remain clinically asymptomatic, thus suggesting that human infection is more common than previously believed but that it may remain subclinical. The development of clinical symptoms appears to be dependent on the number of larvae ingested and the resistance of the host.

Most patients have leukocytosis and eosinophilia. During the acute disease leukocyte counts may range from 30,000 to 90,000 cells/mm^3, with 50% to 90% eosinophils. The eosinophil count is reported frequently to remain elevated for months or even years after the acute infection. There is usually an elevation of serum gamma globulin, especially IgG and IgM, with a normal or slightly decreased serum albumin level. It is of particular interest that anti-A and anti-B blood titers are positive in some children with VLM. This is presumably because toxocara larvae contain surface antigens that stimulate isohemagglutins. More specific laboratory procedures, particularly the enzyme-linked immunosorbent assay (ELISA), can be of great diagnostic importance.

Regardless of the tissue involved, the larvae of *T. canis* produce a pathologic reaction similar to that seen with other parasites. In the early stages each larva is surrounded by eosinophils, producing an eosinophilic abscess. Later there is a focal granulomatous reaction consisting of eosinophils, lymphocytes, epithelioid cells, and giant cells of the foreign body type. The older lesions develop epithelioid cells and dense fibrous tissue. An important aspect of the histopathology of VLM is that the inflammatory reaction around a larva is much larger than the organism itself. Consequently, many histopathologic sections throughout the granuloma may be required to demonstrate the larva or its remnants. In a longstanding granuloma the larva may be totally destroyed, with no remnants identifiable. The Splendore-Hoeppli phenomenon may also be observed around the worm, but this reaction is not specific for *T. canis*.

In many children the infection remains subclinical and no treatment is given.[8] In patients with severe respiratory or myocardial involvement, however, corticosteroids may be lifesaving. Certain antihelmintic drugs such as diethylcarbamazine and thiabendazole have been used. These relieve symptoms and shorten the convalescent time in patients with VLM, although the effectiveness of such drugs is not dramatic. The specific therapeutic modalities that pertain to the ocular involvement will be discussed below.

The prognosis for patients with VLM is usually excellent. Many cases are subclinical and self-limited and the patient has no aftereffects. Clinically manifest cases may leave variable degrees of residual damage in the involved tissues. Except for those that involve the eyes, however, they are of little clinical importance. In rare instances death has occurred, usually secondary to complications of myocarditis or encephalitis.

Ocular. The relationship of ocular toxocariasis to VLM is not entirely clear. The patient with ocular toxocariasis occasionally has a clear-cut prior history of VLM, or the ocular involvement occurs simultaneously with VLM, or in some patients there is no history of VLM.

Helenor Wilder[9] established the fact that nematode larvae can directly invade the intraocular tissues and induce an inflammatory reaction. While serving as Director of the Ophthalmic Branch of the Armed Forces Institute of Pathology, she noted that certain eyes enucleated for suspected retinoblastoma and other conditions actually contained a granulomatous inflammatory process with eosinophilic abscesses. Noting that these lesions resembled those seen in helminth infections elsewhere in the body, she examined more sections of the remaining ocular tissues in hope of finding the responsible organism. Of 46 such eyes sectioned, she was able to demonstrate nematode larvae or their residual capsules in 24 cases. She initially thought that the nematodes were hookworm larvae. Later the parasites were reclassified as the larvae of *T. canis*. Subsequent reports[10,11] supported the fact that *T. canis* and perhaps other nematode larvae can affect the human eye.

Intraocular infestation with *T. canis* typically occurs unilaterally in young children.[1,12] It sometimes occurs bilaterally, however, and in adults. Ocular involvement can assume any of several clinical patterns none of which is pathognomonic, and the ophthalmologist must rely on all available clinical and laboratory data to make the clinical diagnosis. In some cases the child will develop overt signs of ocular inflammation. In others the inflammation may have resolved and the child will be brought in because of strabismus or poor vision detected on a screening test, which prompts further investigation, leading to the diagnosis. In still others the intraocular inflammation will be asymptomatic or nonspecific, making the clinical diagnosis very difficult.

The clinical features of ocular toxocariasis vary, and infection may be manifest in the posterior or peripheral fundus, optic disc, vitreous, cornea, conjunctiva, or lens.[1,12,13] The most commonly recognized ocular site is the fundus. Infection in the posterior pole of the eye often occurs in the center of the macula (Fig. 22-1). It is typically unilateral, although bilateral macular lesions have been found. In the acute stage, retinochoroiditis appears clinically as a hazy, ill defined, white retinal lesion with overlying inflammatory cells in the vitreous. As the acute inflammatory reaction subsides, the lesion appears to be a well-defined, elevated, and white mass ranging from one half to four disc diameters in size. The chronic lesion may have a glistening white or gray appearance with a clear vitreous. Traction bands may extend from the lesion to the optic disc or to the macular area. There is often some associated migration or proliferation of the retinal pigment epithelium.

In chronic granulomas large retinal blood vessels may enter the mass and disappear into its substance. This probably represents a retinochoroidal anastomosis, which may occur in any cicatrized inflammatory or traumatic fundus lesion. The quiescent toxocara granuloma is often recognized in older children as compared to the acute inflammatory variant seen more often in young children.

In the peripheral fundus the toxocara granuloma characteristically appears as a hazy white reaction. It has many of the clinical characteristics of the entity known as idiopathic peripheral uveoretinitis, chronic cyclitis, peripheral uveitis, and pars planitis. In this last entity, however, the inflammation is bilateral in 80% to 90% of cases, whereas ocular toxocariasis is almost always unilateral. In the late stages dragging of the retina toward the inflammatory mass in the periphery produces a falciform fold (Fig. 22-2). In some cases the traction can lead to heterotopia of the macula, resulting in severe loss of vision (Fig. 22-3). It is likely that many cases of "congenital" retinal fold are, in reality, acquired peripheral retinal granulomas of *T. canis.*

The toxocara larva may cause a localized inflammatory reaction in the optic disc. Whether the organism reaches this location through small retinal capillaries from the central retinal artery or via the short posterior ciliary vessels is a matter of controversy. It is characterized by an elevation of the disc with telangiectasis of the blood vessels and sometimes subretinal exudation. If the inflammation is severe, a secondary retinal artery obstruction can occur. It may stimulate primary optic neuritis of any cause or disc edema due to mechanical causes. The overlying vitreous reaction may be minimal or marked. As the inflammation subsides, there may remain a nonspecific peripapillary fibrous nodule similar to those that follow trauma or inflammation from any cause.[14]

Perhaps the best known and most common form of ocular toxocariasis is the inflammatory reaction in the retina and vitreous known as nematode endophthalmitis.[1,15,16] The cases originally described by Wilder were often characterized clinically by a yellow-white mass, retinal detachment, and cells in the vitreous, similar to the findings in many cases of retinoblastoma. In contrast to many other causes of intraocular inflammation, toxocara endophthalmitis does not produce much pain or photophobia. External ocular examination reveals only mild signs of inflammation. During the acute stage of infection, slit-lamp

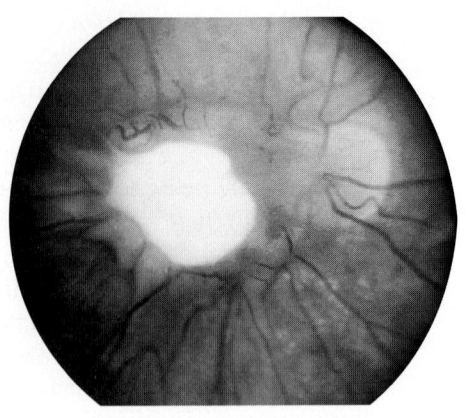

Figure 22-1 Contracted glial nodule in the macula from resolved toxocara granuloma.

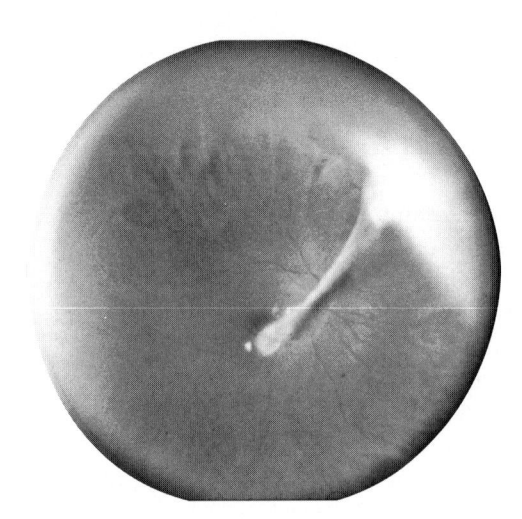

Figure 22-2 Peripheral toxocara granuloma with a falciform fold.

From Shields JA: *Surv Ophthalmol* 28:361-381, 1984.

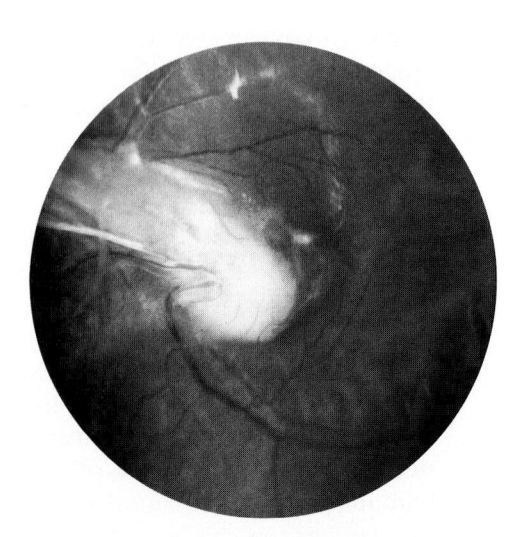

Figure 22-3 Traction on the optic nerve by a peripheral toxocara granuloma.

From Shields JA: *Surv Ophthalmol* 28:361-381, 1984.

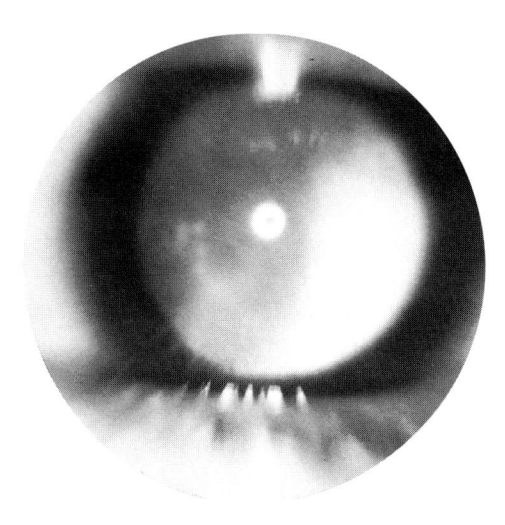

Figure 22-4 Toxocara endophthalmitis with fine diffuse inflammatory cells in the vitreous.

Figure 22-5 White cyclitic membrane in a resolved toxocara endophthalmitis.

From Shields JA: *Surv Ophthalmol* 28:361-381, 1984.

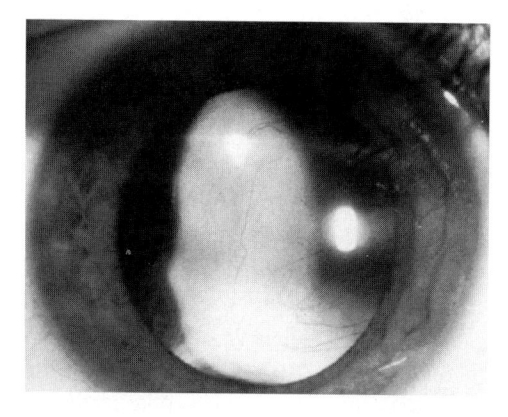

biomicroscopy reveals granulomatous keratic precipitates, aqueous flare and cells, and posterior synechias. A hypopyon may develop in advanced cases. The anterior vitreous usually shows a dense accumulation of white inflammatory cells that obscures a view of the posterior fundus (Fig. 22-4). Through the hazy vitreous one can sometimes see a yellow-white mass, usually in the peripheral retina, that may closely resemble an endophytic retinoblastoma. In some cases the inflammatory reaction may largely subside, leaving a quiet white retrolental mass that represents organization of the inflammatory process into a cyclitic membrane (Fig. 22-5). This cyclitic membrane begins in the quadrant of the most intense peripheral fundus inflammation and progresses across the posterior surface of the lens. In many such cases the patient develops extensive posterior synechias, iris bombe, and posterior subcapsular cataract (which may progress to a totally opaque lens with profound leukokoria and decreased vision). Uncontrollable glaucoma or phthisis bulbi may ensue.

The larvae can occasionally appear in the peripheral cornea lodged in the end arteries near the limbus. They may migrate within the conjunctiva and corneal stroma and can have surprisingly rapid movements. Scleritis and phakitis from nematode larvae is extremely rare.[17]

DIFFERENTIAL DIAGNOSIS

Retinoblastoma

Of the 24 eyes with nematode endophthalmitis studied by Wilder,[9] 20 were enucleated because of suspected retinoblastoma, 3 were diagnosed clinically as having "pseudoglioma," and 1 was believed to have panophthalmitis. All the four cases of larval granulomatosis reported by Ashton were enucleated for the clinical suspicion of retinoblastoma. Numerous other cases of nematode endophthalmitis simulating retinoblastoma have been reported. In our clinical experience, presumed nematode endophthalmitis secondary to *Toxocara canis* is one of the conditions most commonly confused with retinoblastoma. Of 500 children referred to the Oncology Service at Wills Eye Hospital with the diagnosis of possible retinoblastoma, 288 children (58%) had retinoblastoma and 212 (42%) had a simulating condition.[15,16] The three most common pseudoretinoblastomas included persistent hyperplastic primary vitreous (28%), Coats' disease (16%), and presumed ocular toxocariasis (16%).

In contrast to patients with ocular toxocariasis, children with retinoblastoma are usually diagnosed slightly earlier in life, most often before 2 years of age. The family history may be positive for retinoblastoma. The patient with retinoblastoma does not have a history of symptoms and signs of VLM. Examination of the patient with exophytic retinoblastoma usually reveals a quiet anterior segment and a clear lens. There is a retinal detachment overlying the tumor that extends from the retina into the subretinal space. The vitreous is characteristically clear, with no evidence of organizing inflammation or traction that characterizes ocular toxocariasis. Children with endophytic retinoblastoma do have a hazy vitreous, particularly in the region of the tumor, but they do not demonstrate severe vitreous fibrosis or vitreoretinal traction as seen with toxocariasis. The eye is quiet with retinoblastoma and the vitreous cells are indolent soft cotton candy–like tumor cell clumps (Fig. 22-6) whereas in toxocariasis the eye may be inflamed and the cells are diffuse and sticky in a milieu of fibrosis. It is important to stress that patients with retinoblastoma invariably have a clear lens whereas patients with ocular toxocariasis frequently develop cataract secondary to the inflammation. A cyclitic membrane almost never occurs in eyes with retinoblastoma but is a common finding in nematode endophthalmitis.

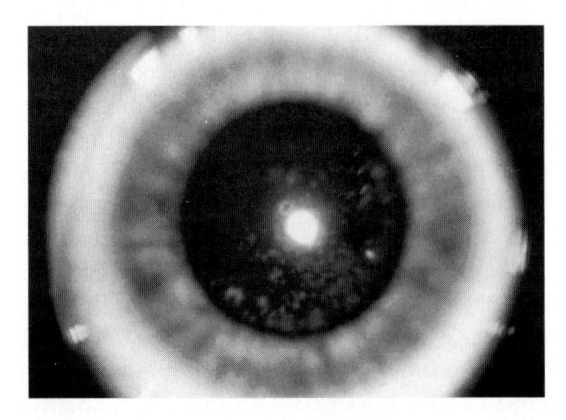

Figure 22-6 Indolent fluffy retinoblastoma tumor seeds in the anterior vitreous.

Ancillary studies may also be helpful in the differentiation of endophytic retinoblastoma from nematode endophthalmitis. Computed tomography and B-scan ultrasonography usually show a typical tumor pattern in retinoblastoma with evidence of calcium in the mass. Nematode endophthalmitis does not usually demonstrate a tumor pattern, but vitreous cells and a funnel-shaped retinal detachment are more likely. When the differential diagnosis is more difficult, aqueous ELISA and cytology may be helpful. Aqueous or vitreal aspiration for cytologic study can reveal tumor cells in cases of endophytic retinoblastoma, but in nematode endophthalmitis eosinophils predominate. This procedure should be used only when the diagnosis is extremely difficult and the suspicion for toxocariasis great. Because of the risk of spreading tumor cells, we do not recommend aqueous or vitreous needle biopsy when the suspicion for retinoblastoma is great. We have seen several patients now who were initially diagnosed elsewhere with toxocariasis and subsequently found by us to have retinoblastoma. Therefore the differentiation can be difficult but is essential because retinoblastoma can be fatal if there is a long delay in diagnosis.

Endophthalmitis

Bacterial, fungal, or sterile endophthalmitis of exogenous or endogenous sources should be differentiated from toxocariasis. Exogenous endophthalmitis typically follows ocular trauma or ocular surgery, so the history is important. Sometimes distant trauma or surgery, especially in an immunosuppressed patient, can result in ocular infection. The clinical features may resemble those of ocular toxocariasis, and for this reason early diagnostic intervention by needle biopsy or vitrectomy helps in establishing the diagnosis. Urgent care is required to preserve the patient's vision and globe.

Persistent Hyperplastic Primary Vitreous (PHPV)

PHPV is a congenital condition usually noted during the first few days or weeks of life. It almost always is unilateral, and the involved eye is usually microphthalmic. In severe cases the anterior chamber is shallow. A characteristic retrolental fibrovascular mass and cataract are present. With the pupil dilated, one may see the ciliary processes pulled into the retrolental mass. If a fundus view can be obtained, a typical hyaloid artery and its associated fibrovascular tissue may be observed passing from the optic disc to the lens. Vascularized pupillary membranes (persistent anterior vascular tunic of the lens) are often present. Nematode endophthalmitis usually appears later in life, is initially associated with a normal-sized eye, and does not demonstrate a persistent thyaloid system or pupillary membranes. Ocular biometry, using ultrasound, may be of particular value in differentiating PHPV from nematode endophthalmitis. The eye with PHPV is often distinctly smaller than the opposite eye, a finding that can be detected with A-scan or B-scan techniques.

Coats' Disease

Coats' disease (retinal telangiectasis with exudation) characteristically occurs unilaterally in boys between the ages of 6 and 12 years who have no prior history of VLM. The anterior segment is usually clear, although cataract and neovascular glaucoma may occur in advanced cases. In early cases ophthalmoscopy reveals typical retinal telangiectasis with yellow intraretinal exudation.

Later a total retinal detachment may occur. In contrast to nematode endophthalmitis, the vitreous characteristically shows little if any inflammatory reaction.

Retinopathy of Prematurity (ROP)

ROP may be almost impossible to differentiate from cicatricial ocular toxocariasis on the basis of ophthalmoscopy alone. Both conditions can produce a falciform fold that extends from the optic disc to a white peripheral retinal mass. Patients with ROP, however, almost always have a history of prematurity; and the condition is almost always bilateral, although asymmetric involvement in the two eyes may occur. Dragging of the retina to produce the falciform fold is usually toward the temporal periphery whereas in nematode disease any quadrant may be involved.

Familial Exudative Vitreoretinopathy

Familial exudative vitreoretinopathy can produce bilateral retinal folds with vitreoretinal traction from the macula to a peripheral mass. It differs from ocular toxocariasis in that it is usually bilateral and more likely to be seen in other family members.

Idiopathic Peripheral Uveoretinitis

Idiopathic peripheral uveoretinitis (pars planitis, chronic cyclitis) is a recurrent inflammation of the peripheral retinal blood vessels and ciliary body. In contrast to ocular toxocariasis, it typically occurs in older children or young adults and is bilateral in 80% to 90% of cases. It is characterized by multiple white exudates on the pars plana, particularly inferiorly, that may be extensive, forming a "snowbank" appearance.

Toxoplasmosis

Acute toxoplasmic retinochoroiditis also produces a white retinal inflammatory lesion with cells in the vitreous. Unlike toxocariasis, it occurs in somewhat older patients and can be bilateral. Fundus examination reveals typical inactive retinochoroidal scars adjacent to the area of acute infection. In the longstanding inactive stage the *Toxoplasma* lesion is flat or depressed whereas the *Toxocara* lesion is slightly elevated. When the differential diagnosis between ocular toxocariasis and toxoplasmosis is uncertain, laboratory tests are helpful in establishing the differentiation.

Histoplasmosis

Ocular histoplasmosis may be associated with a macular disciform process that can resemble larval granulomatosis in the macular area. In contrast to ocular toxocariasis, however, it occurs in adults and has typical peripapillary chorioretinal atrophy and focal peripheral chorioretinal scars that help make the diagnosis.

Optic Neuritis

Inflammation of the optic disc from any cause must be included in the differential diagnosis of ocular toxocariasis. Other granulomatous inflammations of the disc, such as that seen with sarcoidosis, tuberculosis, and syphilis, may be clinically identical to the optic neuritis of toxocariasis, and appropriate laboratory studies are necessary to make the differentiation.[14]

DIAGNOSTIC APPROACH

The clinical diagnosis of ocular toxocariasis can be facilitated by information obtained through a careful history, physical examination, slit-lamp biomicroscopy, and indirect ophthalmoscopy. The diagnosis can be further substantiated by appropriate laboratory tests, although a definitive diagnosis cannot be established without actual demonstration of the larvae in a human eye. Thus the diagnosis of ocular toxocariasis necessarily remains presumptive in most instances.

Clinical Evaluation

History. An accurate history prior to examining the patient may suggest the diagnosis. The patient, or the parents, should be specifically questioned regarding pica and contact with puppies. There appears to be a statistically significant association between ocular toxocariasis and contact with puppies less than 3 months of age. To exclude other causes of leukokoria, particularly retinoblastoma, appropriate questions should be asked regarding family history of ocular disease.

Physical Examination. In most children with ocular toxocariasis, the general physical examination is normal; however, the patient should be evaluated for signs of VLM, since in occasional cases the systemic and ocular diseases occur simultaneously.

Slit-Lamp Biomicroscopy. This examination should be carefully performed to detect findings that might suggest ocular toxocariasis or exclude the diagnosis of other causes of leukokoria or intraocular inflammation. Finding keratic precipitates, aqueous flare and cells, vitreous cells with vitreous traction bands, a cyclitic membrane, and secondary cataract supports the diagnosis of ocular toxocariasis.

Indirect Ophthalmoscopy. Binocular indirect ophthalmoscopy should be performed on all children with suspected ocular toxocariasis. The finding of a posterior pole or peripheral fundus granuloma associated with vitreous traction bands to the macular area or optic disc would support the diagnosis of ocular toxocariasis. Indirect ophthalmoscopy is also useful in detecting an early retinal detachment as a complication of nematode endophthalmitis.

Clinical Laboratory or Other Ancillary Tests

Ultrasonography. Both A-scan and B-scan can be of considerable value in the differential diagnosis of children with leukokoria. In cases of severe nematode endophthalmitis, particularly when the ocular media are hazy or opaque, they have often demonstrated the inflammatory mass and retinal detachment (Fig. 22-7). They also can help exclude the diagnosis of retinoblastoma or PHPV, by failing to demonstrate a tumor with calcification or hyaloid remnants respectively. In addition, computed tomography or magnetic resonance imaging of the orbit may be helpful in eyes with opaque media.

White Blood Cell Count (Eosinophil Count). As previously stated, the patient with VLM usually has leukocytosis and eosinophilia. At the time of diag-

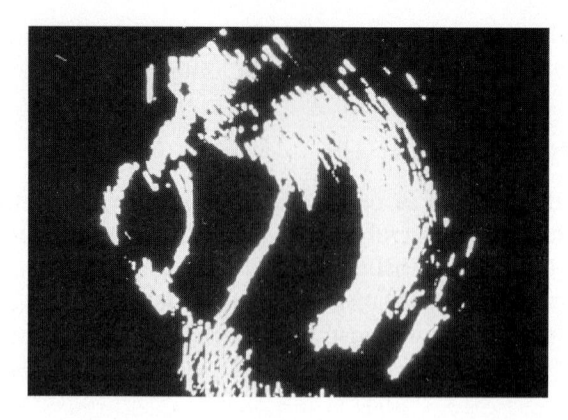

Figure 22-7 B-scan ultrasound demonstrating retinal traction and detachment from a peripheral toxocara granuloma.

From Shields JA: *Surv Ophthalmol* 28:361-381, 1984.

nosis of ocular toxocariasis, however, the white blood count has usually returned to normal and there is no eosinophilia. Therefore the blood count in the peripheral smear is not usually helpful in diagnosing ocular toxocariasis.

Immunodiagnosis. Several laboratory procedures have been used, with limited success, in the diagnosis of VLM and ocular toxocariasis.[18] In the past these included various methods of skin testing, anti-A and anti-B blood titers, Bentonite flocculation, gel diffusion studies, and fluorescent antibody techniques. Most of these had diagnostic limitations with regard to sensitivity and specificity and, in particular, cross reactivity with *Ascaris*. As a result, they are no longer used routinely in the diagnosis of presumed ocular toxocariasis and they will not be further discussed here. The enzyme-linked immunosorbent assay (ELISA), however, is useful in diagnosing a number of parasitic infestations that can involve the eye. It is based on the principle that when an antigen or antibody is chemically (covalently) linked to an enzyme the resultant conjugate retains a large portion of its immunologic and enzymatic activity. In brief, the ELISA uses embryonated egg antigen of *Toxocara canis* larvae adsorbed to wells in a microhemagglutination plate. Serial dilutions of the patient's serum are added, allowed to incubate, and washed. Horseradish peroxidase–goat antihuman IgG is added, incubated, and washed, and a chromagen (e.g., amino antipyrene) is added. The solution is then read in a spectrophotometer.

Although it was initially believed that a titer of 1:32 or greater dilutions was necessary for the diagnosis of VLM, it subsequently became apparent that a serum titer of 1:8 had the greatest sensitivity and specificity for ocular toxocariasis. Consequently, most ophthalmologists today consider a dilution of 1:8 to be positive for ocular toxocariasis if the patient has signs and symptoms compatible with that diagnosis. More recently, ophthalmic clinicians have begun to employ the ELISA on intraocular fluids. High ELISA titers have been found in the vitreous and aqueous humor of patients with presumed ocular toxocariasis. It has recently been pointed out[19] that intraocular fluids may yield a positive result while simultaneous serum samples in the same patient are negative. Therefore, in selected cases, when the diagnosis is uncertain, anterior chamber paracentesis may be carefully employed. Because of the small quantity of aque-

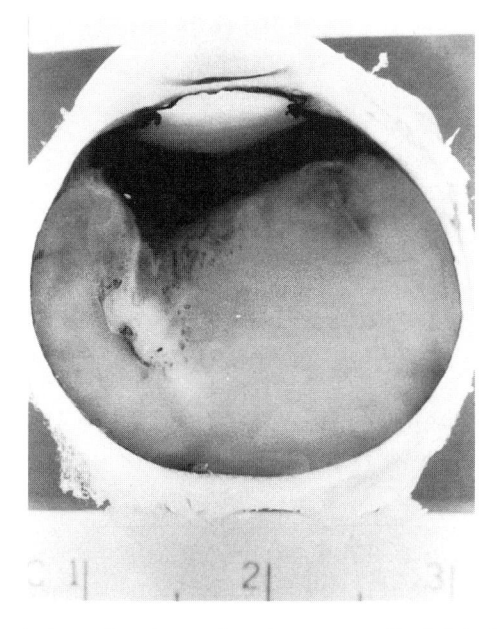

Figure 22-8 Gross pathology showing a chronic serous retinal detachment from toxocariasis.

ous fluid obtained, a microtiter technique facilitates the diagnosis. Vitreous fluid for ELISA can be obtained at the time of vitrectomy.[19,20] ELISA is currently the most reliable laboratory test for the diagnosis of ocular toxocariasis, and it has been shown[13,21] that the titers decrease over time. False-negative and false-positive results may occur.[22] The definitive diagnosis can be made only by histopathologic demonstration of the *T. canis* larvae in ocular tissues.

Aqueous and Vitreous Cytology and Immunology. Cytology and immunologic examination of intraocular fluids can be used to support the clinical diagnosis of ocular toxocariasis.[23] If slit lamp biomicroscopy reveals aqueous cells in a child with intraocular inflammation of uncertain cause, aqueous paracentesis may reveal eosinophils suggesting the diagnosis of a parasitic infestation, most likely toxocariasis. Many other causes of chronic intraocular inflammation would likely demonstrate lymphocytes and plasma cells. Vitreous cytology has also been helpful in the diagnosis of ocular toxocariasis. Vitreous fluid can be obtained by needle aspiration through the pars plana as a pure diagnostic procedure or at the time of therapeutic pars plana vitrectomy for vitreous traction or retinal detachment.[19,20] The demonstration of eosinophils should suggest the diagnosis of ocular toxocariasis. Likewise, the level of immunoglobulin E (IgE) in aqueous humor can be elevated in these cases and again confirm the suspicion of a parasitic infection.[24]

Histopathology. The pathology of ocular toxocariasis varies with the location of the inflammatory process and the severity of the disease. Most of the histopathologically evaluated eyes have been enucleated because they had advanced disease or a mistaken diagnosis of retinoblastoma.

Gross pathology of ocular toxocariasis demonstrates a disorganized eye with a focus of inflammation within a detached retina. (Fig. 22-8). The microscopic

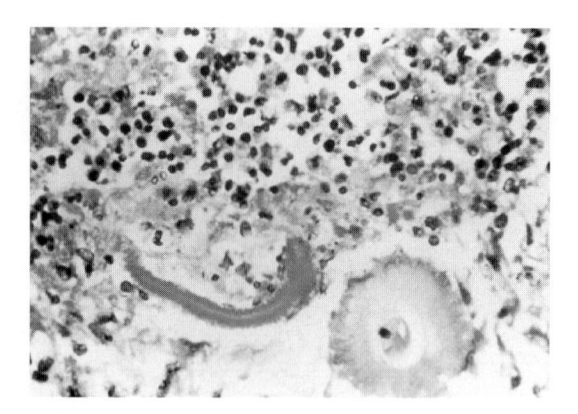

Figure 22-9 Microscopic histopathology demonstrating portions of the *Toxocara* organism surrounded by inflammatory cells. (H&E, ×250.)

findings were described initially by Wilder[9] and later amplified by others. Microscopic examination usually reveals a totally detached retina. Higher magnification demonstrates within the detached retina a focus of granulomatous inflammation composed of an eosinophilic abscess. Surrounding the eosinophilic abscess. are epithelioid cells and granulation tissue infiltrated by eosinophils, lymphocytes, and plasma cells. In the center of the abscess one may see a well-developed larva, the remnants of a degenerated larva, or the residual hyaline capsule (Fig. 22-9). In some eyes a "subretinal tube" surrounded by inflammatory cells has been observed. This probably represents the site where the nematode wandered through the ocular tissues. It may be necessary to make many histologic sections through the granuloma to demonstrate the larva or its remnants.

MANAGEMENT

The treatment of ocular toxocariasis can be frustrating and perplexing.[1,12,25] Accurate assessment of treatment modalities can be particularly difficult because of the variable natural course of the disease. A successful result may be ascribed to a treatment modality when the same result could have been obtained with no treatment at all. Nevertheless, in most cases of severe nematode endophthalmitis the natural course of the disease is characterized by numerous complications, which frequently result in total blindness of the involved eye. Therefore prompt treatment in cases of active nematode endophthalmitis seems justified. Modalities that have been employed include anthelmintics to destroy the larvae and various nonspecific modalities to prevent the severe ocular complications and preserve or restore vision. These latter treatment measures include cycloplegic drugs, corticosteroids, and various types of intraocular surgery.

Anthelmintic Agents

Anthelmintics (e.g., piperazine salts) are usually successful in the treatment of adult worms in the intestinal tract of dogs. Unfortunately, the medical treatment of larvae in canine and human tissues has had more limited success. There are reports of clinical improvement in cases of VLM and ocular toxocariasis after larvicidal treatment with thiabendazole. Others have documented favorable results treating VLM with diethylcarbazine. It has been pointed out, however,[1] that such reported successes are difficult to evaluate because of concurrent use of corticosteroids, failure to confirm the initial diagnosis serologically, and failure to use controls.

Cycloplegic Agents

Cycloplegics are, of course, nonspecific in the management of ocular toxocariasis. They are used in appropriate doses for severe anterior segment inflammation to prevent the development of posterior synechias and secondary glaucoma.

Corticosteroids

Corticosteroids are also nonspecific and are employed primarily to prevent or minimize ocular complications. They can be given as topical drops, by subconjunctival or sub-Tenon injection, or orally depending on the site of the inflammation and its severity. For mild inflammatory processes involving the pars plana region, topical agents may suffice. In most such cases, however, subconjunctival or sub-Tenon injection of a long-acting depocorticosteroid may be preferable. Several authors have reported rather dramatic improvement following this type of therapy.[1] For severe infections or those that threaten vision by proximity to the fovea, oral or systemic corticosteroids are usually justified. Corticosteroids should be tapered and discontinued once the inflammation has subsided.

Ocular Surgery

In the past the severe complications of nematode endophthalmitis frequently led to retinal detachment, cyclitic membrane, and ultimately phthisis bulbi. The development of vitrectomy techniques has provided a method of sometimes preventing these complications.[26] Several investigators have reported success in salvaging the eye in such cases by vitrectomy, retinal detachment surgery, or a combination of the two. Hagler et al.[27] operated on 17 such patients and managed to obtain anatomic reattachment of the retina in 12 cases and stability or improvement in vision in 15. Others[28] have reported an 83% reattachment rate and 58% vision improvement in eyes with toxocara retinal traction treated with vitrectomy. When severe intraocular complications such as a cyclitic membrane or a retinal detachment appear inevitable, it appears that early vitrectomy to eliminate vitreous traction from the surface of the granuloma should be undertaken.[29] Because of the complexities of such cases, this surgery should be performed by experienced vitreoretinal surgeons. We have been referred several patients who had the erroneous diagnosis of toxocariasis made and undergone vitrectomy, only to find retinoblastoma. Because of the very serious consequences of vitrectomy in an eye harboring a neoplasm such as retinoblastoma, one should be sure of the diagnosis of toxocara endophthalmitis in a child before proceeding with vitrectomy.

Other types of intraocular surgery may occasionally be necessary to prevent complications or preserve vision. If a secondary cataract develops and there is a chance at visual recovery, cataract surgery may be considered. If secondary glaucoma cannot be controlled medically, then trabeculectomy or other forms of glaucoma surgery may be undertaken.

SUMMARY

Ocular toxocariasis is recognized to be a cause of childhood blindness. It usually results as a sequela of systemic infestation with the second or third stage larva of *Toxocara canis* (visceral larval migrans). Ocular toxocariasis can assume a variety of clinical forms and must be differentiated from other ocular conditions before the presumed diagnosis of ocular toxocariasis is made. ELISA testing and cytology are important in assisting the diagnosis. Treatment varies depending on the situation, but active inflammatory lesions are usually treated with systemic corticosteroids and sometimes removed by vitrectomy.

References

1. Shields JA: Ocular toxocariasis: a review, *Surv Ophthalmol* 28:361-381, 1984.
2. Sprent JFA: Observations on the development of Toxocara canis in the dog, *Parasitology* 48:184-209, 1958.
3. Beaver PC, Snyder CH, Carrera GM, et al: Chronic eosinophilia due to visceral larval migrans, *Pediatrics* 9:7-19, 1952.
4. Shantz PM, Glickman LT: Current concepts in parasitology-toxocaral visceral larval migrans, *N Engl J Med* 298:436-439, 1978.
5. Vaughn J, Jordan R: Intestinal nematodes in well cared for dogs, *Am J Trop Med Hyg* 9:29-32, 1960.
6. Brog VA, Woodruff AW: Prevalence of infective ova of Toxocara species in public places, *Br Med J* 4:470-472, 1973.
7. Snyder CH: Visceral larva migrans: ten years experience, *Pediatrics* 28:85-91, 1961.
8. Glickman LT, Schantz PM: Epidemiology and pathogenesis of zoonotic toxocariasis, *Epidemiol Rev* 3:230-250, 1981.
9. Wilder HC: Nematode endophthalmitis, *Trans Am Acad Ophthalmol Otolaryngol* 55:99-109, 1950.
10. Parsons HE: Nematode chorioretinitis: report of a case with photographs of a viable worm, *Arch Ophthalmol* 47:799-800, 1952.
11. Irvine WC, Irvine AR: Nematode endophthalmitis—Toxocara canis: report of a case, *Am J Ophthalmol* 47:185-191, 1959.
12. Molk R: Ocular toxocariasis: a review of the literature, *Ann Ophthalmol* 15:216-219, 1983.
13. Watzke RC, Oaks JA, Folk JC: Toxocara canis infection of the eye: correlation of clinical observations with developing pathology in the primate model, *Arch Ophthalmol* 102:282-291, 1984.
14. Cox TA, Haskins GE, Gangitano JL, Antonson DL: Bilateral toxocara optic neuropathy, *J Clin Neuroophthalmol* 3:267-274, 1983.
15. Shields JA, Parsons HM, Shields CL, Shah P: Lesions simulating retinoblastoma, *J Pediatr Ophthalmol Strab* 28:338-340, 1991.
16. Shields JA, Shields CL: *Intraocular tumors: a text and atlas,* Philadelphia, 1992, WB Saunders, pp 350-354.
17. Hemady R, Sainz de la Maza M, Raizman MB, Foster CS: Six cases of scleritis associated with systemic infection, *Am J Ophthalmol* 114:55-62, 1992.
18. Clemett RS, Williamson HJ, Hidajat RR, et al: Ocular Toxocara canis infections: diagnosis by enzyme immunoassay, *Aust N Z J Ophthalmol* 15:145-150, 1987.
19. Sharkey JA, McKay PS: Ocular toxocariasis in a patient with repeatedly negative ELISA titre to Toxocara canis, *Br J Ophthalmol* 77:253-254, 1993.
20. Maguire AM, Green WR, Michels RG, Erozan YS: Recovery of intraocular Toxocara canis by pars plana vitrectomy, *Ophthalmology* 97:675-680, 1990.
21. Pollard ZF: Long term follow up in patients with ocular toxocariasis as measured by ELISA titers, *Ann Ophthalmol* 19:167-169, 1987.
22. Kielar RA: Toxocara canis endophthalmitis with low ELISA titer, *Ann Ophthalmol* 15:447, 1983.

23. Shields JA, Ehya H, Shields CL, et al: Fine needle aspiration biopsy for intraocular tumors and pseudotumors, *Ophthalmology* 100:1677-1684, 1993.
24. Hamel CP, De Luca H, Billotte C, et al: Nonspecific immunoglobulin E in aqueous humor: evaluation in uveitis, *Graefes Arch Clin Exp Ophthalmol* 227:489-493, 1989.
25. Dinning WJ, Gillespie SH, Cooling RJ, Maizels RM: Toxocariasis: a practical approach to management of ocular disease, *Eye* 2:580-582, 1988.
26. Benson WE, Belmont JB, Irvine AR, et al: Vitrectomy for complication of ocular toxocariasis, *Trans Pa Acad Ophthalmol Otolaryngol* 36:25-30, 1983.
27. Hagler WH, Pollard ZF, Jarrett WH, Donnelly EH: results of surgery for ocular Toxocara canis, *Ophthalmology* 88:1081-1086, 1981.
28. Small KW, McCuen BW, de Juan E, Machemer R: Surgical management of retinal traction caused by toxocariasis, *Am J Ophthalmol* 108:10-14, 1989.
29. Rodriquez A: Early pars plana vitrectomy in chronic encophthalmitis of toxocariasis, *Graefes Arch Clin Exp Ophthalmol* 224:218-220, 1986.

23

Cytomegalovirus Infections of the Retina: Retinal and Ophthalmologic Manifestations of AIDS

Emad B. Abboud

The acquired immune deficiency syndrome (AIDS) is caused by infection with a member of the Retrovirus family, the human immunodeficiency virus (HIV). The epidemic has been explosive. In 1982 there were about 300 cases diagnosed in the United States. By late 1991 there was a cumulative total of almost 200,000 cases diagnosed with the syndrome.[9] Sixty-five percent of those have died. Although it is believed that the epidemic has reached a plateau, the number of yearly new cases has steadily increased. In 1989 a total of 35,614 cases were reported to the Centers for Disease Control (CDC); for 1990 this number was 42,442 cases,[6] and almost the same for 1991. The rate is not expected to drop in the coming years, for it is estimated [7,26] that over 1 million people in the United States are seropositive for the HIV, among whom 58,000 to 85,000 will develop full AIDS every year. This is to say that every ophthalmologist is likely to see patients with the ophthalmic manifestations of this disease and particularly that there are suggestions that the epidemic is disproportionately increasing in areas of traditionally low incidence, such as rural areas.[13,19] The main risk groups include homosexual/bisexual men, intravenous drug users, hemophiliacs, sexual partners of infected individuals, and children born to infected mothers.[8] There are four major categories of ophthalmic manifestations in AIDS: (1) microvasculopathy, the commonest being the cotton-wool spots, (2) opportunistic infections, (3) neoplasms, and (4) neuroophthalmic manifestations of intracranial infections and neoplasms. The opportunistic infections are the most visually devastating ophthalmic manifestations of AIDS, and cytomegalovirus (CMV) retinitis is by far the commonest of those infections. That is why the remainder of this chapter will concentrate mainly on this condition.

CMV retinitis is one of the indicator diseases that fulfill the criteria of the Centers for Disease Control (CDC) in the diagnosis of AIDS.[5,4] As the term implies, it is a retinal infection by the human cytomegaloviruses, which are a sub-group of agents within the herpes group of viruses, all with the propensity for remaining latent in humans.

The cytomegaloviruses are ubiquitous. Although the prevalence in the general population increases gradually with age—60% to 90% of adults having experienced infection—manifest clinical disease remains very rare. In an immunodeficiency status, like AIDS, however, these agents do cause significant disease (i.e., retinitis). In the literature CMV retinitis has been reported to occur in 6% to 46% of patients with AIDS and an incidence of 20% to 25% is accepted by most investigators.*

CMV retinitis is usually a late manifestation of AIDS, a the vast majority of patients having already been diagnosed with the syndrome by the time the retinitis develops.[34,54] It is important, however, for the ophthalmologist to know that a small group of patients with AIDS, approximately 1%, will have CMV retinitis as the first indicator disease of the syndrome.[61] None of these patients is free of symptoms (e.g., fever, weight loss, diarrhea, lymphadenopathy). Some of them have preexisting or concurrent conditions, not diagnosed before the development of the retinitis, that fulfill the criteria of the CDC for the diagnosis of AIDS. Very few patients will have CMV retinitis as the first and only condition to fulfill the CDC criteria.†

SYMPTOMS

Presentation can be unilateral or bilateral. The symptoms depend on the location of the focus of retinitis. If the fovea is not involved, the patient usually complains of floaters with little if any visual blur. When the fovea is involved, the patient presents with a variable degree of visual deterioration that has been gradual in onset. Photophobia, pain, and redness, which are the symptoms of iridocyclitis, are very uncommon, since the eye is typically white and quiet in CMV retinitis. Finally, one should add that nowadays, with the increased awareness of CMV retinitis, some cases are diagnosed at routine eye examinations in patients with AIDS.

CLINICAL FEATURES

As mentioned before, the anterior segment is typically quiet, although variable degrees of inflammation have been reported in some cases. An overlying vitreous with minimal to absent reaction is one of the hallmarks of CMV retinitis in AIDS.

The retinitis is a slowly progressive necrotizing one caused by cell-to-cell spread of the virus. It is typically situated around the major retinal blood vessels, and therefore posteriorly located, pointing to the hematogenous spread of the virus. It can, however, occur only in the periphery. The area of active necrosis has a granular yellow-white appearance that has been described as resembling crumbled cheese. There are often retinal hemorrhages, particularly at the border of the lesion, which have made its appearance likened to "pizza"

---

* References 16, 30, 33, 34, 37, 45, 51, 55, 59.
† References 28, 36, 37, 41, 52, 61.

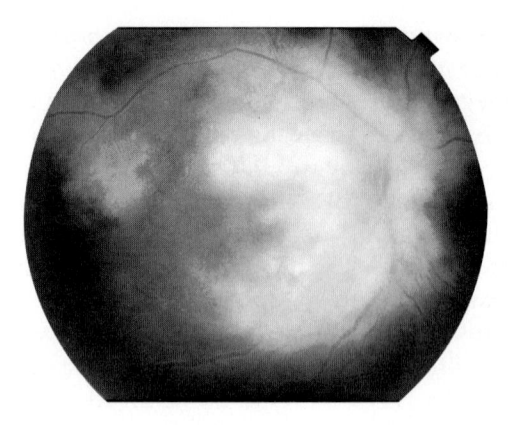

Figure 23-1 Right eye of a 23-year-old homosexual man with AIDS. Note the typical "pizza" appearance with retinal exudates and hemorrhages.

(Fig. 23-1). Retinal vascular sheathing caused by perivascular neutrophilic infiltrates is sometimes present. In a few cases the infiltrates around the arteries and the veins will be dense enough to produce a picture of *frosted branch angiitis.*[62] There is usually a clear demarcation between the area of retinitis and the contiguous normal retina.

In more chronic cases the center of the lesion shows retinal atrophy with widespread retinal pigmentary changes representing healed retinitis.[47] The area of active necrosis, with the characteristics mentioned above, is usually a narrow band at the periphery described in this case as "brush fire border."

The most devastating complication of CMV retinitis is permanent severe visual loss secondary to direct foveal involvement by the necrotizing retinitis. Fortunately, with the advent of different antiretroviral therapies, this is becoming an uncommon occurrence. Rhegmatogenous retinal detachment is another main complication. It is estimated[16,37,60] that retinal detachment will develop in 15% to 29% of these patients, never being present at the time of diagnosis of the retinitis. The literature reports an average of 5 months between the onset of retinitis and the occurrence of retinal detachment. There is a higher risk of detachment with larger lesions as well as lesions reaching the ora serrata.[15,38] Statements have been made[16,60] about the role of antiretroviral therapy in increasing the risk of retinal detachment by decreasing scar formation. As other authors, we believe that retinal detachment is mainly related to the healing of this necrotizing retinitis, regardless of the therapeutic modality used. Furthermore, it should be clear that the benefit of antiretroviral therapy far outweighs any possible theoretic risk of some increased incidence of retinal detachment.

DIFFERENTIAL DIAGNOSIS

There is a long list of agents reported to cause retinitis in patients with AIDS, many of which are single case reports. For practical clinical purposes, four entities are particularly difficult to differentiate from CMV retinitis: acute retinal necrosis (ARN), toxoplasmic retinochoroiditis, syphilitic retinitis, and fungal retinitis. It should be emphasized from the outset that CMV retinitis is far more common in patients with AIDS than any of those entities.

The ARN has been diagnosed in patients with AIDS. Typically, it has a more fulminant course. At presentation patients usually have very poor vision. The anterior segment and vitreous cavity show significantly more inflammatory reaction than in cases of CMV retinitis. There is an occlusive retinal vasculitis with areas of retinal necrosis starting in the far periphery and extending toward the posterior pole. These are areas of flat homogeneous retinal whitening with a sharp demarcation separating them from the posterior uninvolved retina. They typically lack the granular "crumbled cheese" appearance of CMV retinitis. Usually also there are no hemorrhages at the edges of the areas of necrosis. Rhegmatogenous retinal detachment is much more frequent in ARN, occurring in 75% to 84% of the cases. In our experience as well as the experiences of others, these clinical features make the differentiation possible in almost all cases. It is an important differentiation to make, because the herpes simplex and varicella-zoster viruses (HSV, VZV), the causative agents of ARN, are not responsive to ganciclovir but their treatment with intravenous acyclovir is usually beneficial.

Varicella-zoster virus is the causative agent of a distinct entity: outer retinal necrosis.[14] This creates no diagnostic dilemma since the retinitis is clearly deep in the neurosensory retina, without hemorrhages or vascular involvement until late in the disease process.[14,49]

Ocular toxoplasmosis in immune-competent individuals is characterized by a unilateral single focus of intense retinochoroiditis originating at the edge of a pigmented chorioretinal scar. It is clinically different from the ocular toxoplasmosis in AIDS and is not one of the CDC criteria for AIDS diagnosis. It should be differentiated from CMV retinitis because the correct treatment is essential, not only to halt the progression of the retinitis but also to treat the often concurrent life-threatening cerebral toxoplasmosis. The ocular disease can be unilateral or bilateral.[25,32] In contrast to CMV retinitis, it always has a significant anterior chamber and vitreous reaction. Fundus examination reveals single or multifocal discrete foci of retinitis[32] that are yellow-white and edematous with hazy borders. They lack the dry granular "crumbled cheese" appearance of CMV retinitis. Hemorrhages are rarely present. The areas of retinitis are sometimes diffuse. Since there are no reliable laboratory tests, one should start antiparasitic therapy (pyrimethamine, sulfadiazine, clindamycin, and folinic acid) if the clinical picture is suggestive of ocular toxoplasmosis. A favorable response to the therapy will provide a retrospective confirmation of the diagnosis. MRI of the brain with evidence of discrete or diffuse cerebral toxoplasmosis can sometimes be helpful in the diagnosis.

Treponema pallidum is a rare cause of retinitis in patients with AIDS. It can be unilateral or bilateral. Patients usually present with blurred vision of recent onset. Characteristically, there is a significant vitreous cellular reaction. The fundus shows multiple yellow-gray chorioretinal lesions with indistinct borders that are often confluent in the posterior pole or midperiphery. Although superficial flame-shaped retinal hemorrhages are sometimes present, they are different from the larger retinal hemorrhages along the borders of CMV retinitis lesions. Evidence of retinal perivasculitis is often seen elsewhere in the fundus. Most of these patients have the characteristic syphilitic rash on the forearms, palms, and soles.[56] The VDRL and the MHA-TP (microhemagglutination assay for *Treponema pallidum*) or FTA-ABS (fluorescent treponemal antibody absorbed) are positive because most HIV-infected patients have a normal serologic response to *Treponema* infection.[46] It is important to know, however, that the sensitivity of these tests drops from 93% in asymptomatic HIV patients to 63% in symptomatic ones.[24] A high index of suspicion should be maintained for syphilis in patients with AIDS because the conditions have common risk factors. In fact, it is now recommended[58] that tests for both conditions be performed on patients who test positive for either disease. If the diagnosis of syphilitic retinitis is suspected, with negative serologic tests, a course of penicillin can be administered. Most patients will respond favorably to this, providing a retrospective diagnosis of the condition. Acute syphilitic posterior placoid chorioretinitis[20] is not difficult to differentiate from CMV retinitis: there is more vitreous reaction, and the lesion is typically deep (at the level of the RPE and choroid), sparing the inner neurosensory retina.

Candida is an uncommon cause of retinitis in AIDS patients. It is more frequent in patients with other risk factors, particularly intravenous drug abuse. It can be unilateral or bilateral. As in CMV retinitis, patients often present with floaters of gradual onset and some blurring of vision. The fundus picture, however, is quite distinct. The focus of retinitis is a white discrete inner retinal lesion that is usually one disc diameter or smaller in size. There are often multiple foci at the time of diagnosis. Characteristically a hazy cellular reaction overlies the retinitis, with small or large white opacities in the vitreous cavity. Almost all these patients have positive candidemia (i.e., growth of *Candida* from blood cultures).

DIAGNOSTIC APPROACH

In known AIDS patients, because of its frequency and typical appearance, the diagnosis of CMV retinitis can almost always be made solely on the basis of the clinical picture.

In known HIV-positive individuals without other conditions to fulfill the CDC criteria for AIDS, the diagnosis of CMV retinitis is made on the basis of the clinical examination. The diagnosis is confirmed by positive blood cultures for CMV. Urine cultures are of limited diagnostic value since 50% of homosexual men and the majority of patients with AIDS test positive for CMV.

In the few individuals who present with CMV retinitis and who are not known to be HIV infected, the diagnosis is more challenging.

1. The diagnosis is highly suspected on the basis of the typical clinical appearance.
2. You must confirm the HIV infection and investigate the state of immune deficiency, since the latter is always advanced when CMV retinitis is diagnosed:
   a. HIV infection is a high probability when cotton-wool spots are encountered in the ipsilateral or contralateral eye.
   b. Careful history taking will often reveal symptoms (e.g., fever, weight loss and diarrhea) that the patient did not volunteer initially.
   c. An ELISA is ordered to confirm the presence of antibodies against the HIV. This is confirmed by Western Blot analysis.
   d. The CD4 helper count is always less than 50 cells/mm^3.
   e. The helper/suppressor ratio, which is normally between 1 and 2, is often under 0.1 in patients with CMV retinitis, a witness to their extremely advanced immune deficiency.

3. You must confirm the diagnosis of CMV, since you will not only declare this patient HIV-positive but also label him as AIDS, with all the implications that that carries.
   a. Most important is a positive blood culture for CMV.
   b. As mentioned before, urine culture is of limited diagnostic value.
   c. Although a rising titer of complement-fixation antibodies to CMV can sometimes be elicited, these serologic tests are extremely unreliable in patients with AIDS.[16,18]

MANAGEMENT

When CMV retinitis was initially described in patients with AIDS, there was essentially no known treatment to halt the relentless progression of the condition.[34,54] This situation has dramatically changed with the introduction of ganciclovir and then foscarnet. It should be stressed that this is an area in constant evolution, wherein the dosages and regimens mentioned here may be quickly outdated. Also, new therapeutic agents that are now investigative may soon have a place in our daily clinical treatment of this disease. Hence it becomes important for us as ophthalmologists to have some general principles of management before looking into the pharmacologic details of these agents.

1. There is now a consensus that all AIDS patients with CMV retinitis should receive treatment with one of the antiretroviral agents. This has definitely decreased the incidence of blindness, which, in light of the prolonged survival of patients with AIDS, becomes an important improvement in their quality of life.
2. In the management of these patients the ophthalmologist is a member of a team, providing expertise for the diagnosis of retinitis and the important assessment of response to therapy. The choice of the initial agent to use (i.e., ganciclovir vs foscarnet) as well as the monitoring of its effect on the different body functions, is better left to the patient's internist or infectious disease specialist.
3. Constant communication with the different physicians involved in the patient's care cannot be overemphasized.

Ganciclovir

Chemical Structure. Ganciclovir is an acyclic nucleoside analog of deoxyguanosine.

Mechanism of Action. Ganciclovir triphosphate, which is the active form of the drug, acts as an inhibitor and a false substrate to CMV DNA polymerase. It is incorporated in the CMV DNA, altering chain elongation and virus replication. The effect is reversible when ganciclovir is discontinued. That is why it is only *virostatic.*[48,64]

To become converted to the triphosphate active form, ganciclovir is phosphorylated by CMV deoxyguanosine kinase. This intracellular phosphorylation is relatively selective in that levels of ganciclovir triphosphate in CMV-infected cells are much higher than in uninfected cells. It is important to know, however, that bone marrow cells are uniquely sensitive to ganciclovir, which explains the high incidence of neutropenia.[50]

Pharmacokinetics. Ganciclovir is poorly absorbed from the gastrointestinal tract. Therefore it must be given intravenously.

It undergoes virtually no metabolism in the body. Its clearance is totally dependent on renal elimination. Consequently, doses must be adjusted in cases of renal dysfunction.

Toxicity. The most frequent adverse effect is neutropenia, occurring in 40% of patients. Severe dose-limiting neutropenia, however, occurs in only 20% of patients[1] and is usually reversible upon discontinuation of the drug. The use of adjuvant subcutaneous therapy with granulocyte-macrophage colony stimulating factor (GM-CSF) or granulocyte colony stimulating factor (G-CSF) to treat neutropenia is currently under investigation.[23]

It is important to understand the interaction with zidovudine because this drug is the only one proven to prolong survival in AIDS patients.[12] In addition, most patients with CMV retinitis will already be receiving zidovudine at the time of diagnosis. There is a synergistic bone marrow suppression when ganciclovir and zidovudine are used together, causing severe neutropenia. This is always true when the full dose of zidovudine, 1200 mg/day, is used. An alternative approach[3] might be to discontinue zidovudine during induction and restart it with the maintenance therapy at a dose of 300 to 500 mg/day. This regimen has been found to be well tolerated, but its clinical effectiveness is yet to be proven.

Dosage. Currently the recommended dose for induction is 5 mg/kg every 12 hours for 14 to 21 days. This is followed by a permanent maintenance dose of 5 mg/kg/day 7 days a week or 6 mg/kg/day 5 days a week.

Routes of Administration. The vast majority of patients receive ganciclovir intravenously. Most AIDS patients have a permanent indwelling central venous line installed. With the availability of companies providing patients with IV supplies as well as the drug at home, most of the management is now done on an outpatient basis. This has the significant advantage of improving the quality of life of the patients since it gives them a sense of independence.

Intravitreal injection of ganciclovir has been investigated[2,64] and is occasionally used. The recommended dose is 200 µg/0.1 ml. For induction two injections per week are given for 2 to 3 weeks. This is followed by a weekly injection for maintenance. Such administration has many drawbacks, however. In addition to the inherent potential complications, there are logistical difficulties with weekly intravitreal injections administered for an indefinite period. More important, the systemic CMV infection is not treated. Consequently, this route of administration is going to be limited to the few individuals who have visual loss from progressive retinitis and are intolerant of intravenous ganciclovir and foscarnet.

Foscarnet

Chemical Structure. Foscarnet is not a nucleoside analog but a pyrophosphate analog of phosphonoacetic acid.

Mechanism of Action. Foscarnet has a selective noncompetitive inhibitory effect on specific viral DNA polymerases and reverse transcriptases at concentrations that do not affect the cellular DNA polymerases. Because it directly influences the pyrophosphate binding of the polymerases, it does not require phosphorylation. This gives it potential activity against CMV, HSV, and VZV. More importantly, it gives foscarnet an intrinsic anti-HIV effect that ganciclovir lacks.[40,47]

The effect of foscarnet is reversible; and therefore, like ganciclovir, it is *virostatic*.

Pharmacokinetics. Foscarnet is administered intravenously because it is poorly absorbed from the gastrointestinal tract.

It is not metabolized in the body and is cleared via renal elimination.

Toxicity. The most common and serious adverse effect of foscarnet is nephrotoxicity, occurring in 25% of the patients.[43,54] This is reversible, however, on discontinuation of the drug.

Because the drug is eliminated by the kidneys and at the same time is nephrotoxic, constant monitoring of renal function with dose adjustment is mandatory.

Since it does not produce any neutropenia, foscarnet can be used concurrently with the full dose of zidovudine.

Dosage. The recommended induction dose is an intermittent infusion of 60 mg/kg over 1 to 2 hours given every 8 hours for 14 to 21 days. The maintenance dose is 90 to 120 mg/kg/day given over 2 hours indefinitely.

The response of CMV retinitis to induction therapy with ganciclovir or foscarnet has been favorable. Anatomic improvement has been reported[28,31,35,39] in 80% to 100% of patients. The resolution starts within 1 to 2 weeks. The vascular sheathing disappears, the opacification of the edges decreases, and, most important, the lesion stops enlarging. Ultimately, an area of retinal atrophy with diffuse RPE changes remains (Fig. 23-2). This usually requires 3 to 4 weeks. It should be noted that in some patients an opaque white edge remains, without necessarily representing persistent activity, as none of these lesion showed any change when observed over several months.[44]

While on maintenance therapy with ganciclovir or foscarnet, 27% to 50% of patients show evidence of recurrence.[22,29,35,37] This can be in the form of obvious granular white opacification of the edges or a subtle low-grade retinitis detectable only by comparing serial fundus photographs. The patients resume taking an induction dose for 2 weeks, followed by a maintenance dose indefinitely. The vast majority respond favorably,[22,27,42] which indicates that the re-

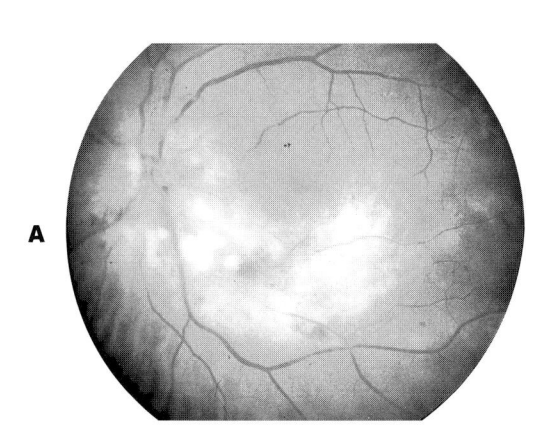

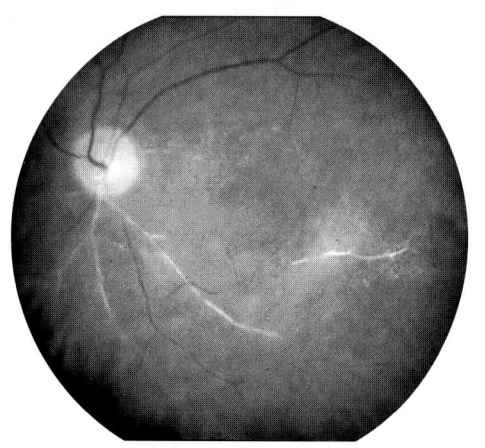

Figure 23-2 A, Active retinitis in the left eye of a 37-year-old man. **B,** Two months after the start of ganciclovir treatment the retinitis has subsided, leaving an area of retinal atrophy.

currence signified not a resistance to the drug but rather that the immune status of the patient had deteriorated to a point rendering the serum levels of ganciclovir insufficient.

AIDS patients with CMV retinitis who are treated with ganciclovir have a mean survival of 5 to 8 months.[27,32,42,52] This contrasts with the 120-day survival reported in untreated patients in 1984.[55] In addition to the antiretroviral therapy, other factors probably contributed to the improved survival: prior treatment with zidovudine and improved prevention and treatment of other opportunistic infections. In the SOCA foscarnet-ganciclovir CMV retinitis trial,[63] foscarnet-treated patients had a mean survival of 12 months, 4 months longer than the ganciclovir group. In the same study, however, foscarnet had more toxicity than ganciclovir. Therefore the answer as to which agent to use initially is not clear yet. As mentioned before, the decision is better left to the patient's internist or infectious disease specialist because there are many nonocular factors to be taken into consideration.

Discussion of the surgical management of retinal detachment complicating CMV retinitis is beyond the scope of this chapter. There are, however, important points to mention. The decision to operate must be tailored to each patient, with consideration taken of visual function before the detachment developed, the condition of the other eye, and the general condition of the patient. Pars plana vitrectomy and silicone oil injection without a lensectomy is the procedure of choice.[17,57] Useful vision is preserved or restored in the majority of patients. This improves the quality of their life, an important consideration since so many are now living longer.

Finally, prophylactic laser photocoagulation around areas of CMV retinitis is not mandatory. It is of little value in preventing the development of retinal detachment.[17]

References

1. Buhles WC Jr, Master BJ, Tinker AJ, et al: Ganciclovir treatment of life-or-sight-threatening cytomegalovirus infection: experience in 314 immunocompromised patients, *Rev Infect Dis* 10(suppl 3):S495-S506, 1988.
2. Cantrill HL, Henry K, Melroe NH, et al: Treatment of cytomegalovirus retinitis with intravitreal ganciclovir: long-term results, *Ophthalmology* 96:367-374, 1989.
3. Causey D: Concomitant ganciclovir and zidovudine treatment for cytomegalovirus retinitis in patients with HIV infection: an approach to treatment, *J Acquired Immun Def Syn* 4(suppl 1):S16-S21, 1991.
4. Centers for Disease Control: Classification system for human T-lymphotropic virus type III/lymphadenopathy-associated virus infections, *MMWR* 35:334, 1986.
5. Centers for Disease Control: Revision of the Centers for Disease Control surveillance case definition for the acquired immunodeficiency syndrome, *MMWR* 36:38, 1987.
6. Centers for Disease Control: HIV, *AIDS Surveill Rep*, p 1, December 1990.
7. Centers for Disease Control: HIV prevalence estimates and AIDS projections for the United States: report based upon a workshop, *MMWR* 39:1, 1990.
8. Centers for Disease Control: Acquired immunodeficiency syndrome: United States, 1981-1990, *MMWR* 40:358, 1991.
9. Centers for Disease Control: Human immunodeficiency virus, *AIDS Surveill Rep*, p 1, November 1991.
10. Cochereau-Massin I, Lehoang P, Lautier-Frau M, et al: Efficacy and tolerance of intravitreal ganciclovir in cytomegalovirus retinitis in acquired immunodeficiency syndrome, *Ophthalmology* 98:1348-1355, 1991.

11. Edwards JE, Foos RY, Mongomerie JZ, Guze LB: Ocular manifestations of Candida septicemia: review of seventy-six cases of hematogenous Candida endophthalmitis, *Medicine* 53:47-75, 1974.
12. Fischl MA, Richman DD, Hansen N, et al: The safety and efficacy of zidovudine (AZT) in the treatment of patients with mildly symptomatic HIV infection: a double-blind, placebo-controlled trial, *Ann Intern Med* 112:727-737, 1990.
13. Fleming DW, Cochi SL, Steece RS, et al: Acquired immunodeficiency syndrome in low incidence areas: how safe is unsafe sex? *JAMA* 258:785, 1987.
14. Forster DJ, Dugel PU, Frangieh GT, et al: Rapidly progressive outer retinal necrosis in the acquired immunodeficiency syndrome, *Am J Ophthalmol* 110:341-348, 1990.
15. Freeman WR, Henderly DE, Wan WL, et al: Prevalence, pathophysiology, and treatment of rhegmatogenous retinal detachment in treated cytomegalovirus retinitis, *Am J Ophthalmol* 103:527, 1987.
16. Freeman WR, Lerner CW, Mines JA, et al: A prospective study of the ophthalmologic findings in the acquired immunodeficiency syndrome, *Am J Ophthalmol* 97:133, 1984.
17. Freeman WR, Freeman WR, Quiceno JI, Crapotta JA, et al: Surgical repair of rhegmatogenous retinal detachment in immunosuppressed patients with cytomegalovirus retinitis, *Ophthalmology* 99:466-474, 1992.
18. Friedman AH, Orellana J, Freeman WR, et al: Cytomegalovirus retinitis: manifestation of the acquired immunodeficiency syndrome (AIDS), *Br J Ophthalmol* 67:372-380, 1983.
19. Gardner LI, Brundage JF, Burke DS, et al: Evidence for spread of the human immunodeficiency virus epidemic into low prevalence areas of the United States, *J Acquir Immune Defic Syndr* 2:521, 1989.
20. Gass JD, Braunstein RA, Chenoweth RG: Acute syphilitic posterior placoid chorioretinitis, *Ophthalmology* 97:1288-1297, 1990.
21. Griffin JR, Pettit TH, Fishman LS, et al: Blood borne Candida endophthalmitis: clinical and pathologic study of 21 cases, *Arch Ophthalmol* 89:450-456, 1973.
22. Gross JG, Bozette SA, Mathews WC, et al: Longitudinal study of cytomegalovirus retinitis in acquired immunodeficiency syndrome, *Ophthalmology* 97:681-686, 1990.
23. Grossberg HS, Bonnem EM, Buhles WC: GM-CSF with ganciclovir for the treatment of CMV retinitis in AIDS, *N Engl J Med* 320:1560, 1989.
24. Hass JS, Bolan G, Larsen SA, et al: Sensitivity of treponemal test for detecting prior treated syphilis during human immunodeficiency virus infection, *J Infect Dis* 162:862-866, 1990.
25. Heinemann MH, Gold JMW, Maisel J: Bilateral toxoplasma retinochoroiditis in a patient with acquired immunodeficiency syndrome, *Retina* 6:224, 1986.
26. Hellinger FJ: Forcasting the medical care cost of the human immunodeficiency virus epidemic 1991-1994, *Inquiry* 28:213, 1991.
27. Henderly DE, Freeman WR, Causey DM, et al: Cytomegalovirus retinitis and response to therapy with ganciclovir, *Ophthalmology* 94:425-434, 1987.
28. Henderly DE, Freeman WR, Smith RE, et al: Cytomegalovirus retinitis as the initial manifestation of the acquired immunodeficiency syndrome, *Am J Ophthalmol* 103:316, 1987.
29. Henderson DK, Fahey BJ, Willy M, et al: Risk for occupational transmission of human immunodeficiency virus type 1(HIV I) associated with clinical exposure: a prospective evaluation, *Ann Intern Med* 113:740-746, 1990.
30. Holland GN: Acquired immunodeficiency syndrome and ophthalmology: the first decade, *Am J Ophthalmol* 114:86-96, 1992.
31. Holland GN, Buhles WC, Mastre B, et al: A controlled retrospective study of ganciclovir treatment for cytomegalovirus retinopathy: use of a standardized system for the assessment of disease outcome, *Arch Ophthalmol* 107:1757-1766, 1989.
32. Holland GN, Engstrom RE, Glasgow BJ, et al: ocular toxoplasmosis in patients with the acquired immunodeficiency syndrome, *Am J Ophthalmol* 106:653-657, 1988.
33. Holland GN, Gottlieb MS, Yee RD, et al: Ocular disorders associated with a new severe acquired cellular immunodeficiency syndrome, *Am J Ophthalmol* 93:393, 1982.
34. Holland GN, Pepose JS, Pettit TM, et al: Acquired immunodeficiency syndrome: ocular manifestations, *Ophthalmology* 90:859, 1983.

35. Holland GN, Sidikaro Y, Kreiger EA, et al: Treatment of cytomegalovirus retinopathy with ganciclovir, *Ophthalmology* 94:815-823, 1987.
36. Holland GN, Sison RF, Jatulis DE, et al: Survival of patients with the acquired immunodeficiency syndrome after development of cytomegalovirus retinopathy, *Ophthalmology* 97:204, 1990.
37. Jabs DA, Enger C, Bartlett JG: Cytomegalovirus retinitis and acquired immunodeficiency syndrome, *Arch Ophthalmol* 107:75, 1989.
38. Jabs DA, Enger C, Haller J, et al: Retinal detachments in patients with cytomegalovirus retinitis, *Arch Ophthalmol 109:794, 1991.*
39. Jabs DA, Newman C, DeBustros G, et al: Treatment of cytomegalovirus retinitis with ganciclovir, *Ophthalmology* 94:824-830, 1987.
40. Jacobson MA, Crowe S, Levy J, et al: Effect of foscarnet therapy on infection with human immunodeficiency virus in patients with acquired immunodeficiency syndrome, *J Infect Dis* 158:862-865, 1988.
41. Jacobson MA, Mills J: Serious cytomegalovirus disease in acquired immunodeficiency syndrome (AIDS), *Ann Intern Med* 108:585, 1988.
42. Jacobson MA, O'Donnell JJ, Brodie HR, et al: Randomized, prospective trial of ganciclovir maintenance therapy for cytomegalovirus retinitis, *J Med Virol* 25:339-349, 1988.
43. Jacobson MA, O'Donnell JJ, Mills J: Foscarnet treatment of cytomegalovirus retinitis in patients with the acquired immunodeficiency syndrome, *Antimicrob Agents Chemother* 33:736-741, 1989.
44. Keefe KS, Freeman WR, Peterson TJ, et al: Atypical healing of cytomegalovirus retinitis, *Ophthalmology* 99:1377-1384, 1992.
45. Kestelyn P, Van de Perre P, Rouvroy D, et al: A prospective study of the ophthalmologic findings in the acquired immunodeficiency syndrome in Africa, *Am J Ophthalmol* 100:230, 1985.
46. Larsen SA: Serological reactions when syphilis and HIV occur as coinfection. In Savage RA (ed): *Summing up.* College of American Pathologists Diagnostic Immunology Resource Committee publication, Autumn 1989.
47. LeHoang P, Girard B, Robinet M, et al: Foscarnet in the treatment of cytomegalovirus retinitis in acquired immunodeficiency syndrome, *Ophthalmology* 96:865-874, 1989.
48. Mar E-C, Cheng Y-C, Huang E-S: Effect of 9-(1,3 dihydroxy-2-propoxymethyl)guanine on human cytomegalovirus replication in vivo, *Antimicrob Agents Chemother* 24:518-521, 1983.
49. Margolis TP, Lowder CY, Holland GN, et al: Varicella zoster virus retinitis in patients with the acquired immunodeficiency syndrome, *Am J Ophthalmol* 112:119-131, 1991.
50. Mathews T, Boehme R: Antiviral activity and mechanism of action of ganciclovir, *Rev Infec Dis* 10(suppl 3):S490-S494, 1988.
51. Newman NM, Mandel MR, Gullett J, et al: Clinical and histologic findings in opportunistic infections: part of a new syndrome of acquired immunodeficiency, *Arch Ophthalmol* 101:396, 1983.
52. Orellana J, Teich SA, Friedmann AH, et al: Combined short- and long-term therapy for the treatment of cytomegalovirus retinitis using ganciclovir (BW B759U), *Ophthalmology* 94:831, 1987.
53. Orellana J, Teich SA, Lieberman RM, et al: Treatment of retinal detachments in patients with the acquired immunodeficiency syndrome, *Ophthalmology* 98:939, 1991.
54. Palestine AG, Polis MA, DeSmet MD, et al: A randomized controlled trial of foscarnet in the treatment of cytomegalovirus retinitis in patients with the acquired immunodeficiency syndrome, *Ann Intern Med* 115:665-673, 1991.
55. Palestine AG, Rodriguez MM, Macher AM, et al: Ophthalmic involvement in acquired immunodeficiency syndrome, *Ophthalmology* 91:1092, 1984.
56. Passo MS, Rosenbaum JT: Ocular syphilis in patients with human immunodeficiency virus infection, *Am J Ophthalmol* 106:1-6, 1988.

57. Regillo CD, Vander JF, Duker JS, et al: Repair of retinitis related retinal detachment with silicone oil in patients with acquired immunodeficiency syndrome, *Am J Ophthalmol* 113:21-27, 1992.
58. Ruffli T: Syphilis and HIV infection, *Dermatologica* 179:113-117, 1989.
59. Schuman JS, Orellana J, Friedmann AH, et al: Acquired immunodeficiency syndrome (AIDS), *Surv Ophthalmol* 31:384, 1987.
60. Sidikaro Y, Silver L, Holland GN, et al: Rhegmatogenous retinal detachment in patients with AIDS and necrotizing retinal infections, *Ophthalmology* 98:129, 1991.
61. Sison RF, Holland GN, McArthur LG, et al: Cytomegalovirus retinopathy as the initial manifestation of the acquired immunodeficiency syndrome, *Am J Ophthalmol* 112:243, 1991.
62. Spaide RF, Vitale AT, Toth ER, et al: Frosted branch angiitis associated with cytomegalovirus retinitis, *Am J Ophthalmol* 113:522-528, 1992.
63. Study of the Ocular Complications of AIDS Research Group, in collaboration with the AIDS Clinical Trial Group: Mortality in patients with the acquired immunodeficiency syndrome treated with either foscarnet or ganciclovir for cytomegalovirus retinitis, *N Engl J Med* 326:213-220, 1992.
64. Tocci MJ, Livelli TJ, Pery HC, et al: Effects of nucleoside analog 2'-nor-2'-deoxyguanosine on human cytomegalovirus replication, *Antimicrob Agents Chemother* 25:247-252, 1984.

24

Acute Retinal Necrosis (ARN) Syndrome

Jay S. Duker

The acute retinal necrosis (ARN) syndrome represents a unique and dramatic posterior segment inflammatory process associated with certain members of the herpes family of viruses. The clinical triad of findings that make it up[1-7] are (1) a full-thickness unilateral or bilateral retinal necrosis that preferentially affects the peripheral retina, (2) a moderate to severe vitritis, and (3) a vasculitis affecting primarily the retinal arteries. Associated findings include iritis, optic neuritis, retinal artery obstructions, macular edema, and exudative retinal detachment. One hallmark of the ARN syndrome is the unusually high incidence of full-thickness retinal breaks, frequently resulting in rhegmatogenous retinal detachment. The retinal detachments typically develop during the healing phase of the infection.

ARN is a recently recognized disease. It was first reported in the Japanese literature in 1971. In the initial report Urayama et al.[8] described five cases of severe unilateral panuveitis that resulted in retinal detachment. Since then there have been over 100 reported cases of ARN. Willerson et al.[9] are credited with reporting the first case of ARN in the English literature, in 1977, although an earlier description of probable ARN syndrome appeared in 1973.[10]

ETIOLOGY

ARN syndrome is the result of an infection of the posterior segment by one of the herpes family of viruses.[1,3] Varicella zoster virus (VZV) and, to a lesser extent, herpes simplex virus (HSV) account for most if not all cases of ARN.[11-21] Another member of the herpes family of viruses, cytomegalovirus (CMV), has been suggested as the cause of ARN in one case report.[22] This association has yet to be confirmed by other investigators.

Both VZV and HSV have been successfully cultured from the vitreous of patients with active ARN.[12,13,15] Other evidence for the viral nature of the disease includes the detection of specific HSV and VZV viral antigens in ocular fluid during active ARN by immunofluorescent antibody techniques as well as rising systemic antibodies to one of the two viruses.[12-21]

In the majority of cases systemic viral titers do not increase in temporal association with an ARN episode. This is explained by the hypothesis that most cases of ARN are due to a local, ocular, secondary reactivation of a latent systemic viral infection. Occasionally a primary viral infection can result in ARN, as is well documented in acute cases of varicella (chickenpox).[23,24]

CLINICAL APPEARANCE

The retinal necrosis associated with ARN is characteristic. It involves the full thickness of the retina and results in a dense whitish opacification. The edges of the necrosis are smooth and geographic, and the border between involved and uninvolved retina tends to be easily discerned. In the typical presentation the retinal necrosis associated with ARN begins in the peripheral retina. In untreated cases the new areas of involvement will include increasingly posterior zones. ARN advances via both cell-to-cell spread and the involvement of noncontiguous new areas (satellite lesions). Advancement is noted over a period of days. As the disease progresses, smaller areas of retinal necrosis coalesce and new lesions develop closer to the posterior pole. With lesional healing the retinal vasculature appears attenuated and retinal pigment epithelial (RPE) changes become prominent. The areas of RPE mottling characteristic of healed ARN usually develop several weeks after the onset of infection.

Initially in the course of ARN a mild to moderate vitreous cellular reaction is present. Rarely the vitritis will precede any sign of retinal necrosis by up to several weeks. More characteristically the vitritis and necrosis are coincident. As the disease progresses, the vitreous reaction becomes increasingly severe. At this stage observation of the posterior pole by ophthalmoscopy can be difficult. Eventually, necrotic retinal cells are shed into the vitreous cavity. As the inflammation subsides, fibrosis of the vitreous with contraction resembling proliferative vitreoretinopathy (PVR) occurs.

Narrowing of the retinal arteries, with inflammatory infiltrates in the vessel walls, is a universal finding in zones of active retinitis. ARN-associated retinal arteritis can be seen outside the areas of necrosis as well. Both central retinal artery obstruction and branch retinal artery obstruction may be associated with the vasculitis. Retinal phlebitis can occur with ARN as well but is less common and less pronounced than the arterial disease. More often there is perivenous hemorrhage. Large zones of hemorrhage akin to those in retinal venous occlusive disease are atypical.

Optic nerve edema is commonly seen in the acute stages of ARN.[25,26] It may be accompanied by evidence of optic neuritis and optic nerve dysfunction. ARN-associated optic neuropathy can be a significant cause of central visual loss.

Other reported findings with the ARN syndrome[1,3,27] include macular edema, exudative retinal detachment, and neovascularization of the retina, disc, and iris. The anterior segment findings are usually mild, often giving no indication of the severity of the posterior segment necrosis. Iritis with fine keratic precipitates is typical. Hypopyon has been reported but is rare. It is not unusual for patients with active ARN to manifest nonspecific systemic complaints such as headache, sinus pain, and stiff neck. Cases in which ARN has developed in close temporal association with herpetic skin lesions (zoster or chickenpox as well as HSV coldsores) have also been reported.[16,28,29] HSV viral keratitis does not usually coexist with the ARN syndrome.

At the onset of symptoms ARN is unilateral in most cases. The incidence of bilaterality at presentation will vary, however, depending on how soon the affected individual seeks treatment. In up to one third of patients bilateral involvement will develop within several weeks of the onset of symptoms[3]; but longer delays between the appearance of ARN in the second eye are well documented, with the longest on record being nearly two decades.[30] There is evidence[31] that the use of acyclovir reduces, but does not completely eliminate, the risk of second eye involvement.

In the initially reported ARN cases all patients had normal systemic immunity. More recently cases of classic ARN syndrome in immune-suppressed individuals, including persons with the acquired immune deficiency syndrome (AIDS), have been recognized.[32-34] Other AIDS patients have been noted to develop a unique form of ARN that begins in the outer retina, tends to spare the tissue immediately surrounding the retinal vessels, and rapidly progresses despite treatment.[35,36] VZV appears to be the cause of this rapidly progressive ARN.

The diagnosis of ARN is a clinical one based on the ophthalmoscopic appearance of the necrosis along with associated signs. Fluorescein angiography is occasionally helpful in sorting out the causes of visual loss but is not needed to secure the diagnosis. Vitreous and/or retinal biopsy are rarely indicated in atypical cases, or in instances in which initial treatment is not successful.[37] Sampling of intraocular fluid for viral antigens, and/or viral antibodies can also be used.[21]

The active stages of an ARN usually last several weeks. Following the inflammatory stage a healing phase occurs. During this time the vitreous tends to contract and fibrose, resulting in a PVR-like appearance. It is during this phase of the disease that retinal tears usually occur. The tears tend to form between involved and uninvolved retina and often are multiple. In most untreated cases retinal detachment ensues. Among the first reported cases of ARN,[38] retinal detachment developed in 75%. Retinal detachment associated with ARN is notoriously difficult to manage.

MEDICAL TREATMENT

The medical treatment of the ARN syndrome has three separate components: (1) antiviral agents (2) antiinflammatory agents, and (3) antithrombotics.

Because of the proven association between ARN and the herpesviruses, VZV, and HSV, the cornerstone of antiviral therapy is acyclovir.[39] Acyclovir is a nucleoside analog that interferes with virally encoded thymidine kinase. Normal cells are unaffected. The recommended dose of acyclovir for active ARN infection is 1500 mg/m^2/day in three divided doses. This typically translates to a dose of 800 to 1000 mg, three times a day. In immunosuppressed patients dosages up to 1500 mg, three times a day have been used. Healing of the retinitis can be seen within 72 hours of the start of acyclovir. Intravenous acyclovir is generally administered for 5 to 10 days followed by a 6- to 12-week course of oral acyclovir. The oral dose is usually 400 to 800 mg, five times per day. Prolonged oral administration appears to reduce significantly, but not eliminate, the risk of bilateral ARN in cases that begin unilaterally.[31]

Ganciclovir is also effective against VZV and HSV. Because of its greater systemic toxicity and need for intravenous administration, its use in ARN syndrome should be restricted to cases that have failed acyclovir. In suspected instances of viral resistance to acyclovir, intravenous foscarnet should be considered as an alternative treatment.

In an effort to reduce the inflammatory complications of ARN, systemic and/or local corticosteroids are generally used. Topical corticosteroids help alleviate the anterior segment inflammation. It is recommended that systemic corticosteroids be used in conjunction with antiviral therapy, since they do have immunoinhibitory effects that at least theoretically may potentiate the damage from the virus.

Patients with ARN syndrome have been shown[40] to have systemic platelet aggregation abnormalities. These may play a role in ARN's propensity for causing retinal and choroidal vascular occlusions. The aggregation abnormalities are correctable with aspirin and corticosteroids. Systemic anticoagulation with heparin and/or coumadin has also been used. Since these agents are not without potential systemic complications, however, their use should be discouraged.

SURGICAL TREATMENT

The currently accepted surgical therapy of ARN syndrome has two components: (1) prophylaxis against retinal detachment and (2) treatment of the detachment when it occurs. Other clinicians have suggested a role for two additional surgical approaches[25,41-43]: (1) optic nerve sheath decompression (ONSD) in instance of ARN-associated optic neuritis and (2) prophylactic vitrectomy and endolaser, with or without intravitreal infusion of acyclovir, for cases in which media opacity prevents transpupillary laser application.

Laser therapy in an effort to prevent retinal detachment is advised in cases of ARN.[44,45] Retrospective data imply that the application of laser confluently, posterior to the zones of necrosis, will help decrease the risk of detachment. Unfortunately, the cases with the most severe media opacity from vitreous debris and opacification, which are probably at highest risk for retinal detachment, cannot be treated by transpupillary laser.

If retinal detachment occurs with ARN, pars plana vitrectomy is usually indicated for repair.[46-48] The use of vitrectomy enables the surgeon to deal with the contracted vitreous, intravitreal inflammation, and the often multiple posterior retinal breaks better than scleral buckling alone can. It has been suggested[48] that vitrectomy without scleral buckling leads to a better visual prognosis in ARN detachments. With currently available microsurgical techniques, endolaser, and the use of long-acting vitreous substitutes, over 80% of ARN-associated retinal detachments can now be repaired. Visual acuity may be limited, however, by damage caused by the infection or the detachment.

DIFFERENTIAL DIAGNOSIS

In general, any unilateral or bilateral ocular inflammatory condition that produces retinal whitening and vitreous cells should be considered in the differ-

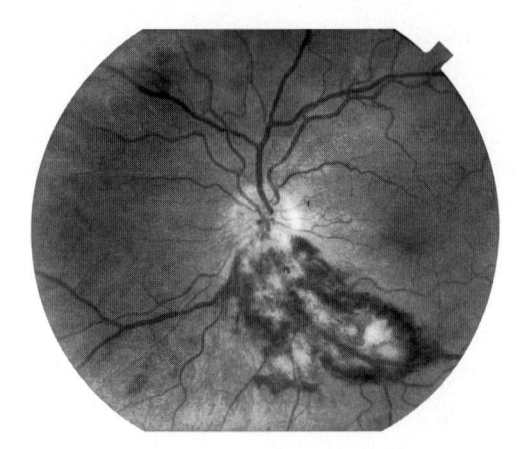

Figure 24-1 Typical CMV retinitis in an AIDS patient. Note the clarity of the media, the perivenous posterior location, and the relatively large amount of hemorrhage.

ential diagnosis for ARN. Practically speaking, however, only several of these conditions bear enough similarity to make differentiation challenging.[1]

CMV retinitis can usually be differentiated from ARN by both its clinical appearance and its clinical course. With CMV a mild vitreous reaction is seen but almost never reaches the proportion of the ARN syndrome (Fig. 24-1). *Toxoplasmosis* can usually be differentiated on an ophthalmoscopic basis; however, in cases with a severe vitreous reaction a trial of medication may be indicated. *Large cell lymphoma* (reticulum cell sarcoma syndrome) tends to have a more protracted course than the ARN syndrome. Vitreous biopsy will usually assist in the diagnosis.

Behçet's disease and *sarcoidosis* should also be in the differential diagnosis for ARN. If the ophthalmoscopic appearance does not help differentiate, then the systemic evaluation should. Finally, in young patients, *retinoblastoma, pars planitis,* and *toxocariasis* should all be considered.

References

1. Duker JS, Blumenkranz MS. Diagnosis and management of the acute retinal necrosis syndrome, *Surv Ophthalmol* 35:327-343, 1991.
2. Culbertson WW, Clarkson JG, Blumenkranz M, et al: Acute retinal necrosis, *Am J Ophthalmol* 96:683-685, 1983.
3. Duker JS, Fischer DH: Acute retinal necrosis syndrome. In Tasman WS, Jaeger EA (eds): *Duane's Clinical ophthalmology,* Philadelphia, 1990, JB Lippincott, vol 4, chapter 38.
4. Fisher JP, Lewis ML, Blumenkranz M, et al: The acute retinal necrosis syndrome. I. Clinical manifestations, *Ophthalmology* 89:1309-1316, 1982.
5. Gass JDM: *Stereoscopic atlas of macular diseases,* ed 3, St Louis, 1987, Mosby, vol 2, pp 490-495.
6. Gorman BD, Nadel AJ, Coles RS: Acute retinal necrosis, *Ophthalmology* 89:809-814, 1982.
7. Nussenblatt RB, Palestine AG: *Uveitis: fundamentals and clinical practice,* Chicago. 1989, Year Book, pp 407-415.
8. Urayama A, Yamada N, Sasaki T, et al: Unilateral acute uveitis with periarteritis and detachment, *Jpn J Clin Ophthalmol* 25:607-619, 1971.
9. Willerson D, Aaberg TM, Reeser FH: Necrotizing vasoocclusive retinitis, *Am J Ophthalmol* 84:209-219, 1977.

10. Brown RM, Mendis U: Retinal arteritis complicating herpes zoster ophthalmicus, *Br J Ophthalmol* 57:344-346, 1973.
11. Culbertson WW, Blumenkranz MS, Haines H, et al: The acute retinal necrosis syndrome. II. Histopathology and etiology, *Ophthalmology* 89:1317-1325, 1982.
12. Culbertson WW, Blumenkranz MS, Pepose JS, et al: Varicella zoster virus is a cause of the acute retinal necrosis syndrome, *Ophthalmology* 93:559-569, 1986.
13. Duker JS, Nielsen J, Eagle RC, et al: Rapidly progressive, acute retinal necrosis (ARN) secondary to herpes simplex virus, type 1, *Ophthalmology* 97:1638-1643, 1990.
14. Freeman WR, Thomas EL, Rao NA, et al: Demonstration of herpes group virus in acute retinal necrosis syndrome, *Am J Ophthalmol* 102:701-709, 1986.
15. Lewis ML, Culbertson WW, Post JD, et al: Herpes Simplex virus type 1: a cause of the acute retinal necrosis syndrome, *Ophthalmology* 96:875-878, 1989.
16. Ludwig IH, Zegarra H, Zakov ZN: The acute retinal necrosis syndrome: possible herpes simplex retinitis, *Ophthalmology* 91:1659-65, 1984.
17. Margolis T, Irvine AR, Hoyt WF, et al: Acute retinal necrosis syndrome presenting with papillitis and arcuate neuroretinitis, *Ophthalmology* 95:937-940, 1988.
18. Matsuo T, Date S, Tsuji T, et al: Immune complex containing herpesvirus antigen in a patient with acute retinal necrosis, *Am J Ophthalmol* 101:368-374, 1986.
19. Sarkies N, Gregor Z, Forsey T, et al: Antibodies to herpes simplex type 1 in intraocular fluids of patients with acute retinal necrosis, *Br J Ophthalmol* 70:81-84, 1986.
20. Soushi S, Ozawa H, Matsuhashi M, et al: Demonstration of varicella-zoster virus antigens in the vitreous aspirates of patients with acute retinal necrosis syndrome, *Ophthalmology* 95:1394-1398, 1988.
21. Suttorp-Schulten MS, Zaal MJ, Luyendijk L, et al: Aqueous humor tap and serology in acute retinal necrosis, *Am J Ophthalmol* 108:327-328, 1989.
22. Rungger-Brandle E, Roux L, Leuenberger PM: Bilateral acute retinal necrosis (BARN): identification of the presumed infectious agent, *Ophthalmology* 91:1648-1657, 1984.
23. Culbertson WW, Brod RD, Flynn HW, et al: Chickenpox-associated acute retinal necrosis syndrome, *Ophthalmology* 98:1641-1646, 1991.
24. Kelly SP, Rosenthal AR: Chickenpox chorioretinitis, *Br J Ophthalmol* 74:698-699, 1990.
25. Sergott RC, Anand R, Belmont JB, et al: Acute retinal necrosis neuropathy: clinical profile and surgical therapy, *Arch Ophthalmol* 107:692-696, 1989.
26. Sergott RC, Belmont JB, Savino PJ, et al: Optic nerve involvement in the acute retinal necrosis syndrome, *Arch Ophthalmol* 103:1160-1162, 1985.
27. Wang CL, Kaplan HJ, Waldrep JC, et al: Retinal neovascularization associated with acute retinal necrosis. *Retina* 3:249-252, 1983.
28. Browning DJ, Blumenkranz MS, Culbertson WW, et al: Association of varicella zoster dermatitis with acute retinal necrosis syndrome, *Ophthalmology* 94:602-606, 1987.
29. Yeo JH, Pepose JS, Stewart JA, et al: Acute retinal necrosis syndrome following herpes zoster dermatitis, *Ophthalmology* 93:1418-1422, 1986.
30. Rabinovitch T, Nozik RA, Varenhorst MP: Bilateral acute retinal necrosis syndrome, *Am J Ophthalmol* 108:735-736, 1989.
31. Palay DA, Sternberg P, Davis J, et al: Decrease in the risk of bilateral acute retinal necrosis by acyclovir treatment, *Am J Ophthalmol* 112:250-255, 1991.
32. Chambers RB, Derick RJ, Davidorf FH, et al: Varizella-zoster retinitis in human immunodeficiency virus infection, *Arch Ophthalmol* 107:960-961, 1989.
33. Chess J, Marcus DM: Zoster-related bilateral acute retinal necrosis syndrome as presenting sign in AIDS, *Ann Ophthalmol* 20:431-435, 438, 1988.
34. Friberg TR, Jost BF: Acute retinal necrosis in an immunosuppressed patient, *Am J Ophthalmol* 98:515-519, 1984.
35. Forster DJ, Dugel PU, Frangieh GT, et al: Rapidly progressive outer retinal necrosis in the acquired immune deficiency syndrome, *Am J Ophthalmol* 110:341-347, 1990.
36. Margolis TP, Lowder CY, Holland GN, et al: Varicella-zoster virus retinitis in patients with the acquired immune deficiency syndrome, *Am J Ophthalmol* 112:119-131, 1991.
37. Freeman WR, Wiley CA, Gross JG, et al: Endoretinal biopsy in immunosuppressed and healthy patients with retinitis, *Ophthalmology* 96:1559-1565, 1989.

38. Clarkson JG, Blumenkranz MS, Culbertson WW, et al: Retinal detachment following the acute retinal necrosis syndrome, *Ophthalmology* 91:1665-1668, 1984.
39. Blumenkranz MS, Culbertson WW, Clarkson JG, et al: Treatment of the acute retinal necrosis syndrome with intravenous acyclovir, *Ophthalmology* 93:296-300, 1986.
40. Ando F, Kato M, Goto S, et al: Platelet function in bilateral acute retinal necrosis, *Am J Ophthalmol* 96:27-32, 1983.
41. Carney MD, Peyman GA, Goldberg MF, et al: Acute retinal necrosis, *Retina* 6:85-94, 1986.
42. Peyman GA, Goldberg MF, Uninsky E, et al: Vitrectomy and intravitreal antiviral drug therapy in acute retinal necrosis syndrome, *Arch Ophthalmol* 102:1618-1621, 1984.
43. Immonen I, Laatikainen L, Linnanvuori K: Acute retinal necrosis syndrome treated with vitrectomy and intravenous acyclovir, *Acta Ophthalmol* 67:106-108, 1989.
44. Sternberg P, Han DP, Yeo JH, et al: Photocoagulation to prevent retinal detachment in acute retinal necrosis, *Ophthalmology* 95:1389-1393, 1988.
45. Han DP, Lewis H, Williams GA, et al: Laser photocoagulation in the acute retinal necrosis syndrome, *Arch Ophthalmol* 105:1051-1054, 1987.
46. Blumenkranz M, Clarkson J, Culbertson WW, et al: Visual results and complications after retinal reattachment in the acute retinal necrosis syndrome, *Retina* 9:170-174, 1989.
47. Blumenkranz M, Clarkson J, Culbertson WW, et al: Vitrectomy for retinal detachment associated with the acute retinal necrosis syndrome, *Am J Ophthalmol* 106:426-429, 1988.
48. McDonald HR, Lewis H, Kreiger AE, et al: Surgical management of retinal detachment associated with the acute retinal necrosis syndrome, *Br J Ophthalmol* 75:455-458, 1991.

25

Pars Planitis

James F. Vander

Pars planitis (also known as *intermediate uveitis, chronic cyclitis,* and *peripheral uveitis*) is a form of uveitis with characteristic features in the peripheral fundus that make it a distinct clinical entity. Its hallmark peripheral changes were first described by Schepens[1] in 1947. The entity is characterized by inflammatory exudation in the region of the pars plana and ora serrata. In addition, there are often numerous associated features and a wide-ranging clinical presentation, making diagnosis and management of the condition a challenge.[2-8]

FINDINGS

Pars planitis typically occurs in the second and third decades; however, presentations early in childhood occur in about 10% of cases and, rarely, older adults can become afflicted.[8] The sexes are affected, and there is no known racial predilection. Rarely, cases with "familial" pars planitis will occur.[9,10] Although external and anterior chamber findings of acute nongranulomatous uveitis may occur, the typical presentation is a quiet white eye.[1-8] The classic symptoms are floaters and decreased visual acuity. Involvement may be in one or both eyes, with 80% of cases bilateral, although there may be a considerable delay before the second eye becomes involved. The onset may be abrupt or, more often, fairly gradual. In general, the younger the patient at the time of diagnosis, the more severe will be the course of the disease. The etiology is unknown. On examination, vision is usually mildly reduced, although in severe cases there may be profound visual loss. As noted above, there is frequently an absence of anterior segment pathology. In more severe longstanding cases, considerable cellular reaction can appear in the anterior chamber, sometimes with fibrin formation. In cases of longer duration posterior synechiae may form and there may be cataract, especially posterior subcapsular in nature.

The characteristic features of pars planitis are detected at posterior segment ophthalmoscopy. There is generally cellular reaction with prominent floaters in the anterior and posterior vitreous. The hallmark features of pars planitis are *snowbanking* and *snowballs*. The presence of at least one of these features is

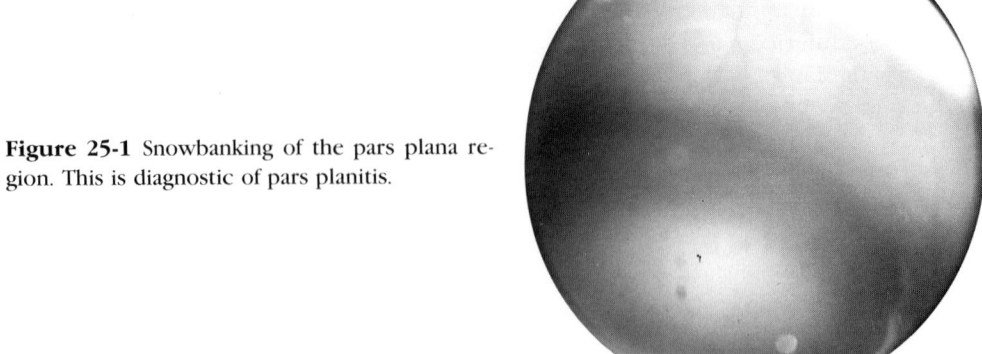

Figure 25-1 Snowbanking of the pars plana region. This is diagnostic of pars planitis.

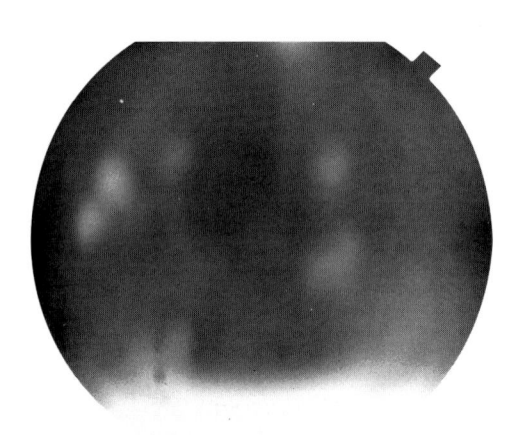

Figure 25-2 Snowballs floating in the vitreous cavity near the vitreous base. These are highly suggestive of pars planitis.

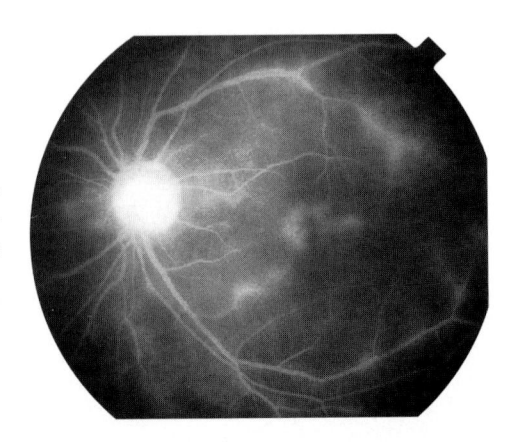

Figure 25-3 Fluorescein angiogram showing diffuse cystoid macular edema with hyperfluorescence of the optic disc. Note also staining of the retinal veins.

required to make the diagnosis of pars planitis. Snowbanking is a white raised sheet of inflammatory material present over the pars plana, most often involving the inferior pars plana region first (Fig. 25-1). When present, it is diagnostic of pars planitis[8,11] although it may be absent in over 10% of cases. Snowbanking may extend across the ora serrata and over the peripheral retina in severe cases. Also frequently noted are snowballs, which are creamy white intravitreal fluffy opacities generally found near the ora serrata (Fig. 25-2). They are suggestive of pars planitis, although similar vitreous opacities can be seen in other conditions, such as fungal endophthalmitis. The optic nerve is usually normal but can be slightly hyperemic and swollen. Severe swelling is unusual, however. Cystoid macular edema (CME) occurs in up to 80% of patients and is the most common cause of long-term visual loss with pars planitis. It may occur in patients with very little midvitreous and posterior vitreous inflammation. As such, patients with CME of unknown etiology should have indirect ophthalmoscopy performed with scleral depression to rule out the possibility of pars planitis as the cause for their edema. The retinal vessels are usually normal in mild to moderate cases of pars planitis.

Significant perivasculitis, particularly involving the retinal veins, may occur. This may be identifiable as sheathing at ophthalmoscopy but is more readily appreciated angiographically. In severe cases peripheral retinal neovascularization can develop. There may be recurrent vitreous hemorrhage or tractional retinal detachment as the cause for severe visual loss.[12] Other reported findings include cataract, glaucoma, band keratopathy, and disc neovascularization.

Fluorescein Angiography

Fluorescein angiography in patients with pars planitis will often show CME, even when vision is well preserved and there is no grossly apparent edema at ophthalmoscopy.[13] Late hyperfluorescent staining of the optic nerve head is seen as well (Fig. 25-3). Scanning views of the periphery may show staining along vessel walls, especially the veins. Peripheral retinal capillary nonperfusion, sometimes associated with leakage from retinal neovascularization, may also be detected. The angiographic features of pars planitis are not unique but may be seen in many other types of inflammatory ocular conditions.

PATHOGENESIS

The origin of pars planitis is uncertain. Although associations have been made with other clinical entities the majority of cases are idiopathic in nature. Breger and Leopold[14] first reported a link between pars planitis and multiple sclerosis. Chester et al.[15] found that 8% of patients with pars planitis developed multiple sclerosis. More recently Zierhut and Foster[16] have reported an 11% incidence of multiple sclerosis in pars planitis patients. Either condition may occur first, and there can be a delay of many years before onset of the second condition. The mechanism of any possible association between these two entities is uncertain, although some data[17] suggest they may share certain genetic markers, with the HLA-DR2 and DQw1 having been linked to both diseases.

Landers,[18] Crick,[19] and Chester et al.[15] have all reported an association between pars planitis and sarcoidosis. Zierhut and Foster[16] found that almost 10%

of their pars planitis patients had sarcoidosis. In most cases this developed years after the diagnosis of pars planitis was made. There were no ophthalmologic features found to be helpful in predicting who would develop sarcoidosis, and the typical features of sarcoid uveitis (e.g., "candle wax drippings" and choroidal granulomas) were not observed.

Winward et al.[20] and, more recently, Breeveld et al.[21] have reported an association between pars planitis and Lyme disease. This association is of particular interest since Lyme disease is a potentially treatable and curable condition. In the report of Breeveld et al.[21] the ophthalmologic condition improved promptly, despite 10 years of prior activity, once treatment for Lyme disease was given. This information awaits confirmation by other investigators.

CLINICAL COURSE

The clinical course of pars planitis is highly variable and often difficult to predict at the time of presentation. Many patients with minimal disease will maintain excellent vision and require no therapy.[6] Sometimes patients will have alternating periods of exacerbation and remission lasting between several weeks and several years. After many years of this pattern the disease may go into a more permanent remission for reasons that are unclear.

TREATMENT

Not all patients with pars planitis require continual medical therapy. Treatment is indicated when there is increasing vitreous debris leading to decreased vision or, more often, decreased vision on the basis of CME. Development of secondary neovascularization is also an important indication for treatment.

The mainstay of pars planitis treatment is corticosteroids.[7] Although patients with anterior uveitis may benefit from topical therapy, most with pars planitis will require treatment via a different route. This may be systemic steroids or a periocular steroid injection. At the time of initial presentation, especially for patients with bilateral disease, I prefer the systemic route of administration. This allows for greater flexibility in terms of duration and dosage and also avoids some of the psychologic stress of a periocular injection. Initial therapy may be between 40 and 80 mg daily of prednisone. The dose is maintained until a clinical response is obtained and then is slowly tapered. Recurrences during tapering are not infrequent. As the duration of systemic therapy increases and the potential for severe side effects develops, patients frequently will benefit from a periocular injection. Long-acting compounds are ideally suited for this condition. Multiple injections are usually necessary, with the interval between injections determined by the clinical course. The goal of treatment is to minimize opacification of the media and maximize visual acuity with resolution of edema. Peripheral neovascularization may show regression in response to antiinflammatory therapy as well. Additional complications include cataract and glaucoma, which may result from the disease process or the corticosteroids necessary to treat it. Treatment in patients with steroid-responsive intraocular pressure can be particularly challenging.

Additional medical regimens have been tried for pars planitis, with variable success. Medications studied include chlorambucil, cyclophosphamide, and cyclosporin.[22,23] For refractory cases some success has been achieved with cryotherapy.[24,25] This is performed with a double freeze-thaw application transconjunctivally in the region of pars plana snowbanking. It may produce long-lasting resolution of the inflammation. In addition to reducing inflammatory exudation, cryotherapy is helpful in the treatment of peripheral neovascularization, lowering the risk of vitreous hemorrhage and tractional retinal detachment.

In cases of severe retinal neovascularization, if there is evidence of retinal capillary nonperfusion, panretinal photocoagulation to these areas may help prevent or reverse neovascularization. In cases with severe inflammatory infiltration or tractional retinal detachment, pars plana vitrectomy remains an option.[7] Vitrectomy may help reduce the "antigenic load," which seems to be a factor in the inflammatory process. In general, a stepwise approach to therapy is most appropriate.

The role of intraocular lenses in managing the cataracts that often occur in pars planitis is controversial. Many patients with burned-out disease that is quiescent at the time of surgery will tolerate a posterior chamber lens fairly well, with visual acuity of 20/40 or better having been obtained in 60% of patients in one series.[26] Multiple YAG laser or surgical procedures to maintain a clear visual axis may be necessary, however. Patients with more than a trace of inflammatory activity at the time of cataract extraction are probably not good candidates for implant surgery.

References

1. Schepens CL: A new ophthalmoscopic demonstration, *Trans Acad Ophthalmol Otolaryngol* 51:298-301, 1947.
2. Brockhurst RJ, Schepens CL, Okamura ID: Uveitis. II. Peripheral uveitis: clinical description and differential diagnosis, *Am J Ophthalmol* 49:1257-1260, 1960.
3. Brockhurst RJ, Schepens CL, Okamura ID: Uveitis. III. Peripheral uveitis. Pathogenesis, etiology and treatment, *Am J Ophthalmol* 51:19-26, 1961.
4. Welch RB, Maumenee AE, Wahlen HE: Peripheral posterior segment inflammation, vitreous opacities, edema of the posterior pole, *Arch Ophthalmol* 64:540-549, 1960.
5. Hogan MJ, Kamura SJ, O'Connor GR: Peripheral retinitis and chronic cyclitis in children, *Trans Ophthalmol Soc UK* 85:39-51, 1965.
6. Smith RE, Godfrey SA, Kamura SJ: Chronic cyclitis. I. Course in visual prognosis, *Trans Am Acad Ophthalmol Otolaryngol* 77:760-768, 1973.
7. Henderly DE, Genstler AJ, Rao NA, Smith RE: Pars planitis, *Trans Ophthalmol Soc UK* 105:227-232, 1986.
8. Henderly DE, Haoiman RS, Rao NA, Smith RE: Significance of the pars plana exudate in pars planitis, *Am J Ophthalmol* 103:669-671, 1987.
9. Culbertson WW, Giles CL, West C, Stafford T: Familial pars planitis, *Retina* 3:179-181, 1983.
10. Augsburger JJ, Annesley WH, Sergott RC, et al: Familial pars planitis, *Ann Ophthalmol* 13:553-557, 1981.
11. Smith RE: Intermediate uveitis: What is the significance of the pars plana exudate in "pars planitis"? *Develop Ophthalmol* 23:48-49, 1992.
12. Brockhurst RJ, Schepens CL: Uveitis. IV. Peripheral uveitis: complications of retinal detachment, *Arch Ophthalmol* 80:747-753, 1968.
13. Pruett RC, Brockhurst RJ, Letts N: Fluorescein angiography of peripheral uveitis, *Am J Ophthalmol* 77:448-453, 1974.
14. Breger BC, Leopold IH: The incidence of uveitis in multiple sclerosis, *Am J Ophthalmol* 62:540-545, 1966.

15. Chester GH, Blach RK, Cleary PE: Inflammation in the region of the vitreous base, *Tarns Ophthalmol Soc UK* 96:151-197, 1976.
16. Zierhut M, Foster CS: Multiple sclerosis, sarcoidosis and other diseases in patients with pars planitis, *Develop Ophthalmol* 23:41-47, 1992.
17. Davis J: HLA in intermediate uveitis. In Proceedings of an international workshop on intermediate disease. Gütersloh West Germany, 1990.
18. Landers PH: Vitreous lesions observed in Boeck's sarcoid, *Am J Ophthalmol* 32:1740-1741, 1949.
19. Crick RP: Ocular sarcoidosis, *Trans Ophthalmol Soc UK* 75:189-206, 1955.
20. Winward KE, Smith JL, Culbertson WW, et al: Ocular lyme borreliosis, *Am J Ophthalmol* 108:651-657, 1989.
21. Breeveld J, Rothova A, Kuiper H: Intermediate uveitis and lyme borreliosis, *Br J Ophthalmol* 76:181-182, 1992.
22. Nussenblatt RB, Palestine AG: Cyclosporin (Sandimmun®) therapy: experience and treatment of pars planitis in present therapeutic guidelines, *Develop Ophthalmol* 23:177-184, 1992.
23. Buckley CE III, Giles JP Jr: Cyclophosphamide therapy of peripheral uveitis, *Arch Intern Med* 124:29-35, 1969.
24. Aaberg TM, Cesarz TJ, Flickinger R: Treatment of peripheral uveoretinitis by cryotherapy, *Am J Ophthalmol* 75:685-688, 1973.
25. Okinami S, Sunakawa M, Arai I, et al: Treatment of pars planitis with cryotherapy, *Ophthalmologica* 202:180-186, 1991.
26. Michelson JB, Friedlaender MH, Nozak RA: Lens implant surgery in pars planitis, *Ophthalmology* 97:1023-1026, 1990.

26

Diffuse Unilateral Subacute Neuroretinitis

Arunan Sivalingam

Diffuse unilateral subacute neuroretinitis (DUSN) is a clinical syndrome characterized by insidious visual loss. It was originally reported on by Donald Gass and associates in a group of young healthy patients with unilateral severe visual loss, optic atrophy, vitritis, retinal pigment epithelial changes, narrowing of retinal vessels, and an abnormal electroretinogram.[1-3]

In the early stages of the disease, visual loss is often severe and out of proportion to the retinal findings.[2] There is usually vitreous inflammation, and almost always an afferent pupillary defect is detected. In addition, there is swelling of the optic nerve in the early stages with multifocal crops of gray-white lesions involving the retinal pigment epithelium and deep retina, often sparing the macular area. The evanescent lesions may fade over several days and reappear nearby. These crops of lesions usually involve the deep or external layers of the retina as well as the retinal pigment epithelium. They typically fade within several days, leaving minimum ophthalmoscopic evidence of the underlying retinal pigment epithelium.[2] Successive crops of lesions may occur from week to week, and over periods of months diffuse retinal pigment epithelial alteration takes place. In the early stages one almost always finds vitreous inflammation with or without anterior chamber cells and flare.

Late-stage DUSN, originally termed the "unilateral wipeout syndrome," is characterized by severe monocular visual loss, optic atrophy with marked narrowing and sheathing of the retinal vasculature, and diffuse atrophy of the retinal pigment epithelium.[2] In general, the optic disc pallor and retinal arteriolar narrowing parallel central visual loss.

The hallmark of DUSN is the presence of a motile nematode in association with the previously mentioned clinical features.[1,2,4-6] Most of the time the worm is observed either within or beneath the retina (Fig. 26-1). Very rarely it may be seen in the anterior vitreous cavity. To find it, a careful search with a Goldmann three-mirror lens is required. The nematode is found most frequently in the midperiphery of the fundus. Its length may vary anywhere from 400 to 2000 μm, with the longest diameter being 1/20 its length.[1,2,7,8] It propels itself by a

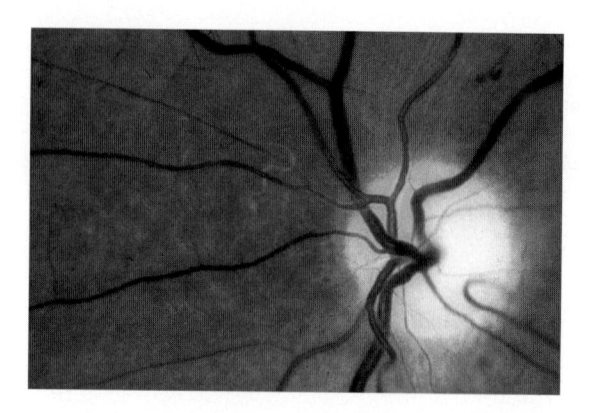

Figure 26-1 Left eye with a nematode near the nasal aspect of the optic nerve. In addition, there is evidence of optic nerve pallor and mild attenuation of the retinal arterioles.

series of coiling and uncoiling movements. The worm can be found in either the early or the late stages of the disease.

Fluorescein angiography during the early stages may demonstrate leakage of dye from the optic nerve head. In addition, the gray-white area of retinal lesions is sometimes nonfluorescent early in the angiography but stains during the later phases. In the late stages of the disease, because of the loss of retinal pigment epithelium, there are marked transmission defects. The electroretinogram may be abnormal at any stage of the disease, but the b-wave is usually affected to a much greater degree than the a-wave. In the unaffected eye the ERG is always small.

The mechanism of retinal damage in DUSN appears to be related to an inflammatory toxic reaction to the nematode. Although the gray-white retinal pigment epithelial changes might also be a result of local changes secondary to the migrating worm, the more severe visual loss with minimum fundus findings is likely a diffuse toxic reaction to the worm.

Many types of nematodes have been postulated to be the cause of DUSN, but to date the exact species acting as the etiologic factor is still unknown.

In the early stages DUSN can mimic acute multifocal posterior placoid pigment epitheliopathy, choroiditis, multiple evanescent white dot syndrome, Behçet's disease, or toxoplasmosis. By contrast, the later stages of the disease are sometimes diagnosed as retrobulbar neuritis, unilateral optic atrophy secondary to intracranial lesions, unilateral retinitis pigmentosa, or posttraumatic choroidopathy.

Photocoagulation is an effective mode of therapy that does not cause significant ocular inflammation. At the present time it is the preferred mode of therapy using argon laser. Oral treatment with thiabendazole and diethylcarbamazine has been shown to be an ineffective.

References

1. Gass JDM, Braunstein RA: Further observations concerning the diffuse unilateral subacute neuroretinitis syndrome. *Arch Ophthalmol* 101:1689-1697, 1983.
2. Gass JDM, Gilbert WR Jr, Guerry RK, Scelfo R: Diffuse unilateral subacute neuroretinitis, *Ophthalmology* 85:521, 1978.
3. Gass JDM, Scelfo R: Diffuse unilateral subacute neuroretinitis, *JR Soc Med* 71:95, 1978.
4. Kazacos KR, Raymond LA, Kazacos EA, Vestre WA: The raccoon ascarid: a probable cause of human ocular larva migrans, *Ophthalmology* 92:1735, 1985.
5. Kazacos KR, Vestre WA, Kazacos EA, Raymond LA: Diffuse unilateral subacute neuroretinitis syndrome: probable cause, *Arch Ophthalmol* 102:967, 1984.
6. Parsons HE: Nematode chorioretinitis: report of a case, with photographs of a viable worm, *Arch Ophthalmol* 47:799, 1952.
7. Price JA Jr, Wadsworth JAC: An intraretinal worm: report of a case of macular retinopathy caused by invasion of the retina by a worm, *Arch Ophthalmol* 83:768, 1970.
8. Raymond LA, Gutierrez Y, Strong LE, et al: Living retinal nematode (filarial-like) destroyed with photocoagulation, *Ophthalmology* 85:944, 1978.

27

Sarcoidosis of the Posterior Segment

Jay S. Duker

Sarcoidosis is a chronic idiopathic granulomatous disease of multiple organ systems.[1-3] The eyes and adnexal structures are commonly affected. Nonocular sites of involvement typically include the lungs, skin, liver, and central nervous system. The diagnosis is based on a combination of clinical, laboratory, and biopsy information.

It is estimated[1,4] that the incidence of sarcoidosis is between 10 and 200 per 100,000 population. Sarcoidosis is worldwide in distribution but is more common in certain countries such as Scandinavia. In the United States it is more common in the Southeast and frequently is seen in African-Americans. Children under the age of 16 years are rarely afflicted.[5] Women are affected more often than men, by a 2:1 margin.

Sarcoidosis has a particular affinity for the eye and its adnexa. Two recent reports[3,6] have documented a rate of ophthalmic involvement in patients with chronic sarcoidosis of slightly greater than 25%. As stated, ophthalmic involvement among Americans appears to be more common in those of African descent.[6]

The lacrimal glands and conjunctiva are probably the most common sites of ocular involvement, although an anterior granulomatous uveitis is said to be the "hallmark" of the ocular disease.[2,3] Posterior segment manifestations, once believed rare, are now noted in an increasing percentage of cases.[6] In the report by Jabs and Johns[6] the incidence of posterior segment involvement was 7% in their population of 183 patients with chronic sarcoidosis who were followed for 5 years or greater.

NONOCULAR MANIFESTATIONS AND DIAGNOSIS

The hallmark pathologic lesion of sarcoidosis is the noncaseating granuloma. The clinical syndrome of sarcoidosis is due to multiple organ involvement by these granulomas. The clinical course is highly variable, with rapidly progressive, chronic remittent, and stable courses all possible.

The pulmonary system is the most frequently affected in sarcoidosis (> 90%).[1-3,7] Lymphadenopathy, especially hilar adenopathy, is typical (with or without pulmonary infiltrates). In most cases chest radiographs will be diagnostic. Chest computed tomography (CT) and gallium scanning are also useful adjuncts. Pulmonary function testing will reveal functional deficits in most affected patients, and the clinical response to therapy can be assessed by serial testing.

Other commonly noted systemic abnormalities in patients with sarcoidosis include peripheral lymphadenopathy, skin lesions, hepatosplenomegaly, arthritis, cardiac abnormalities, cranial nerve palsies, and central nervous system (CNS) abnormalities.

The diagnosis of sarcoidosis is a clinical one, since there is no single test that can absolutely confirm it.[7] Aside from the typical constellation of clinical findings, laboratory parameters backing up the diagnosis include abnormal blood count, calcium levels, lysozyme, and angiotensin converting enzyme (ACE) levels. ACE levels are elevated in over 50% of patients regardless of disease activity.[7] In patients with uveitis the ACE level is both sensitive and specific for sarcoidosis when highly elevated.[8] It is an excellent study for following the activity of the disease since it will fall to normal with treatment. Aside from blood studies, skin testing is helpful in sarcoidosis since many patients will be anergic to intradermal mumps, *Candida,* and *Trichophyton.* The Kveim test, which consists of the subcutaneous administration of heat sterilized human sarcoid antigenic material followed by biopsy looking for noncaseating granulomas 6 weeks later, is of mostly historical interest. Although both sensitive and specific, it is of limited availability at the present time.

Biopsy of involved organ tissue with histopathologic confirmation of noncaseating granulomas is helpful in confirming the diagnosis. Typical sites of biopsy include involved suspicious skin lesions, enlarged subcutaneous lymph nodes, mediastinal lymph nodes, lung tissue, and liver. One of the most accessible areas to biopsy is conjunctiva. Areas of follicle formation should be biopsied if present. *Blind* conjunctival biopsy (i.e., biopsy of a clinically normal site) is said[8] to be positive in greater than 50% of true cases of sarcoidosis, provided multiple, serial, thin sections are examined. An enlarged lacrimal gland can easily be biopsied in an office setting as well.

ADNEXAL AND ANTERIOR SEGMENT FINDINGS

The most common ocular manifestations of sarcoidosis are granulomas affecting the lacrimal gland and conjunctiva.[2,6,10] In approximately half the patients with ocular sarcoidosis, lacrimal gland enlargement will be diagnosed clinically or by gallium scan. Conjunctival granulomas can be detected in about half as well.

Anterior uveitis develops in anywhere from 28% to 74% of patients with ophthalmic involvement.[2,6,7,10] Of these, nearly half will have only one or two isolated episodes of anterior uveitis and chronic problems will not occur. Bilateral involvement is the rule, although not necessarily simultaneous. Keratic precipitates, either fine or muttonfat, are usually seen. Iris nodules may develop.

As in any type of chronic uveitis, band keratopathy can occur in the cornea. Glaucoma, both open angle and closed angle, is not uncommon. Closed-angle glaucoma can be synechial (anterior or posterior) or neovascular. Alternatively, in severe cases hypotony and even phthisis can develop. Cataract formation is quite common.

POSTERIOR SEGMENT FINDINGS

Approximately 7% of patients with chronic sarcoidosis will develop posterior segment ocular manifestations.[3,6] The inflammation can occur in all areas of the posterior segment. In some cases posterior segment inflammation will occur in the absence of active anterior segment disease. For this reason all sarcoid patients with visual complaints should receive a dilated fundus examination. The posterior segment findings can be widely variable and nonspecific, with all three ocular coats involved to varying degrees.

In the vitreous, inflammatory cellular infiltration is the usually noted finding. Spillover from an anterior uveitis can be seen in the anterior vitreous, without true posterior segment involvement. More posteriorly collections of cells and fibrin (called descriptively *snowballs* and *strings of pearls*) may be seen.[11] Pars plana exudation resembling the classic snowbanks seen in pars planitis may develop. For this reason sarcoidosis should be ruled out in any patient presenting with an intermediate uveitis. In severe cases the vitreous may become so opacified that vision is decreased considerably. Therapeutic vitrectomy can be considered in such cases, but the natural course of the inflammatory disease does not appear to be altered by surgical removal of the vitreous.

A retinal vasculitis that affects primarily the retinal veins occurs in a relatively small percentage of patients with ophthalmic sarcoidosis.[10,12-14] (Fig. 27-1). Retinal periphlebitis, given the descriptive term "candle wax drippings," can lead to branch retinal vein obstruction (BRVO) in severe cases. Capillary nonperfusion and secondary macular edema can also be seen, even in the absence to true BRVO. Healed vasculitis may produce perivenular chorioretinal alterations.

Posterior segment neovascularization is an infrequent complication of the chronic severe inflammation that sarcoidosis may induce.[15-17] It can occur in the subretinal space (both in the peripapillary and in the macular areas), on the optic disc, and in any zone of the retina. Peripheral retinal neovascularization appears to be due to capillary nonperfusion associated with chronic retinal vasculitis and is occasionally seen in eyes with minimal or no antecedent or concurrent anterior segment involvement[15] (Fig. 27-2). The fact that neovascularization of the disc (NVD) has been documented to regress following corticosteroid treatment lends support to the theory that inflammation alone, without capillary dropout, can produce NVD. Subretinal new vessel growth may result around previous choroidal inflammation or in the peripapillary area associated with prior optic disc edema.[18]

Granulomas involving either the optic disc or the choroid can develop in the posterior segment. The choroidal granulomas seen in sarcoidosis are typically pale yellow raised lesions accompanied by subretinal fluid. They can vary in size from very small (100 μm) to massive (several millimeters), simulating a choroidal metastatic carcinoma (Fig. 27-3). Large choroidal granulomas may be isolated findings in patients who later develop systemic sarcoidosis.[19] Choroidal and optic nerve involvement can occur without concurrent retinal vascular lesions.[20] Fluorescein angiography of the choroidal lesions typically shows initial blockage of fluorescence followed by late staining.[19] The optic disc granulomas can simulate other lesions such as optic disc edema (Fig. 27-4). Longstanding lesions can result in profound optic atrophy.

Sarcoidosis of the posterior segment 351

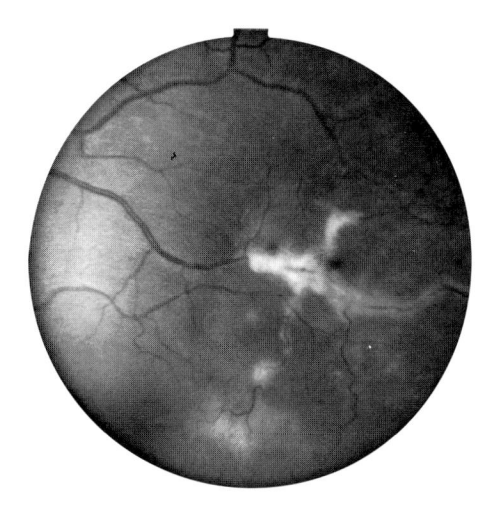

Figure 27-1 Retinal periphlebitis in a case of posterior segment sarcoidosis.

Figure 27-2 Retinal neovascularization with fibrovascular proliferation of the posterior hyaloid and retinal capillary nonperfusion in the periphery. Vision was 20/20, and the patient was asymptomatic. Because of a vitreous hemorrhage in the other eye from proliferative sarcoid retinopathy, this eye was treated prophylactically with peripheral panretinal photocoagulation.

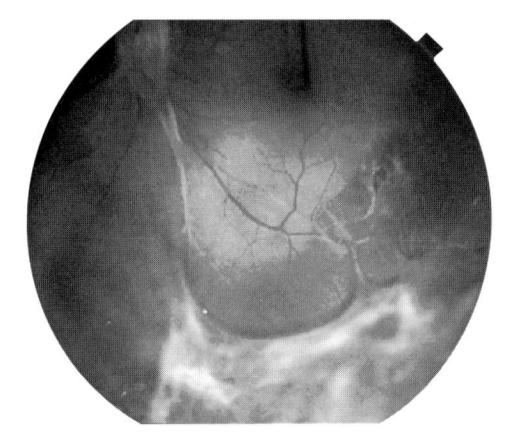

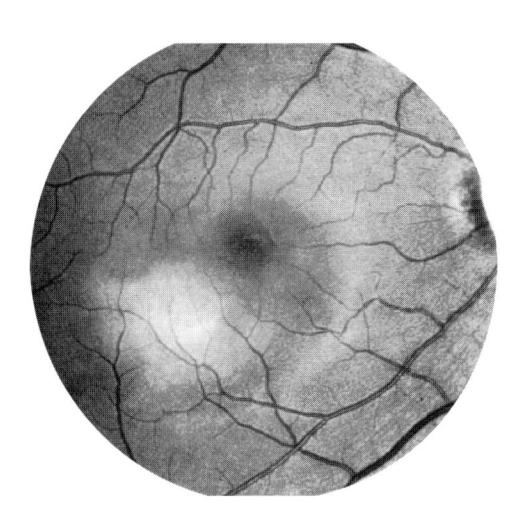

Figure 27-3 Submacular choroidal granuloma associated with sarcoidosis.

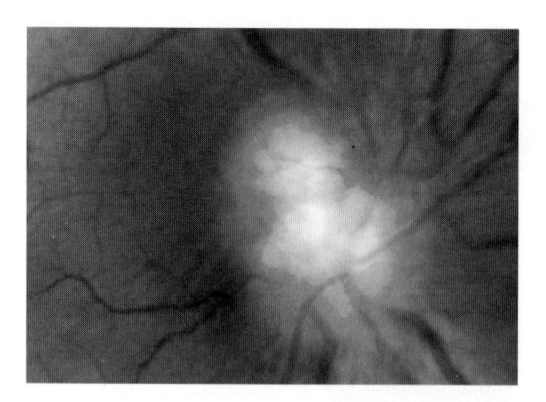

Figure 27-4 Optic nerve granuloma in a patient with sarcoid. This lesion resolved completely following oral corticosteroids.

TREATMENT

Corticosteroid therapy is the cornerstone of ocular sarcoidosis treatment. The severity, duration, and (most important) location of involvement will typically dictate its dosage, route, and length. Generalizations about treatment are difficult to make since many acute inflammatory episodes prove to be self-limiting and the chronic course can be highly variable. In general, corticosteroid treatment is withheld in chronic situations unless vision-threatening complications are occurring. Treatment of the chronic disease is important, however, because long-term ocular inflammation from sarcoidosis can lead to severe visual morbidity.

Topical therapy is usually employed for anterior segment inflammation. Posterior segment complications (e.g., vitritis and macular edema) are rarely improved by topical therapy alone. In such cases sub-Tenon injections of depot steroids should be considered. Oral corticosteroids can be used as well. In severe cases unresponsive to corticosteroids, or to limit corticosteroid side effects, immunosuppression has been used on a limited basis, with some success.

Retinal periphlebitis alone does not require treatment unless it is severe and/or impairs visual acuity. Capillary nonperfusion associated with it can lead to neovascularization, however. Laser treatment should be performed to ischemic areas when neovascularization occurs.[15,17] Photocoagulation of subretinal neovascularization should be entertained in vision-threatening lesions that are amenable to such therapy.[18] In cases of subretinal neovascular membranes associated with inflammatory granulomas, corticosteroid therapy should be considered as well. Oral and/or local depot corticosteroids are generally effective for optic disc and choroidal granulomas.

References

1. James DG, Neville E, Siltzbach LE, et al: A worldwide review of sarcoidosis, *Ann NY Acad Sci* 278:321-329, 1976.
2. Crick RP, Hoyle C, Smellie H: The eye in sarcoidosis, *Br J Ophthalmol* 45:461-471, 1961.
3. Karma A, Huhti E, Poukkula A: Course and outcome of ocular sarcoidosis, *Am J Ophthalmol* 106:467-472, 1988.
4. Siltzbach LE, James DG, Neville E, et al: Course and prognosis of sarcoidosis around the world, *Am J Med* 57:847-852, 1974.
5. Hoover DL, Khan JA, Giangiacomo J: Pediatric ocular sarcoidosis, *Surv Ophthalmol* 30:215-228, 1986.
6. Jabs D, Johns C: Ocular involvement in chronic sarcoidosis, *Am J Ophthalmol* 102:297-301, 1986.
7. Weinreb RN, Tessler H: Laboratory diagnosis of ophthalmic sarcoidosis, *Surv Ophthalmol* 28:653-664, 1984.
8. Baarsma GS, La Hey E, Glasius E, et al: The predictive value of serum angiotensin converting enzyme and lysozyme levels in the diagnosis of ocular sarcoidosis, *Am J Ophthalmol* 104:211-217, 1987.
9. Nichols CW, Eagle RC, Yanoff M, Menocal NG: Conjunctival biopsy as an aid in the evaluation of the patient with suspected sarcoidosis, *Ophthalmology* 87:287-291, 1980.
10. Obenauf C, Shaw H, Sydnor C, Klintworth G: Sarcoidosis and its ophthalmic manifestations, *Am J Ophthalmol* 86:648-655, 1978.
11. Landers H: Vitreous lesions seen in Boeck's sarcoid, *Am J Ophthalmol* 32:1740, 1949.
12. Spalton DJ, Sanders MD: Fundus changes in histologically confirmed sarcoidosis, *Br J Ophthalmol* 65:348-358, 1981.
13. Gould H, Kaufman H: Sarcoid of the fundus, *Arch Ophthalmol* 65:161-164, 1961.
14. Chumbley L, Kearns T: Retinopathy of sarcoidosis, *Am J Ophthalmol* 73:123-131, 1972.
15. Duker JS, Brown GC, McNamara JA: Proliferative sarcoid retinopathy, *Ophthalmology* 95:1680-1686, 1988.
16. Asdourian GK, Goldberg MF, Busse BJ: Peripheral retinal neovascularization in sarcoidosis, *Arch Ophthalmol* 93:787-791, 1975.
17. Hirose S, Ohno S: Argon laser treatment of retinal neovascularization associated with sarcoidosis, *Jpn J Ophthalmol* 28:356-361, 1984.
18. Gragoudas ES, Regan CDJ: Peripapillary subretinal neovascularization in presumed sarcoidosis, *Arch Ophthalmol* 99:1194-1197, 1981.
19. Campo RV, Aaberg TM: Choroidal granuloma in sarcoidosis, *Am J Ophthalmol* 97:419-427, 1984.
20. Marcus DF, Bovino JA, Burton TC: Sarcoid granuloma of the choroid, *Ophthalmology* 89:1326-1330, 1982.

Index

A

Abetalipoproteinemia, treatment of, 58
Acquired immunodeficiency syndrome
　ocular toxoplasmosis in, 295
　retinal/ophthalmologic manifestations of, 320-328; *see also* Cytomegalovirus retinitis
Acute retinal necrosis syndrome, 332-336
　clinical appearance of, 333-334
　cytomegalovirus retinitis differentiated from, 322
　differential diagnosis of, 335-336
　etiology of, 332-333
　medical treatment of, 334-335
　ocular toxoplasmosis differentiated from, 298-299
　surgical treatment of, 335
Acyclovir for acute retinal necrosis, 334-335
Adenopathy, hilar, in sarcoidosis of posterior segment, 348-349
Adult-onset foveomacular vitelliform dystrophy, 132
Adult vitelliform macular dystrophy, 39, *40*, 41
Age-related macular degeneration, 78-91
　central serous chorioretinopathy differentiated from, 107
　complications and sequelae of, treatment of, 89-91
　etiology of, 80
　exudative, 84-86, 87
　　choroidal neovascularization in, 87-89
　　natural course of, 84-86
　　pigment epithelial detachments in, 84, 85
　　treatment of, 86, 87
　nonexudative, 80-84
　　atrophy in, 83-84
　　drusen in, 80-81, *81-82*, 83
　pathogenesis of, 78-79
　retinal arterial macroaneurysms differentiated from, 257
　symptoms of, 80-89

Italicized number denotes a page with an illustration; *italicized t* a page with a table.

Alpha-interferon for age-related macular degeneration, 91
Amaurosis, Leber's, 32-33
Aminoglycoside toxicity, retinal arterial obstructive disease differentiated from, 168
Anemia, sickle cell, 211-218; *see also* Sickle cell anemia
Angiitis, frosted branch, in cytomegalovirus retinitis, 322
Angiography, fluorescein, 3-24; *see also* Fluorescein angiography
Angiomatosis retinae, Coats' disease differentiated from, 207, *208*
Anterior chamber paracentesis for retinal arterial obstructive disease, 170
Anthelmintic agents for ocular toxocariasis, 316-317
Antiangiogenic factors for age-related macular degeneration, 91
Aortic arch syndrome, ocular ischemic syndrome differentiated from, 282
Aqueous, cytologic and immunologic examination of, in ocular toxocariasis diagnosis, 315
Areolar choroidal sclerosis, central, 43, *44*, 45
Argon laser photocoagulation for neovascularization in sickle cell retinopathy, 218-219
Arterial macroaneurysms, retinal, 253-259; *see also* Retinal arterial macroaneurysms
Arteriolar occlusion of retinal vessels in sickle cell anemia, 215
Arteriolar-venular anastomoses in sickle cell anemia, 215
Arteriosclerosis, hypertension and, 190, *191*
Arteriovenous anastomoses in sickle cell anemia, 215
Arteritis, associated with acute retinal necrosis, 333
Artery
　cilioretinal, obstruction of, 171-172
　ophthalmic, obstruction of, acute, retinal arterial obstructive disease differentiated from, 168, *169*, 169t
　retinal, obstruction of, 163-173; *see also* Retinal arterial obstructive disease

Atherosclerosis, ocular ischemic syndrome and, 277
Autosomal dominant drusen, 42-43

B

Bactrim for ocular toxoplasmosis, 296
Behçet's disease, acute retinal necrosis differentiated from, 336
Best's disease, 38-39, 132, *133-134*, 135
Biomicroscopy, slit-lamp, in ocular toxocariasis diagnosis, 313
Biopsy of ocular tissue ocular toxoplasmosis diagnosis, 295
Block-Sulzberger syndrome, retinopathy of prematurity differentiated from, 231, *232*
Blood vessels
  in ocular toxoplasmosis, 290, *291-292*
  retinal, diseases of, 139-353; see also Retina, vascular diseases of
Bone marrow transplantation, radiation retinopathy and, 267
Branch retinal artery obstruction, 170, *171*
  in sickle cell anemia, 214
Branch retinal vein occlusion, 182-189; see also Retinal branch vein occlusion
Bruch's membrane dystrophies, 135
Bullous central serous chorioretinopathy, 113
Bull's-eye dystrophies, 45-46
Bull's eye maculopathy, 131, 131*t*
Butterfly pigment dystrophy, 132, *133*

C

Calcific emboli in retinal arterial obstructive disease, 165, *166*
Candida
  endophthalmitis from, ocular toxoplasmosis differentiated from, 299, *301*
  retinitis from, cytomegalovirus retinitis differentiated from, 324
Carotid endarterectomy for ocular ischemic syndrome, 284
Cavernous hemangioma of retina
  Coats' disease differentiated from, 207, *208*
  retinal arterial macroaneurysms differentiated from, 257
Central areolar choroidal dystrophy, *134*, 135
Central areolar pigment epithelial dystrophy, 136
Central retinal artery occlusion in sickle cell anemia, 214-215
Central retinal artery/vein obstruction, retinal arterial obstructive disease differentiated from, 168, *169*
Central retinal vein obstruction, 175-180
  clinical presentation of, 175
  diabetic retinopathy differentiated from, 143
  histopathology of, 175-180
Central retinal vein obstruction
  ischemic, 176, *177-178*, 179, *179*, 180
  nonischemic, 176, *177*
  ocular ischemic syndrome differentiated from, 283*t*, 283-284

Central retinal vein obstruction—cont'd
  pathophysiology of, 175-180
  treatment of, 180
Central serous chorioretinopathy, 103-113
  bullous, 113
  chronic, 112-113
  clinical features of, 103-106
  differential diagnosis of, 107-109
  etiology of, 106
  hyperfluorescence in, 14, *14*
  natural course of, 106-107
  pathogenesis of, 109-111
  symptoms of, 106
  treatment of, 111-112
  variants of, 112-113
Central serous choroidopathy, choroidal neovascularization associated with myopic macular degeneration differentiated from, 100
Chemotherapy, radiation retinopathy and, 267
Cholesterol emboli in retinal arterial obstructive disease, 165
Chorioretinal atrophy, paravenous pigmented, in retinitis pigmentosa, 31-32
Chorioretinal degeneration, helicoid peripapillary, in retinitis pigmentosa, 32
Chorioretinopathy, central serous, 103-113; see also Central serous chorioretinopathy
Choroid
  dystrophies of, *134*, 135
  fluorescein angiography of, 5, 7
  folds in, hypofluorescence in, 24, *24*
  granuloma of, in sarcoidosis of posterior segment, 350, *351*
  hemangioma of, hyperfluorescence in, 14, *16*
  inflammatory disease of, central serous chorioretinopathy differentiated from, 108
  melanoma of, hyperfluorescence in, 14, *17*, 19
  metastatic lesions of, hyperfluorescence in, 14, *18*, 19
  nevus of, hypofluorescence in, *22*, 24
  in sickle cell anemia, 213
  tumors of, central serous chorioretinopathy differentiated from, 108
  vascular disease of, central serous chorioretinopathy differentiated from, 108
Choroidal filling, delayed, in ocular ischemic syndrome, 277, 280
Choroidal neovascularization
  in age-related macular degeneration, 87-89
  associated with myopic macular degeneration, 95-101
    differential diagnosis of, 99-100
    findings in, 95, *96*, 97, *98-99*, 99
    treatment of, 100-100
  in ocular toxoplasmosis, 290, *292*
Choroideremia, 36-37
Choroiditis striata in retinitis pigmentosa, 32

Choroidopathy
  central serous choroidal neovascularization associated with myopic macular degeneration differentiated from, 100
  hypertensive, *194*, 195
Cilioretinal artery obstruction, 171-172
Clindamycin for ocular toxoplasmosis, 297
Coats' disease, 204-209
  clinical findings in, 204-206
  differential diagnosis of, 206-209
  idiopathic parafoveal telangiectasis differentiated from, 202
  ocular toxocariasis differentiated from, 311-312
  presenting signs and symptoms of, 204
  treatment of, 209
Color vision, defective, 47-48
Computed tomography in Coats' disease diagnosis, 206
Concentric annular dystrophy, benign, 131
Cone defects, 47-48
Cone disorders, 128-129
Congenital optic nerve pits, central serous chorioretinopathy differentiated from, 108
Congenital receptor defects, 47-51
Congenital stationary night blindness, 48-49
Conjunctiva in sickle cell anemia, 212
Corticosteroids
  for acute retinal necrosis, 335
  for ocular toxocariasis, 317
  oral, for ocular toxoplasmosis, 297
  for pars planitis, 342
  for sarcoidosis of posterior segment, 352
Cotton-wool spots, 172-173
Cryotherapy
  for Coats' disease, 209
  for neovascularization in sickle cell retinopathy, 128
  for ocular toxoplasmosis, 298
  panretinal, for proliferative diabetic retinopathy, 158
  for pars planitis, 343
  for retinopathy of prematurity, 233-237
Cyclitis, chronic, 339; *see also* Pars planitis
Cycloplegics for ocular toxocariasis, 317
Cystoid macular edema, 129-130
  in pars planitis, 341
Cytology, aqueous and vitreous, in ocular toxocariasis diagnosis, 315
Cytomegalovirus retinitis, 320-328
  acute retinal necrosis differentiated from, 336
  clinical features of, 321-322
  diagnostic approach to, 324-325
  differential diagnosis of, 322-324
  management of, 325-328
  symptoms of, 321

Italicized number denotes a page with an illustration; *italicized t* a page with a table.

D

Daraprim (Pyrimethamine), 296-297
Dark adaptation, prolonged, 49-51
Deuteranomaly, 47
Deuteranopia, 47
Diabetes mellitus, radiation retinopathy and, 266-267
Diabetic retinopathy
  cotton-wool spots in, 173
  nonproliferative, 141-151
    clinical findings in, 141-142
    diagnostic approach to, 143-144
    differential diagnosis of, 142-143
    Early Treatment Diabetic Retinopathy Study and, 143-144
      results of, 147-150
    management of, 144-146, *145-147*
    patient presentation with, 141
    retinal branch vein occlusion differentiated from, 183
    symptoms of, 141-142
    ocular ischemic syndrome differentiated from, 282-283, 283*t*
  proliferative, 152-158
    clinical findings in, 152-153
    differential diagnosis of, 153
    patient presentation with, 152
    symptoms of, 152-153
  radiation retinopathy differentiated from, 266
Diathermy for neovascularization in sickle cell retinopathy, 218
Diethylcarbazine for ocular toxocariasis, 317
Diffuse unilateral subacute neuroretinitis, 345-346
Dominant drusen, *134*, 135
Doyne's honeycomb dystrophy, 43
Drusen
  autosomal dominant, 42-43
  dominant, *134*, 135
  hyperfluorescence in, 19, *20*
  in nonexudative age-related macular degeneration, 80-81, *81-82*, 83

E

Electrooculography in retinitis pigmentosa, 35
Electroretinography
  in ischemic central retinal vein obstruction diagnosis, 179
  in ocular ischemic syndrome, 282
  in retinitis pigmentosa, 34
Emboli in retinal arterial obstructive disease, 165, *165-166*
Endarterectomy, carotid, for ocular ischemic syndrome, 284
Endophthalmitis
  Candida, ocular toxoplasmosis differentiated from, 299, *301*
  nematode, in ocular toxocariasis, 307, 309
  ocular toxocariasis differentiated from, 311
Enhanced S cone syndrome, 129
Enzyme-linked immunosorbent assay in ocular toxocariasis diagnosis, 314-315

Eosinophil count in ocular toxocariasis diagnosis, 313-314
Eosinophilia in ocular toxocariasis, 305
Exudate, intraretinal, in retinal arterial macroaneurysms, 253, *254*

F

Familial exudative vitreoretinopathy
  ocular toxocariasis differentiated from, 312
  retinopathy of prematurity differentiated from, 231, *231-232*
Fenestrated sheen macular dystrophy, 131
Fibrin-platelet emboli in retinal arterial obstructive disease, 165, *166*
Fleck retina of Kandori, 51
Fluid, subretinal, in choroidal neovascularization associated with myopic macular degeneration, 95, *96*
Fluorescein angiography, 3-24
  anatomic considerations for, 7-8
  in central serous chorioretinopathy, 105-106
  in choroidal neovascularization associated with myopic macular degeneration, 97-99
  in diffuse unilateral subacute neuroretinitis, 346
  dye for, 3-7
  in idiopathic macular hole, *118*, 119
  in idiopathic parafoveal telangiectasis, 199-200
  interpretation of, 9
  in ocular ischemic syndrome, 277, *278-279*, 280, *281*, 281t
  in ocular toxoplasmosis, 293
  in pars planitis, *340*, 341
  patterns in
    abnormal, 12-13, *13-14*, 14, *15-19*, 19, *20-24*, 24
    hyperfluorescence as, 13-14, *13-14*, *15-19*, 19, *20*
    hypofluorescence as, 19, *21-24*, 24
    normal, 5-6, 9-10, *10*, *11-12*, 12
  photographic equipment for, 8
  of radiation retinopathy, 264, *265*
  in retinal branch vein occlusion, 185-186
  in sickle cell anemia, *216*
Fluorescein dye, 3-7
  administration of, 4-6
  chemical properties of, 4
  historical perspective on, 3-4
  physical properties of, 4
  toxicity of, 6-7
Foscarnet for cytomegalovirus retinitis, 326-328
Foveomacular vitelliform dystrophy, adult-onset, 132
Frosted branch angiitis in cytomegalovirus retinitis, 322
Fuchs' spot in myopia, 99, *99*
Fundus albipunctatus, 50-51
Fundus examination in retinal branch vein occlusion, 184
Fundus flavimaculatus, *44*, 45, 130-131
Fungal retinitis, cytomegalovirus retinitis differentiated from, 324

G

Ganciclovir
  for acute retinal necrosis, 335
  for cytomegalovirus retinitis, 325-326
Glaucoma
  in sarcoidosis of posterior segment, 349
  secondary to hyphema, 218
Granulomas
  in sarcoidosis of posterior segment, 348, 349, 350, *351-352*
  toxocara, 307, *308*
Gyrate atrophy, treatment of, 58-59

H

Helicoid peripapillary chorioretinal degeneration in retinitis pigmentosa, 32
Hemangioma
  choroidal, hyperfluorescence in, 14, *16*
  retinal
    cavernous
      Coats' disease differentiated from, 207, *208*
      retinal arterial macroaneurysms differentiated from, 257
    congenital, retinal arterial macroaneurysms differentiated from, 257
Hemoglobinopathies, 211-221
  glaucoma secondary to hyphema as, 218
  sickle cell anemia as, 211-218; *see also* Sickle cell anemia
Hemorrhage
  retinal, in ocular ischemic syndrome, 277, *278*
  in retinal arterial macroaneurysms, 253, *254*
  subretinal, in choroidal neovascularization associated with myopic macular degeneration, 95, *96*
  vitreous, in sickle cell retinopathy, *216*, 217
    treatment of, 219-220
Herpes simplex virus, acute retinal necrosis from, 332
Hilar adenopathy in sarcoidosis of posterior segment, 348-349
Histopathology in ocular toxocariasis diagnosis, 315-316
Histoplasmosis
  ocular, hyperfluorescence in, 14, *15*
  ocular toxocariasis differentiated from, 312
Hyperfluorescence, 13-14, *13-14*, *15-19*, 19, *20*
  in central serous chorioretinopathy, 14, *14*, 105-106
  in choroidal hemangioma, 14, *16*
  in choroidal melanoma, 14, *17*, 19
  in choroidal neovascularization associated with myopic macular degeneration, 97-99
  in drusen, 19, *20*
  in heredodegeneration of retinal pigment epithelium, 19, *19*
  in metastatic lesions of choroid, 14, *18*, 19
  in ocular histoplasmosis, 14, *15*
  in retinal branch vein occlusion, 186
  in retinal pigment epithelium detachment, 13, *13*

Macula—cont'd
  holes in—cont'd
    idiopathic—cont'd
      treatment of, 122-123
      from known causes, idiopathic macular holes differentiated from, 122
Macular branch retinal vein occlusion, retinal branch vein occlusion differentiated from, 183
Macular dystrophies, 125-136
  of Bruch's membrane, 135
  of choroid, *134*, 135
  clinical presentations of, 125
  diagnostic approach to, 125-127
  of neurosensory retina, 127-130
  pattern, 131-135
Macular retina in sickle cell anemia, 213-214
Malattia levantinese, 43
Malignant hypertension, diabetic retinopathy differentiated from, 142-143
Melanoma, choroidal, hyperfluorescence in, 14, *17*, 19
Membrane(s)
  Bruch's, dystrophies of, 135
  choroidal neovascular, in age-related macular degeneration, 87-89
Metabolic storage diseases, retinal arterial obstructive disease differentiated from, 168
Metastatic lesions, choroidal, hyperfluorescence in, 14, *18*, 19
Minocycline for ocular toxoplasmosis, 297
Monochromatism, 48
Myopic macular degeneration, choroidal neovascularization associated with, 95-101; *see also* Choroidal neovascularization associated with myopic macular degeneration

N

Necrotizing retinitis complicating cytomegalovirus retinitis, 322
Nematode endophthalmitis in ocular toxocariasis, 307, 309
Nematode in diffuse unilateral subacute neuroretinitis, 345-346
Neovascularization
  choroidal; *see* Choroidal neovascularization
  iris, in retinal arterial obstructive disease, 164
  in ocular ischemic syndrome, 277, *279*
  posterior segment, in sarcoidosis of posterior segment, 350
  in proliferative diabetic retinopathy, 152-153
  in retinal branch vein occlusion, 186
  in sickle cell retinopathy, 215-216
  treatment of, 218-219
Nerve, optic; *see* Optic nerve
Neuritis, optic, ocular toxocariasis differentiated from, 312-313
Neuroretinitis, diffuse unilateral subacute, 345-346
Neurosensory retina, dystrophies of, 127-130
Nevus, choroidal, hypofluorescence in, *22*, 24
Night blindness
  congenital stationary, 48-49
  in retinitis pigmentosa, 33
North Carolina macular dystrophy, 46-47, 131

O

Ocular histoplasmosis, hyperfluorescence in, 14, *15*
Ocular ischemic syndrome, 276-284
  clinical findings in, 277, *278-279*, 280, 280*t*, 281*t*, *281-282*, 282
  diabetic retinopathy differentiated form, 143
  differential diagnosis of, 282-284
  presenting symptoms of, 276-277
  treatment of, 284
Ocular syphilis, ocular toxoplasmosis differentiated from, 299, *300*
Ocular toxocariasis, 304-318
  background on, 304-309
  clinical evaluation of, 313
  clinical features of, 305-307, *308-309*, 309
  clinical laboratory/ancillary tests for, 313-316
  diagnostic approach to, 313-316
  differential diagnosis of, 310-313
  epidemiology of, 304-305
  management of, 316-317
  ocular features of, 306-307, *308-309*, 309
  systemic features of, 305-306
Ocular toxoplasmosis, 289-302
  acute retinal necrosis differentiated from, 336
  clinical diagnosis of, 289-290, *291-293*, 293, *294*
  cytomegalovirus retinitis differentiated from, 323
  differential diagnosis of, 298-299, *300-301*, 301
  laboratory diagnosis of, 295
  ocular toxocariasis differentiated from, 312
  therapy for, 295-298
Oguchi's disease, 49-50
Ophthalmic artery obstruction, acute, retinal arterial obstructive disease differentiated from, 168, *169*, 169*t*
Ophthalmoscopy
  in central serous chorioretinopathy, 103-105
  indirect, in ocular toxocariasis diagnosis, 313
  radiation retinopathy on, 261-264
Optic disc
  in acute hypertension, 195
  granulomas of, in sarcoidosis of posterior segment, 350, *352*
Optic nerve
  disease of, central serous chorioretinopathy differentiated from, 109
  edema of, in acute retinal necrosis syndrome, 333
  granuloma of, in sarcoidosis of posterior segment, *352*
  pits of, central serous chorioretinopathy differentiated from, 108
  in sickle cell anemia, 212-213
Optic neuritis, ocular toxocariasis differentiated from, 312-313

Hypertension, 190-196
  acute, 193-195
  arteriosclerosis and, 190, *191*
  malignant, diabetic retinopathy differentiated from, 142-143
  pregnancy-induced, 195-106
  retinal vascular changes in, 191-193
Hyphema, glaucoma secondary to, 218
Hypofluorescence, 19, *21-24*, 24
  in choroidal folds, 24, *24*
  in choroidal nevus, *22*, 24
  in coloboma, 19, *21*, 24
  in focal hypertrophy of retinal pigment epithelium, *22*, 24
  in hemorrhagic detachment of retinal pigment epithelium, *23*, 24
  in retinal branch vein occlusion, 186
  in Stargardt's disease, *23*, 24

I

Immunodiagnosis of ocular toxocariasis, 314-315
Immunoglobulin G (IgG) antibody, serum levels of, in ocular toxoplasmosis, 295
Immunology, aqueous and vitreous, in ocular toxocariasis diagnosis, 315
Incontinentia pigmenti, retinopathy of prematurity differentiated from, 231, *232*
Inflammatory disease, 287-353
  acute retinal necrosis syndrome as, 332-336; *see also* Acute retinal necrosis syndrome
  choroidal, central serous chorioretinopathy differentiated from, 108
  cytomegalovirus retinitis as, 320-328; *see also* Cytomegalovirus retinitis
  ocular toxocariasis as, 304-318; *see also* Ocular toxocariasis
  ocular toxoplasmosis as, 289-302; *see also* Ocular toxoplasmosis
Intraretinal exudate in retinal arterial macroaneurysms, 253, *255*
Ionizing ocular irradiation
  dose of, occurrence and severity of radiation retinopathy and, 266-267
  radiation retinopathy from, 264-265
Iris in sickle cell anemia, 212
Iris neovascularization in retinal arterial obstructive disease, 164

J

Juvenile retinoschisis, 127-128

L

Lacquer cracks in choroidal neovascularization associated with myopic macular degeneration, *96*, 97
Laser photocoagulation
  for acute retinal necrosis, 335
  for background radiation retinopathy, 270, *271*

Italicized number denotes a page with an illustration; *italicized t* a page with a table.

Laser photocoagulation—cont'd
  for central serous chorioretinopathy, 111-112
  for choroidal neovascularization associated with myopic macular degeneration, 100-101
  for diffuse unilateral subacute neuroretinitis, 346
  for exudative age-related macular degeneration, 89-90
  for idiopathic parafoveal telangiectasis, 203
  for neovascularization in sickle cell retinopathy, 218-219
  for nonproliferative diabetic retinopathy, 144-145
  for pigment epithelial detachments, 86, *87*
  of pigment epithelial detachments, 86, *87*
  for retinal branch vein occlusion, 187-188
  for retinopathy of prematurity, 237-241
  for sarcoidosis of posterior segment, 352
Leber's amaurosis, 32-33
Leukocytosis in ocular toxocariasis, 305
Lymphadenopathy in sarcoidosis of posterior segment, 348-349
Lymphoma, large cell, acute retinal necrosis differentiated from, 336

M

Macroaneurysms, retinal arterial, 253-259; *see also* Retinal arterial macroaneurysms
Macula
  degeneration of
    age-related, 78-91; *see also* Age-related macular degeneration
    myopic, choroidal neovascularization associated with, 95-101; *see also* Choroidal neovascularization associated with myopic macular degeneration
  diseases of, 27-138
    age-related macular degeneration as, 78-91; *see also* Age-related macular degeneration
    congenital receptor defects as, 47-51
    dystrophies as, 125-136; *see also* Macular dystrophies
    retinal photoreceptor dystrophies as, 29-47; *see also* Retinal photoreceptor dystrophies
  dystrophy of
    adult vitelliform, 39, *40*, 41
    pseudoinflammatory, 41-42
  edema of
    cystoid, in pars planitis, 341
    in nonproliferative diabetic retinopathy, 141
  holes in
    central serous chorioretinopathy differentiated from, 109
    idiopathic, 117-123
      differential diagnosis of, 121-122
      findings in, 117, *118*, 119
      pathogenesis of, 119, *120-121*

P

Pain in ocular ischemic syndrome, 276-277
Panretinal cryotherapy for proliferative diabetic retinopathy, 158
Panretinal photocoagulation
  for central retinal vein obstruction, 180
  for pars planitis, 343
  for proliferative diabetic retinopathy, 154-158
    complications of, 157
    mechanism of efficacy of, 157-158
    studies on, 156-157
    technique of, 154-156
  for retinal arterial obstructive disease, 170
Papilledema in malignant hypertension, 93, *94*, 95
Papillopathy, radiation, 262, *263*, 264
Paracentesis, anterior chamber, for retinal arterial obstructive disease, 170
Parafoveal telangiectasis, idiopathic, 198-203
  clinical description of, 198-201
  differential diagnosis of, 202
  etiology of, 201-202
  pathology of, 201-202
  treatment of, 203
Paravenous pigmented chorioretinal atrophy in retinitis pigmentosa, 31-32
Pars plana vitrectomy
  for complications of age-related macular degeneration, 90, *91*
  for idiopathic macular holes, 122-123
  for retinal detachment in acute retinal necrosis, 335
Pars planitis, 339-343
  clinical course of, 342
  findings in, 339, *340*, 341
  pathogenesis of, 341-342
  treatment of, 342-343
Pattern dystrophies, 131-135
Peripapillary crescent in choroidal neovascularization associated with myopic macular degeneration, 96, *97*
Peripheral uveoretinitis, idiopathic, ocular toxocariasis differentiated from, 312
Peripherin in pathogenesis of retinal photoreceptor dystrophies, 55-56
Perivasculitis in pars planitis, 341
Persistent hyperplastic primary vitreous, ocular toxocariasis differentiated from, 311
Phlebitis, retinal, in acute retinal necrosis syndrome, 333
Photocoagulation
  laser; *see* Laser photocoagulation
  panretinal
    for central retinal vein obstruction, 180
    for pars planitis, 343
    for proliferative diabetic retinopathy, 154-158; *see also* Panretinal photocoagulation for proliferative diabetic retinopathy

Photocoagulation—cont'd
  panretinal—cont'd
    for retinal arterial obstructive disease, 170
    for proliferative radiation retinopathy, 270, *271*, 272
    for retinal arterial macroaneurysms, 259
Photographic equipment for fluorescein angiography, 8
Photoreceptor dystrophies, 128-129
Pigment epithelial detachment in exudative age-related macular degeneration, 84, 85
Piperazine salts for ocular toxocariasis, 316-317
Pregnancy-induced hypertension, 195-196
Prematurity, retinopathy of, 224-250; *see also* Retinopathy of prematurity
Protanomaly, 47
Protanopia, 47
Pseudoinflammatory macular dystrophy, 41-42
Pseudomacular hole, idiopathic macular hole differentiated from, 121
Pyrimethamine for ocular toxoplasmosis, 296-297

R

Radiation retinopathy, 261-273
  background, 262
    treatment of, 270, *271*
  clinical features of, 261-264
  as complication/side effect, 272
  development of, mechanism of, 266
  diabetic retinopathy differentiated from, 142
  differential diagnosis of, 266
  fluorescein angiography of, 264, *265*
  history of ionizing ocular irradiation and, 264-265
  incidence of, 267-268, *269*
  management of, 270
  natural history of, 269
  occurrence of, factors influencing, 266-267
  ophthalmoscopic features of, 261-264
  preproliferative, 262, *263*
  prevention of, 272
  proliferative, 262, *263*
    treatment of, 270, *271*, 272
  severity of, factors influencing, 267
  symptoms of, 261
  treatment of, 270-272
Radiation tumor vasculopathy, 267
Reflexes, tapetal, in retinitis pigmentosa, 33
Refsum's syndrome, treatment of, 59
Reticular pattern dystrophy, 132, *133*
Retina
  cytomegalovirus infections of, 320-328; *see also* Cytomegalovirus retinitis
  detachment of
    central serous chorioretinopathy differentiated from, 108
    rhegmatogenous, complicating cytomegalovirus retinitis, 322
    in sickle cell retinopathy, 217
    treatment of, 220-221
  dystrophies of, 129-130

Italicized number denotes a page with an illustration; *italicized t* a page with a table.

Retina—cont'd
    fleck, of Kandori, 51
    fluorescein angiography of, 8
    hemangioma of
        cavernous
            Coats' disease differentiated from, 207, *208*
            retinal arterial macroaneurysms differentiated from, 257
        congenital, retinal arterial macroaneurysms differentiated from, 257
    hemorrhage in, in ocular ischemic syndrome, 277, *278*
    macular, in sickle cell anemia, 213-214
    necrosis of, acute, 332-336; *see also* Acute retinal necrosis syndrome
    neurosensory, dystrophies of, 127-130
    peripheral, in sickle cell anemia, 214-218
        nonproliferative changes in, 214-215
        proliferative changes in, 215-218
    vascular diseases of, 139-285
        central retinal vein obstruction as, 175-180; *see also* Central retinal vein obstruction
        Coats' disease as, 204-209
        diabetic retinopathy as, 141-158; *see also* Diabetic retinopathy
        hemoglobinopathies as, 211-221; *see also* Hemoglobinopathies
        hypertensive, 190-196
        idiopathic parafoveal telangiectasis as, 198-203; *see also* Parafoveal telangiectasis, idiopathic
        ocular ischemic syndrome as, 276-284; *see also* Ocular ischemic syndrome
        radiation retinopathy as, 261-273; *see also* Radiation retinopathy
        retinal arterial macroaneurysms as, 253-259; *see also* Retinal arterial macroaneurysms
        retinal arterial obstructive disease as, 163-173; *see also* Retinal arterial obstructive disease
        retinal branch vein occlusion as, 182-189; *see also* Retinal branch vein occlusion
        retinopathy of prematurity as, 224-250; *see also* Retinopathy of prematurity
Retinal arterial macroaneurysms, 253-259
    clinical findings in, 253, *254-256*, 256
    differential diagnosis of, 256-257
    treatment of, 257-259
Retinal arterial obstructive disease
    ancillary studies in, 168
    background features of, 163
    branch, 170, *171*
    clinical characteristics of, 163-168
    clinical findings in, 163-164, *164-166*
    differential diagnosis of, 168, *169*, 169*t*
    disease entities associated with, 167*t*
    historical background of, 163
    management of, 168, 170
    symptoms of, 163
    systemic associations with, 167*t*, 168

Retinal branch vein occlusion
    clinical examination in, 183-185
    diagnostic approach to, 183-186
    differential diagnosis of, 183
    laser therapy for, 187-188
    management of, 187-189
    medical therapy for, 187
    retinal arterial macroaneurysms differentiated from, 257
    vitrectomy for, 189
Retinal photoreceptor dystrophies, 29-47
    adult vitelliform macular dystrophy as, 39, *40*, 41
    central, 38-47
        autosomal dominant drusen as, 42-43
        Best's disease as, 38-39
        bull's-eye, 45-46
        central areolar choroidal sclerosis as, 43, *44*, 45
        fundus flavimaculatus as, *44*, 45
        North Carolina, 46-47
        pattern, *40*, 41
        Sorsby's fundus dystrophy as, 41-42
    implications of advances in molecular biology for, 60-61
    management of, 57-60
        counseling in, 60
        disease identification in, 57
        inheritance identification in, 58
        treatment in, 58-60
    pathogenesis of, 51-56
        peripherin in, 55-56
        rhodopsin in, 52-55
    peripheral, 30-38
        Bietti's crystalline dystrophy as, 38
        choroideremia as, 36-37
        retinitis pigmentosa as, 30-36; *see also* Retinitis pigmentosa
Retinal pigment epithelium
    detachment of
        hemorrhagic, hypofluorescence in, 23, 24
        hyperfluorescence in, 13, *13*
    dystrophies of, 130-131
    fluorescein angiography of, 7-8
    focal hypertrophy of, hypofluorescence in, *22*, 24
    heredodegeneration of, hyperfluorescence in, 19, *19*
Retinal vein, central, obstruction of, 175-180
Retinitis
    cytomegalovirus, 320-328; *see also* Cytomegalovirus retinitis
    viral, ocular toxoplasmosis differentiated from, 298-299
Retinitis pigmentosa, 30-36
    clinical genetic studies in, 30
    diffuse, 31
    electrophysiologic studies of, 34-35
    functional studies in, 30-34
    genomic studies in, 35-36
    management of, 59-60

Retinitis pigmentosa—cont'd
  paravenous pigmented chorioretinal atrophy in, 31-32
  regional, 31
  sector, 31
  unilateral, 34
  X-linked, 33-34
Retinoblastoma
  Coats' disease differentiated from, 206-207
  ocular toxocariasis differentiated from, 310-311
Retinochoroiditis
  in ocular toxocariasis, 307
  toxoplasmic, 289-290, *291*, *293*, 293
    cytomegalovirus retinitis differentiated from, 323
Retinopathy
  diabetic, nonproliferative, 141-151; *see also* Diabetic retinopathy, nonproliferative
  hypertensive, 191-193
  of prematurity, 224-250
    classification of, 225-228, *229*
    cryotherapy for, 233-237
    diagnostic approach to, 232-233
    differential diagnosis of, 231-232
    incidence of, 224-225
    laser photocoagulation for, 237-241
    management of, 233-250
    ocular toxocariasis differentiated from, 312
    regression patterns in, 228, *230*, 230*t*
    scleral buckle for, 241-246
    vitrectomy for, 246-250
  radiation, 261-273; *see also* Radiation retinopathy
  sickle cell, 214-221; *see also* Sickle cell retinopathy
Retinoschisis, juvenile (X-linked), 127-128
  retinopathy of prematurity differentiated from, 232
Rhodopsin in pathogenesis of retinal photoreceptor dystrophies, 52-55
Rod-cone disorders, 129
Rod defects, 48-51
  congenital stationary night blindness from, 48-49
  prolonged dark adaptation as, 49-51
Rubeosis iridis in ocular ischemic syndrome, 277, *278*

S

S cone system dysfunction, 129
Sarcoidosis
  acute retinal necrosis differentiated from, 336
  of posterior segment, 348-352
    adnexal findings in, 349
    anterior segment findings in, 349
    diagnosis of, 348-349
    nonocular manifestations of, 348-349

Sarcoidosis—cont'd
  of posterior segment —cont'd
    posterior segment findings in, 350, *351-352*
    treatment of, 352
Scleral buckle for retinopathy of prematurity, 241-246
Sclerosis, choroidal, central areolar, 43, *44*, 45
Sickle cell anemia, 211-218
  anterior segment in, 212
  orbital swelling in, 212
  posterior segment in, 212-218; *see also* Sickle cell retinopathy
Sickle cell retinopathy
  nonproliferative, 214
  proliferative, 214-221
    treatment of, 218-221
Slit-lamp biomicroscopy in ocular toxocariasis diagnosis, 313
Snowballs
  in pars planitis, 339, *340*, 341
  in sarcoidosis of posterior segment, 350
Snowbanking in pars planitis, 339, *340*, 341
Sorsby's fundus dystrophy, 41-42
Sorsby's pseudoinflammatory macular dystrophy, 135
Stargardt's disease, 130-131
  hypofluorescence in, *23*, 24
"Strings of pearls" in sarcoidosis of posterior segment, 350
Subretinal fluid in choroidal neovascularization associated with myopic macular degeneration, 95, 96
Sulfadiazine for ocular toxoplasmosis, 296, 297
Surgery, ocular, for ocular toxocariasis, 317
Syphilis, ocular
  cytomegalovirus retinitis differentiated from, 323-324
  ocular toxoplasmosis differentiated from, 299, *300*

T

Tapetal reflexes in retinitis pigmentosa, 33
Telangiectasis
  congenital retinal, retinal arterial macroaneurysms differentiated from, 257
  parafoveal, idiopathic, 198-203; *see also* Parafoveal telangiectasis, idiopathic
Thiabendazole for ocular toxocariasis, 316-317
Toxocariasis, ocular, 304-318; *see also* Ocular toxocariasis
Toxoplasmosis, ocular, 289-302; *see also* Ocular toxoplasmosis
Transplantation, bone marrow, radiation retinopathy and, 267
Tumors, choroidal, central serous chorioretinopathy differentiated from, 108

U

Ultrasonography in ocular toxocariasis diagnosis, 313, *314*

Italicized number denotes a page with an illustration; *italicized t* a page with a table.

Unilateral wipeout syndrome, 345
Uveitis
　anterior, in sarcoidosis of posterior segment, 349
　intermediate, 339; *see also* Pars planitis
　peripheral, 339; *see also* Pars planitis
Uveoretinitis, idiopathic peripheral, ocular toxocariasis differentiated from, 312

V

Varicella zoster virus, acute retinal necrosis from, 332
Vasculitis
　in ocular toxoplasmosis, 293, *294*
　retinal, in sarcoidosis of posterior segment, 350
Vasculitis syndrome, ocular toxoplasmosis differentiated from, 299, 301
Vasculopathy, radiation tumor, 267
Viral retinitis, ocular toxoplasmosis differentiated from, 298-299
Visceral larval migrans, 304-306
Visual acuity
　in ocular ischemic syndrome, 276
　in retinal arterial obstructive disease, 163-164
Vitelliform dystrophy, 132, *133-134*, 135
　foveomacular, adult-onset, 132
Vitrectomy
　for complications of age-related macular degeneration, 90, *91*
　for ocular toxocariasis, 317
Vitrectomy—cont'd
　for ocular toxoplasmosis, 298
　pars plana
　　for idiopathic macular holes, 122-123
　　for retinal detachment in acute retinal necrosis, 335
　for retinal branch vein occlusion, 189
　for retinopathy of prematurity, 246-250
Vitreoretinal dystrophies, 127-128
Vitreoretinopathy, familial exudative
　ocular toxocariasis differentiated from, 312
　retinopathy of prematurity differentiated from, 231, *231-232*
Vitreous
　cytologic and immunologic examination of, in ocular toxocariasis diagnosis, 315
　hemorrhage in, in sickle cell retinopathy, *216*, 217
　　treatment of, 219-220
　persistent hyperplastic primary, ocular toxocariasis differentiated from, 311
Vitritis in acute retinal necrosis, 333

W

White blood cell count in ocular toxocariasis diagnosis, 313-314

X

X-linked retinoschisis, retinopathy of prematurity differentiated from, 232